Practical Guide to Cardiac CT

Armin Arbab Zadeh • John Hoe
Editors

Practical Guide to Cardiac CT

Springer

Editors
Armin Arbab Zadeh
Department of Medicine
Johns Hopkins University
Baltimore, MD, USA

John Hoe
Department of Radiology
Mount Elizabeth Hospital
Singapore, Republic of Singapore

ISBN 978-981-97-6918-6 ISBN 978-981-97-6919-3 (eBook)
https://doi.org/10.1007/978-981-97-6919-3

This Springer imprint is published by the registered company Springer Nature Singapore Pte Ltd.
The registered company address is: 152 Beach Road, #21-01/04 Gateway East, Singapore 189721, Singapore

Preface

Over the past few decades, cardiac CT has emerged as the test of choice for addressing critical cardiovascular disease questions and guiding many cardiac procedures. The technology continues to advance with major refinements in image resolution and decreased radiation doses to patients. Cardiac CT is poised to attain a more dominant role among the options for cardiovascular imaging, given its speed of acquisition, widespread availability, modest cost, and low toxicity.

The field of coronary artery disease will be particularly affected, where we are witnessing a shift from stress testing to coronary CT angiography, supported by robust clinical trial data demonstrating improved patient outcome. Coronary artery disease is a leading cause of mortality and morbidity in the world. The growing role of cardiac CT in this context will require massive expansions of our imaging infrastructure to meet the anticipated demand.

The UK was one of the earliest adapters of routine CT coronary angiography for patients presenting with chest pain. While they observed a decrease in mortality associated with greater utilization of cardiac CT, they struggle to provide the service across the country. Cardiology and radiology training programs have not yet adequately adapted to the demand for cardiac CT training. Reimbursement for cardiac CT services in many countries remains disproportionally low when long reading times are taken into consideration.

Artificial intelligence has had and will continue to have a major impact on cardiac CT. Workflow will improve and interpretation times will decrease. Fully automated analyses and interpretations are no longer a vision for the distant future. The provider will be moving towards a supervisory role, overseeing analyses and correcting, when needed. Thus, reader experience and provider input will remain indispensable.

These are exciting times for the rapidly growing field of cardiac CT. This book aims to guide healthcare providers on the process of acquiring and interpreting cardiac CT images. While background information is provided, we focused on a concise style to convey the most pertinent information—without burdening the reader with excessive text or unessential data. This book thus differentiates itself from other, more voluminous texts in the field. We hope readers will find this approach useful for quickly attaining relevant, clinically applicable, information in their busy schedules.

This book covers the practice of cardiac CT, written by experts in the field from around the world, who have many years of experience reading and teaching cardiac CT. We are proud that chapters were written by professionals from various specialties and includes a balanced representation of cardiologists and radiologists. A collaborative approach among medical specialties is vital for better patient care, research, and education.

New applications and technologic advances emerge constantly but typically require years to find acceptance in routine clinical care. This book provides the reader with a comprehensive text covering all aspects of cardiac CT, relevant to today's clinical practice. This book may also serve as an excellent source of preparation for the cardiac CT board examination, which is offered in many countries.

We are deeply grateful to the contributing authors of this book, who spent endless hours conceptualizing, drafting, and editing chapters. As always, we would like to thank our families for allowing us to carve out time from our busy days to take on this endeavor. Lastly, we thank the publisher for accepting our book proposal and for working with us through the process. We are most excited about the release of this book, and we hope it will be of great use to many.

Baltimore, MD, USA
Singapore, Republic of Singapore
October 14, 2024

Armin Arbab Zadeh
John Hoe

Contents

Contributors

Abdullah Al Khalifah, M.D. Johns Hopkins Aramco Healthcare, Al-Hasa, Saudi Arabia

Johns Hopkins University, Baltimore, MD, USA

Armin Arbab Zadeh, M.D., Ph.D., M.P.H. Department of Medicine, Johns Hopkins University, Baltimore, MD, USA

Richard J. Bloomingdale, M.D. Corewell Health, Royal Oak, MI, USA

Roger S. Blumenthal, M.D. Department of Medicine, Johns Hopkins School of Medicine, Johns Hopkins Ciccarone Center for the Prevention of Cardiovascular Disease, Baltimore, MD, USA

Thomas Boyle, M.D. Department of Medicine, Johns Hopkins School of Medicine, Johns Hopkins Ciccarone Center for the Prevention of Cardiovascular Disease, Baltimore, MD, USA

Rhanderson N. Cardoso, M.D., M.H.S. Division of Cardiovascular Medicine, Harvard Medical School, Brigham and Women's Hospital, Boston, MA, USA

Omar Chehab, M.D., M.Sc. Division of Cardiology, Department of Medicine, The Johns Hopkins University School of Medicine, Baltimore, MD, USA

Kavitha M. Chinnaiyan, M.D. Oakland University William Beaumont University, Corewell Health, Royal Oak, MI, USA

Julianna Czum, M.D. Johns Hopkins University, Baltimore, MD, USA

Carlo N. De Cecco, M.D., Ph.D. Department of Radiology, Emory University School of Medicine, Emory University, Atlanta, GA, USA

Henrique Doria De Vasconcellos, M.D., M.Sc. Division of Cardiology, Department of Medicine, The Johns Hopkins University School of Medicine, Baltimore, MD, USA

David I. Feldman, M.D., M.P.H. Division of Cardiology, Harvard University, Boston, MA, USA

Department of Medicine, Johns Hopkins School of Medicine, Johns Hopkins Ciccarone Center for the Prevention of Cardiovascular Disease, Baltimore, MD, USA

Cristina Fuss, M.D., Ph.D. Yale University, New Haven, CT, USA

John Hoe, MBBS Department of Radiology, Mount Elizabeth Hospital, Singapore, Republic of Singapore

Jin Hur, M.D., Ph.D. Department of Radiology and Research Institute of Radiological Science and Center for Clinical Image Data Science, Severance Hospital, Yonsei University College of Medicine, Seoul, Republic of Korea

James Iwaz, M.D. University of California, Irvine, Irvine, CA, USA

Veterans Affairs Long Beach Healthcare System, Long Beach, CA, USA

Division of Cardiology, Tibor Rubin VA Medical Center, Long Beach, CA, USA

Eun-Ju Kang, M.D., Ph.D. Department of Radiology/Cardiovascular Imaging, College of Medicine, Dong-A University, Busan, Republic of Korea

Klaus Fuglsang Kofoed, M.D., Ph.D. Cardiac CT Research Unit, Rigshospitalet, University of Copenhagen, Copenhagen, Denmark

Department of Cardiology, Copenhagen University Hospital Rigshospitalet, Copenhagen, Denmark

Jongmin John Lee Department of Radiology, School of Medicine, Kyungpook National University, Daegu, Republic of Korea

Shuai Leng, Ph.D. Department of Radiology, Mayo Clinic, Rochester, MN, USA

Bruno B. Lima, M.D., PH.D. Division of Cardiology, Harvard Medical School, Boston, MA, USA

Division of Cardiovascular Medicine, Harvard Medical School, Brigham and Women's Hospital, Boston, MA, USA

Division of Cardiovascular Medicine, Vanderbilt Heart and Vascular Institute, Nashville, TN, USA

Joao A. C. Lima, M.D., M.B.A. Division of Cardiology, Department of Medicine, The Johns Hopkins University School of Medicine, Baltimore, MD, USA

Yuen Li Ng, MBBS Department of Radiology, Mount Elizabeth Hospital, Singapore, Republic of Singapore

Kristian Altern Øvrehus, M.D., Ph.D. Division of Cardiology, Odense University Hospital, Odense, Denmark

Michael Huy Cuong Pham, Ph.D. Division of Cardiology, University of Copenhagen, Copenhagen, Denmark

Department of Cardiology, Copenhagen University Hospital Rigshospitalet, Copenhagen, Denmark

Alexander C. Razavi, M.D., PhD, MPH Division of Cardiology, Emory University, Atlanta, GA, USA

Department of Medicine, Emory University School of Medicine, Atlanta, GA, USA

Edward P. Shapiro, M.D. Johns Hopkins Bayview Medical Center, Johns Hopkins University, Baltimore, MD, USA

Division of Cardiology, John Hopkins University, Baltimore, MD, USA

Muhammad Umair, M.D. Johns Hopkins University, Baltimore, MD, USA

Seamus P. Whelton, MD Department of Medicine, Johns Hopkins School of Medicine, Baltimore, MD, USA

Johns Hopkins Ciccarone Center for the Prevention of Cardiovascular Disease, Baltimore, MD, USA

Dong Hyun Yang, M.D. Asan Medical Center, University of Ulsan College of Medicine, Seoul, Republic of Korea

Jeannie Yu, M.D. University of California, Irvine, Irvine, CA, USA

Veterans Affairs Long Beach Healthcare System, Long Beach, CA, USA

Division of Cardiology, Tibor Rubin VA Medical Center, Long Beach, CA, USA

Stefan L. Zimmerman, M.D. Johns Hopkins University, Baltimore, MD, USA

1 Computed Tomography (CT) Fundamentals

Shuai Leng

Abstract

CT acquires data with an X-ray tube rotating around the patient, from which an image reconstruction process generates tomographic images of the patient's cross-section. CT images, presented as CT numbers (Hounsfield Unit, HU), represent the intrinsic property of the human body interacting with X-ray photons. CT scanner is a sophisticated system including various components with different functionality to enable data acquisition and image reconstruction, with numerous parameters selectable by operators that impact image quality and radiation dose. In cardiac CT, ECG gating is required to image the beating heart. Both prospective and retrospective gating have been used in cardiac CT, together with various scan modes such as axial, sequential, helical/spiral, and Flash, depending on the scanner type and hardware.

Keywords

CT number · Generations of CT scanner Sinogram · Image reconstruction · Major components · Scan mode · ECG gating Prospective · Retrospective · Image quality Radiation dose

S. Leng (✉)
Department of Radiology, Mayo Clinic, Rochester, MN, USA
e-mail: Leng.Shuai@mayo.edu

Abbreviations

AI	Artificial intelligence
CNR	Contrast-to-noise ratio
DAS	Data acquisition system
ECG	Electrocardiogram
EID	Energy-integrating detectors
FBP	Filtered back projection
FOV	Field of view
HU	Hounsfield unit
kV	Kilovolt
MTF	Modulation transfer function
PCD	Photon-counting detector
UHR	Ultra-high resolution

1.1 Basic Principles and Image Formation

- The principle of CT imaging is similar to other X-ray imaging techniques, i.e., the generation of images based on the radiodensity of structures [1, 2].
- A CT image represents the distribution of linear attenuation coefficients, which represent the interaction of X-ray photons with the human body.
- Radiodensity in CT imaging is given as CT number on the Hounsfield scale (HU = Hounsfield Unit), which is defined as:

$$\text{CT Number}(\text{HU}) = \frac{(\mu - \mu_{\text{water}})}{\mu_{\text{water}}} \times 1000$$

A. A. Zadeh, J. Hoe (eds.), *Practical Guide to Cardiac CT*,
https://doi.org/10.1007/978-981-97-6919-3_1

μ is the linear attenuation coefficient of a given object or image pixel, and μ_{water} is the linear attenuation coefficient of water.
By definition, the CT number of water is 0 HU and the CT number of air is −1000 HU. Soft tissue is in the tens HU (e.g., 30–60 HU), while fat has a negative CT number (e.g., −120 to −40 HU) due to lower density than water. Calcified plaques are usually >130 HU (minimal HU number for Agatston score).

- The raw data acquired in CT need to go through an image reconstruction process to generate tomographic images representing the cross-section of a patient's body part (orthogonal to the head-to-toe (z-axis) orientation). Reconstruction algorithms such as filtered back projection (FBP) and iterative reconstruction (IR) have been used. Details of reconstruction techniques are discussed in Chap. 2.

1.2 CT Scanner Design

- The gantry is a ring-shaped housing that holds major components of a CT scanner. A modern CT scanner rotates 360° at a sub-second (e.g., 0.23 s) with thousands of pounds of components while acquiring data.
- Slip ring transmits high or low voltage power to the rotating gantry and passes detector data to the computer system. The introduction of the slip ring method eliminates the need to "rewind" the cable and was a major breakthrough for multi-slice, helical (spiral) data acquisition.
- X-ray tube generates X-ray photons used in CT imaging, with high power provided by the generator (e.g., 120 kV). Modern X-ray tubes have a high heat capacity and long tube life, with a small focal spot (<1 mm) maintaining high spatial resolution.
- X-ray collimators shape the X-ray beam to the target area, reducing the unnecessary dose for patients.
- Flat filters are used to remove very low-energy photons that cannot penetrate through patients. These photons do not contribute to image quality but add to the patient radiation dose.
- Bow-tie filter is a special part of CT (not in general radiography), with the center of the filter thinner than the peripherals. This is to compensate for the attenuation difference between the center (high) and peripheral (low) of the human body. This provides a more balanced photon flux on the detector.
- Early CT scanner had only a single detector row along the z-direction. Modern CT scanners have multiple detector rows along the z-direction (head to toe), which is referred to as multi-slice, multi-row, or multi-detector CT scanners. These scanners are commonly labeled based on the number of slices, e.g., 64 slice or 640 slice CT scanners. *Note that the number of slices may differ from the number of physical detector rows when multiple data acquisitions occur on one detector row, e.g., flying focal spot.* For example, the 640 slice CT scanner consists of 320 detector rows but acquiring 640 channels/slices of data along the z-direction. Adding to the confusion, the literature is inconsistent with labeling CT scanners according to their physical detector rows or data channels, though the former is generally preferred.
- Data acquisition system (DAS) consists of electronics and computers to perform corrections and calibrations before the image reconstruction.
- The actual image reconstruction system (IRS) involves high-power computers and workstations to perform image reconstruction within seconds after data acquisition. Reconstruction times depend on the complexity of reconstruction algorithms and the amount of data to handle. For example, data sets using very thin slices and some model-based iterative reconstruction algorithms may take longer reconstruction time.
- Dual energy CT refers to image acquisition using more than one beam spectrum. Various approaches have been explored, including dual source, dual layer detector, fast-kV switching, two consecutive scans, and the use

of beam filters [3]. Potential applications of dual energy CT include:

- Use low keV virtual monoenergetic/monochromatic images (VMI) to enhance iodine contrast, which can be used to reduce iodine contrast dose, reduce radiation dose, and rescue suboptimal exams with poor contrast enhancement.
- Use high keV VMI to reduce beam hardening and metal artifacts, e.g., for patients with pacemakers.
- Assess myocardium perfusion based on iodine map generated through dual energy material decomposition.

1.3 Energy-Integrating Detector vs. Photon-Counting Detector

- Most current CT scanners use conventional energy-integrating detectors (EID), which are typically made of scintillating materials, i.e., certain types of rare-earth ceramics (e.g., $CdWO_4$, Gd_2O_2S).
- When X-ray photons interact with the scintillating materials, visible light is generated (step 1), which is subsequently converted into electric signals by the photodiode (step 2).
- Because this is a 2-step process, EID-based image generation is commonly referred to as *indirect* conversion technique.
- The detected signal is proportional to the total energy deposited by all photons (i.e., energy-integrating mode), without information from each individual photon.
- A major limitation of the EID method is the need for insulation of detector cells (using septa) to avoid spread of visible light to other cells, which would reduce spatial resolution. As a consequence, fill factor and geometric efficiency are reduced due to the dead space occupied by the septa (Fig. 1.1a) [4].
- Photon-counting detector (PCD) CT technology has emerged as a commercially available option in 2021 [5].
- PCD overcomes key limitations of EID by *directly* converting the absorbed X-rays into electron–hole pairs (without the interim step generating visible light as with EID).
- The electron–hole pairs are separated by the strong electric field created with high voltage bias. As electrons travel to the anode, they induce electric signals with each individual photon counted instead of integrating them together (Fig. 1.1b) [4].
- The pulse height of the electric signal is proportional to the X-ray energy of each photon, enabling intrinsic multi-energy capability. Since no visible light is created, there is no need of septa in PCD, resulting in a higher fill factor and dose efficiency compared to that of EID.
- Comparing to conventional EID-CT, PCD-CT offers the benefits of reduced electronic noise (beneficial for low-dose exams and large body parts, e.g., shoulder and pelvis), increased contrast-to-noise ratio (CNR), higher spatial resolution, reduced radiation dose, simultaneous ultra-high-resolution and multi-energy

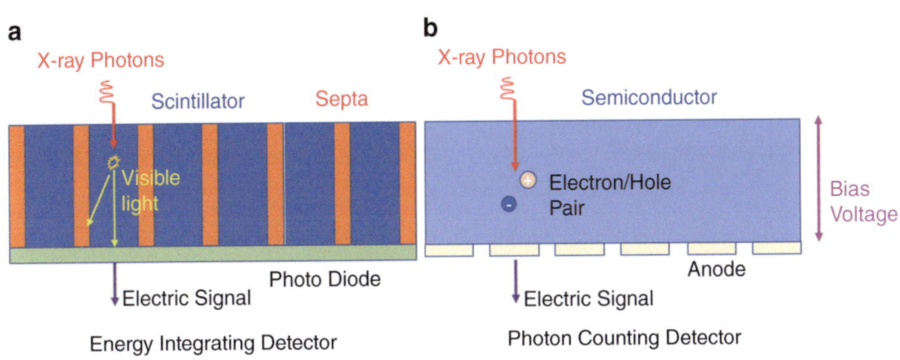

Fig. 1.1 Overview of X-ray photon processing using EID (**a**) and PCD (**b**) technology

capabilities, artifact reduction, and k-edge and multi-contrast imaging [4].

1.4 General Characteristics of CT Scanning in Cardiac Imaging

- ECG gating is required in cardiac imaging to target quasistatic cardiac phases, e.g., end systole or diastasis, where cardiac motion is least.
- High temporal resolution facilitates avoidance of motion artifacts and can be achieved with faster gantry rotation, certain acquisition techniques, and/or more use of more than one X-ray source.
- Cardiac imaging requires high spatial resolution given the interest in small structures, e.g., coronary atherosclerotic plaques, which can be achieved with specific detector designs, configuration, and image reconstruction techniques.
- 64 or more slice multi-detector CT scanners are preferred for cardiac imaging to maintain acceptable scan times and breath-hold periods for patients.
- Certain CT scanners hold specific benefits for cardiac imaging:
  - Wide area detector CT (*z* coverage up to 16 cm) allows fast, whole heart imaging during one gantry rotation, thus avoiding table motion and "stitch" artifacts from fusing image slabs.
  - Dual-source CT scanner provides better temporal resolution compared to single source CT and may reduce or even eliminate motion artifacts as well as the need for heart rate reducing medications.

1.5 Factors Influencing Image Quality in Cardiac CT

- The overall image quality in cardiac CT depends on the interplay of multiple image quality metrics, such as temporal resolution, spatial resolution, and contrast-to-noise ratio (CNR). All these metrics are impacted by both system hardware (e.g., focal spot size, detector size, and rotation time) and image reconstruction (e.g., pixel size and reconstruction kernel/algorithm).
- *Temporal Resolution*
  - Temporal resolution in CT is defined as the data acquisition time to form a given image. It has a major impact on the risk of motion artifacts, particularly in cardiac CT [6].
  - In cardiac CT, a short scan (half rotation, about 180 degrees) is used for image acquisition, resulting in temporal resolution approximately equal to half gantry rotation time (Fig. 1.2).
  - Temporal resolution can be improved by increasing gantry rotation speed (reducing gantry rotation time) or using multiple-sources, e.g., dual-source CT which has temporal resolution approximately equals to quarter rotation time by combining projection data from the two X-ray sources that are offset by ~90° (Fig. 1.3).
  - Multi-segment image reconstruction has been used to improve temporal resolution. Instead of completing data acquisition of a

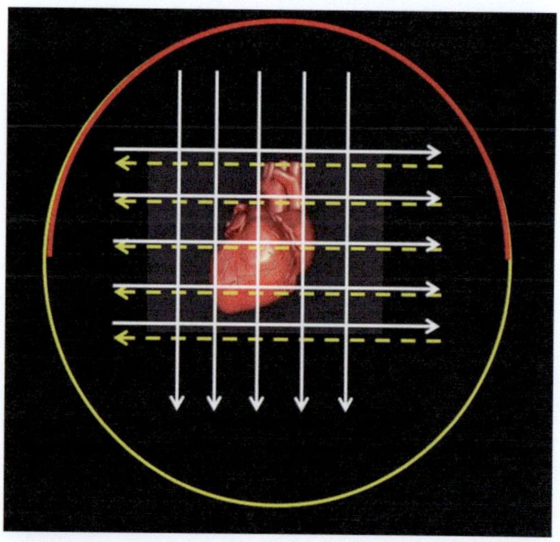

Fig. 1.2 Illustration of short scan in cardiac CT with parallel beam geometry. Half rotation (180 degree) provides sufficient data for accurate image reconstruction, noted as the redundant measurements from the two projections in the horizontal direction (solid lines from left to right, and dashed lines from right to left). This results in temporal resolution of cardiac CT approximately half gantry rotation time

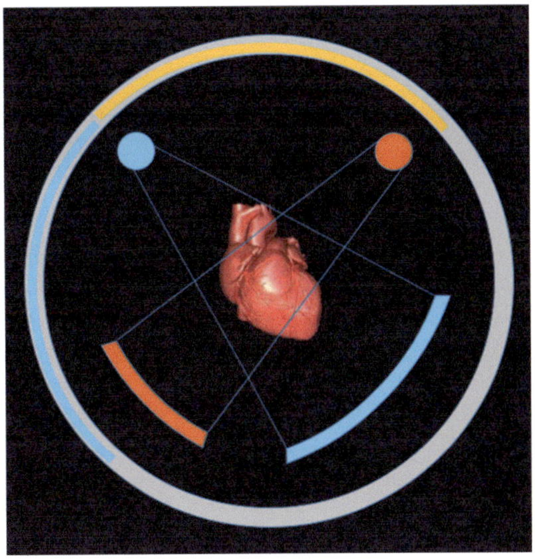

Fig. 1.3 In dual-source CT, two X-ray tubes/detectors are approximately 90° offset. By combining projection data from the two sources, temporal resolution in dual-source CT is approximately quarter gantry rotation time

given image in one heartbeat using half gantry rotation, it separates data acquisition into several segments using one quarter or less rotation over multiple heartbeats. Temporal resolution is thus improved because individual images are acquired within less time. However, limitations include the need for multi-cycle acquisition (often increasing radiation dose) and synchronization of heartbeat rate and gantry rotation time (details are discussed in Chap. 2).

  - Software algorithms (including artificial intelligence [AI] methods) are available to correct motion which essentially improves temporal resolution without altering image acquisition, but the improvements are typically modest and patient specific.
  - *Note the difference between temporal resolution and total data acquisition time*. For example, more detector rows generally increase *z*-axis coverage which reduces overall data acquisition time, but it does not impact temporal resolution which is determined by the factors discussed above.
- *Spatial Resolution*
  - Spatial resolution is a measurement of the smallest features that can be differentiated. It is important in cardiac CT given the small size of the imaging targets, e.g., atherosclerosis.
  - Spatial resolution can be measured using bar pattern phantoms (in terms of line pairs/cm), point spread function, or modulation transfer function (MTF).
  - Given the tomographic nature of CT, spatial resolution in CT is usually characterized by in-plane (x–y) spatial resolution and longitudinal (z) resolution, although modern CT scanners can provide isotropic resolution in all directions.
  - Spatial resolution is determined by both hardware (e.g., focal spot size, detector pixel size, sampling pattern) and image reconstruction (e.g., reconstruction kernel and pixel size).
  - Typical focal spot size is 0.4–1.1 mm. Small focal spot (e.g., 0.4 mm) is needed for high spatial resolution. One trade-off of a small focal spot is its limited tube power (tube current, mA).
  - Conventional CT scanning operates with detector width/pixel size of 0.5–0.625 mm (at the isocenter), while ultra-high resolution (UHR) CT provides a detector width of 0.25 mm or below.
  - Note that pixel size impacts sampling frequency and should be small enough to support the system resolution. After that, a further decrease in pixel size will not increase spatial resolution.
  - *Partial volume effect* occurs when an imaging object (e.g., calcium chunk) is smaller than the image pixel size due to overrepresentation of very dense structures vs. other signals allocated to one pixel. As result, the object appears larger ("blooming artifact") but with lower density due to the limits in spatial resolution.
- *Signal, Contrast, Noise, and Contrast-to-Noise Ratio (CNR)*
  - In CT, *signal* refers to the CT number in the target pixel of object and *contrast* refers to CT number difference between two imaging objects.

- Image contrast intrinsically depends on the attenuation properties of the imaging targets. Imaging targets with different attenuations, e.g., bone vs. soft tissue, tend to have higher contrast, while ones with similar attenuation properties, e.g., gray and white matters, have lower contrast.
- Tube potential (kV) has a substantial impact on image contrast. Lower kV tends to provide higher contrast, especially when iodine contrast is used.
- *Noise* is measured as the standard deviation of CT numbers inside a uniform region of interest (ROI). Many factors influence image noise, such as tube potential, tube current, reconstruction algorithm, reconstruction kernel, and slice thickness.
- *Contrast-to-noise ratio (CNR)* is the ratio between image contrast and noise and is an important indicator of image quality. In general, higher CNR is preferred, and sufficient CNR is needed for specific clinical tasks.
- Multiple factors could impact CNR. As iodinated contrast is commonly used in cardiac CT, CNR is influenced by the contrast enhancement which can be impacted by the contrast injection protocol including volume and rate. Suboptimal exam could result from poor contrast enhancements.
- Increasing radiation dose could reduce image noise and consequently enhance CNR, which needs to be balanced between image quality and radiation dose (Fig. 1.4).
- Lower kV has been used as a CNR improvement (or radiation dose reduction) technique, especially with contrast-enhanced exams such as coronary CTA.
- Iterative reconstruction or AI algorithms have been used to reduce image noise and improve CNR.

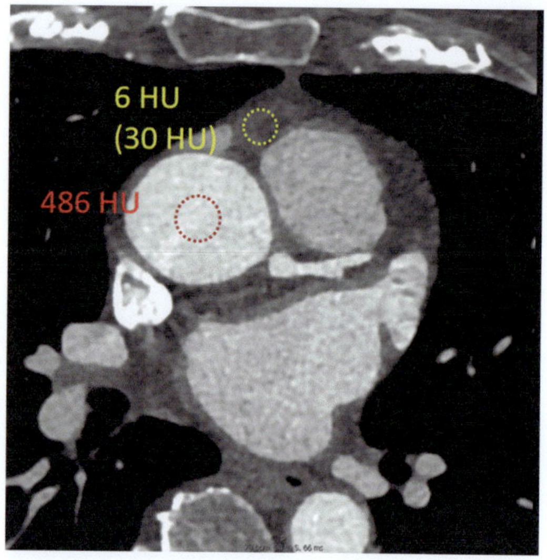

Fig. 1.4 Sample case of contrast, noise, and CNR measurements. CT number difference between the target (red ROI) and background (yellow ROI) provides the contrast of 486 HU—6HU = 480 HU. The standard deviation of CT numbers in the background provides the noise of 30 HU. CNR is the ratio between the contrast and noise, i.e., 480 HU/30 HU = 16

1.6 Scan Acquisition Components and Features

- CT localizer radiograph (also known as Topogram/Scout/SureView/Scanogram) provides a radiographic view of the patient, which can be used for patient positioning, scan range prescription, and patient size estimation for the purpose of automatic exposure control.
- Axial mode (also referred to as Volume mode) scan acquisition is performed with a single rotation at a fixed table location. *Z* coverage is determined by the detector width.
- Cine or dynamic CT acquisition consists of continuous axial scans with multiple rotations, without table translation, thus imaging the same region over time. This is mainly used for perfusion imaging and CT fluoroscopy to guide interventions.

- Sequential acquisition mode can be considered as multiple scans of axial mode at different table locations, with acquisition paused during the table motion.
- Helical (or spiral) mode is performed with continuous data acquisition during table motion and X-ray tube rotating around the patient. Note that the scan range is not limited by detector width as it is in axial mode.
- *Helical pitch* is defined as the ratio of table motion per rotation over the total detector collimation. Higher helical pitch is associated with higher scan speed given the same rotation time and detector collimation.
- For multi-slice (or multi-row detector) CT, various detector configurations exist by combining different detector channels (e.g., 320 × 0.5 mm, 60 × 3.0 mm, 64 × 0.625 mm, 24 × 1.2 mm, etc.).
- Rotation time has a significant impact on temporal resolution and scanning speed, which is important for cardiac imaging. Faster rotation time is associated with a better temporal resolution with reduced risk of motion artifacts.
- Tube potential (e.g., 80, 100, 120, 140 kV) has a large impact on image quality and radiation dose. As X-ray attenuation is energy dependent, lower tube potentials provide better image contrast, especially with iodine contrast on board. However, lower tube potential also has less penetration which could be problematic for large patients, body parts, or patients with high attenuating substances. Tube potential should be appropriately selected based on patient size and imaging tasks.
- Tube current (mA) determines photon flux, i.e., how many photons are being emitted from the tube in a unit of time. A couple of related parameters include mAs (tube current x rotation time) and effective mAs (mAs/pitch). As mAs increase, image noise decreases (inverse square root), and patient dose increases.

1.7 Reconstruction Parameters

- Image reconstruction algorithms play a critical role for image quality and indirectly influence radiation dose because noise reductions allow lower X-ray tube settings.
  - Traditional, analytical reconstruction algorithm, e.g., filtered backprojection (FBP), has been the main model for decades but is being increasingly replaced by iterative reconstruction. FBP allows fast reconstruction but lacks good noise properties.
  - Iterative reconstruction can model system geometry, spectrum, and statistical noise. Noise reduction, image quality improvement, and dose reduction have been observed using iterative reconstruction compared to FBP. It requires more computational power than FBP but with recent advances in hardware and algorithms, it has reached reconstruction speeds suitable for routine clinical practice [7].
  - Artificial intelligence (AI) or deep learning-based reconstruction algorithms are now available, which potentially require even greater time and computation power. This approach involves training a neural network (mostly a convolutional neural network) to obtain high-quality images from low-dose (noisy) data. Future models likely will use more AI-based image reconstruction.
- The slice thickness greatly impacts spatial resolution (in the *z*-axis) and the partial volume effect (see above). Thinner slices provide higher *z*-resolution but come with the limitation of higher image noise as the number of photons in the slice decreases. To maintain the same image noise at a thinner slice, the radiation dose may need to be increased or image processing further optimized.
- Slice interval/increment determines the overlap/gap between image slices along the z-direction for image reconstruction. Typically, particularly for 3D display purposes, some overlap between slices (i.e., slice increment < slice thickness) is preferred to optimize visualization.
- Reconstruction field of view (FOV) can be adjusted and does not need to be the same as scanning FOV. For example, a smaller FOV centered around the heart is commonly used for cardiac CT.
- Display window maps a certain range of CT numbers of interest to the gray scale of the

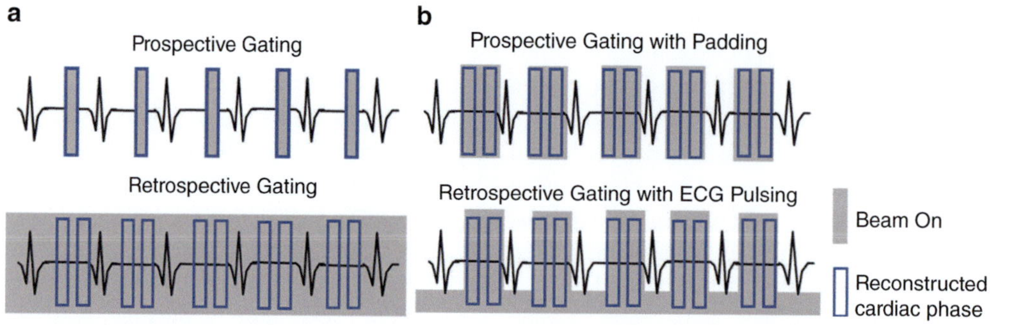

Fig. 1.5 (**a**) Illustration of prospective and retrospective gating. Prospective gating triggers data acquisition (X-ray beam on) only at a predetermined cardiac phase or phases. Retrospective gating acquires all data, then sort out the corresponding reconstructed phases of interest (e.g., systolic and diastolic) afterward. (**b**) Padding in prospective gating and ECG pulsing in retrospective gating

monitor to provide appropriate visual contrast and brightness for the imaging task.

- Reconstruction techniques are discussed in detail in Chap. 2.

1.8 ECG Gating in Cardiac CT Imaging

- ECG gating is an essential component of cardiac CT to synchronize data acquisition with cardiac motion [8].
- *Retrospective Gating*: All data are being acquired throughout the cardiac cycle and image reconstruction then focuses on phases of interest after scan completion, e.g., during motion-free periods (Fig. 1.5a). The benefit of this approach is the availability of many data points for image section and the option to synchronize data which may have gotten affected by ectopic heartbeats. The key limitation is unnecessary radiation during much of the cardiac cycle not used for image reconstruction.
- *Prospective Gating (or Prospective Triggering):* Data acquisition (X-ray on) occurs only at a predetermined cardiac phase or phases (Fig. 1.5a). The benefit is typically much lower radiation dose compared to retrospective gating, but fewer data are available for reconstruction [9, 10].
- ECG pulsing or tube current modulation technique is used to reduce radiation dose in conjunction with retrospective gating, typically applied to phases within the cardiac cycle where there is excessive motion, e.g., systole, and thus not utilized for image reconstruction. It maintains regular tube current output at the target cardiac phases for high image quality while reducing mA outside of the target cardiac phases where the requirement of image quality is not as high as the phases inside the pulsing window (Fig. 1.5b). The width and height of the pulsing window determine how much radiation dose can be achieved.
- In prospective gating, the so-called padding technique can be used to expand the duration of data acquisition, allowing imaging the heart at multiple phases (Fig. 1.5b). The increase of the width however increases radiation dose. Therefore, a practical trade-off between data acquisition flexibility and radiation dose needs to be appropriately balanced.

1.9 Scan Modes in Cardiac CT

- Depending on the hardware and scanner type, various scan modes, in combination with either prospective or retrospective ECG gating can be used in cardiac CT [8, 11].
- Here we differentiate between 3 principal scan modes:
  - *Helical (Spiral)*:

    Helical (spiral) mode uses continuous tube rotation and table motion while acquiring data. Compared to non-cardiac applications, cardiac imaging in helical mode is usually performed with lower pitch (e.g., 0.2–0.35) to avoid data gap between heartbeats. The specific pitch value depends on heart rates, with higher heart rates requiring lower pitch. This mode requires multiple rotations and multiple heartbeats to complete the data acquisition of the whole heart. The number of heartbeats depend on the scanner's z-axis coverage, typically 3–5 for cardiac applications.

A special helical/spiral mode is the *high pitch spiral* (up to 3.4) mode, commonly referred to as Flash mode. It is available with dual-source CT technology. In standard CT, the highest helical pitch is around 1.5 to ensure sufficient data acquisition without data gap between rotations. In dual-source CT, with projection data acquired from the two sources filling in gaps of each other, it enables a high pitch (>1.5) during a spiral scan, resulting in a very fast scanning speed (up to 747 mm/s). With sufficiently low heart rates, this may allow scanning the whole heart in a short time (e.g., 160 ms), enabling single heartbeat cardiac CT with spiral mode. It is a very low-dose scan mode at the expense of very few data available for image reconstruction.

- *Volume (Or Also Called "Axial Mode")*:

  This refers to the scan mode where the detector is wide enough to cover the whole heart along the *z*-direction which typically allows to acquire all images with one rotation and one heartbeat. This applies to scanners with 12–16 cm *z*-axis coverage. Scan time is very short with this kind of acquisition, limiting breath-hold.

- *Sequential (Or Also Called "Step and Shoot")*:

  This refers to the image mode where data are acquired at multiple stationary table positions, with table translation in between. At each table position, part of the heart (along *z*-direction) is imaged with table stays stationary during the data acquisition (similar as the volume mode). Table is then translated to the next position to image another part of the heart. Data acquisition is paused during the table translation. This process is repeated until data acquisition is complete for the whole heart. The number of acquisitions depends on the scanner's *z*-axis coverage, typically 3–5 for cardiac applications. Limitations include the need for fusing image slabs, which may introduce artifacts. Irregular heart rhythm could represent a major challenge.

• Terminology used for different scan mode may vary from different manufacturers and in the literature. For example, "axial mode" in some literatures may include "sequential mode." It is therefore important to have terminology clearly defined and self-consistent in the same context.

• ECG gating needs to be paired with the scan mode in cardiac CT. Historically, helical (spiral) mode was usually associated with retrospective gating, and sequential/ volume mode was associated with prospective gating. However, with the introduction of ECG pulsing in retrospective gating and padding in prospective gating, the distinction between these two becomes less prominent (Fig. 1.5b). Right now, there is prospective-gated helical/spiral mode and retrospective-gated volume/sequential mode available.

• Shuttle mode, either sequential or helical, can be used in acquiring dynamic information, e.g., myocardium perfusion. Data acquisition is performed with scanner going back and forth along the scan range of z-direction for a given a period time to capture images in the same region over time.

References

1. Jiang H. Computed tomography: principles, design, artifacts, and recent advances. Bellingham, WA: SPIE; 2009.
2. Kalender WA. Computed tomography: fundamentals, system technology, image quality, applications. Hoboken, NJ: Wiley; 2011.

3. McCollough CH, et al. Dual-and multi-energy CT: principles, technical approaches, and clinical applications. Radiology. 2015;276(3):637–53.
4. Leng S, et al. Photon-counting detector CT: system design and clinical applications of an emerging technology. Radiographics. 2019;39(3):729–43.
5. Rajendran K, et al. First clinical photon-counting detector CT system: technical evaluation. Radiology. 2022;303(1):130–8.
6. Kalisz K, et al. Artifacts at cardiac CT: physics and solutions. Radiographics. 2016;36(7):2064–83.
7. Beister M, Kolditz D, Kalender WA. Iterative reconstruction methods in X-ray CT. Phys Med. 2012;28(2):94–108.
8. Abbara S, et al. SCCT guidelines for the performance and acquisition of coronary computed tomographic angiography: a report of the society of cardiovascular computed tomography guidelines committee: endorsed by the north American Society for Cardiovascular Imaging (NASCI). J Cardiovasc Comput Tomogr. 2016;10(6):435–49.
9. Halliburton SS, et al. SCCT guidelines on radiation dose and dose-optimization strategies in cardiovascular CT. J Cardiovasc Comput Tomogr. 2011;5(4):198–224.
10. Leipsic J, et al. SCCT guidelines for the interpretation and reporting of coronary CT angiography: a report of the Society of Cardiovascular Computed Tomography Guidelines Committee. J Cardiovasc Comput Tomogr. 2014;8(5):342–58.
11. Halliburton S, et al. State-of-the-art in CT hardware and scan modes for cardiovascular CT. J Cardiovasc Comput Tomogr. 2012;6(3):154–63.

2 Image Reconstruction and Postprocessing in Cardiac CT

Rhanderson N. Cardoso and Bruno B. Lima

Abstract

Technological advancements in cardiac CT imaging, coupled with robust data to support evidence-based practices in the field, have established cardiac CT as a first-line test in many coronary and structural applications. Cardiac motion and heart rate variability during image acquisition pose significant challenges for imaging acquisition and interpretation. Understanding these factors and meticulous attention to reconstruction methods and post-processing techniques allow improved visualization of the cardiac anatomy and enhanced diagnostic accuracy of cardiac CT. This chapter covers the fundamental aspect of cardiac CT imaging reconstruction and post-processing.

R. N. Cardoso (✉)
Division of Cardiovascular Medicine, Harvard Medical School, Brigham and Women's Hospital, Boston, MA, USA
e-mail: rcardoso2@bwh.harvard.edu

B. B. Lima
Division of Cardiovascular Medicine, Harvard Medical School, Brigham and Women's Hospital, Boston, MA, USA

Division of Cardiovascular Medicine, Vanderbilt Heart and Vascular Institute, Nashville, TN, USA
e-mail: bruno.lima@vumc.org

Keywords

Imaging reconstruction · Slice thickness
Field of view · Reconstruction filters
Post-processing

Abbreviations

CAC	Coronary artery calcium
CCTA	Coronary CT angiography
CT	Computed tomography
FoV	Field of view
HU	Hounsfield units
MIP	Maximum intensity projection
MPR	Multiplanar reformation
SCCT	Society of Cardiovascular Computed Tomography
TAVR	Transcatheter aortic valve replacement

2.1 Understanding CT Imaging Reconstruction

- As X-ray photons penetrate the patient, they will be affected by tissue properties.
- At the detector array, an X-ray attenuation profile is created for each detector row, as discussed in Chap. 1.
- Attenuation data are collected from multiple scan angles as the gantry rotates, allowing for

A. A. Zadeh, J. Hoe (eds.), *Practical Guide to Cardiac CT*,
https://doi.org/10.1007/978-981-97-6919-3_2

calculation of attenuation in different structures within the body.

- The raw projection data are reprocessed via a mathematical algorithm into a cross-sectional CT image, creating digital images in which each voxel is assigned a digital numerical value (CT value) expressed in Hounsfield units (HU).
- Back projection is the process by which the projections and the angles at which the projections were obtained are used to reconstruct images, each pixel representing the X-ray attenuation at the respective location.
- Standard, conventional reconstruction methods use filtered back projection, in which a filter is applied in the detector domain to remove blurring and to improve edge definition (Fig. 2.1).
- Increasing computational power has allowed for rapid processing of iterative reconstruction techniques, which add to filtered back projection by maximizing the consistency between the measured projection and the simulated projections from the reconstructed images, significantly decreasing image noise.
- This iterative process of image reconstruction and denoising is repeated multiple times until an optimal image is achieved.
- Lower image noise and improved signal-to-noise ratio allow image acquisition with lower X-ray tube power, thus reducing radiation dose while maintaining diagnostic quality [1, 2].
- Reconstruction algorithm, filters, field of view, slice thickness, and other reconstruction parameters will affect image quality, artifacts, edge enhancement, and resolution [3].

2.2 Acquired vs. Reconstructed Slice Thickness

- The *z*-axis (head-to-toe orientation) resolution is determined by the detector width. A thin detector width allows better z-axis resolution, at the expense of increased image noise.
- Conventional cardiac CT scanner detector widths typically range from 0.5 to 6.25 mm. Ultra-high-resolution CT systems provide detector width of <0.5 mm, e.g., 0.1–0.25 mm.
- Acquisition and reconstruction with thinner slices improve signal detection and decrease the partial volume effect (Fig. 2.2); however, image noise generally increases.
- Collimation refers to the restriction of X-rays to certain areas on the detector and activation of different detector channels (see Chap. 1), which may lead to acquisition with larger slice thickness than available, e.g., 10 × 3 mm instead of 64 × 0.5 mm for a 64-detector row CT scanner.
- The smallest *reconstructed* slice is limited/dependent on the smallest *acquired* slice, whereas larger slices may be reconstructed from smaller acquired slices.
- The smallest slice thickness reconstruction is generally recommended for interpretation of

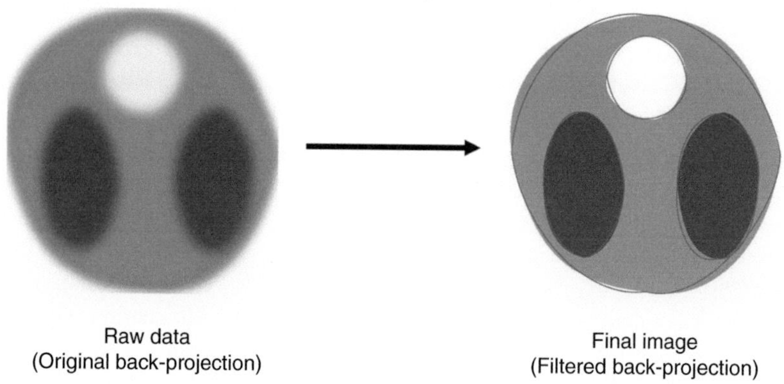

Fig. 2.1 Filtered back projection applies a filter to remove blurring with conventional back projection

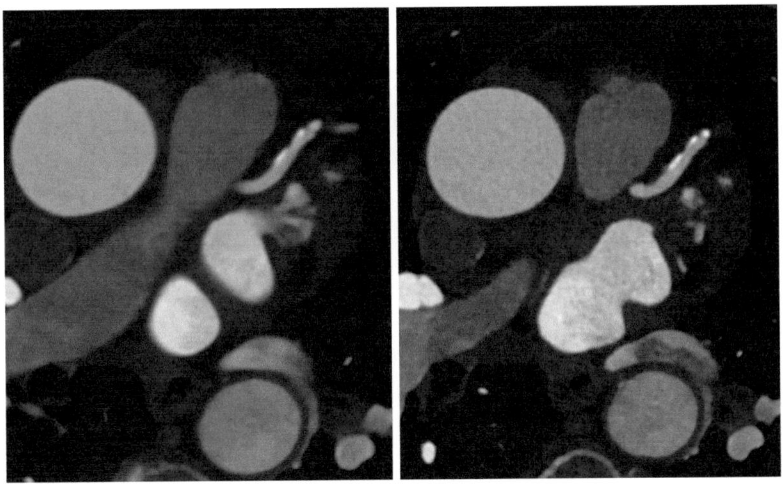

Fig. 2.2 Reconstruction with 1.5 mm slices (left) leads to more blurring and less image noise, whereas the reconstruction with 0.5 mm slices (right) yields better edge-to-edge definition at the expense of increased image noise

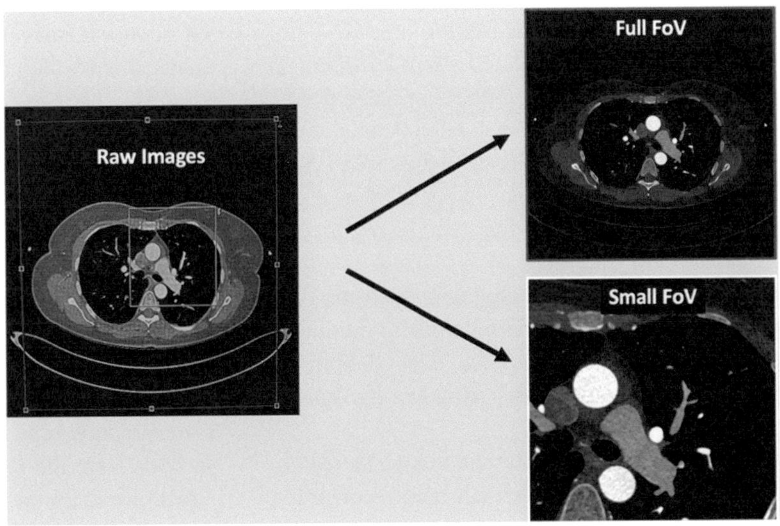

Fig. 2.3 Cardiac CTs are reconstructed in (1) the full scanned field of view for evaluation of incidental findings and (2) in a smaller field of view to maximize resolution for evaluation of cardiac anatomy

most cardiac CT indications, including coronary CT angiography.

- Coronary artery calcium (CAC) scans are an exception as reconstruction is performed with 3-mm slice thickness by convention for standardization of the Agatston score.

2.3 Field of View and Image Matrix

- The term field of view (FoV) may refer to the *scanned* FoV (also known as scan range) or the *reconstructed* FoV. The reconstructed FoV is always a subset of or the entire scanned FoV, but not larger.
- The typical reconstructed field of view for the heart is approximately 250–300 mm (Fig. 2.3).
- The matrix size refers to the grid of pixels along both in-plane dimensions. Typically, the matrix has 512 × 512 pixels. Ultra-high resolution may use 1024 × 1024 or even greater matrices.
- The pixel size is given by the size of the reconstructed FoV divided by the matrix size, e.g., for a 512 × 512 matrix and a reconstructed FoV of 250 mm, each pixel size will be ~0.5 mm.
- To maximize resolution, i.e., smallest pixel size, the reconstructed FoV should be as small as possible.

- An important goal is the creation of isotropic voxels of ~0.5 mm in the *x*-, *y*-, and *z*-axis, which allows for multiplanar reformatting while maintaining image resolution in all planes—a distinct advantage to other imaging modalities, e.g., MRI.

2.4 Reconstruction Kernels

- Data received at the scanner detectors undergo a processing step, called filtering, before they are back-projected to form an image to address noise and edge detection. This filter is also called a kernel or convolution kernel, essentially consisting of a small matrix processing data before forming the image.
- Kernels may be considered *sharp*, *medium*, or *soft,* depending on their effect on edge detection. Sharp filters increase edge details at the expense of allowing more image noise. Soft filters make the image "smooth," i.e., they decrease image noise but also decrease edge details (Fig. 2.4).
- Calcified coronary plaques and stents are better evaluated with a sharp kernel, to minimize blooming artifact, improve edge definition, and consequently, better visualize the lumen [4, 5].
- Images in obese patients tend to have increased image noise and may benefit from reconstruction with *soft* filters to reduce image noise (smoothen image). Nomenclature for specific kernels is vendor-specific, but principles are similar.

2.5 Cardiac Phase Selection for Image Acquisition and Reconstruction

- Appropriate cardiac phase selection for scanning and reconstruction is critical for obtaining high-quality analyzable data [6].
- The optimal cardiac phase is variable and dependent on indication (e.g., TAVR, coronary, cardiac function, etc.) and patient-related factors, such as rhythm irregularity and heart rate.
- Of *acquired* images, reconstructions may be selected according to lack of motion or other specific characteristics. Commonly, reconstructions are performed at ~5% intervals within the available phases to provide a selection, e.g., 65, 70, 75, and 80% for a scan obtained 65–80% of the R-R interval (starting with 0% at the peak of the R wave).
- Specific indications determine need for timing of phases, e.g., phase with largest annular dimensions for TAVR guidance [7].
- Instead of using percentage of the R-R cycle, reconstructions can also be identified in milliseconds from the R wave. Time-based reconstructions may be particularly helpful for systolic reconstructions with irregular rhythms,

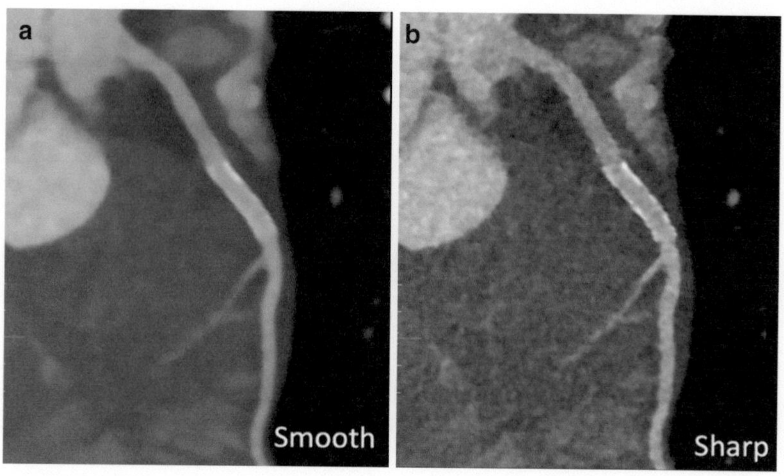

Fig. 2.4 Curved multiplanar reformation (MPR) with smooth (**a**) versus sharp (**b**) reconstruction filters for assessment of stent patency. Note the better edge definition with the sharp filter, at the expense of increased image noise

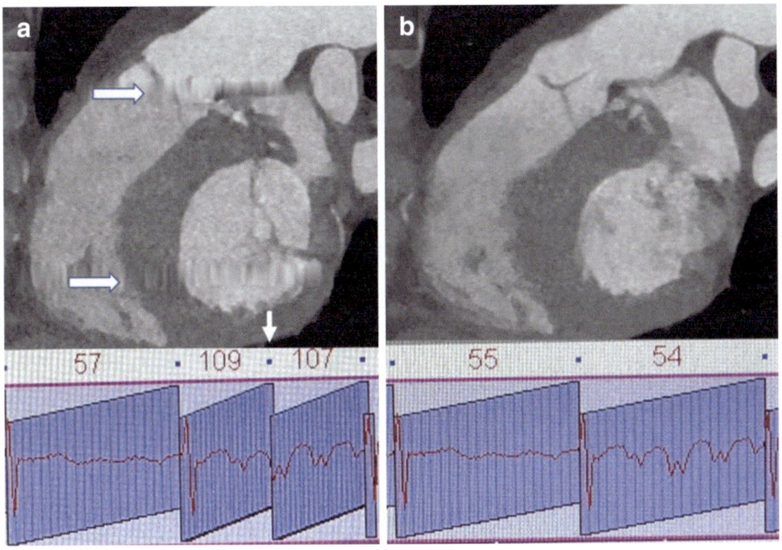

Fig. 2.5 Banding artifact (horizontal arrows) from incorrect ECG data (**a**). Note the incorrect synchronization triggered by artifact in the ECG tracing (vertical arrow). The artifact disappears after ECG editing and removal of the artifactual synchronization (**b**)

given that the duration of systole is much less affected than diastole with irregular and/or fast heart rates, e.g., 300–400 ms for atrial fibrillation.

- At lower heart rates (< 65–70 bpm), mid-diastole (65–80% of the R-R cycle) is typically the ideal window for reduced cardiac motion and optimal coronary interpretation. At higher heart rates (>65–70 bpm), the optimal phase is variable and may lie within late systole or mid-diastole (30–80% of the R-R cycle), thus typically requiring a larger exposure window. The ideal phase may also be different for different coronary segments [6].

2.6 ECG Editing

- Cardiac CT image acquisition occurs while concomitantly recording ECG data to allow registering images to specific phases in the cardiac cycle.
- With retrospective ECG-gating, both ECG and image data are acquired throughout the cardiac cycle and reconstructed images are assigned retrospectively to different portions of the cardiac cycle based on the ECG data.
- Given the plentitude of data, this scanning mode facilitates editing of the ECG synchronization data after image acquisition, which may be helpful in the presence of arrhythmias or artifacts in the ECG data [8].
- With ECG editing, the interpretation of an R wave by the ECG dataset can be corrected, e.g., removed, or shifted to align more accurately with the actual timing of the QRS complex. This can often salvage what would otherwise be an uninterpretable scan in the setting of artifacts (Fig. 2.5).

2.7 Post-Processing Techniques

- Multiple post-processing techniques are regularly utilized in cardiac CT, including multiplanar reformation (MPR); curved MPR; thicker slices with maximum intensity projection (MIP), minimum-intensity projection (MinIP), or average-intensity projection; and volume rendering.
- In cardiac CT, isotropic voxels (i.e., with equal dimensions in all three planes) allow for MPR with preserved image resolution in all planes, facilitating unlimited viewing options throughout the dataset.
- Interpretation of CCTA with MPR is commonly performed using two long-axis views and one short-axis view of the structure of interest. The alignment of two planes (perpendicular to each other) with the long axis of the

vessel results in a short-axis image of the structure on the third plane (Figs. 2.6 and 2.7).

- A limitation of MPR is that it can only evaluate short segments of the coronary arteries at a time before their tortuous course moves out of the image plane, requiring multiple adjustments of the imaging planes along the curved course of an artery (also called the "vessel walk").
- A separate type of image reconstruction, called *curved* planar reformation or curved MPR, can circumvent this issue by tracking the vessel centerline and displaying the anatomy center around the vessel's entire course (Fig. 2.8).
- Given the involved image processing, curved MPR is vulnerable to artifacts (creating false stenoses) when the centerline does not track

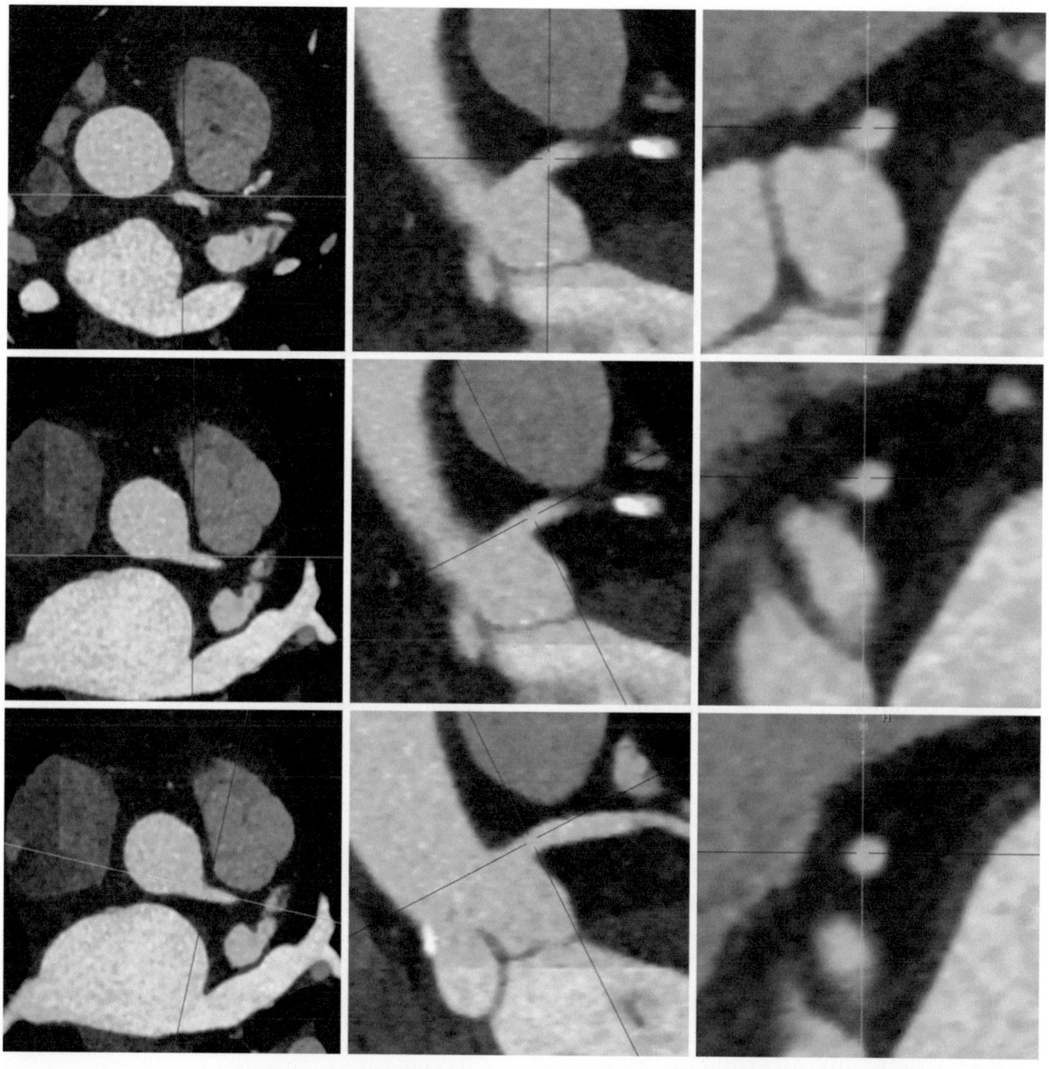

Fig. 2.6 Multiplanar reconstruction to obtain a short-axis image of the left main coronary artery. The first row has images in axial (left), coronal (center), and sagittal (right) planes. In the second row, the blue plane (center) is adjusted in the long axis of the left main coronary artery. In the third row, the green plane (left) is also adjusted in the long axis of the vessel. With two images aligned on long axis, the third plane (third row, right image) is now in a true short axis of the left main coronary artery

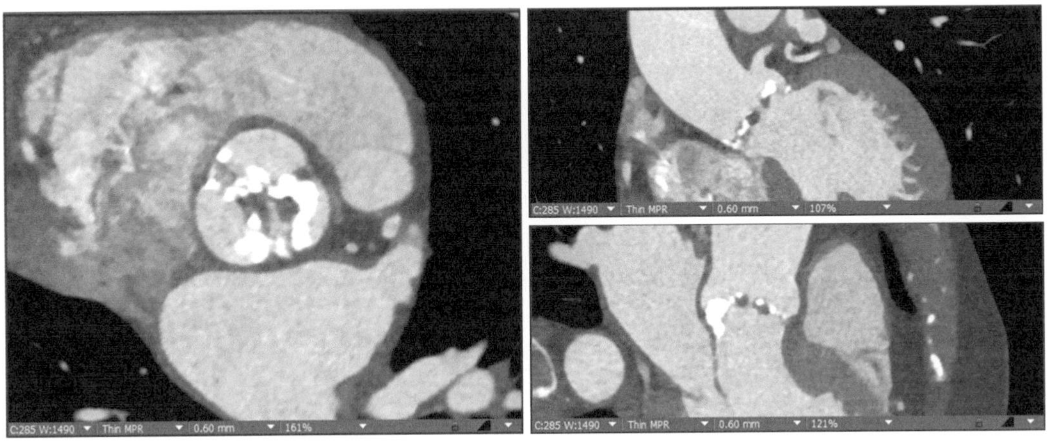

Fig. 2.7 Multiplanar reconstruction images demonstrating a heavily calcified aortic valve in the short-axis (left) and two orthogonal long-axis planes (right)

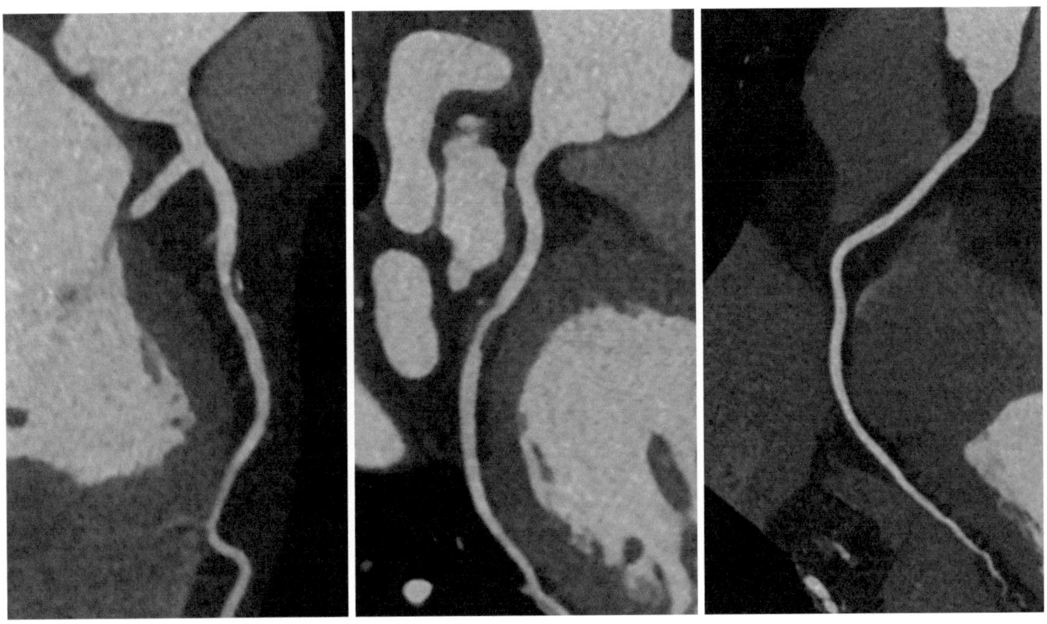

Fig. 2.8 Coronary CT angiography reconstructed in curved multiplanar reformation. From left to right, images show (1) calcified and noncalcified plaque in the mid left anterior descending artery with mild stenosis; (2) noncalcified plaque in the mid circumflex with moderate stenosis; and (3) right coronary artery without plaque or stenosis

well with the lumen. Therefore, curved MPR images should be interpreted with caution and in conjunction with regular MPR.

- Creating image slabs with several slices (e.g., 5–6 mm) using MIP is effective for obtaining an overview of the anatomy. MIP implies greatest representation of structures with highest attenuation value within the slice (Fig. 2.9).
- MIP may be used to visualize small structures, such as septal branches, but it may worsen "blooming" artifacts of high-density structures and miss subtle findings, e.g., noncalcified plaque.

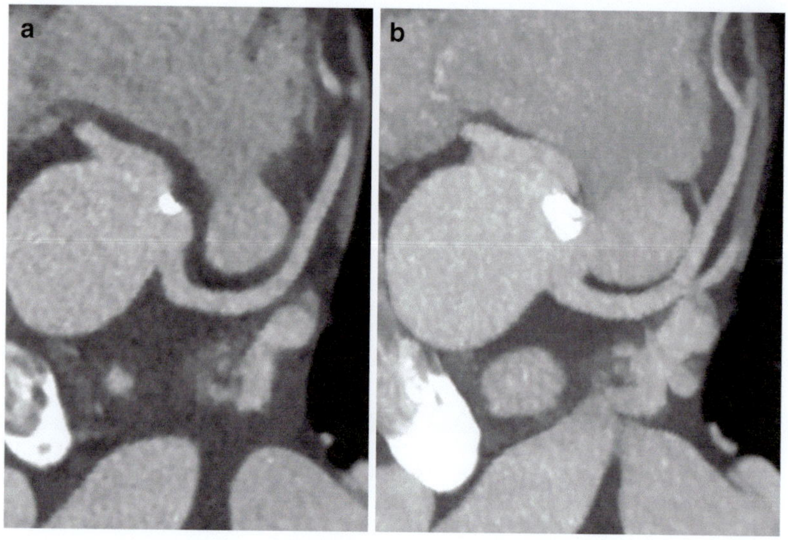

Fig. 2.9 Thin multiplanar reformation images with 0.5 mm slice thickness (**a**) versus 6-mm slice thickness with maximum intensity projection (**b**)

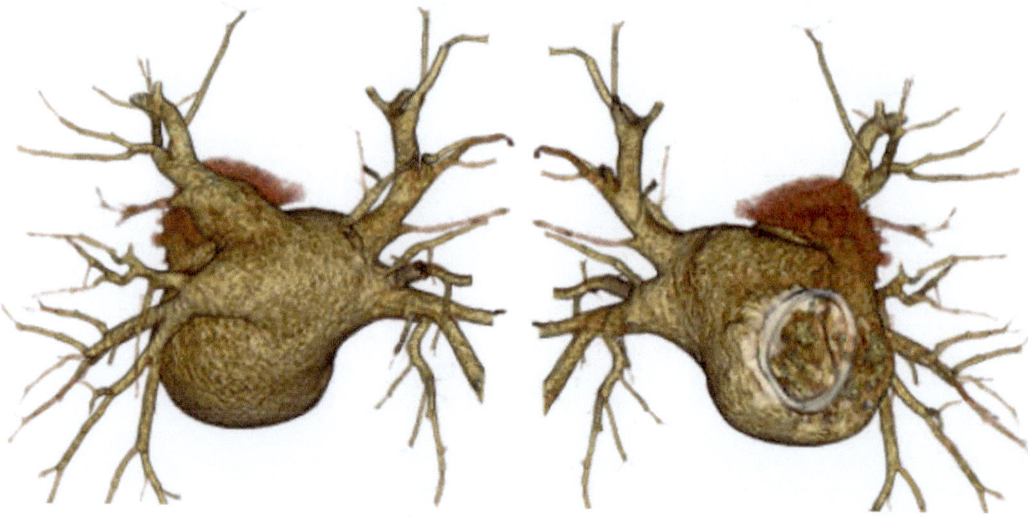

Fig. 2.10 Volume-rendering 3D reconstructed CT images provides added value in the assessment of pulmonary vein anatomy prior to catheter ablation of atrial fibrillation

- Volume rendering is a post-processing technique that creates a three-dimensional representation of data. A rendering algorithm of color, texture, shadowing, and transparency is applied to the volumetric CT data to create a 3D projection of an organ or structure (Fig. 2.10).
- Volume rendering allows for interactive rotation and can help in visualization of complex 3D structural relationships. It is effective for displaying congenital and structural abnormalities. Given the complex data processing, caution should be used for the interpretation of coronary arteries.
- The Society of Cardiovascular Computed Tomography Guidelines for the Interpretation and Reporting of Coronary CT Angiography recommends post-processing of CCTA with axial, MPR, MIP, and (optional) curved MPR reconstructions (Table 2.1) [9].

Table 2.1 Recommended image post-processing formats for coronary assessment [9]

Axial image review	Recommended
Multiplanar reformation (MPR) image review	Recommended
Maximum intensity projection (MIP) image review	Recommended
Curved multiplanar reformation (MPR) image review	Optional
Volume-rendered reconstructions	Consider under limited circumstances

References

1. Deseive S, Chen MY, Korosoglou G, et al. Prospective randomized trial on radiation dose estimates of CT angiography applying iterative image reconstruction: the PROTECTION V study. JACC Cardiovasc Imaging. 2015;8:888–96.
2. Yin W-H, Lu B, Gao J-B, et al. Effect of reduced x-ray tube voltage, low iodine concentration contrast medium, and sinogram-affirmed iterative reconstruction on image quality and radiation dose at coronary CT angiography: results of the prospective multicenter REALISE trial. J Cardiovasc Comput Tomogr. 2015;9:215–24.
3. Abbara S, Blanke P, Maroules CD, et al. SCCT guidelines for the performance and acquisition of coronary computed tomographic angiography: a report of the society of cardiovascular computed tomography guidelines committee: endorsed by the north American Society for Cardiovascular Imaging (NASCI). J Cardiovasc Comput Tomogr. 2016;10:435–49.
4. Ammon F, Moshage M, Smolka S, et al. Influence of reconstruction kernels on the accuracy of CT-derived fractional flow reserve. Eur Radiol. 2022;32:2604–10.
5. Achenbach S, Boehmer K, Pflederer T, et al. Influence of slice thickness and reconstruction kernel on the computed tomographic attenuation of coronary atherosclerotic plaque. J Cardiovasc Comput Tomogr. 2010;4:110–5.
6. Yang C-C, Law W-Y, Lu K-M, Wu T-H. Relationship between heart rate and optimal reconstruction phase in coronary CT angiography performed on a 256-slice multidetector CT. Br J Radiol. 2019;92:20180945.
7. Blanke P, Weir-McCall JR, Achenbach S, et al. Computed tomography imaging in the context of transcatheter aortic valve implantation (TAVI)/transcatheter aortic valve replacement (TAVR): an expert consensus document of the Society of Cardiovascular Computed Tomography. J Cardiovasc Comput Tomogr. 2019;13:1–20.
8. Matsumoto H, Kondo T, Watanabe S, et al. ECG-edited middiastolic phase reconstruction improves image quality at 64-MDCT coronary angiography of patients with atrial fibrillation. AJR Am J Roentgenol. 2008;191:1659–66.
9. Leipsic J, Abbara S, Achenbach S, et al. SCCT guidelines for the interpretation and reporting of coronary CT angiography: a report of the Society of Cardiovascular Computed Tomography Guidelines Committee. J Cardiovasc Comput Tomogr. 2014;8:342–58.

Introduction to the Cardiac CT Imaging Workstation

3

Edward P. Shapiro

Abstract

Isovolumetric image acquisition opens vast opportunities for image display which is fully realized on dedicated workstations, including three-dimensional rendering. Although individual features and organization are found on different proprietary platforms, there is a common approach to display and analyze images. This chapter will provide a general overview of cardiac CT display and analysis using dedicated imaging workstations.

Keywords

CT image interpretation · Workstation
Image display · Image analysis

Abbreviations

AV	Atrioventricular
cMPR	Curved MPR
EP	Electrophysiology
HU	Hounsfield unit
KVp	Kilovolt peak
LAD	Left anterior descending artery
LCx	Left circumflex artery
LV	Left ventricular
MESA	Multi-Ethnic Study of Atherosclerosis
MIP	Maximum intensity projection
MPR	Multiplanar reformation
PACS	Picture Arching and Communication System
PDA	Posterior descending artery
RCA	Right coronary artery
TAVR	Transcutaneous aortic valve replacement
TMVR	Transcutaneous mitral valve replacement

E. P. Shapiro (✉)
Johns Hopkins Bayview Medical Center, Johns Hopkins University, Baltimore, MD, USA
e-mail: eshapiro@jhmi.edu

3.1 Background

- Although the standard radiology user interfaces for interpretation of axial CT scans provide measurement tools and display options, the use of advanced software is required for interpretation of cardiac CT, allowing 3D display of structures, fine control of oblique planes, varied image display protocols, easy visualization of structures through the cardiac cycle, automatic tracking of arteries, and automatic measurements.
- Different system architectures for these workstations exist, using either a stand-alone computer, or thin clients which rely on a central server for processing.
- The workstations offered by the major vendors have similar basic tools, displays, and

A. A. Zadeh, J. Hoe (eds.), *Practical Guide to Cardiac CT*,
https://doi.org/10.1007/978-981-97-6919-3_3

capabilities, but these are accessed using different buttons, keystrokes, and screens.
- Detailed training on any particular workstation can be transferred to another with some instruction and practice.

3.2 Workflow

- Patient data are acquired on the scanner console and are then reconstructed into images.
- Reconstructed images are sent directly to the designated workstation and also to storage in a picture arching and communication system (PACS) or can be recalled from the PACS to the workstation at a later time.
- Raw data are saved on the scanner console for only a limited period of time before they are overwritten by new patient data. Some facilities have raw data servers, in which the raw data can be stored indefinitely. While the raw data are available, new images can be reconstructed using different protocols or at different phases of the cardiac cycle, at the request of the interpreter.
- Local regulation may mandate form and period of data storage.
- Images are manipulated and interpreted on the workstation. Snapshots, cines, and other data can be saved on the workstation and/or added to long-term storage in PACS.

3.3 Recommended Steps for Cardiac CT Analysis

- The different applications of cardiac CT require specific protocols and tools for analysis, and these are available for calcium scoring, coronary artery analysis, cardiac structure and functional analysis, myocardial perfusion analysis, electrophysiological procedure planning, and transcutaneous aortic valve replacement (TAVR) analysis. The images that are loaded into the workstation may contain metadata that allow the software to select the proper protocol automatically, or it may have to be designated by hand.

3.3.1 For Coronary Calcium Scoring

- Coronary calcium scores are predominantly used to provide risk prediction in asymptomatic patients. The scans are acquired using prospectively gated protocols designed to be similar to those of the original electron beam scanners so that the results can be historically compatible. The slice thickness used is 3 mm, and the voltage used is 120 kVp, with mA varying based on overall chest attenuation. The workstation software automatically highlights pixels with HU $\geq$ 130, which can be selected in each slice and assigned to specific arteries with automatic determination of Agatston and volume scores. Mass scores can be calculated if a calibration phantom containing varying concentrations of calcium hydroxyapatite has been scanned.
- The workstation software may incorporate reference data from clinical studies, most commonly from the MESA study [1], which allows comparison of the patient with age, gender, and ethnicity matched peers. The absolute calcium score is the best predictor of a coronary event over a 10-year period. The percentile score compares a patient's score to that of the population and therefore supplies information about lifetime risk. Both should be reported.

3.3.2 For Coronary Artery Analysis

- Loading of multiple volumes is recommended to distinguish findings from potential artifacts, particularly motion artifacts. Motion artifacts vary within the cardiac cycle, even within the two "sweet spots" for imaging, diastasis, and isovolumic relaxation. 3D images or automatically derived curved MPR images at different phases, i.e., 70, 75, and 80% may be quickly perused to evaluate gross image clarity. We begin our coronary analysis with the best appearing volume (no or least artifacts).
- The workstation's starting screen contains a 3D volume-rendered image, presented as a lit/shaded surface display, and three 2D tomo-

graphic views, displaying the scanned volume in the axes of the body, the axial, coronal, and sagittal planes (Fig. 3.1).

- Review the 3D volume-rendered image.
  - The workstation typically provides presets for specific applications, e.g., coronary CTA, which uses display algorithms that automatically sculpt the non-cardiac components of the 3D image, such as the chest wall, spine, and diaphragm. Further efforts to "clean up" the image can be achieved by carving away any remnants of these extraneous structures, but this is generally time consuming and usually not necessary unless images are being prepared for a presentation or formal display.
  - A brief survey of the 3D reconstruction helps to alert the reader to gross anatomic findings, including coronary dominance or anomalies. As the 3D image is rotated, subtle artifacts that are otherwise difficult to detect may become visible. Coronary calcium and stenotic lesions may be evident. The absence of contrast where a coronary artery should be located, with clearly seen tell-tale deposits of calcium, suggests total coronary occlusion (Fig. 3.2).
  - However, the 3D display should not be used to ultimately determine the extent of coronary disease since it is a shaded display of the surface of the heart and coronary arteries and does not visualize the lumen.
- Review of the 2D axial images.

  It is recommended to quickly scan each coronary artery from superior to inferior and back again. Most coronary segments are oblique to the axial views, but with experience atherosclerotic plaque and significant stenoses can be detected. Anomalous coronary arteries are easily detected and characterized in the axial planes (Fig. 3.3). These views are also useful for evaluating non-cardiac pathology (i.e.,

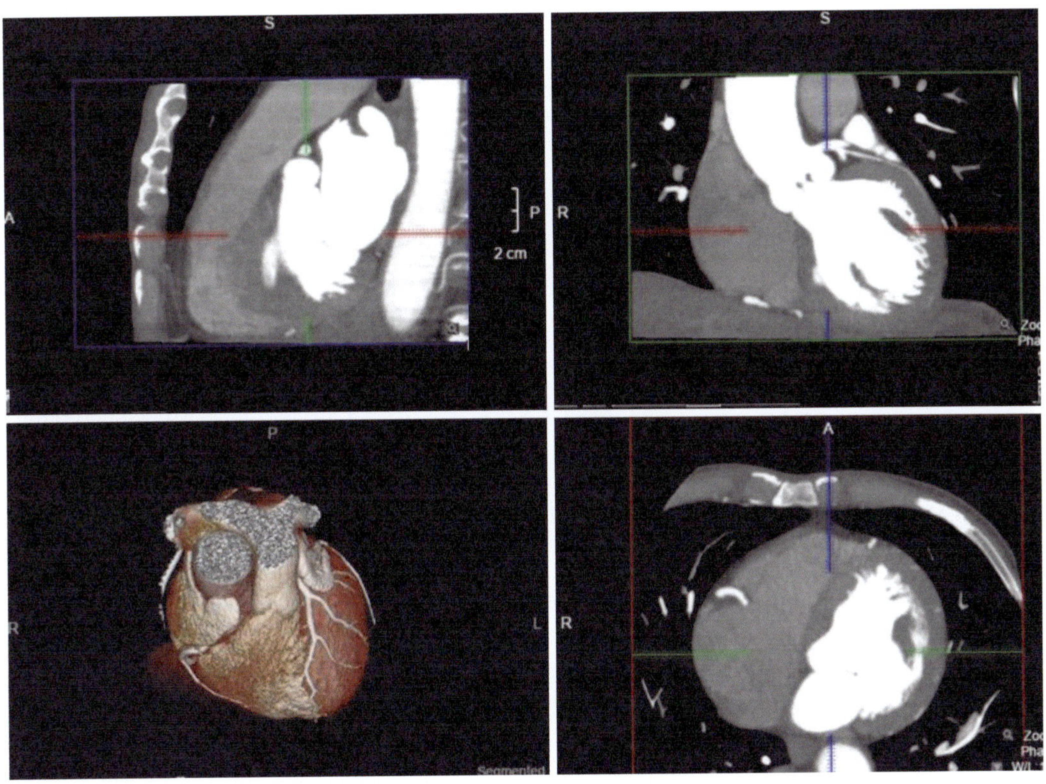

Fig. 3.1 Typical arrangement of an imaging workstation view using four windows, including one dedicated to 3D image rendering and three 2D tomographic views in the axial, coronal, and sagittal planes

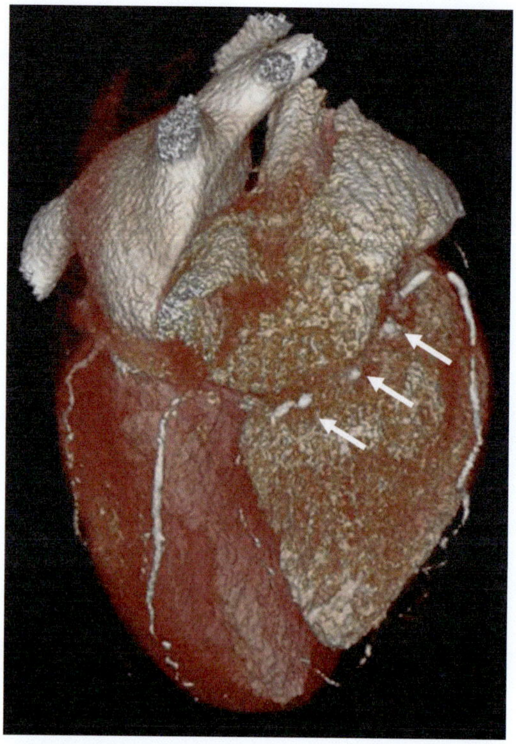

Fig. 3.2 3D view showing the absence of an arterial vessel in the AV groove where the RCA typically travels. This is not due to suboptimal image quality, as spots of calcium can be seen along the track of the vessel (arrows), suggesting artery occlusion

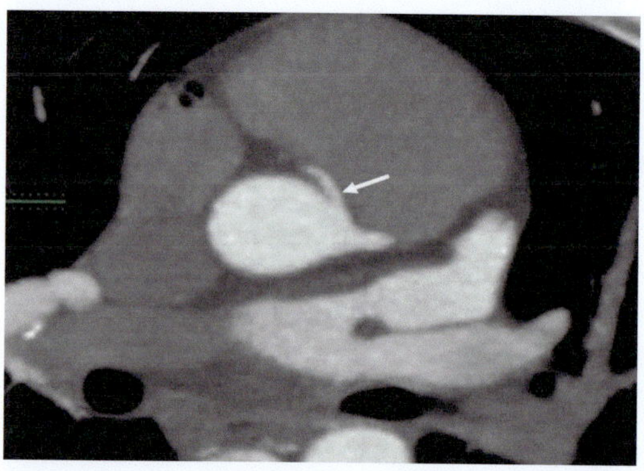

Fig. 3.3 Axial image showing anomalous RCA from the left sinus of Valsalva (arrow)

lung nodules, esophageal abnormalities, pulmonary emboli, bone lesions, or aortic disease). Changes in the window/level settings are necessary for viewing lung and bone.

- Review of the multiformat reformation (MRP) or maximum intensity projection (MIP) images in oblique planes.

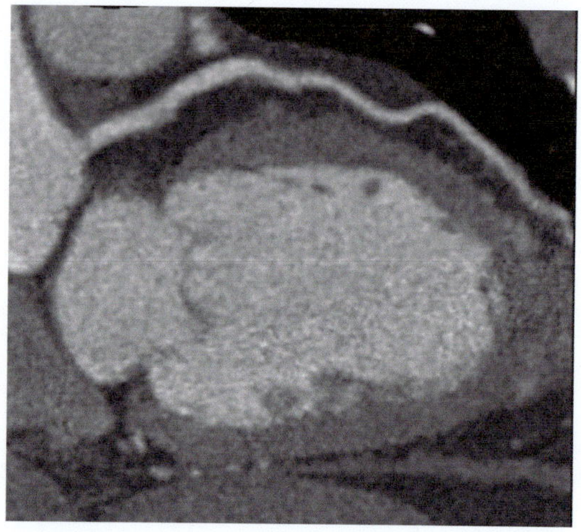

Fig. 3.4 Curved MRP (cMPR), able to accurately represent the 3D course of a vessel in a 2D image

- Finally, using 2D images, it is recommended to manipulate the views of each segment of each coronary artery and its secondary branches into oblique planes such that each portion of artery can be seen in its longitudinal and cross-sectional orientation along each artery until its size tapers to about 1.5 mm. There are four different approaches to this task that can be utilized. These are listed below:
  - The Curved MPR (cMPR).

    This approach uses software that automatically tracks the centerline of a vessel along its course. cMPR images are created by defining a "virtual" plane along that centerline. Workstations vary with respect to how these are generated. Some use a single "seed point" in the artery of interest and propagate along the 3D volume from there. Others use a seed point that originates in the aortic root. Others connect two points that are identified by hand.

    The cMPR converts a 3D representation into a 2D representation and thus accomplishes the objective of visualizing a long longitudinal segment of artery (Fig. 3.4).

    Readers should be aware that automatic vessel centerline algorithms may fail to adequately track the vessel if the image quality is not optimal.

The cMPR should be rotated so that multiple viewpoints are available. Regions that contain plaque may be further assessed in a cross-sectional view of the artery. Workstation tools that allow automatic or semi-automatic calculation of "percent stenosis" can be accessed from these views. However, the edges that are detected and used for this calculation should be examined closely since these might not correspond to edges that seem appropriate visually. Lesions are better reported in broad ranges (1–24%, 25–49%, 50–69%, 70–99%), as described in the CAD-RADS system for uniform reporting [2], rather than with an exact percent stenosis.

The cMPR can be displayed in a MIP format, which simulates an angiographic view (Fig. 3.5).

– The Vessel "Oblique Walk".

Segments of the coronary artery are visualized along their long axes using oblique planes.

The disadvantage of using these real planes in space (as compared to their respective cMPRs) is that the arteries do not run for long distances in any single plane, so only short segments can be visualized at any one time.

The advantages include no degradation due to improper centerline tracking, and easy manipulation of the image format (i.e., maximum intensity projection [MIP], etc.), rendering oblique images more tolerant of suboptimal study quality than curved MPRs. An "oblique walk" is accomplished by finding the plane that best displays the arterial segment along its long axis (usually beginning with the axial plane).

A second, perpendicular plane is defined along the apparent long axis of the vessel segment, allowing the artery to be viewed in this resulting second plane, followed by a third plane along its long axis, etc. (Fig. 3.6).

Several iterations of this process are typically necessary to be able to display the vessel in a long segment.

The vessels are often viewed as a "slab," i.e., combining several layers of voxels (e.g., 6 × 0.5 mm = 3 mm slice thickness) for overview and then as thin slices for more detail.

An image may be displayed using the average density of the pixels within the slab, the maximal density within the slab (MIP), or minimal density within the slab (MinIP).

To evaluate stents and regions of heavy calcification, the thinnest possible slice should always be used. Thin slices should also be used in evaluation of arterial cross section, and in any situation where the density of a structure in Hounsfield Units is being measured.

– The "Pivot"

A single point within a coronary artery can be used as a pivot, with movement of the mouse used to tilt the currently visualized plane into another arbitrary plane that displays a substantial length of coronary artery (Fig. 3.7).

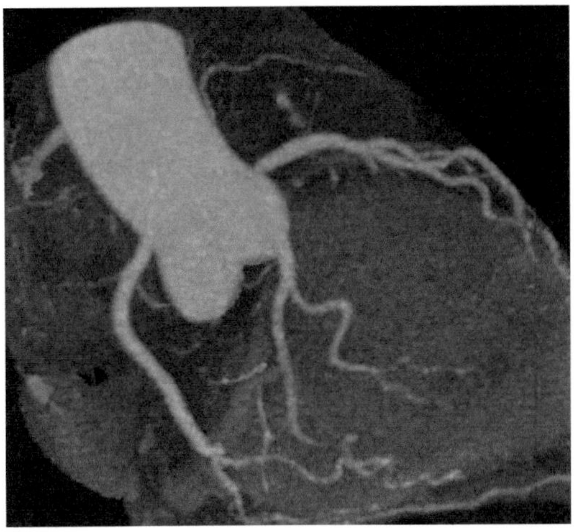

Fig. 3.5 An automatically generated series of cMPRs displayed in a view that simulates the appearance of an invasive angiogram

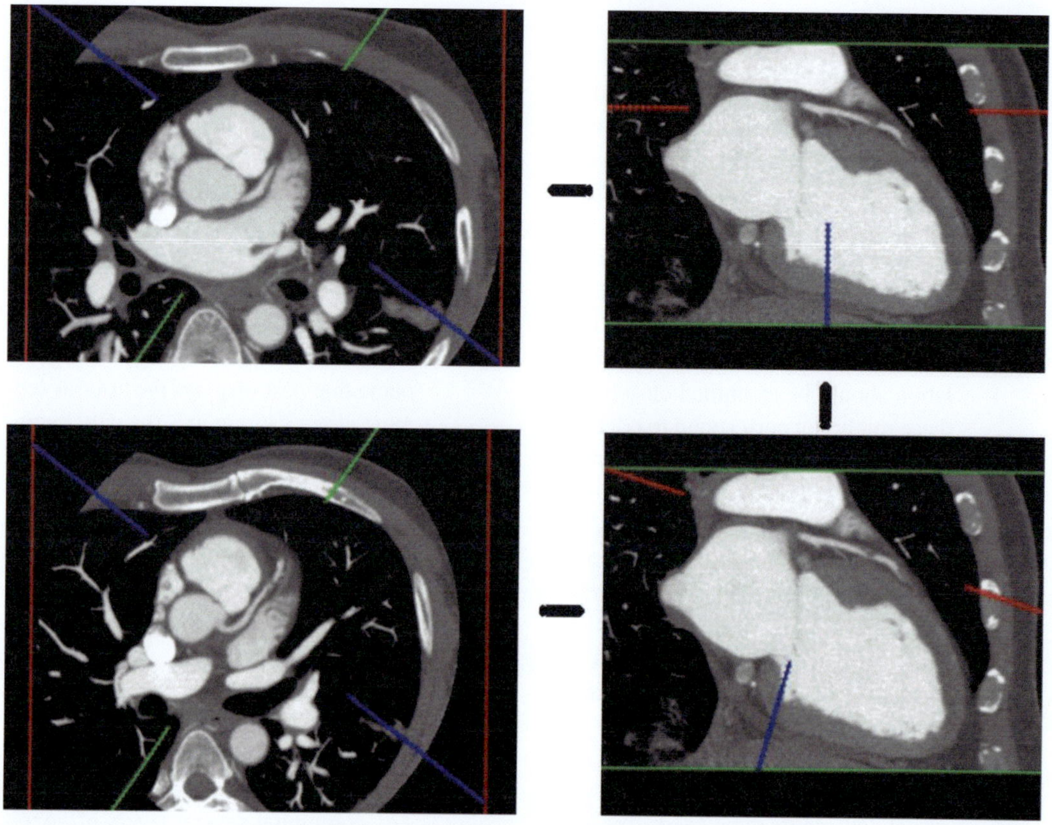

Fig. 3.6 The vessel "oblique walk". Series of images are shown illustrating the "oblique walk," a method for visualizing longitudinal segments of coronary arteries by repetitive aligning of orthogonal planes

Fig. 3.7 The "pivot". Illustration of how a pivot method allows the tilting of a plane in space to visualize cardiac structures. The 2D plane, given as a red parallelogram, can be adjusted, pivoting on the point of the red arrow

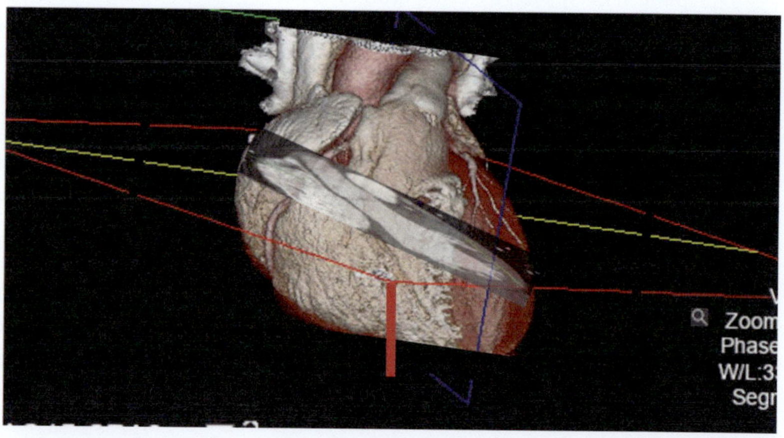

The location of the pivot point is then updated to a location more distal in the coronary, and the plane is tilted further. In this way, the visualized plane can be "rolled" around the surface of the heart, quickly following the coronaries.

This method is among the fastest and most popular methods to visualize the entire coronary tree.

– "Special Planes": This nickname describes planes that can be identified quickly using ventricular anatomy, which provide excellent starting points for tracking segments of the coronary arteries known to run in those planes. The most useful are:

Right-Sided AV Groove Plane for Evaluating a Dominant RCA: This is sometimes referred to as the "C" plane. The RCA makes a sharp curve and may be difficult to track using methods described above. Given that the RCA and its distal continuation (as the posterolateral branch) usually run in or close to the AV groove, the latter may be identified quickly by manipulating planes using easily identified cardiac anatomy. When placing a crosshair intersection in the visible portion of the RCA in a plane that cuts along the AV groove in the two other planes, the RCA should be well visualized (Fig. 3.8). A similar procedure can be used to track a dominant circumflex, which runs in the AV groove on the left side.

Planes for Evaluating the PDA: Starting from the AV grove plane above, defining a new plane along the distal RCA will show the PDA well. If not easily seen in that view, a simple axial plane at the inferior aspect of the heart may show the PDA well or at least provide a starting point for its evaluation.

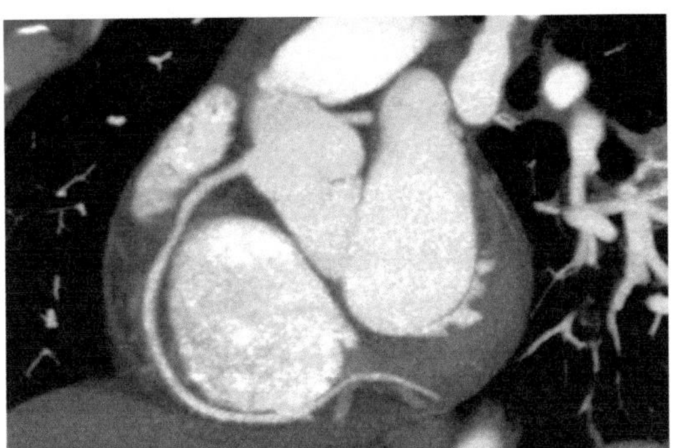

Fig. 3.8 Specific planes in which segments of coronary artery tend to run can be identified by ventricular anatomy. In this example, a plane has been aligned along the AV groove resembling a "C." Most of the RCA is visible within this plane

3.3.3 For LV Function Analysis

If retrospective, continuous, or dose-modulated CT has been used for acquisition, a time series of 2D or 3D images can be displayed in cine loops, and left ventricular function can be accurately measured. The workstation can automatically adjust the planes so that instead of displaying the orthogonal planes of the body (axial, coronary, and sagittal), the orthogonal planes of the heart, similar to the 4-chamber, 2-chamber, and short-axis views in echocardiography, are visualized. The endocardial edge is automatically tracked, and volumes are calculated at each phase using Simpson's rule. The largest volume is assigned to represent end diastole, and the smallest to represent end systole. Parameters of global LV function including ejection fraction, end diastolic volume, end systolic volume, stroke volume, cardiac output, and left ventricular mass are readily displayed. Playing a loop of these images permits assessment of regional function, which can also be shown using a typical bulls-eye display.

3.3.4 For EP Procedure Planning

Percutaneous methods for electrically isolating the pulmonary veins are now commonly performed to treat atrial fibrillation. The anatomy of the pulmonary veins is highly variable, and an understanding of left atrial anatomy prior to ablation procedures is important for procedural success. Dedicated software allows corresponding catheter positions with previously recorded CT images. The CT workstation may contain "EP planning" modules which automatically display pulmonary vein anatomy and facilitate measurements.

3.3.5 For Myocardial Perfusion

Myocardial perfusion studies at rest and after vasodilator stress can be aligned and displayed side-by-side for visual and color-coded assessment of perfusion defects (see Chap. 18).

3.4 Formats Used by Specific Vendors

- The four major manufacturers of CT scanners are Canon, General Electric, Philips, and Siemens. Each makes their own workstation, and each can accept DICOM images from multiple vendors. TeraRecon is a popular workstation that is independent of scanner manufacturers. Additional platforms such as 3Mensio and Circle target advanced measurements needed for TAVR or TMVR.
- The workstations that are used for interpreting cardiac CT all have similar tools. In general, there is a connection to the PACS system where reconstructed images are stored, so that multiple volumes (each consisting of a stack of images) for each patient can be downloaded.
- The volumes may differ with respect to the phase of the cardiac cycle (reconstructed by either absolute milliseconds from the QRS or percentage of the RR interval). They may vary with respect to the kernel used in reconstruction, the thickness of the slice, and the field of view in which the data is displayed.
- Each patient's multiple images appear in a study directory. As each set of images is loaded into active memory, the workstation determines which application is most appropriate, i.e., for coronaries, for LV function, for TAVR analysis, for myocardial perfusion, for EP planning, etc., based on metadata embedded in the image.
- Most workstations start coronary analysis by displaying 3D images, then axial, coronary, and sagittal planes which are easily obliqued to follow the coronary arteries. Curved MRPs for the major arteries are automatically generated.

3.4.1 General Electric

See Fig. 3.9.

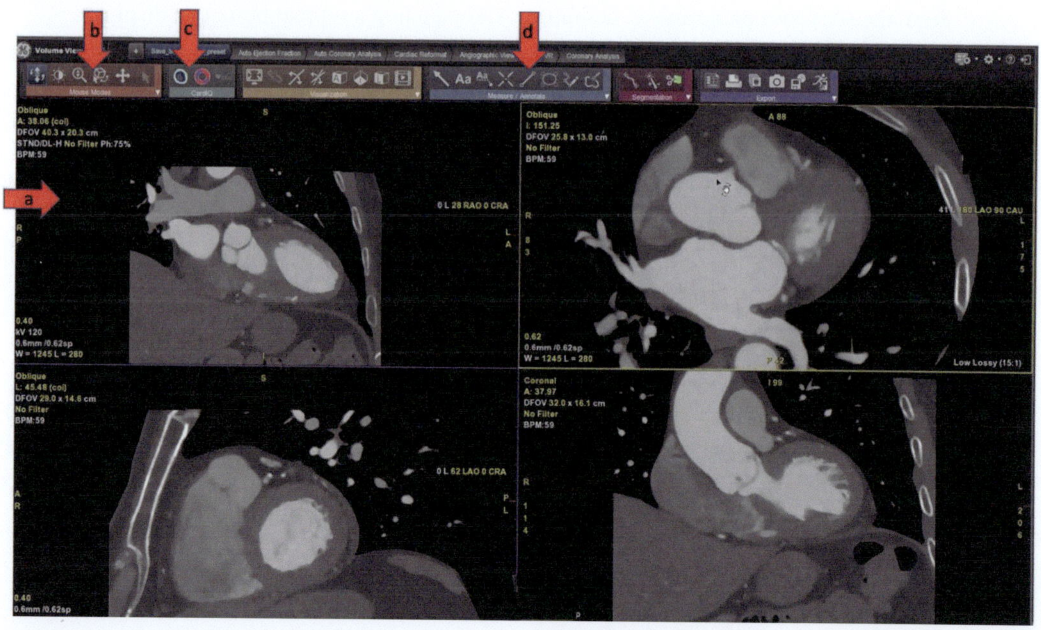

Fig. 3.9 A home screen of General Electric's AW workstation that illustrates some of many features available to analyze cardiac CT images. (**a**) A quad screen consisting of a coronal and three oblique MPRs that can be positioned to track the coronary arteries. (**b**) Various functions of mouse motions and buttons can be defined here. (**c**) The CardiQ Suite refers to an array of functions for 3D analysis of cardiac structural and functional images. (**d**) A set of tools is available for quick measurements

3.4.2 Philips

See Fig. 3.10.

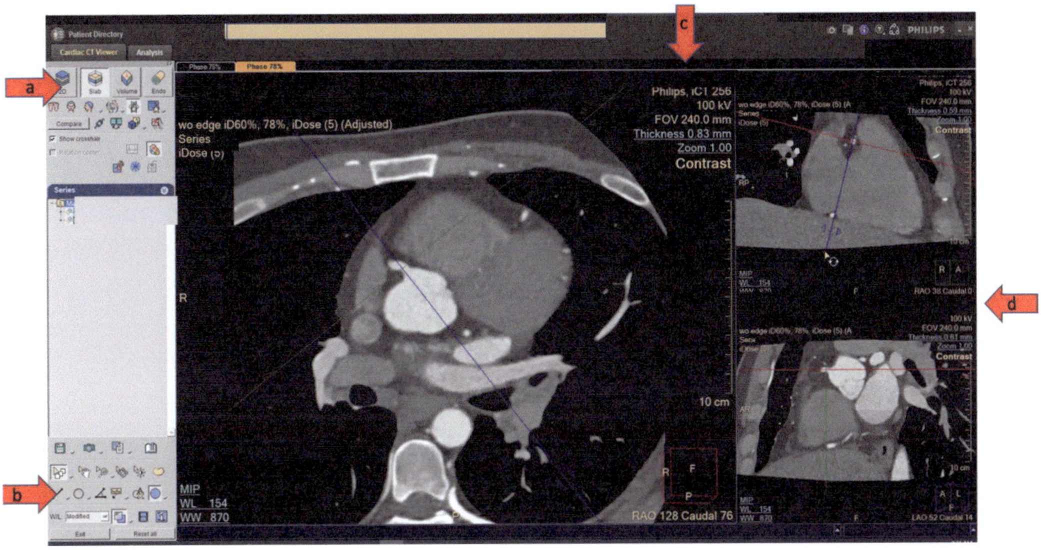

Fig. 3.10 A home screen of Philips workstation that illustrates some of the functions available. (**a**) Controls for image display are shown. (**b**) Multiple image measurements can be made. (**c**) Images from the Philips 256 slice scanner are seen. (**d**) Oblique planes and a sagittal MRP views are shown

3.4.3 Siemens

See Fig. 3.11.

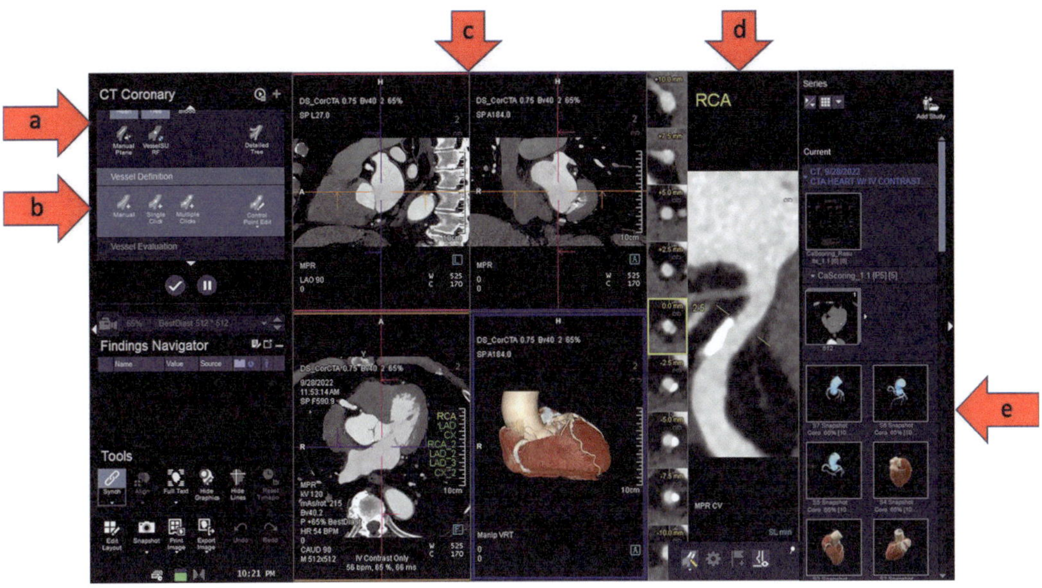

Fig. 3.11 A home screen of Siemens' Syngo-Via workstation that illustrates some of the many available tools for analysis of cardiac CT angiography. (**a**) Oblique planes can be generated manually using the "manual plane" tool, a method described in the text here as the "oblique walk." The "pivot method" described here is invoked using the tool labeled "vessel surf." (**b**) Curved MPRs can be generated automatically or manually using one or multiple clicks. (**c**) The initial planes shown are axial (lower left), sagittal (upper left), and coronal (upper left). The planes are color-coded. A 3D-shaded surface display is shown in the fourth pane. (**d**) An automatically derived curved MPR of RCA is shown. (**e**) Multiple 3D displays are available, including those that show a simulation of the invasive angiogram

3.4.4 TeraRecon

See Fig. 3.12.

3.4.5 Vital Images/Canon

See Fig. 3.13.

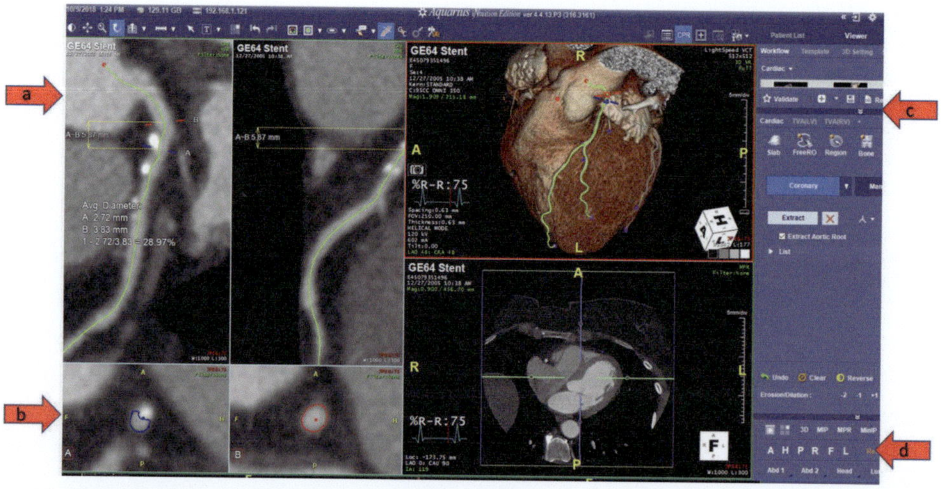

Fig. 3.12 A home screen of the TeraRecon workstation, a platform that is independent of CT scanner manufacturer that has been popular for many years is shown. (**a**) A curved MPR is shown, seen in two perpendicular virtual planes. (**b**) The lesion is quantified based on image analysis. (**c**) Tools for measurement are shown. (**d**) Tools for image angle and presentation are shown

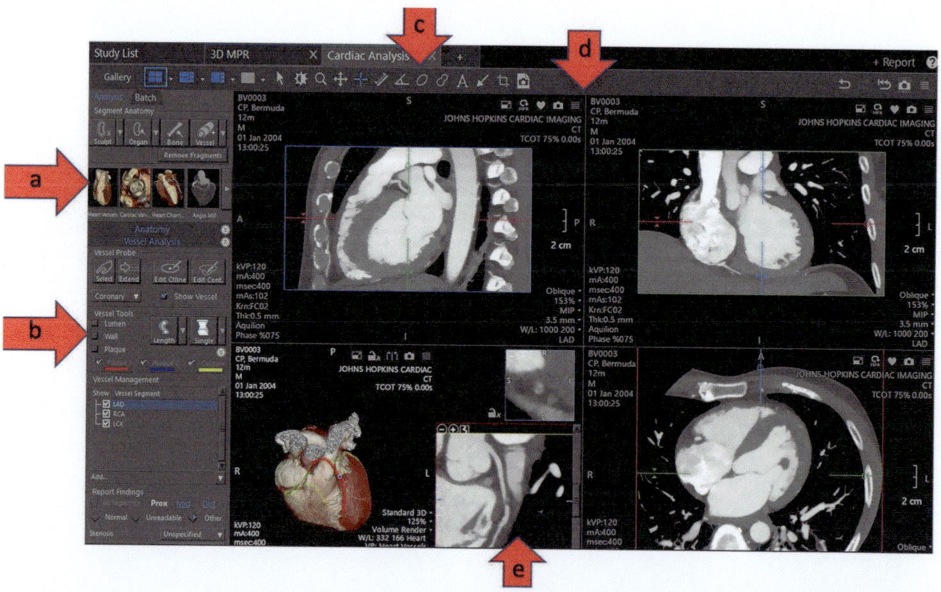

Fig. 3.13 A home screen of Canon's' Vitrea workstation that illustrates some of the many available tools for analysis of cardiac CT angiography. (**a**) Multiple 3D displays are available, including those that show a simulation of the invasive angiogram, here labeled "angio MIP." (**b**) Tools are available for automatically defining the lumen, the coronary wall, and the plaque. (**c**) Multiple tools are available for adjusting and manipulating the images. (**d**) The initial planes shown are axial (lower right), sagittal (upper left), and coronal (upper right). Oblique images to perform the "oblique walk" are derived by rotating the lines representing the color-coded planes. A 3D-shaded surface display is shown in the lower left pane. (**e**) Curved MPRs can be generated automatically or manually. Shown here is the LAD, containing a severe stenosis

References

1. Detrano R, Guerci AD, Carr JJ, Bild DE, Burke G, Folsom AR, Liu K, Shea S, Szklo M, Bluemke DA, O'Leary DH, Tracy R, Watson K, Wong ND, Kronmal RA. Coronary calcium as a predictor of coronary events in four racial or ethnic groups. N Engl J Med. 2008;358(13):1336–45.
2. Cury RC, Abbara S, Achenbach S, Agatston A, Berman DS, Budoff MJ, Dill KE, Jacobs JE, Maroules CD, Rubin GD, Rybicki FJ, Schoepf UJ, Shaw LJ, Stillman AE, White CS, Woodard PK, Leipsic JA. CAD-RADS(TM) Coronary Artery Disease—Reporting and Data System. An expert consensus document of the Society of Cardiovascular Computed Tomography (SCCT), the American College of Radiology (ACR) and the North American Society for Cardiovascular Imaging (NASCI). Endorsed by the American College of Cardiology. J Cardiovasc Comput Tomogr. 2016;10(4):269–81.

4 Indications for Cardiac CT Imaging

Armin Arbab Zadeh

Abstract

Application of cardiac CT is rapidly expanding because of its excellent image resolution, rapid acquisition time, relatively low cost, widespread availability, and decreasing radiation exposure. Conversely, cardiac CT imaging does involve some risks and costs. Indications for imaging should be restricted to cases for which imaging information is associated with improved patient outcome. Clinical practice guidelines and appropriate use criteria are tasked with weighing the evidence for and against indications for imaging. This chapter summarizes recommendations from major clinical and scientific societies and outlines discrepancies along with emerging evidence from recent investigations.

Keywords

Coronary CT · Coronary CT angiography Cardiac CT · Practice guideline · Appropriate use criteria

Abbreviations

AHA	American Heart Association
AUC	Appropriate use criteria
CAC	Coronary artery calcium
CAD	Coronary artery disease
CCS	Coronary calcium scanning
CCTA	Cardiac computed tomography angiography
CPG	Clinical practice guidelines
CT-FFR	CT with fractional flow reserve
ESC	European Society of Cardiology
ETT	Exercise treadmill testing
GDMT	Guideline directed medical therapy
ICA	Invasive coronary angiography
MPR	Multi-planar reformation
NSTEMI	Non-ST-elevation myocardial infarction
PCI	Percutaneous coronary intervention
PTP	Pretest probability
SCCT	Society of Cardiovascular Computed Tomography

A. A. Zadeh (✉)
Department of Medicine, Johns Hopkins University, Baltimore, MD, USA
e-mail: arminzadeh@jhu.edu

A. A. Zadeh, J. Hoe (eds.), *Practical Guide to Cardiac CT*,
https://doi.org/10.1007/978-981-97-6919-3_4

4.1 Introduction

- Cardiac CT has evolved into an established imaging modality for cardiac testing.
- This chapter summarizes the status of endorsement by major scientific or clinical societies for the appropriate use of cardiac CT.
- Given the rapid evolution of this technology paired with decreasing radiation exposure, it is expected that indications for cardiac CT will continue to expand over the upcoming years.
- Clinical practice guidelines (CPG) and appropriate use criteria (AUC) are the main sources of appraisal for clinical indications, but they often lag behind the most current evidence.
- CPG require rigorous review of the available data and provide graded consensus recommendations, but they commonly are subject to political influence among competing societies.
- AUC statements largely rely on expert opinion and tend to be more supportive of the test in question, particularly, if the AUC is dedicated to a single modality.

4.2 Appropriate Use Criteria

- The last iteration of a consensus statement by multiple societies solely addressing the appropriate use of cardiac CT stems from 2010 [1].
- While some of the recommendations may be questioned in lieu of more current evidence, most statements are still valid today.
- A document by largely the same medical societies focused on multi-modality imaging in the setting of stable chest pain was released in 2014 [2], however, these AUC have lost significance since the release of the 2021 Chest Pain Guideline [3].

Relative contraindications for coronary CTA expressed by Appropriate Use Criteria Consensus Document:

- Irregular heart rhythm (atrial fibrillation, frequent ectopy).
- Heart rate > 70 bpm despite medication.
- Renal failure (AUC use creatinine > 1.8 mg/dL as threshold).
- Very severe coronary artery calcification (commonly defined as > 1000 CACS).
- Morbid obesity (BMI > 40).
- Metal implants which may interfere with imaging.
- Inability of the patient to cooperate with the exam instructions.
- Intolerance of vasodilators and heart rate controlling medication.
- History of severe contrast allergy.

Note that coronary CTA in clincal practice is often performed accepting these limitations, particularly, after careful consideration of individual factors (e.g., patient preferences, lack of alternative options, etc.).

4.2.1 Assessment of Pretest Probability

- Pretest probability (PTP) assessment is based on the Bayes' theorem postulating poor test performance in situations of very low or very high disease probability.
- PTP has focused on the probability of *obstructive* coronary artery disease (CAD) typically defined as the presence of at least one ≥50 or ≥70% coronary artery stenosis.
- CPG and AUC require pretest probability for determining appropriateness of testing.
- CPG and AUC from different societies use different PTP scoring systems leading to vastly different recommendations in some cases.
- Older PTP schemes, e.g., using merely symptom characteristics, age, and sex, overestimate disease, while newer systems allow a much smaller testing window.
- In the US, institutions may be granted establishment of local algorithms for determining testing eligibility of patients, supported by

Table 4.1 Traditional PTP assessment used by the CCTA appropriateness use criteria document released in 2010 [1]

Age	Sex	Typical angina	Atypical angina	Nonanginal pain
<39	Women	Intermediate	Very low	Very low
	Men	Intermediate	Intermediate	Low
40–49	Women	Intermediate	Low	Very low
	Men	High	Intermediate	Intermediate
50–59	Women	Intermediate	Intermediate	Low
	Men	High	Intermediate	Intermediate
>60	Women	High	Intermediate	Intermediate
	Men	High	Intermediate	Intermediate

Table 4.2 PTP assessment by the European Society of Cardiology Chest Pain Guideline released in 2019 [4]

Age	Sex	Typical angina	Atypical	Nonanginal	Dyspnea
30–39	Women	5	3	1	3
	Men	3	4	1	0
40–49	Women	10	10	2	3
	Men	22	6	3	12
50–59	Women	13	6	3	9
	Men	32	17	11	20
60–69	Women	16	11	6	14
	Men	44	26	22	27
70+	Women	27	19	10	12
	Men	52	34	24	32

Given are the probabilities (%) for obstructive CAD. The guideline suggests individual considerations for testing in patients ≤15% PTP, e.g., ECG findings, CACS, risk factors, or imaging findings suggestive of CAD

Medicare under the Clinical Decision Support Mechanism (CDSM) program.

- The evolving focus on *nonobstructive* CAD rather than the traditional emphasis on obstructive CAD may diminish the role of PTP testing.
- PTP schemes used by the major societies are shown in Tables 4.1, 4.2, and 4.3.

Key Points: While PTP testing is required by most CPG and AUC, there is no consensus on how to best determine PTP and available grading systems vary widely in their categorization, rendering their application cumbersome in clinical practice. PTP testing is likely to lose significance with our transition from focusing on obstructive to detecting nonobstructive CAD.

Table 4.3 PTP assessment used by the Multi-Society 2021 Chest Pain Guideline [3]

Age	Sex	Chest pain	Dyspnea
30–39	Women	≤5	3
	Men	≤4	0
40–49	Women	≤10	3
	Men	≤22	12
50–59	Women	≤13	9
	Men	≤32	20
60–69	Women	≤16	14
	Men	≤44	27
70+	Women	≤27	12
	Men	≤52	32

Given are the probabilities (%) for obstructive CAD. The guideline considers ≤15% as low PTP and >15% as intermediate to high PTP

4.2.2 Specific Indications for Coronary CTA According to Appropriate Use Criteria

- Cardiac AUC support CCTA in patients with *stable CAD without history of known CAD* in the following situations:

ECG/exercise capability	Pretest probability		
ECG interpretable AND able to exercise	Low: uncertain	Intermediate: appropriate	High: inappropriate
ECG uninterpretable OR unable to exercise	Low: appropriate	Intermediate: appropriate	High: inappropriate

- Other specific endorsements of CCTA use are:
  - Discrepant or equivalent results from stress testing.
  - New heart failure and reduced ejection fraction (unless high PTP).
  - Noncoronary cardiac surgery (unless high PTP).
  - Assessment of CABG graft patency.
  - Evaluation of patients without history of CAD and ACUTE chest pain in the absence of high-risk features, e.g., biomarker elevation or ST segment changes.

- Specific conditions WITHOUT support for CCTA are:
  - Assessment of stent patency (except for left main stents).
  - Asymptomatic individuals (except for left main stent assessment).
  - Symptomatic patients with high PTP.

4.3 Chest Pain Guidelines

4.3.1 Stable Chest Pain Without History of CAD

- Both ESC and Multi-Society Chest Pain Guidelines support the use of CCTA in patients with stable chest pain and without history of known CAD *as first-line test (class I recommendation)*, particularly in patients with intermediate PTP [3, 4].
- The Multi-Society Chest Pain Guideline discourages *any* testing in patients of low PTP, while the ESC document encourages *individual* considerations.
- Both guidelines are less supportive of CCTA in patients with high PTP (favoring invasive angiography in this setting).
- An overview of chest pain evaluation according to the Multi-Society Chest Pain Guideline is shown in Fig. 4.1.

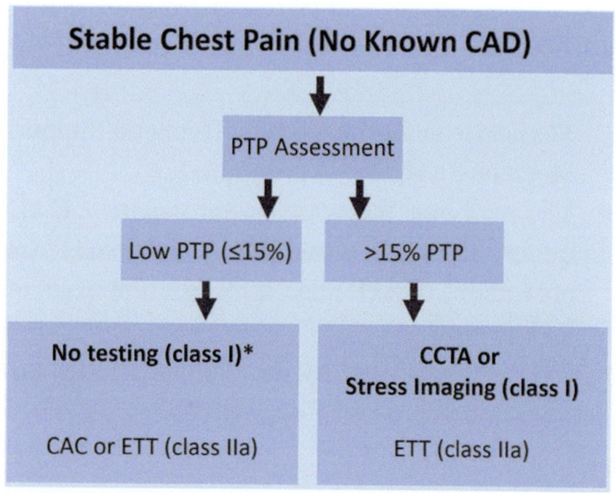

Fig. 4.1 Overview of recommended testing in patients with stable chest pain and *without* history of coronary artery disease. (Modified after Gulati et al. [3]). *Note the deviation from the ESC Stable Ischemic Heart Disease Guideline which encourages individualization based on additional risk features. *CAC* coronary artery calcium, *CAD* coronary artery disease, *CCTA* coronary CT angiography, *ESC* European Society of Cardiology, *ETT* exercise treadmill testing, *PTP* pretest probability

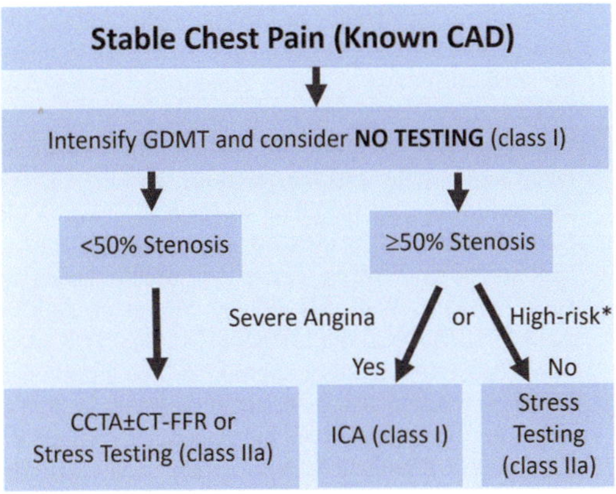

Fig. 4.2 Overview of recommended testing in patients with stable chest pain and *with* history of coronary artery disease. (Modified after Gulati et al. [3]). *Defined as left main stenosis ≥50% or obstructive CAD with FFR-CT ≤0.80. *CAD* coronary artery disease, *CCTA* coronary CT angiography, *CT-FFR* CT with fractional flow reserve, *GDMT* guideline-directed medical therapy, *ICA* invasive coronary angiography

4.3.2 Stable Chest Pain *With* History of CAD

- The role of CCTA in this setting is poorly defined.
- There is broad consensus for the role of CCTA in evaluating for coronary bypass graft patency by all guidelines and appropriate use criteria.
- Assessment of stent patency is generally discouraged except for left main stents.
- A potential role of CCTA is emerging for ruling out significant left main disease after the negative results of ISCHEMIA [5].
- The multi-Society Chest Pain Guideline algorithm is shown in Fig. 4.2, but it should be noted that current evidence for the recommended steps shown is weak and subject to controversy.

4.3.3 Acute Chest Pain

- CCTA is generally indicated in the absence of high-risk features:

  - Abnormal cardiac troponin levels.
  - ST segment changes suggestive of acute myocardial ischemia.
  - Moderate to severe abnormal CAD test within 12 months.
  - History of PCI.
  - History of ≥50% coronary artery stenosis.

- Testing is *not* indicated with a normal CCTA <2 years or normal stress test <1 year.
- Notwithstanding above recommendations, recent data suggest utility of CCTA in patients with NSTEMI for identifying patients with obstructive CAD and the indications for CCTA will likely expand over the upcoming years [6, 7].
- Similarly, there is a growing demand for identifying patients with known CAD presenting with recurrent chest pain who can be safely discharged from the emergency department. CCTA, possibly paired with myocardial perfusion imaging or other hemodynamic assessment, may grow into this new role.

4.3.4 Coronary Calcium Scanning

- Coronary calcium scanning (CCS) currently is largely confined to applications in *asymptomatic* individuals for advanced risk stratification, while its role in *symptomatic* patients is poorly defined—though likely expanding given the evolving supporting evidence in this setting.

- There is consensus for the use of CCS in asymptomatic patients considered of intermediate risk of adverse events (≥7.5% to <20% 10 year risk) for advanced risk stratification [8].
- A detailed discussion on the indications of CCS is provided in Chap. 9.
- The Multi-Society Chest Pain Guideline does see a role of CCS in low-risk patients with stable chest pain—see Fig. 4.1.

4.3.5 Noncoronary Cardiac CT

- There is broad support for the use of cardiac CT for the assessment of cardiac structure, morphology, and function.
- While not limited to these indications, common applications of cardiac CT include evaluation of:
  - Pericardium, e.g., thickness, calcification, effusion.
  - Myocardium, e.g., mass, thickness, structure, function.
  - Valves, e.g., thickness, calcification, anatomy, structure, function.
  - Chambers, e.g., size, volume, morphology, function.
  - Epicardiac, pericardiac, perivascular fat, e.g., mass, structure.
- The use of CT myocardial perfusion imaging follows guidelines for stress testing.

References

1. Taylor AJ, Cerqueira M, Hodgson JM, et al. ACCF/SCCT/ACR/AHA/ASE/ASNC/NASCI/SCAI/SCMR 2010 appropriate use criteria for cardiac computed tomography: a report of the American College of Cardiology Foundation appropriate use criteria task force, the society of cardiovascular computed tomography, the American College of Radiology, the American Heart Association, the American Society of Echocardiography, the American Society of Nuclear Cardiology, the north American Society for Cardiovascular Imaging, the society for cardiovascular angiography and interventions, and the society for cardiovascular magnetic resonance. J Am Coll Cardiol. 2010;56(22):1864–94.
2. Multimodality Writing Group for Stable Ischemic Heart Disease, Wolk MJ, Bailey SR, et al. ACCF/AHA/ASE/ASNC/HFSA/HRS/SCAI/SCCT/SCMR/STS 2013 multimodality appropriate use criteria for the detection and risk assessment of stable ischemic heart disease: A report of the American College of Cardiology Foundation Appropriate Use Criteria Task Force, American Heart Association, American Society of Echocardiography, American Society of Nuclear Cardiology, Heart Failure Society of America, Heart Rhythm Society, Society for Cardiovascular Angiography and Interventions, Society of Cardiovascular Computed Tomography, Society for Cardiovascular Magnetic Resonance, and Society of Thoracic Surgeons. J Card Fail. 2014;20(2):65–90.
3. Writing Committee Members, Gulati M, Levy PD, et al. 2021 AHA/ACC/ASE/CHEST/SAEM/SCCT/SCMR guideline for the evaluation and diagnosis of CHEST pain: a report of the American College of Cardiology/American Heart Association joint committee on clinical practice guidelines. J Cardiovasc Comput Tomogr. 2022;16(1):54–122.
4. Knuuti J, Wijns W, Saraste A, et al. ESC guidelines for the diagnosis and management of chronic coronary syndromes. Eur Heart J. 2019;2019:ehz425.
5. Maron DJ, Hochman JS, Reynolds HR, et al. Initial invasive or conservative strategy for stable coronary disease. N Engl J Med. 2020;382:1395–407. https://doi.org/10.1056/NEJMoa1915922.
6. Kofoed KF, Engstrom T, Sigvardsen PE, et al. Prognostic value of coronary CT angiography in patients with non-ST-segment elevation acute coronary syndromes. J Am Coll Cardiol. 2021;77(8):1044–52. https://doi.org/10.1016/j.jacc.2020.12.037.
7. Linde JJ, Kelbaek H, Hansen TF, et al. Coronary CT angiography in patients with non-ST-segment elevation acute coronary syndrome. J Am Coll Cardiol. 2020;75(5):453–63. https://doi.org/10.1016/j.jacc.2019.12.012.
8. Arnett DK, Blumenthal RS, Albert MA, et al. ACC/AHA guideline on the primary prevention of cardiovascular disease. Circulation. 2019;2019:e596. https://doi.org/10.1161/CIR.0000000000000678.

5 Patient Preparation and Image Acquisition in Cardiac CT

Michael Huy Cuong Pham,
Kristian Altern Øvrehus,
and Klaus Fuglsang Kofoed

Abstract

In this chapter, we provide an overview of the processes in performing a cardiac CT scan, organized in chronological order from patient preparation to scan image acquisition. Meticulous attention to details of patient preparation and scan acquisition is critical for appropriate and safe application of cardiac CT as well as for acquiring images of diagnostic quality. Patient preparation and scan acquisition should follow a detailed protocol to optimize conditions for excellent image quality and to avoid errors.

Keywords

Cardiac CT · Coronary CT angiography · CT patient preparation · CT image acquisition · CT scan methods · Cardiac CT guide

Abbreviations

ALARA	As low as reasonably achievable
BMI	Body mass index
CACS	Coronary artery calcium scoring
CCTA	Coronary computed tomography angiography
CIN	Contrast-induced nephropathy
CT	Computed tomography
ECG	Electrocardiogram
eGFR	Estimated glomerular filtration rate
ICD	Implantable cardioverter-defibrillator
kV	Kilovoltage
kVp	Kilovoltage peak
mA	Milliampere
mAs	Milliampere seconds
PO	Per oral administration
ROI	Region of interest
SL	Sublingual administration
SOP	Standard of procedure

5.1 Introduction

To ensure that CT scan images are acquired at the highest quality and the lowest possible radiation dose, a dedicated sequence of steps including patient selection, patient preparation, scanner acquisition procedures, and post-processing reconstruction techniques are required. In this

M. H. C. Pham · K. F. Kofoed (✉)
Department of Cardiology, Copenhagen University Hospital Rigshospitalet, Copenhagen, Denmark
e-mail: Michael.Huy.Cuong.Pham@regionh.dk; Klaus.Kofoed@regionh.dk

K. A. Øvrehus
Department of Cardiology, Odense University Hospital, Odense, Denmark
e-mail: Kristian.Altern.Ovrehus@rsyd.dk

A. A. Zadeh, J. Hoe (eds.), *Practical Guide to Cardiac CT*,
https://doi.org/10.1007/978-981-97-6919-3_5

chapter, we review the processes of adult patient preparation and image acquisition for a high-quality cardiac CT examination.

5.2 Patient Preparation

- Several steps of preparation and pre-scan assessments may be performed to optimize scan image quality.
- Note that most instructions provided here relate to preparation of *coronary* CT angiography, whereas *noncoronary* cardiac CT typically does *not* require extensive preparation, i.e., heart rate control.
- An individualized approach to patient preparation is needed depending on the scan indication and clinical setting (elective or acute/subacute). The steps of CT patient preparation until the CT image acquisition are illustrated in Fig. 5.1.

A flowchart is provided illustrating a step-by-step guide for the preparation of patients undergoing coronary CT angiography examination. The work processes are divided into two phases, in which Phase 1 takes place in a separate preparation room before entering the imaging suite, and Phase 2 occurs in the CT scanner room just before image acquisition.

5.2.1 Patient History and Instructions

- Patient preparation is typically provided in a separate preparation room to avoid workflow interruption within the scanner room (Phase 1 of the CT patient preparation in Fig. 5.1).
- Patients should be made aware ahead of arrival that preparation may take between 15 min and 3 h depending on heart rate on presentation and heart rate goals.
- Every step of patient preparation and CT examination should be explained thoroughly in a calm manner and in a relaxed atmosphere to avoid anxiety and associated heart rate increase.
- Patients should be advised to not consume caffeine for 12 h before scanning, e.g., coffee, tea, cola, cocoa or chocolate, as it interferes with heart rate control and, considered in select patients, with vasodilator challenge (adenosine, etc.).
- Patient fasting is no longer recommended for routine contrast examination [1]; however, some sites still maintain a 4-h fasting rule. Fasting facilitates quicker onset of medications which may be necessary for heart rate control.
- Adequate hydration is important and patient should be encouraged to drink plenty of water prior to arrival. Intravenous hydration may be provided if hydration is inadequate.
- The patient's history should be reviewed, including current medications and allergies. This ideally occurs prior to patient arrival to avoid cancellation of cases after presentation, e.g., for allergies without premedication.
- Particular attention should be placed to symptoms and history of heart failure, reactive airway disease, and cardiac arrhythmia, as these may interfere with administration of medications for heart rate control and vasodilation.
- Local policies regulate the management of patients with prior life-threatening reactions to iodine contrast, i.e., cardiac arrest, laryngeal edema requiring intubation, etc., but such reactions are commonly reason to withhold repeated exposure for *elective* procedures.
- Patients with history of non-critical reactions to iodine contrast, e.g., rash, typically receive a combination of corticosteroids and antihistamine drugs. The specific dosing varies, but a common prescription is the regimen of oral prednisone 50 mg given 13, 7, and 1 h together with a histamine-1 receptor blocker 1 h prior to contrast exposure.
- All patients undergoing contrast-enhanced CT imaging, i.e., coronary and noncoronary CT angiography, should be screened for risk factors for kidney failure, e.g., diabetes, age 75 or older, heart failure, or preexisting renal insufficiency.
- Patients at increased risk of contrast-associated acute kidney injury typically undergo testing

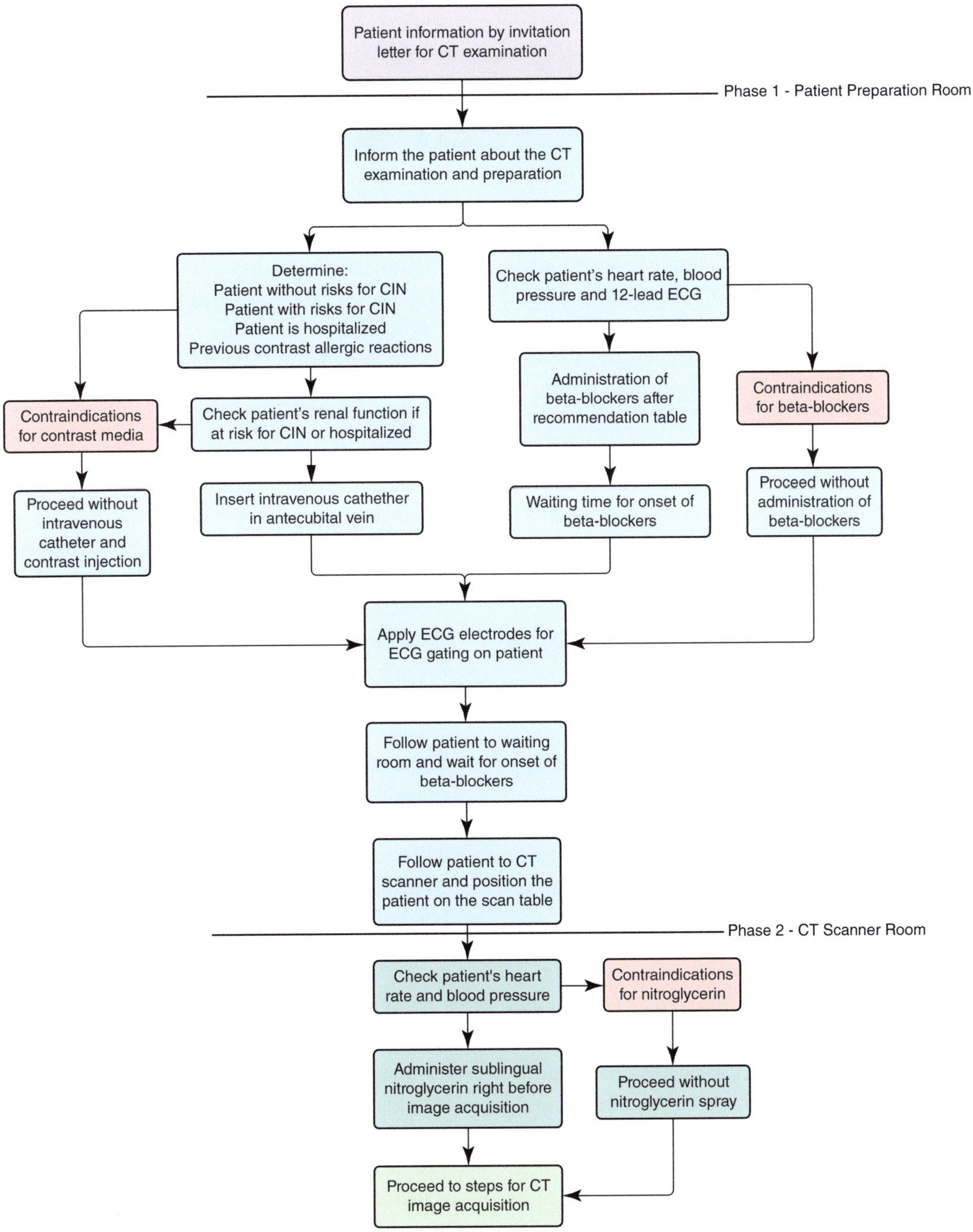

Fig. 5.1 Overview of patient preparation and coronary CT angiography scan acquisition

for serum creatinine level and estimated glomerular filtration rate (eGFR).

- All patients are advised to avoid nephrotoxic drugs, e.g., nonsteroidal anti-inflammatory drugs, within 48 h prior to contrast exposure to minimize risk of kidney injury.
- Metformin does not need to be withheld prior to contrast exposure, but it may be held after contrast if there is concern for contrast-associated acute kidney injury. In this case, metformin should be resumed only after such injury is ruled out.

- The patient should be instructed in the correct breathing techniques and adequate breath-hold duration, e.g., avoiding Valsalva maneuver.

5.2.2 Patient Attire in the Imaging Suite

- A hospital gown is commonly worn to allow easy application of ECG leads and to avoid potential interferences from metal buttons, belts, etc.
- Necklaces or underwired bras, etc. should be removed.
- Metal accessories outside the scan field of view, such as glasses and watches, may be kept on during CT examination without affecting the scan.
- Cardiac devices, such as pacemakers, do not pose problems for cardiac CT image acquisition, but may impact image interpretation for affected areas.

5.2.3 Heart Rate and Blood Pressure Assessment

- Ideally, heart rate control is commenced prior to patient arrival at the imaging suite but this is often logistically difficult.
- Patients undergoing *coronary* CT angiography must be monitored for heart rate and blood pressure because of the common need for heart rate control and coronary vasodilation.
- Heart rate control is typically required to reduce the risk of motion artifacts and nondiagnostic image quality.
- Even with a high temporal resolution, e.g., 40–60 ms, which is not available with most contemporary CT technology, heart rates >60 bpm will result in some coronary artery motion artifacts [2].
- The patient's blood pressure should be sufficiently high to allow administration of beta-blockers and nitroglycerin for vasodilation prior to the CT scan.
- Coronary vasodilation facilitates greater diagnostic accuracy (vs. scanning without vasodilation) for coronary artery disease detection, largely by allowing better visualization of smaller blood vessels and branches.

5.2.4 Heart Rhythm Assessment

- Electrocardiogram (ECG) recording should be obtained on patient arrival to verify sinus rhythm and to identify arrhythmias that would affect image acquisition and administration of medication.
- At minimum, a 3-lead rhythm analysis is performed, but a 12-lead ECG recording is preferred.
- Irregular heart rhythms, conduction abnormalities, and/or bradycardia should be reviewed by the attending medical provider to determine whether the patient is eligible for administration of heart rate controlling medication.
- Patients with atrial fibrillation or frequent premature ectopic beats may present particular challenges to scan acquisition—as discussed below.
- The attending physician must decide if conditions for study indication, pretest probability, and patient characteristics are met to proceed with scanning—with or without heart rate control.
- For cardiac gating, three electrodes will be placed to allow reliable identification of R waves, which the scanner will use for scan triggering.
- ECG electrodes should be rated for minimal/no interference with scanner function and should be placed outside the scan range to avoid interference with image interpretation.
- The lead with the highest, unambiguous R waves should be used for scan triggering.

5.3 Administration of Heart Rate Lowering Medication

5.3.1 General Principles and Considerations

- A low and stable heart rate increases the probability of achieving optimal image quality and high diagnostic accuracy of coronary CT angiography.

- Heart rate may typically be lowered by administering oral or intravenous beta-blockers and/or oral ivabradine.
- Non-dihydropyridine calcium channel blockers, e.g., verapamil, can also be used, but they are less effective than beta-blockers or ivabradine.
- Contraindications for beta-blockers and ivabradine should be reviewed for each patient.
- Beta-blockers are considered contraindicated in the setting of active airway disease, e.g., asthma, severe heart failure, or advanced atrioventricular block (second or third degree) without a pacemaker in place (Table 5.1).
- Metoprolol is attractive for heart rate control because of its beta-1 receptor selectivity and relatively short onset of action (approximately 30–60 min after oral administration) with peak effects after 90–120 min [3].
- Common doses of metoprolol are 25–150 mg, based on heart rate, systolic blood pressure, and body weight.
- Administration of oral beta-blockers should take place at least 1 h before the CT scan to ensure optimal pharmacological effect.
- Intravenous beta-blockers can be administered alone or in combination with oral beta-blockers.
- The use of intravenous beta-blockers is typically limited by the small approved doses and slow administration, e.g., 5 mg IV metoprolol at a time over 2 min for a total of 15 mg initially. Peak effect is expected after 20 min, and heart rate and blood pressure should be carefully monitored.
- If target heart rate is achieved, additional intravenous metoprolol may be given but most institutions do not allow total doses of more than 30 mg, some up to 50 mg.
- Given an approximately 60% bioavailability, more effective heart rate control can be achieved with 100 mg or more of *oral* metoprolol.
- Short infusions of intravenous esmolol have shown effectiveness, but the drug is uncommonly given because of its high cost [4].
- Patients should be informed of possible side effects to the medications, e.g., temporary fatigue, orthostatic hypotension, lightheadedness, and dizziness [5].
- We generally advise patients to not drive (a car) after drug administration if they have never taken beta-blockers before and thus are not familiar with their effect on them.
- Administration of oral metoprolol should not exceed the 200–400 mg a day and doses for patients already taking beta-blockers should be adjusted accordingly. Table 5.2 lists equivalent doses of common beta-blockers.
- An alternative or addition to beta-blockers is ivabradine, which is a hyperpolarization-activated cyclic nucleotide-gated (HCN) channel blocker and acts by selectively inhibiting the cardiac (I_f) pacemaker current.
- Ivabradine may be favored over beta-blockers in patients with active airway disease and heart failure given the absence of effects related to beta-receptors.
- Different regimens of ivabradine administration have been proven effective, e.g., 5.0–7.5 mg twice daily on 1–5 days before or 10–15 mg 1–2 h before the examination [6, 7].
- The key limitation of ivabradine is its fairly long time to onset, which is approximately 90–120 min. Potentially faster onset may be

Table 5.1 Contraindications to beta-blockers and nitroglycerin

Contraindications		
Beta-blockers		Nitroglycerin
1. Hypotension, systolic BP <100 mmHg 2. Active reactive airway disease 3. Severely reduced systolic ventricular function	4. Decompensated or acute heart failure 5. 2nd/3rd degree heart block, sick sinus syndrome 6. Critical aortic stenosis	1. Critical aortic stenosis 2. Hypotension, systolic BP <100 mmHg 3. Recent PDE-5 inhibitor intake

Table 5.2 Beta-blocker equivalent dose conversion table

Medication	Dose
Metoprolol	100 mg
Carvedilol	25 mg
Propranolol	80 mg
Bisoprolol	5 mg
Atenolol	50 mg
Labetalol	200 mg

Table 5.3 Typical dosing of metoprolol (or equivalent) for heart rate control (60 bpm or less)

	Systolic blood pressure (mmHg)					
		111–120 mmHg		>120 mmHg		
Heart rate (bpm)	≤110 mmHg	<65 kg	≥65 kg	<65 kg	≥65 kg	Waiting time
>65	None	50 mg	100 mg	100 mg	150 mg	1½ h
61–65	None	25 mg	75 mg	75 mg	100 mg	1 h
55–60	None	0 mg	25 mg	50 mg	50 mg	
<55	None	None	None	None	None	

achieved with chewing rather than swallowing tablets.

- Ivabradine is not effective in the setting of atrial fibrillation and is associated with a small risk of triggering atrial fibrillation in patients with paroxysmal atrial fibrillation.
- Ivabradine is contraindicated in patients with sick sinus syndrome and without pacemaker in place, and it is not supposed to be combined with non-dihydropyridine calcium channel blockers, e.g., diltiazem.
- In contrast to metoprolol, ivabradine uncommonly leads to hypotension.

5.3.2 Common Heart Rate Control Prescriptions

- Heart rate control goal for coronary CTA depends on several factors, including scanner technology and available spatial resolution, pretest probability, and patient characteristics. For example, heart rate control should be tighter in patients with other challenging features, e.g., severe obesity and/or high pretest probability of CAD vs. those with otherwise optimal characteristics and lower probability of CAD.
- Using common 64-detector CT technology, heart rates of 50–60 bpm generally allow image acquisition with little or no cardiac motion artifacts. Accordingly, heart rate of 60 or lower is often targeted for heart rate control.
- Typical dosing of metoprolol for heart rate control is presented in Table 5.3. Please note that the recommendations are based primarily on Caucasians. Doses may be adjusted in other populations.
- Note that elderly patients are often more sensitive to beta-blockers and smaller doses may be adequate.
- When ivabradine is being combined with metoprolol, beta-blocker doses should be adjusted. An example of combined prescriptions is provided in Table 5.4.

Table 5.4 Example for combined administration of ivabradine and metoprolol

Heart rate	Ivabradine (mg)	Metoprolol PO (mg)
>70	15	50–75
66–70	15	25
61–65	None	50

5.3.3 Poor Heart Rate Control Despite Medications or in Case of Contraindications

- If heart rate control is not feasible, an individualized approach is recommended for deciding whether or not to proceed with imaging. In some patients, a diagnostic scan may be achieved without the administration of medication.

- The likelihood of answering the clinical question without heart rate control should be determined, and the risks of the procedures, e.g., radiation and contrast, should be considered.
- Adjustments of the scan acquisition protocol to accommodate high heart rates depend on the available technology. CT scanners with fast temporal resolution and/or wide coverage will be better positioned to deal with higher heart rates.
- The two principal options for adjusting the scan protocol to high heart rates are: (1) widening the exposure window to include end-systole and (2) multi-cycle acquisition. Both can be used in combination and both increase radiation exposure compared with narrow window prospective scan triggering.
- A widened exposure window can be obtained by prospectively increasing X-ray time, e.g., 40–80% of the R-R cycle or by full R-R cycle exposure and retrospective gating—see next section.

5.4 Contrast Application and Safety

5.4.1 General Principles

- Contrast application is essential for CT coronary angiography because the coronary arteries and non-calcified atherosclerotic plaque provide little X-ray attenuation and are poorly visualized without contrast.
- Patients should be informed ahead of arrival that the scan involves the application of iodine contrast and a detailed history of prior exposure should be taken.
- Importantly, any history of allergic/hypersensitivity reactions to iodine contrast should prompt considerations on the value of exposure in the given setting.
- Patients should be made aware that they will experience a warm sensation throughout the body with contrast injection. Some experience a metallic taste and few feel some nausea.
- Iodinated contrast media are available in two types as ionic and nonionic contrast media.
- Ionic contrast media were introduced first and defined as iodinated contrast agents that can dissociate into cations and anions when used in a solution, whereas nonionic contrast media are defined as iodinated contrast agents that do not dissociate into cations and anions.
- Ionic contrast media are less expensive and have high osmolarity, but they are associated with a higher incidence of adverse reactions than nonionic contrast media [8].
- Nonionic iodinated contrast media used in CT are typically either of low-osmolar or iso-osmolar concentration.
- Commonly used low-osmolar iodinated contrast media are iohexol (Omnipaque), iopamidol (Isovue), iopromide (Ultravist), ioversol (Optiray), and ioxilan (Oxilan).
- The most commonly used iso-osmolar iodinated contrast media is iodixanol (Visipaque).
- Differences in properties of nonionic iodinated contrast media are presented in Table 5.5.

Table 5.5 Properties of common iodinated contrast agents in CT

Iodinated contrast medium	Concentration (mg/mL)	Viscosity (cP at 37 °C)	Osmolarity (mOsm/kgH_2O)
Nonionic monomer			
Iohexol (Omnipaque)	140–350	1.5–10.4	322–844
Iopamidol (Isovue)	200–370	2.0–8.6	413–796
Iopromide (Ultravist)	150–370	1.5–9.5	328–774
Ioversol (Optiray)	160–350	1.9–9.0	355–792
Ioxilan (Oxilan)	300–350	5.1–8.1	610–721
Nonionic dimer			
Iodixanol (Visipaque)	270–320	6.3–11.8	290

5.4.2 Hypersensitivity Reactions to Contrast Agents

- Contrast media safety profile differs depending on the specific medium used.
- Overall incidence of hypersensitivity reactions to iodinated contrast media is 0.5–1.0%, and severe reactions occur in approximately 0.02% of cases [9].
- The distribution of symptoms by organ systems is presented in Table 5.6.
- Adverse drug reactions to iodinated contrast media can be divided into two types of reactions: hypersensitivity reactions and chemotoxic events [10].
- According to ACR Manual on Contrast media and ESUR Guideline [11], the adverse reactions are categorized into three grades: mild, moderate, and severe (Table 5.7).
- Hypersensitivity reactions are divided into immediate hypersensitivity reaction (<1 h) and delayed hypersensitivity reaction (>1 h).
- Activation of mast cells and basophils with release of histamine, tryptase, and other mediators is implicated in immediate hypersensitivity reactions.
- Delayed hypersensitivity is likely mediated via activation of T-cells and associated pathways.
- High-osmolarity iodinated contrast media have been largely replaced by low-osmolarity agents, as the former show more frequent associations with adverse reactions.
- In patients with prior contrast reactions, steroid and antihistamine prophylaxis before administration of iodinated contrast media are typically administered, although the evidence for the effectiveness of premedication is not well established.
- The American College of Radiology recommends premedication for elective cases using 50 mg prednisone orally 13 h, 7 h, and 1 h before contrast use plus 50 mg diphenhydramine orally 1 h before exposure.
- Please note that diphenhydramine may cause drowsiness and should preclude driving while under its effect.
- Patients should be examined and monitored for allergic reactions and all reactions must be documented.
- Patients should be advised that late (>60 min) adverse reactions may occur and to seek immediate medical attention in this setting.

Table 5.6 Symptoms of iodinated contrast media adverse effects by organ system

Organ system	Iodinated contrast media %
Skin and appendages	63.4
Gastrointestinal system	13.7
Respiratory system	8.0
Body as a whole—General	5.6
Central and peripheral nervous system	5.1
Vascular (extracardiac)	1.3
Cardiovascular	0.9
Vision	0.8
Heart rate and rhythm	0.3
Application site	0.3
Urinary system	0.3
Others	0.5

5.4.3 Contrast-Associated Acute Kidney Injury

- Iodinated contrast exposure is frequently being implicated in acute kidney injury among hospitalized patients.
- Nephrotoxicity of iodinated contrast media is ascribed to the combination of cytotoxic effects on the renal tubular epithelial and endothelial cells, and an impairment of intrarenal blood flow [12].
- High iodinated contrast osmolarity, viscosity, and volume are associated with greater toxicity.
- Most data on contrast toxicity, however, stem from in vitro studies and investigations with older generation contrast media.
- While many studies found associations of contrast application with acute kidney injury, recent analyses of pooled data did not find evidence of a causal link when data were compared to controls [13].
- Current recommendations only caution for contrast administration in selected groups,

Table 5.7 Categories and grades of acute adverse reactions to iodinated contrast media

Grade	Hypersensitivity	Chemo-toxic
Mild	Limited urticaria/pruritus Cutaneous edema Limited itchy/scratchy throat Nasal congestion Conjunctivitis/rhinorrhea	Limited nausea/vomiting Transient flushing/warmth/chills Headache/dizziness/anxiety/altered taste Mild hypertension Vasovagal reaction that resolves spontaneously
Moderate	Diffuse urticarial/pruritus Diffuse erythema, stable vital signs Facial edema without dyspnea Throat tightness or hoarseness without dyspnea Wheezing/bronchospasm, mild or no hypoxia	Protracted nausea/vomiting Hypertensive urgency Isolated chest pain Vasovagal reaction that requires and is responsive to treatment
Severe	Diffuse edema, or facial edema with dyspnea Diffuse erythema with hypotension Laryngeal edema with stridor and/or hypoxia Wheezing/bronchospasm, significant hypoxia Anaphylactic shock (hypotension and tachycardia)	Vasovagal reaction resistant to treatment Arrhythmia Convulsions, seizures Hypertensive emergency

i.e., those with acute kidney injury or those with advanced chronic kidney failure (eGFR<30 mL/min) [13].

- Patients should be screened for risk factors of kidney failure.
- Low-risk outpatients without known risk factors of contrast-induced nephropathy may be scanned without assessment of kidney function.
- For patients with risk factors (diabetes, age ≥75 years, heart failure, prior kidney failure), a recent (<30 days) assessment of kidney function is recommended.
- Iodixanol and Iohexol are commonly used for CT angiography, preferably with high iodine concentration to ensure high vascular contrast opacification.
- The vascular contrast enhancement and image quality are not impaired when comparing different iodinated contrast agents or different concentrations of iodine [14].
- Current guidelines (e.g., ESUR Guidelines on Contrast Agents) recommend hydration of patients at risk (eGFR <30) with either intravenous sodium bicarbonate or with intravenous isotonic saline.
- Recommendations for administering contrast agents are summarized in Table 5.8.

5.4.4 Contrast Injection

- An intravenous (IV) catheter in the antecubital vein is the preferred vascular access site for contrast administration.
- Contrast is injected via a power injector at rates typically ranging between 3.5 and 7 mL/s. Such high flow rates place high demands on the IV access with poorly placed IVs leading to rapid infiltration of contrast into the surrounding tissue.
- For this reason, we recommend against IV access in forearms or hands as they have little space to accommodate contrast infiltration and thus may lead to greater discomfort or even tissue damage (compartment syndrome).
- Recommended IV size for contrast media injection is 14–18 G. Smaller IVs may limit flow rates, unless they are equipped with side holes rated for higher flow.
- To ensure that the intravenous catheter is placed correctly in a large vein, repeated and rapid saline flushes should be applied to test the IV and to ensure that the volume is not deposited subcutaneously.
- On the scanner table, the injection syringe catheter is connected to the patient and a test

Table 5.8 Recommendations for precautions with administering intravenous iodine contrast media

Condition	eGFR	Contrast	Medication
Patients with no risk factors for CIN[a]	Not required	Normal contrast dosing	
Patients with risk factors for CIN[a] History with kidney disease Diabetes Previous urinary tract surgery Proteinuria Hypertension Increased serum uric acid History with cardiovascular disease Prescribed nephrotoxic medication	>30 mL/min within 3 months	Normal contrast dosing	Continue metformin per usual
	<30 mL/min within 3 months	No contrast media or lower contrast dosing	Discontinue metformin from time of contrast media administration[b]
Hospitalized patients	>30 mL/min within 7 days	Normal contrast dosing	Continue metformin per usual
	<30 mL/min within 7 days	No contrast media or lower contrast dosing	Discontinue metformin from time of contrast media administration[b]

Please note that these recommendations do not apply to emergent use of contrast application for which imaging may outweigh the risk of acute kidney injury

[a]Contrast-induced nephropathy

[b]Measure eGFR 48 h post-CT examination and continue metformin if renal function is habitual

injection of 20 mL of saline using the desired injection rate of, e.g., 4–7 mL/s, is performed.

- If the patient complains of pain or discomfort at the peripheral catheter site in the elbow or back of the arm, it may indicate that the bevel of the catheter is against the wall of the vein and there is likelihood of an extravasation of contrast occurring during the scan acquisition.
- Straightening the patients elbow by padding up with sponges or asking the patient to touch the gantry housing may help avoid IV infiltration.
- Extravasation of contrast into the arm is the most common complication of CT angiography examinations due to the high injection rates required and its incidence may be used as quality performance measure for programs (goal of <1/1000).

5.5 Administration of Nitroglycerin

- Administration of nitroglycerin sublingually immediately prior to the cardiac CT examination is highly recommended and associated with increased diagnostic accuracy [15].
- Nitroglycerin results in coronary artery dilatation and improved visualization of the coronary arteries, especially in peripheral, smaller arteries.
- Contraindications to administration of nitroglycerin are listed in Table 5.1 (aortic stenosis, hypotension, recent intake of sildenafil or other PDE-5 inhibitors). Duration of the washout period of PDE-5 inhibitors depends on their half-lives, ranging between 24 and 72 h.
- Nitroglycerin is typically administered via sublingual spray or tablet with doses of 0.4–1.2 mg.

- The peak effect is typically observed after 2–3 min, but effects may last for up to 30 min.
- Patients should be advised about potential side effects, e.g., headache, flushing, dizziness, and nausea.
- The most common side effects of nitroglycerin are hypotension and headache. If headache occurs due to vasodilatation, the patient may benefit from caffeine intake to counteract the vasodilatory effect or a mild analgesic.
- Nitroglycerin may increase heart rate, which may warrant a brief delay until return to baseline.

5.6 Scan Acquisition

5.6.1 Overview of Scan Modes

- Cardiac CT scanning can be performed using different scan modes (also see Chap. 1). The optimal scan mode depends on hardware as well as patient characteristics.
- Scan modes are commonly categorized by the form of gating, i.e., prospective scan triggering vs. retrospective gating, and the way X-rays are being delivered, i.e., helically vs. axially.
- Figure 5.2 provides an overview of common CCTA scan modes.

5.6.2 Helical Scanning

- Characteristics of helical acquisition (also known as spiral acquisition) depend on collimation and pitch.
- The beam collimation refers to the thickness of the X-ray beam, whereas the pitch represents the table feed or table increment (the table speed per rotation of the X-ray beam) divided by the beam collimation.
- Low-pitch helical acquisition, the traditional CT scanning mode, refers to a pitch of <1, often approximately 0.2.
- The scan mode leads to some overlap of X-ray imaging for a given anatomical region to avoid missing data (Fig. 5.2a).
- High-pitch helical acquisition refers to scanning with pitch >1.0.

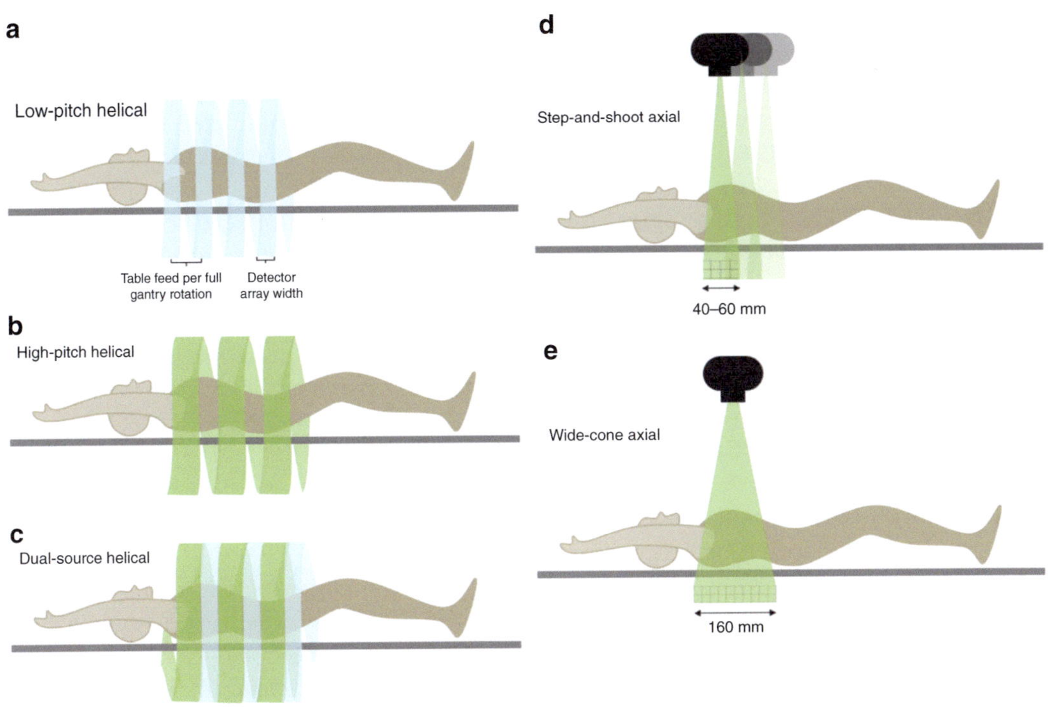

Fig. 5.2 Illustration of different CT scan modes. Note that the *z*-axis is the horizontal plane from head to toe

- High-pitch helical acquisitions include both single- and dual-source tube systems. Some scanners have two X-ray tubes and two detectors which are commonly referred to as 2T2D (dual-source) systems, which provide high temporal resolution (Fig. 5.2b, c).
- Helical scan acquisition can be performed using either prospective scan triggering or retrospective gating (see below for further details).

5.6.3 Axial Scanning

- In axial scanning, images are being obtained with X-rays penetrating perpendicularly to the z-axis.
- Depending on the detector coverage, the table either moves after each acquisition (step-and-shoot or multi-slab axial mode) or stays stationary (wide-cone axial or volume scanning).
- Common 64-detector row CT technology provides coverage of 40–60 mm, requiring 3–4 slabs to cover 120–160 mm (typically required to cover the entire heart). An example is shown in Fig. 5.2d.
- Wide-cone or volume scanning (120–160 mm coverage) typically allows scanning of the heart without table movement (one gantry rotation) and thus facilitates dynamic imaging (scanning the same structure over time).
- Axial scan acquisition can be performed using either prospective scan triggering or retrospective gating (see below for further details).
- Figure 5.2e illustrates the wide-cone axial scan mode.

5.6.4 Overview of ECG Gating

- Synchronizing scanning to the patient's ECG allows obtaining and selecting images associated with no or least cardiac motion.
- The selected phase within the cardiac cycle may be expressed as either percentage of the RR interval or absolute milliseconds after the last R wave.
- ECG gating techniques that are used for cardiac CT include two essential methods: retrospective ECG gating and prospective ECG triggering. The principles of different ECG gating techniques are illustrated in Fig. 5.3.

5.6.5 Retrospective Gating

- In retrospective ECG gating, the cardiac CT imaging data is continuously obtained throughout the entire cardiac cycle. For multi-beat acquisition, scan time spans over all phases of the cardiac cycles, as shown in Fig. 5.3a–c, enabling reconstruction of images in systole and diastole, for functional cardiac assessment.
- The central advantage of this scan mode is the availability of substantial image data for selecting those with least motion.
- The central disadvantage is much greater radiation exposure compared to prospective scan triggering.
- Radiation dose can be reduced (30–50%) in this mode by applying tube current modulation, i.e., reducing X-ray tube current during parts of the cardiac cycle, e.g., systole.
- Figure 5.3b, c shows the principles of retrospective gating with tube modulation, in which the tube current is lowered outside the specific targeted cardiac phase of the examination. Depending on whether the focus of the cardiac CT examination is in diastole or systole, the retrospective ECG-gated images are acquired typically during 70–80% or 35–55% of the RR interval, respectively. Some CT systems are able to target both systole and diastole during the same cycle.

5.6.6 Prospective Scan Triggering

- With prospective scan triggering, the X-ray tube is switched on only during pre-specified parts of the cardiac cycle.
- The period of scanning during the cardiac cycle is referred to as exposure window.

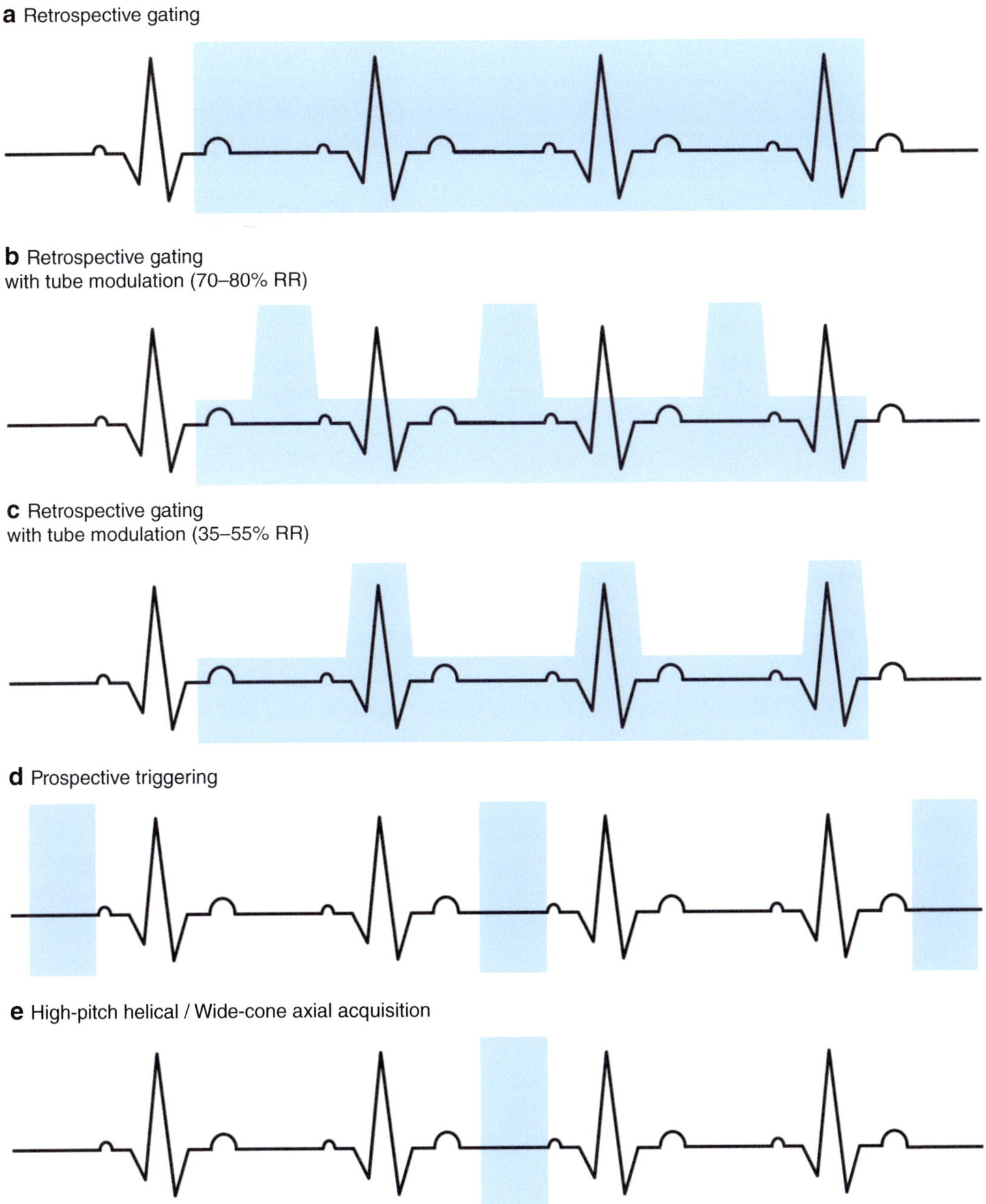

Fig. 5.3 Retrospective gating vs. prospective scan triggering. Illustration of the ECG (black line) and tube current with or without tube modulation during different acquisition methods (blue area). Panel **a** shows constant tube current output during a retrospective gated acquisition. Panels **b** and **c** illustrate the options of tube current modulation during a retrospective gated acquisition. The cardiac phase where there is least coronary artery motion can be typically identified in the 70–80% RR interval or the 35–55% RR interval (where the tube current is at its peak) while providing sufficient image quality for assessing cardiac function during the remaining phases (where the tube current is reduced). The helical acquisitions depicted in panels **a–c** facilitate cardiac function assessment. Panel **d** shows a prospective image acquisition using a 64-row CT scanner, requiring data collection over multiple heartbeats given its limited coverage. The different scans are separated by at least one heartbeat to allow for moving the table. Panel **e** shows a whole-heart high-pitch helical (possible only with low heart rate) or volumetric wide-cone axial image acquisition during diastole of a single RR interval, which can be achieved with a dual-source energy CT system (high-pitch helical) or a wide-detector array CT scanner (e.g., 16 cm coverage)

- The exposure window may be short, e.g., focusing on only a specific phase, or may encompass a wider portion of the cycle, e.g., 40–80%.
- The range around a target exposure is called "padding," e.g., 70% target exposure ±20%. Prospective scan triggering can be applied with both helical and axial acquisition.
- In the so-called step-and-shoot method, scan images are acquired in a sequential and axial manner during a predefined phase of the RR interval, e.g., 65–75% of the RR interval as shown in Fig. 5.3d. After one set of images has been obtained, the table moves to a new position and stops for image acquisition of the next portion and so forth.
- Large coverage scanners (12–16 cm) allow prospectively triggered scan acquisition of the entire heart within a single heartbeat, as illustrated in Fig. 5.3e (also known as volume scan).
- The high-pitch image acquisition requires a dual-source CT scanner with a pitch of >1.5 and low heart rates (e.g., <60 bpm) to allow acquisition in one heartbeat.
- The central advantage of prospective scan triggering is the much lower radiation dose compared to retrospective gating.
- The key drawback is the limited dataset, typically not allowing functional assessment.
- Prospective scan triggering is particularly feasible with regular and low heart rates; however, volume CT may also facilitate prospective scan triggering with high rates when focused on systolic image acquisition.
- Scan acquisitions over more than one cardiac cycle are more vulnerable to cardiac arrhythmias vs. single heartbeat acquisition.

5.6.7 Sequence of Scanning Steps

- An overview of the workflow in scanning of patients with cardiac CT is illustrated in Fig. 5.4.
- The patient is placed on the CT scanner table in a supine position with the arms above the head (Fig. 5.5). The patient should be lying comfortably.
- ECG leads are being connected and continuous ECG recording is displayed on the ECG monitor visible to the operators in the control room. ECG signal should be adjusted to display the largest possible R-wave amplitudes since they will be used for the ECG gating as shown in Fig. 5.5.

5.6.8 Breathing and Instructions Immediately Prior to Scanning

- Breathing practice is important to assure consistent heart level positioning between scanning steps and to avoid artifacts related to breathing.
- Patient is instructed to "breathe-in, breathe-out, breathe-in, and hold it."
- Breath holding for 15–20 s should be practiced while monitoring the heart rate. If done correctly, the heart rate should decrease and stabilize during the breath hold.
- If heart rate increases during breath hold, the patient should be coached to take a deeper or shallower breath.
- The patient should be reminded that they will feel a warm sensation from the contrast typically starting in the head traveling down to the groin.
- Any pain sensation should be communicated immediately.

5.6.9 Scout Image Acquisition: Scan Set Up

- The scan table position should be moved so the patient is in the isocenter of the CT scanner gantry as shown in Fig. 5.6.
- To set up the scan, initial localizer images are being obtained to identify landmark anatomic structures, also called "scout images," "topogram," or "scanogram." These images are being obtained not for diagnostic purposes but to assist the radiographer in planning the scan range and position the patient.

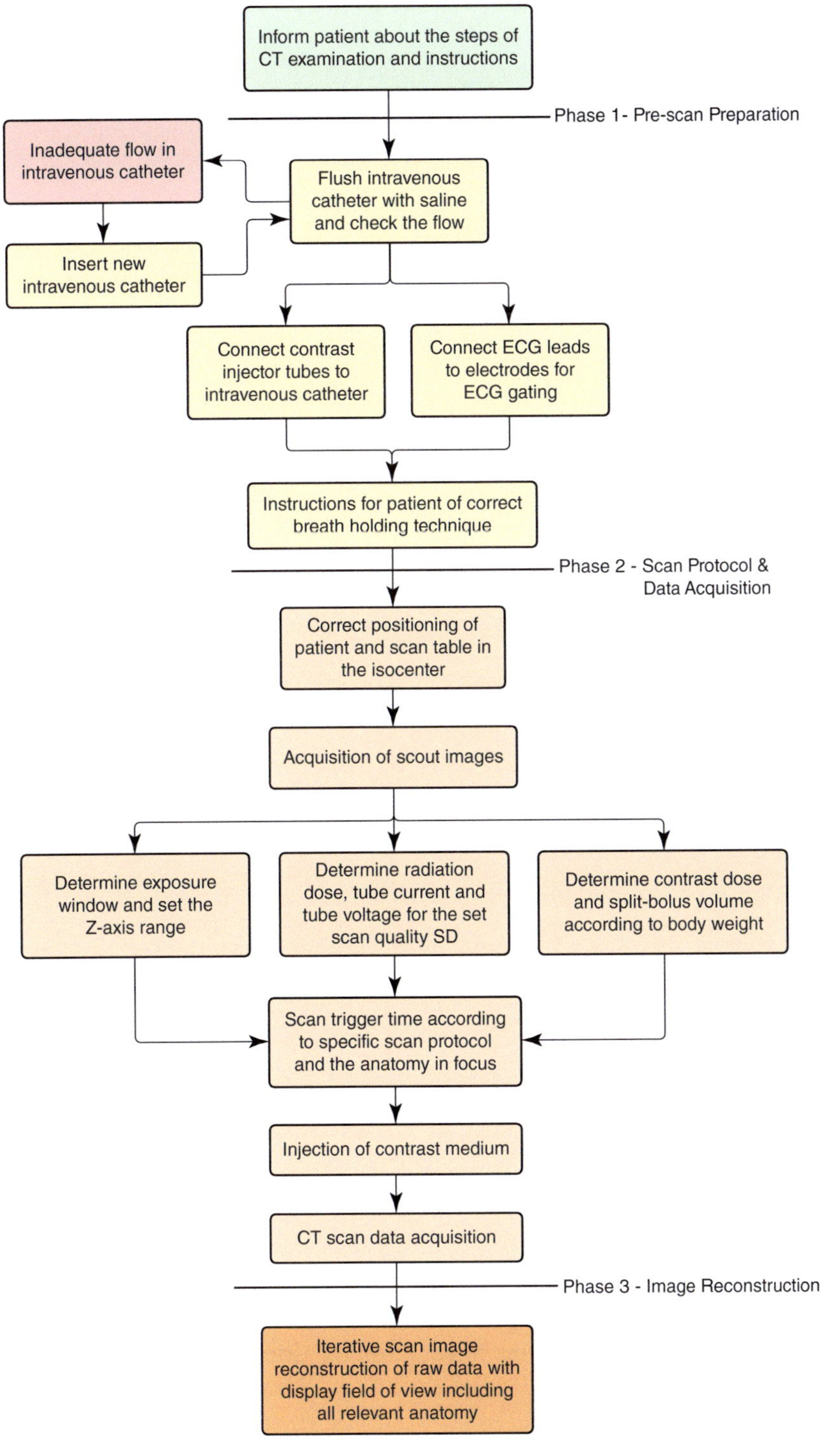

Fig. 5.4 Overview of the sequence of scanning steps. Flowchart illustrating a step-by-step guide for the pre-scan preparations and image data acquisition. The work processes are divided into three phases: Pre-scan preparation, scan protocol and data acquisition, and image reconstruction

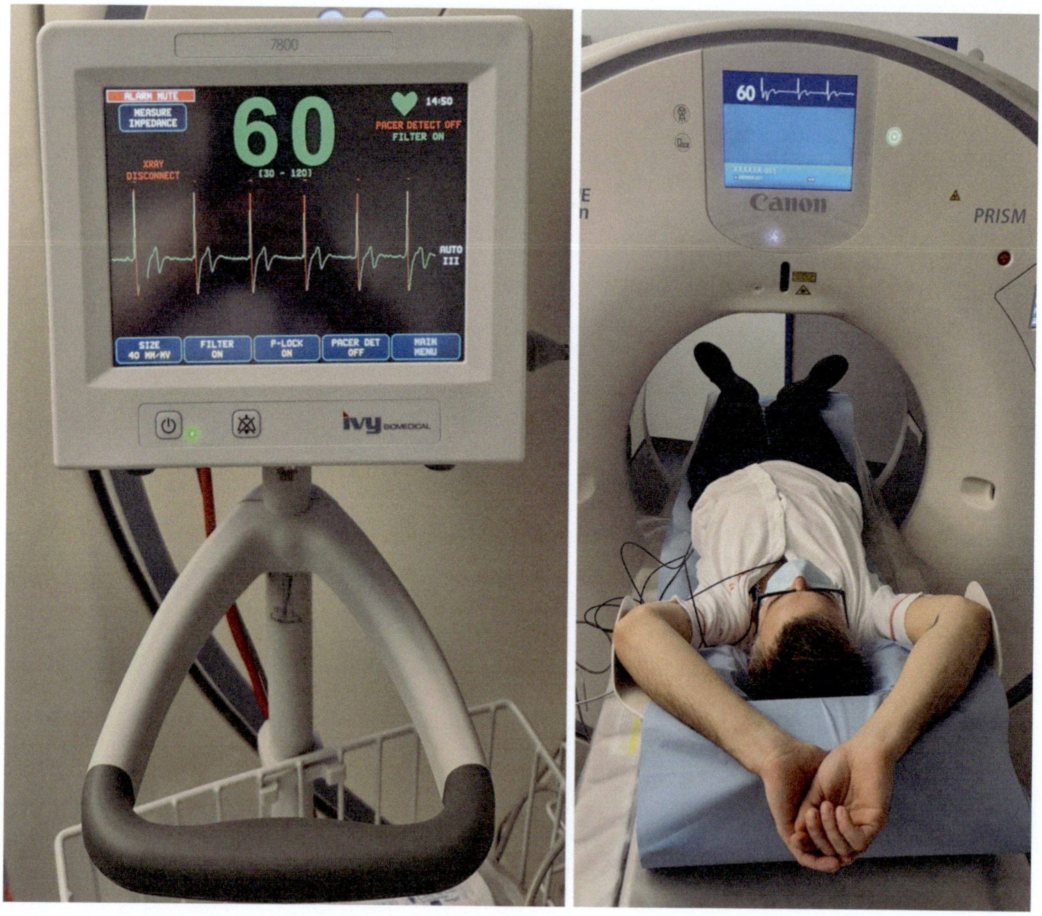

Fig. 5.5 Patient positioning for cardiac CT Scanning. Display of the ECG monitor with large and appropriate R-wave amplitude and correct positioning of the patient on the scan table in the supine position with arms above the head

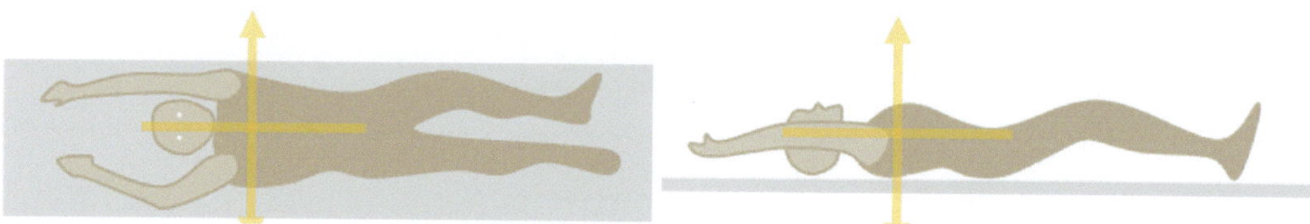

Fig. 5.6 Patient positioning. Correct positioning of the patient in the isocentric position of the scanner gantry. Lines with arrows indicate the adjustable positioning axes to correctly position the patient in the isocenter

The cylindrical scan area made of the three axes is also referred to as the exposure window.

- For most cardiac CT acquisition, the scan range is from the carina to just below the apex of the heart. The scan range should be as small as possible to minimize the radiation dose (Fig. 5.7).

5.6.10 Coronary Artery Calcium Scan Acquisition

- The non-contrast images are acquired for the assessment of coronary artery calcium scoring (CACS). In some centers, calcium calibration rods are placed under the patient on the scan table. Calcium calibration instruments are

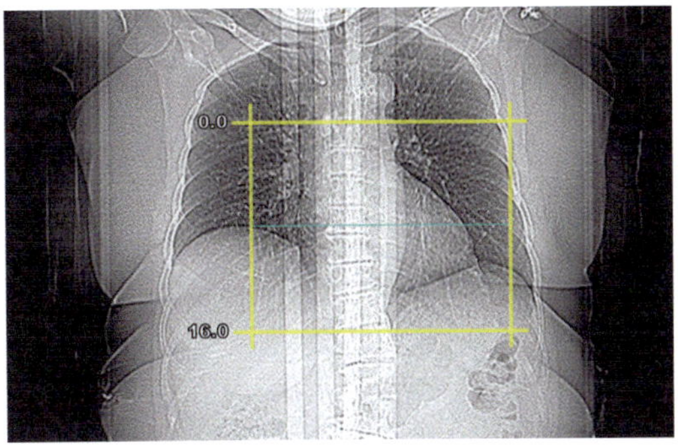

Fig. 5.7 Scan set up. Placement of a 16 cm Z-axis scan range on a scout image including all relevant cardiac anatomy in the scan field

used to calibrate the Hounsfield units of the different tissues appearing in the CT scan images.

- Depending on clinical indication and patient profile, the CACS image acquisition may be omitted, to reduce radiation dose (0.3–2 mSv).
- Note that the scan parameters used for Agatston calcium scoring are:
  - Tube voltage: 120 kVp.
  - Scan or reconstruction slice thickness: 3 mm.
  - Threshold for calcium to be scored as positive is 130 HU (software is typically programmed to use this threshold).
- Some sites scan using 100 kVp to reduce radiation dose, but the calcium score by Agatston is likely to be different with lower than 120 kVp.

5.6.11 Automated Exposure Control and X-Ray Tube Settings

- Current-generation CT scanners offer automated radiation dose reduction algorithms, adjusting X-ray tube output according to the tissue depth, and operating filters to reduce scatter radiation.
- Doses may also be adjusted based on newer iterative image reconstruction algorithms and tube voltage selection based on patient size and shape, scan area, and user-defined acceptable image quality.
- Individual adjustments are necessary to optimize settings for individual patients, especially in younger patients (e.g., lower kVp) and very large patients (maximize tube settings though there is no benefit of greater than 120 kVp).
- In patients with stents and/or heavily calcified vessels, 120 kVp instead of 100 kVp usually leads to better image quality.
- In general, 100 kVp tube voltage is chosen for normal weight patients, while 120 kVp is used for obese patients.
- In very thin patients, 80 kVp may be used.
- Tube current selection (mAs) is usually selected automatically by the scanner based on various factors such as selected kVp, image noise during scanogram, and use of reconstruction options to reduce image noise.

5.6.12 Contrast Dosing and Timing

- Contrast dosing depends on patient weight/size, heart rate, z-axis scan range, and scan duration.
- A general formula for total contrast dose is: (scan time + [5–10]) × injection rate.
- Typical contrast dose for cardiac CT ranges between 50 and 120 mL.
- Contrast trigger timing depends on the anatomical structure in focus for the CT examination—primarily left sided (arterial), primarily right sided (venous), or both.
- The optimal timing of contrast enhancement in cardiac CT is important to visualize the target anatomy at the peak of contrast enhancement. This can be achieved by using either the bolus-tracking or test bolus technique.
- Bolus tracking is conducted by placing a region of interest (ROI) in a predefined intracardiac or intravascular region depending on the target anatomy. The scan is initiated once the ROI reaches a preset threshold, e.g., 180 HU in the descending aorta (Fig. 5.8).
- The test bolus technique uses a test bolus (e.g., 10–20 mL) to estimate the travel time of contrast to the ROI (placed in a similar manner as described for bolus tracking). The entire

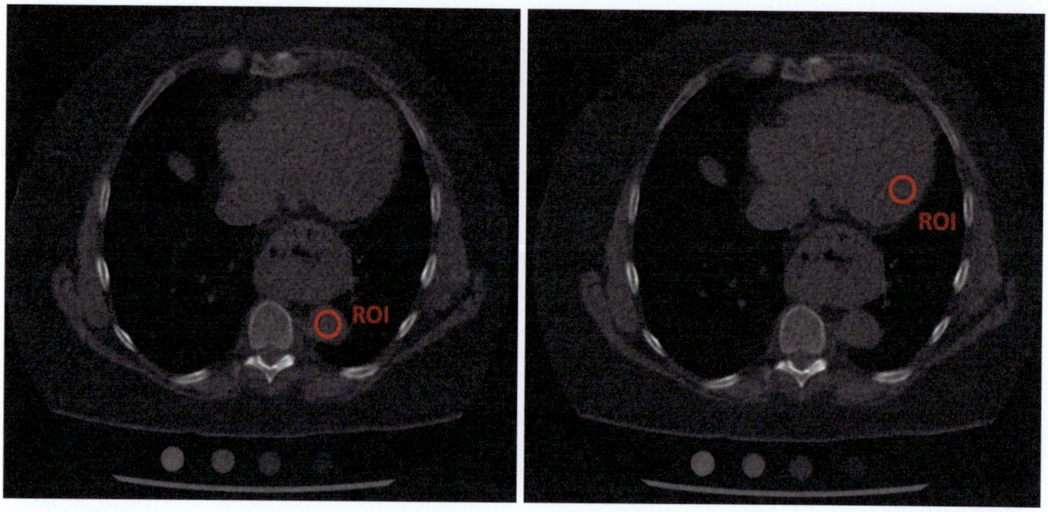

Fig. 5.8 Scan triggering using contrast bolus tracking. Placement of ROI in the descending aorta or left ventricle on the non-contrast images

contrast bolus (typically 60–70 mL) is then injected, and the scan is triggered after the determined travel time of the test bolus.

- The ROI is commonly set in the descending aorta but also can be in any cardiac chamber. The trigger threshold depends on the scan time and may range between 150 and 375 HU.
- The operator must not be reliant on using the selected threshold as sometimes the target threshold is not reached if too low of a contrast volume or rate is chosen. In this situation, the scan may be triggered manually at peak enhancement.
- A two- or three-phase contrast injection protocol may be used for standard cardiac CT.
- A two-phase contrast protocol consists of an initial injection of 50–70 mL contrast followed by a 30–50 mL saline chaser.
- A three-phase protocol consists of an initial injection of 50–70 mL contrast followed by a 20–30 mL of a contrast-saline mix (30/70 or 20/80), followed by a 30–50 mL saline chaser. The advantage of the three-phase protocol is the reduction of contrast enhancement artifacts compared to the two-phase protocol. Figure 5.9 provides an example of a split-bolus contrast dosing protocol.
- In cardiac CT examinations focusing on both right-sided and left-sided heart chambers (biventricular contrast) or other vascular structures, the contrast media injection duration should be sustained over a longer period of time (thus requiring a greater contrast volume).
- Mild side effects of iodinated contrast media include nausea, headache, itching, flushing, and skin rash or hives. The patient should be informed of the side effects of contrast media and instructed to seek immediate medical attention when experiencing allergic symptoms (see Sect. 5.8 below).
- Table 5.7 provides an overview of symptoms of adverse effects related to iodinated contrast media.

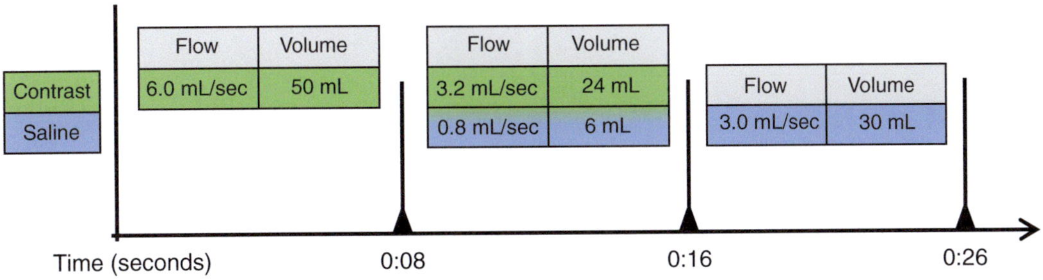

Fig. 5.9 Example of a split-bolus contrast dosing for a cardiac CT protocol in patients with a body weight of 80–100 kg

5.7 Image Reconstruction

- After the injection of contrast media and CT scan acquisition, the steps of image reconstruction begin. This is referred to as "Phase 3" in Fig. 5.4.
- The initial data acquisition creates the so-called raw data. Raw data are no actual images but rather all the acquired attenuation data from the detectors during the scan.
- Raw data need to be reconstructed into images by using mathematical algorithms and filtering.
- The traditional mode of image reconstruction has been based on filtered back projection, but it has been largely replaced by iterative reconstruction algorithms.
- More recently, advanced deep learning image reconstruction algorithms have been introduced for greater noise reduction.
- Specific reconstruction protocols are specific for each manufacturer—please also see Chap. 2 for a detailed discussion on this subject.
- In addition, there are algorithms for specific situations, e.g., metal artifact reduction algorithms in patients with metal devices.
- It is advisable for the patient to remain on the scanner table after scan acquisition until initial image reconstruction is completed to assure diagnostic data.
- Typically, the first dataset to be post-processed is in diastasis, e.g., 75% of the RR interval, but systolic phases may be selected if the heart rate was >70–75 bpm during acquisition.
- The first reconstructions should be reviewed for completeness of acquisition and image quality.
- Images affected by ectopic beats during scan acquisition may be improved by ECG editing (re-assigning R waves) if sufficient data are available (Chap. 2).
- Figure 5.10 presents an example of how image reconstructions in different cardiac phases can enhance the visibility of coronary structures.
- If the images are not diagnostic, repeat scan acquisition should be considered.

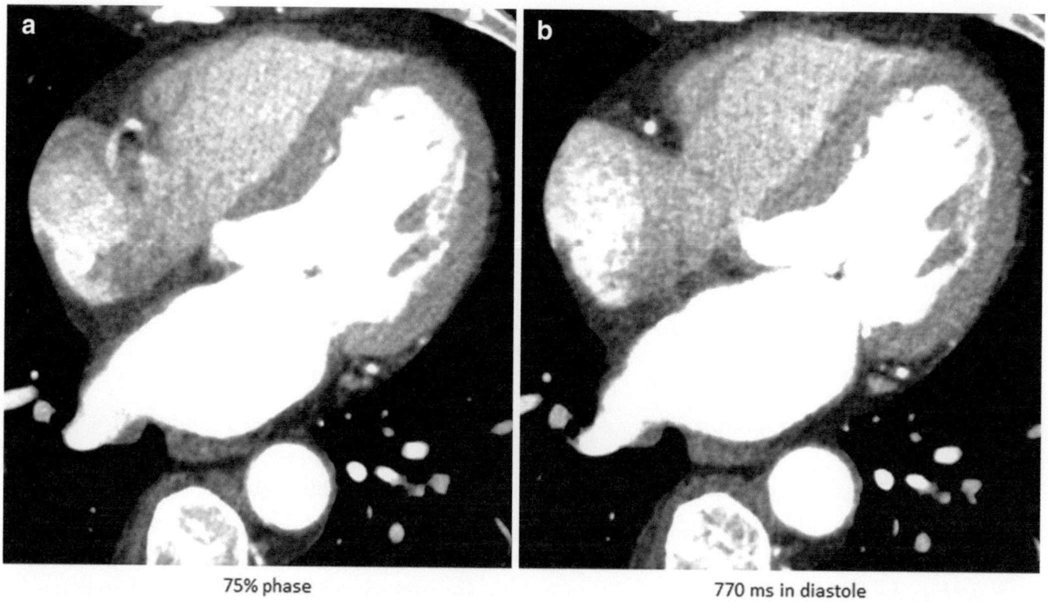

Fig. 5.10 Case example of the impact of phase selection. Patient scanned with low heart rate 53 bpm. Panel **a** shows initial image reconstruction using the 75% phase with the RCA slightly blurred. Panel **b** shows image reconstruction from a slightly different cardiac phase (770 ms in diastole) resulting in motion-free images of the RCA

5.8 Complications

- When conducted with appropriateness and care, cardiac CT is a safe diagnostic test with very rare associated adverse events.
- Nevertheless, the procedure involves radiation to the patient, contrast exposure, and often administration of medications.
- Every precaution should be taken—in accordance with the ALARA principle—that the total radiations dose is kept low yet maintaining a diagnostic accuracy relevant to the severity of the pertinent clinical question.
- Furthermore, stringent guidelines should be implemented when conducting clinical cardiac CT to avoid unwanted side effect related to medication and/or contrast media administrated during the procedure.
- In the rare event that a patient becomes acutely unwell during a cardiac CT procedure, the patient should be immediately assessed for anaphylaxis or other life-threatening conditions and the emergency team should be alerted without delay.
- A resuscitation cart with adrenaline should be readily available in the scanner room.
- Acute complications include:
  - Contrast reactions (discussed above).
  - Adverse events from medications (discussed above).
  - Contrast infiltration.
- Contrast infiltration into the tissue surrounding the IV may have medicolegal implications, and each imaging center should have a standard operating procedure (SOP) for such event.
- Patients who suffer contrast infiltration should be examined for the extent of swelling, pain level, and function of the affected muscles, blood vessels, and nerves.
- The amount of contrast infiltrated into tissue should be estimated. As there is often saline also extravasated, a simply scout view of the patient's arm using the CT scanner or a conventional X-ray of the elbow may help estimating the amount of contrast extravasated (Fig. 5.11).

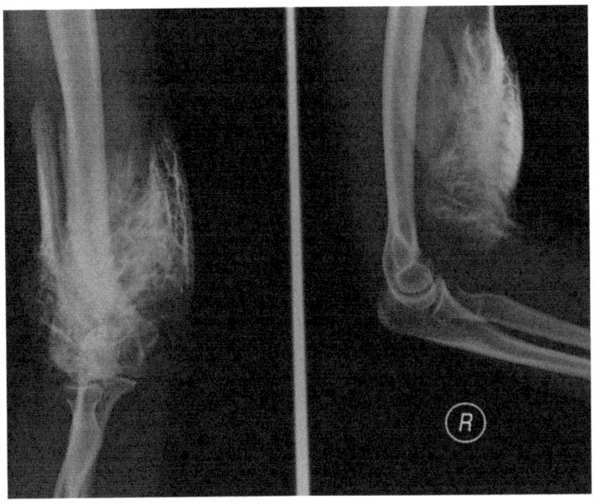

Fig. 5.11 Imaging contrast infiltration. Example of X-ray picture taken after extravasation of contrast media

- If amount of infiltrated contrast is estimated to be <50 mL, the following steps are recommended:
  - Apply compression with ice packs and elevate arm.
  - Observe patients for 1–2 h for swelling and pain. If the patient is comfortable and no functional deficits are noted, the patient can be discharged with instructions to seek immediate medical attention if there is altered sensation in arm, persistent pain, skin blistering, or discoloration.
  - Compression with ice packs three times a day for 10–15 min may be continued until swelling has subsided.
- If amount extravasated is estimated to be >50 mL:
  - Consult with orthopedic or plastic surgeon for further care and management.
  - This may entail injection of saline into the arm to dilute the contrast concentration [16].

5.9 Specific Cardiac CT Acquisition Protocols

- Cardiac CT may allow visualization of various cardiovascular structures and thoracic anatomy. Depending on the focused anatomy, specific image acquisition protocols are needed to adjust contrast timing and tube settings for optimal visualization of structures. In this section, we provide some examples of cardiac CT protocols for a range of clinical indications.
- As different vendors provide different CT systems with specific properties and terms, the presented protocols are *general* examples. Specific protocols need to be established at sites using local equipment and experience.
- Specific image acquisition settings will depend on the available CT technology, and consultation with the respective vendor representation is strongly advised.
- Well-defined CT acquisition protocols may allow the CT technologist to conduct the entire CT examination without the need of a physician during most routine examinations.

5.9.1 Coronary Angiography

- Purpose: Visualizing of coronary arteries to detect and estimate severity and extent of coronary artery or other disease, e.g., dissection, aneurysm, etc.
- Scan range: Below carina of trachea to below cardiac apex for native coronary arteries; include the subclavian arteries for bypass evaluations.
- Medications: 0.4–1.2 mg SL NTG for coronary vasodilation.
- Collimation: Smallest available slice thickness, e.g., 64 × 0.5 mm.

- Gantry rotation: Fastest rotation synchronized with heart rate.
- Tube settings: Optimized for high signal-to-noise ratio (>30).
- Scan method: Dependent on heart rate, rhythm, and scanner technology. Prospective scan triggering is recommended whenever possible, e.g., with regular heart rate <60 bpm.
- Consider including end-systole in the image acquisition if heart rate > 70–75 bpm.
- ROI setting: ROI placed in descending aorta.
- Contrast volume: 40–120 mL depending on patient size and heart rate.
- Triggering threshold for bolus tracking: Typical range 180–375 HU depending on patient size and scanner technology.

5.9.2 Cardiac Function

- Purpose: Cine visualizing of left and right ventricle contractile function and delineation of end-systolic and end-diastolic frames for assessment of ventricular volumes and ejection fraction.
- Scan range: Below carina of trachea to below cardiac apex, may be expanded depending on clinical indication.
- Medications: Not usually necessary.
- Collimation: Smallest available slice thickness or slightly higher if no concomitant coronary evaluation is performed.
- Gantry rotation: Fastest rotation synchronized with heart rate.
- Tube settings: Optimized for high signal-to-noise ratio (>30), though less stringent as with coronary evaluation.
- Scan method: Full R-R scan acquisition with retrospective gating, with or without tube modulation.
- ROI setting: ROI placed in descending aorta or ascending aorta.
- Triggering threshold: 150–375 HU or use test bolus technique.
- Contrast volume: 60–100 mL depending on patient size and heart rate.

5.9.3 Combined Cardiac Chambers, Coronary Arteries, and Aorta

- Purpose: Visualizing of cardiac chambers, coronary arteries, and aortic arch in chest pain patients who also have suspected aortic dilatation and/or ascending aortic dissection.
- Scan range: From aortic arch or carina to below cardiac apex or whole range of aorta.
- Medications: 0.4–1.2 mg SL NTG for coronary vasodilation and beta-blockers/ivabradine as needed for heart rate control.
- Collimation: Smallest available slice thickness.
- Gantry rotation: Fastest rotation synchronized with heart rate.
- Tube settings: Optimized for high signal-to-noise ratio (>30).
- Scan method: Preferable prospective scan triggering to minimize radiation.
- ROI setting: ROI placed in left cardiac ventricle or descending aorta.
- Triggering threshold: 200–375 HU or use test bolus technique.
- Contrast volume: 60–120 mL depending on patient size and heart rate.

5.9.4 Pre-Atrial Fibrillation Ablation Scan with Exclusion of Left Atrial Appendage Thrombus

- Purpose: Visualizing left atrial appendage anatomy, exclusion of filling defects, and delineation pulmonary vein anatomy for planning pulmonary vein isolation.
- Scan range: 1 cm above carina of trachea to below cardiac apex. This can be narrowed into only including left atrium, left atrial appendage, and pulmonary veins to reduce radiation dose.
- Medications: None.
- Collimation: Smallest available slice thickness or slightly greater given that less spatial resolution is needed.
- Gantry rotation: Fastest rotation synchronized with heart rate.

- Tube settings: Optimized for high signal-to-noise ratio (>30).
- Scan method: Prospective scan triggering in end-systole (e.g., 40% of R-R cycle) with repeated scan after 30-s delay focused on the left atrial appendage.
- ROI setting: ROI placed in left atrium or descending aorta.
- Triggering threshold: 180–375 HU or use test bolus technique.
- Contrast volume: 40–80 mL depending on patient size and heart rate.

5.9.5 Pre-Procedure Transcatheter Aortic Valve Replacement (TAVR)

- Purpose: Visualization of aortic valve and coronary arteries for TAVR valve sizing and procedure planning, including evaluation of access site (aortic arch, subclavian and femoral arteries).
- Scan range: Below carina of trachea to below cardiac apex (ECG-gated cardiac component), above the subclavian artery to trochanter minor (ungated spiral acquisition, access site component).
- Medications: Ivabradine and/or beta-blockers for heart rate control, as needed.
- Collimation: Smallest available slice thickness.
- Gantry rotation: Fastest rotation synchronized with heart rate.
- Tube settings: Optimized for high signal-to-noise ratio (>30).
- Scan method: Calcium score (for valve and aortic root calcification), CTA retrospective gated (with or without tube modulation for systolic aortic root sizing and diastolic coronary artery visualization).
- ROI setting: ROI placed in left cardiac ventricle.
- Triggering threshold: 180–350 HU or use test bolus technique.
- Contrast volume: 80–120 mL depending on patient size and heart rate.

References

1. ACR Guidelines. ACR–NASCI–SPR practice parameter for the performance and interpretation of cardiac computed tomography. 2021.
2. Otton JM, Phan J, Feneley M, et al. Defining the mid-diastolic imaging period for cardiac CT—lessons from tissue Doppler echocardiography. BMC Med Imaging. 2013;13:5.
3. Krumpl G, Domanovits H, Stix G, et al. Esmolol in cardiology, emergency and critical-care medicine. J Kardiologie. 2012;19:2–8.
4. Wang J-D, Zhang H-W, Xin Q, et al. Safety and efficacy of intravenous esmolol before prospective electrocardiogram-triggered high-pitch spiral acquisition for computed tomography coronary angiography. J Geriatr Cardiol. 2014;11:39–43.
5. BC Guidelines. Heart failure care, Appendix B—Beta blockers. 2008.
6. Lambrechtsen J, Egstrup K. Pre-treatment with a sinus node blockade, ivabradine, before coronary CT angiography: a retrospective audit, vol. 68. Clin Radiol; 2013. p. 1054.
7. Celik O, Atasoy MM, Erturk M, et al. Comparison of different strategies of ivabradine premedication for heart rate reduction before coronary computed tomography angiography, vol. 8. J Cardiovasc Comput Tomogr; 2014. p. 77.
8. Baerlocher MO, Asch M, Myers A. The use of contrast media. Can Med Assoc J. 2010;182:697.
9. An J, Jung H, Kwon OY, et al. Differences in adverse reactions among iodinated contrast media: analysis of the KAERS database. J Allergy Clin Immunol Pract. 2019;7:2205.
10. Chiu T-M, Chu S-Y. Hypersensitivity reactions to iodinated contrast media, vol. 10. Biomedicines; 2022. p. 1036.
11. ESUR Guidelines on Contrast Agents v10.0. 2018.
12. Faucon A-L, Bobrie G, Clément O. Nephrotoxicity of iodinated contrast media: from pathophysiology to prevention strategies. Eur J Radiol. 2019;116:231.
13. Davenport MS, Perazella MA, Yee J, et al. Use of intravenous iodinated contrast media in patients with disease: consensus statements from the American College of Radiology and National Kidney Foundation, vol. 2. Radiology; 2020. p. 85.
14. Honoris L, Zhong Y, Chu E, et al. Comparison of contrast enhancement, image quality and tolerability in coronary CT angiography using 4 contrast agents: a prospective randomized trial. Int J Cardiol. 2015;186:126.
15. Takx RAP, Suchá D, Park J, et al. Sublingual nitroglycerin administration in coronary computed tomography angiography: a systematic review. Eur Radiol. 2015;25:3536.
16. Bellin M-F, Jakobsen JA, Tomassin I, et al. Contrast medium extravasation injury: guidelines for prevention and management. Eur Radiol. 2002;12:2807.

6 Radiation Risks and Safety in Cardiac CT

Armin Arbab Zadeh

Abstract

X-ray imaging is associated with exposure to ionizing radiation which has the potential to cause harm. Risk from radiation is commonly categorized as deterministic (or non-stochastic) vs. stochastic. Non-stochastic risk from CT imaging is exceedingly low, typically stemming from major human errors. Estimating stochastic risk from CT imaging, on the other hand, is controversial. The general assumption is that there is a linear non-threshold relationship between radiation dose and cancer risk. While such risk is very low for a given individual, the risk is considerable on a population level due to the many studies performed. Furthermore, it is conceivable that repeated exposure from medical imaging increases the probability of cancer development in a person. Radiation safety is critical to minimize radiation exposure and to reduce risk. This chapter covers fundamental principles of radiation dose concepts, estimation of dose, measures to reduce dose, and appropriate monitoring/reporting.

Keywords

Radiation · Dose · Exposure · X-ray risk · Dose-length-product · Cancer risk

Abbreviations

ALARA	As low as reasonable achievable
BMI	Body mass index
CABG	Coronary artery bypass grafting
CTDI	Computed tomography dose index; product
DLP	Dose-length-product
Gy	Gray
PE	Pulmonary embolism
Sv	Sievert

A. A. Zadeh (✉)
Department of Medicine, Johns Hopkins University, Baltimore, MD, USA
e-mail: arminzadeh@jhu.edu

A. A. Zadeh, J. Hoe (eds.), *Practical Guide to Cardiac CT*,
https://doi.org/10.1007/978-981-97-6919-3_6

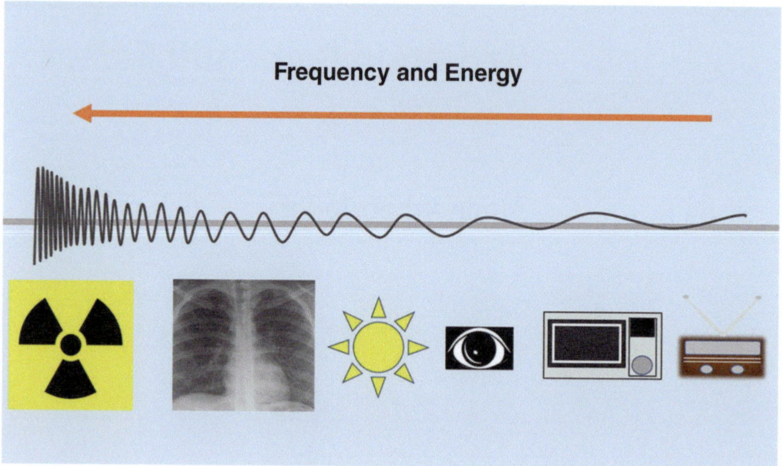

Fig. 6.1 The electromagnetic spectrum

6.1 The Concept of Radiation Dose

- Radiation refers to energy emitted from a source, e.g., from the sun or radioactive material. On the electromagnetic spectrum, X-rays are on the high energy, high frequency end (Fig. 6.1).
- In contrast to low energy radiation, e.g., visible light, X-rays may display electrons from their orbit (hence called ionizing radiation) which is potential harmful to living tissue.
- The radiation dose refers to the amount of energy absorbed by a given mass of tissue, given in Gray (Gy).
- Adjusted for the destructive potency of the type of radiation, the *equivalent* dose is given in Sievert (Sv). The adjustment factor for X-rays is 1, rendering the same value for dose and equivalent dose.
- In radiation safety, the equivalent dose is most commonly used and thus doses are given in Sievert or Millisievert (mSv).
- An X-ray examination typically leads to radiation exposure confined to a certain body area (also known as non-uniform radiation exposure). To be able to compare the dose and associated risk in persons with different body area exposure, the concept of *effective* dose was introduced, which integrates the organ doses and weights them according to organ sensitivity equivalent to an exposure of the entire body.
- Since most of the radiation risk data initially came from atomic bomb survivors, who received uniform exposure to the entire body, the effective dose estimate has been an effective tool for comparing risk in populations.
- Note that the effective dose is *not* intended for accurate dose or risk estimation in an individual—although it is widely misused for this purpose [1].

6.2 Radiation Dose Estimates by CT

- In CT imaging, radiation dose is crudely estimated using the CT dose index (CTDI), which integrates the dose profile of a scan producing one tomographic image (Fig. 6.2).
- The CTDI is typically weighted for the higher peripheral doses than the center ($CTDI_w$) and for the pitch (CTDI volume or $CTDI_{vol}$).
- The $CTDI_{vol}$ is readily available from the scanner based on the scan settings, e.g., X-ray tube voltage and current, pitch, etc. (Fig. 6.2).
- The $CTDI_{vol}$ is NOT derived from actual dose measurements but from modeling and assumptions (e.g., body shape) and thus is crude estimate of radiation dose, given in mGy. As such, the CTDI does not reflect an accurate assessment of the actual radiation dose.
- The $CTDI_{vol}$ multiplied by the scan range in the z-axis gives the dose-length-product (DLP,

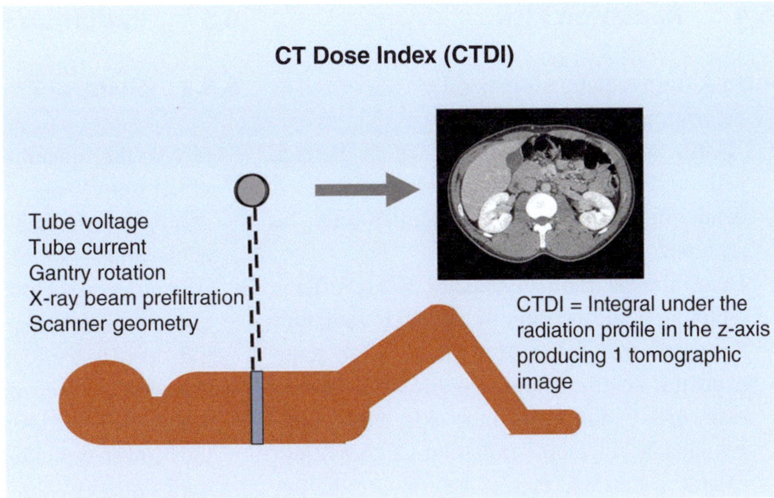

Fig. 6.2 The CT Dose Index integrates the dose profile of one tomographic scan

Table 6.1 Common radiation doses in cardiovascular medicine

Test	CXR	CACS	Chest CT	CT PE	CT heart	SPECT	PET heart	Cardiac cath	PCI
Typical dose	0.1	2	7	10	9	12	8	7	23
Typical range	0.02–0.2	0.5–3	5–8	0.2–14	1–30	7–24	2–13	3–12	10–100

Sources: Vano E, et al., Insights Imaging 2021, Lin EC Mayo Clin Proc 2010, Mettler FA, Radiology 2020, Einstein A, Circ 2007 [3–6]

CACS coronary artery calcium scanning, *CXR* chest X-ray, *Cath* catheterization, *PCI* percutaneous coronary intervention, *PE* pulmonary embolism, *PET* positron emission tomography, *SPECT* single-photon emission computed tomography

mGy/cm), a key metric for estimating radiation dose in CT imaging, yet subject to the same limitation as the CTDI.

- The radiation dose for an entire CT scan is commonly estimated by multiplying the DLP with a conversion factor k (for the body region imaged):

> – **DLP = $CTDI_{vol}$ × scan range. The DLP is given in mG/cm.**
> – **Estimated Dose = DLP × *k*. Dose is given in mSv.**

- For cardiac CT, a conversion factor *k* of 0.014 has been widely used to estimate the effective dose. However, several studies demonstrated severe underestimation of more accurate dose estimates and a *k* factor of 0.026 has been proposed instead [2].
- At this time, no consensus has been reached on the most appropriate conversion factor for cardiac CT. Current dose estimates are prone to substantially underestimate dose and risk in cardiac CT.

6.3 Typical Radiation Doses in Medical Imaging

- Table 6.1 lists radiation dose estimates for common medical imaging tests.
- For comparison, the annual background radiation from natural sources is approximately 3 mSv.
- Similar to CT imaging, radiation dose estimates from fluoroscopy and nuclear imaging are crude and estimated values only provide a general sense of the respective orders of magnitude.
- Furthermore, there is considerable dose variability for each test based on equipment and handling.

6.4 Radiation Risk

- Risk from radiation is generally categorized as deterministic vs. stochastic.
- X-rays are ionizing radiation which damage cells and their DNA. The result may be cell death or injury which generally can be repaired.
- Deterministic (non-stochastic) X-ray effects on living tissue are directly related to radiation dose and manifest within hours after acute exposure or after months/years with chronic exposure. Examples include skin burns, nausea, headaches (acute radiation sickness) and cataract, sterility, cancer (chronic radiation sickness). Deterministic effects predictably occur with certain doses.
- Stochastic effects, on the other hand, are those which may potentially but not necessarily occur. These effects are likely related to the probability of unsuccessful DNA repair and resulting mutations which may go on and develop malignancies and/or gene defects transmitted to offspring.
- Current models assume that *any* level of radiation poses risk of cancer, with the probability increasing linearly with the dose.
- In CT imaging, deterministic radiation effects are very rare and typically result from errors in scan acquisition. Most of the concern arises over stochastic effects.
- The risk from stochastic effects are very difficult to estimate given the long latency after exposure and the many covariates. Data consistently show greater cancer risk with increasing dose, however.
- Current models assume a 0.1% increased risk of cancer development per life time with a 10 mSv exposure. Such risk may appear small in context of an approximately 20% life time risk of cancer, but individuals may have many similar exposures, which likely further increases risk. Furthermore, many millions of patients undergo X-ray imaging each year, with models associating many thousands of cancers on a population level.

6.5 Radiation Safety

6.5.1 General Principles

- Given the uncertain but potential harmful effect from X-ray radiation, the general rule of dosing in imaging is "as low as reasonably achievable"—or ALARA.
- Advances in cardiac CT technology and acquisition techniques have allowed substantial dose reductions. Most CT systems now use sophisticated noise reduction algorithms which allows lower X-ray tube settings, and thus lower radiation dose, while maintaining image quality.
- Key factors influencing the radiation dose in cardiac CT are listed in Table 6.2. Of note, the radiation dose changes approximately with the square of the tube voltage and thus lowering tube voltage is particularly effective in reducing dose.

6.5.2 Adjusting X-Ray Tube Settings to Reduce Radiation Exposure

- Adjustment of X-ray tube settings is central to balancing image quality with radiation dose and has a profound effect on the radiation dose to the patient.
- Image noise generally decreases with higher peak tube voltage and tube current due to reduced tissue attenuation, while radiation dose increases with higher X-ray tube settings.
- Increasing peak tube voltage, however, also decreases contrast, i.e., attenuation differ-

Table 6.2 Comparison of image characteristics and radiation dose according to peak tube voltage

Metric	120 kV	80 kV
Image noise	24 ± 4	40 ± 6
Image contrast	472 ± 55	714 ± 88
CNR	20 ± 3	18 ± 4
Radiation dose (mSv)	14 ± 1	6 ± 1

Adapted after Oda et al. [7]
CNR contrast-to-noise ratio, *kV* kilovolt, *mSv* milli-Sievert

ences between tissues, which may hinder identification of structures and processes. A balance between image noise and contrast is critical for achieving good image quality.

- The peak tube voltage is adjusted according to patient size, with higher voltage required for larger patients due to the need for higher energy X-rays to achieve adequate penetration.
- Most patients can be imaged with a peak tube voltage of 80–120 kilovolt (kV).
- A peak tube voltage of >120, e.g., 130–140 kV, may be considered in very large patients but a better balance of image noise and contrast is typically achieved with 120 kV even in large patients.
- Patients with body mass index (BMI) of <30 may be scanned using 100 kV (instead of 120) and patients with BMI <25 may be suitable for 80 kV imaging.
- Tube current adjustments may be considered as "fine-tuning" after the tube voltage is set. The effect of tube current adjustment on radiation dose is generally smaller than the result of changing the tube voltage (linear vs. exponential relationship).
- Individual X-ray tube settings or noise targets should be adjusted according to the purpose of imaging and disease pretest probability.
- Coronary CT angiography generally requires optimal image quality, given the small size of atherosclerotic plaques and vessel lumen. However, greater noise level may be acceptable in younger individuals with low pretest probability of disease in whom radiation risk is greater than in older patients.

6.5.3 Exposure Window Adjustments

- The largest reduction in radiation dose may be achieved by prospective scan triggering with narrow exposure window as opposed to retrospective gating (up to 80–90% dose reduction).
- Whenever feasible, prospective scan triggering is the desired acquisition mode to keep radiation doses low.
- Aside from CT hardware, optimal heart rate control facilitates prospective scan triggering because motion-free images can then be obtained among a small selection of diastolic frames, thus limiting exposure (see Chap. 5).
- A minimal exposure window (e.g., 75–75% of the R-R cycle) is often sufficient with regular heart rates (e.g., in the 50's).
- If the heart rate is less than optimal, the exposure window may be widened at the expense of radiation dose.
- Unless functional information is required, an exposure window of more than 40–80% of the R-R cycle is rarely needed even with higher, regular heart rates.
- In the setting of irregular heart rates, however, retrospective gating may be necessary unless a wide detector scanner with whole heart coverage is used (see Chap. 5).

6.5.4 Scan Range

- The scan range is adjusted in the z-axis and should contain only organs of interest while sparing all other tissue, if possible.
- For cardiac imaging without bypass graft assessment, the scan typically starts at the level of the pulmonary artery and ends just distal to the cardiac apex (Fig. 6.3).

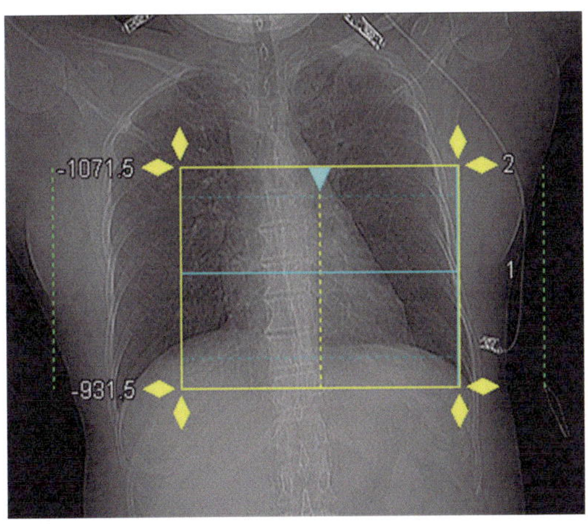

Fig. 6.3 Typical scan range for cardiac CT

- Minimizing the scan range has been associated with 30% radiation dose reduction compared to liberal scan range selection.
- Unless extended scan range is necessary, e.g., CABG or PE protocol, cardiac scans typically range from the mid pulmonary artery to 2 cm below the diaphragm. For every 1 cm reduction of scan length, radiation dose may be reduced by up to 10%.

6.5.5 Image Noise Reduction Software

- Iterative scan reconstruction (IR) and newer artificial intelligence-based algorithms allow image noise reduction such that scans can be acquired with lower radiation dose while maintaining diagnostic image quality.
- IR algorithms facilitate dose reduction by allowing lower tube current settings (typically reduced from 300–400 mAs to 30–50 mAs) which otherwise would result in increased image noise.
- Some IR and deep learning algorithms require large computing power and may be available on higher end systems.
- Contemporary CT systems allow the selection of acceptable image noise ranges for which the scanner automatically will adjust its acquisition settings, i.e., peak tube voltage and current.
- The extent of noise reduction from these algorithms is vendor specific but all offer similar options.

6.5.6 Monitoring and Reporting Radiation Dose

- Regulatory requirements for reporting radiation doses vary for each country and state but it becomes increasingly mandatory.
- Radiation doses also should be monitored internally for quality control.
- Radiation doses should be recorded and reported using the dose-length-product (DLP) in mGy*cm.
- Estimated dose in mSv may be provided only in conjunction with the DLP estimate such that the conversion factor is disclosed.

6.5.7 Relating Radiation Doses to Patients

- Life time cancer risk is approximately 1 in 5 or 20% for each person.
- An X-ray exposure of 10 mSv increases cancer risk by approximately 0.1%.
- Thus, a person's life time cancer risk increases from 20% to 20.1% with one 10 mSv exposure.
- Annual radiation from natural sources (background radiation) is approximately 3 mSv.
- A coronary CTA may give less than the annual background radiation or several-fold more, depending on the protocol and settings (current technology average 3–12 mSv or up to four times the annual background radiation).
- A transatlantic flight corresponds for approximately 0.8 mSv.
- A banana exposes a person to approximately 0.0001 mSv.
- Most coronary CT angiograms can be performed with radiation doses equivalent to less than 10 transatlantic flights and therefore less than 1:1000 increase of cancer risk.

References

1. Martin CJ, Harrison JD, Rehani MM. Effective dose from radiation exposure in medicine: past, present, and future. Phys Med. 2020;79:87–92. https://doi.org/10.1016/j.ejmp.2020.10.020.
2. Trattner S, Halliburton S, Thompson CM, et al. Cardiac-specific conversion factors to estimate radiation effective dose from dose-length product in computed tomography. JACC Cardiovasc Imaging. 2018;11(1):64–74. https://doi.org/10.1016/j.jcmg.2017.06.006.
3. Lin EC. Radiation risk from medical imaging. Mayo Clin Proc. 2010;85(12):1142–6; quiz 1146. https://doi.org/10.4065/mcp.2010.0260.
4. Mettler FA, Mahesh M, Bhargavan-Chatfield M, et al. Patient exposure from radiologic and nuclear medicine procedures in the United States: procedure volume and effective dose for the period 2006-

2016. Radiology. 2020;295(2):418–27. https://doi.org/10.1148/radiol.2020192256.

5. Vano E, Frija G, Loose R, et al. Dosimetric quantities and effective dose in medical imaging: a summary for medical doctors. Insights Imaging. 2021;12(1):99–2. https://doi.org/10.1186/s13244-021-01041-2.
6. Einstein AJ, Moser KW, Thompson RC, Cerqueira MD, Henzlova MJ. Radiation dose to patients from cardiac diagnostic imaging. Circulation. 2007;116(11):1290–305.
7. Oda S, Utsunomiya D, Funama Y, et al. A low tube voltage technique reduces the radiation dose at retrospective ECG-gated cardiac computed tomography for anatomical and functional analyses. Acad Radiol. 2011;18(8):991–9. https://doi.org/10.1016/j.acra.2011.03.007.

7 Difficult Cardiac CT Scan Conditions

Jin Hur

Abstract

CT coronary angiography (CCTA) has become a widely accepted test for non-invasive evaluation of the heart and coronary arteries. Despite numerous technical advances, scan acquisition in the setting of high heart rate, arrhythmia, severe obesity, devices, or inability to cooperate, may be associated with artifacts and/or poor image quality. In this chapter, we discuss several difficult scan conditions and possible solutions to improve image quality.

Keywords

CT coronary angiography · Calcium score
Coronary artery stents · Heart rate
Arrhythmia · Obesity

Abbreviations

CCTA	CT coronary angiography
CT	Computed tomography
HR	Heart rate
ISR	In-stent restenosis
TR	Temporal resolution

7.1 Introduction

- Because of rapid cardiac motion and small structures to be imaged, CT coronary angiography (CCTA) is one of the most challenging clinical applications of computed tomography (CT) [1, 2].
- Advancements in CT technology, e.g., faster gantry rotation and larger z-axis coverage, have facilitated diagnostic image quality in most patients but challenges remain [3].

J. Hur (✉)
Department of Radiology and Research Institute of Radiological Science and Center for Clinical Image Data Science, Severance Hospital, Yonsei University College of Medicine, Seoul, Republic of Korea
e-mail: khuhz@yuhs.ac

A. A. Zadeh, J. Hoe (eds.), *Practical Guide to Cardiac CT*,
https://doi.org/10.1007/978-981-97-6919-3_7

Table 7.1 Difficult scan condition causes and possible solutions

Difficult scan condition	Problem	Possible solutions
Severe coronary artery calcification	Blooming artifact	• High spatial resolution • Smallest slice collimation • Noise reduction software • Sharp convolution kernel • Spectral imaging • Digital subtraction • Heart rate control
Presence of coronary artery stent	Blooming artifact; beam-hardening artifact	• High spatial resolution • Smallest slice collimation • Noise reduction software • Sharp convolution kernel. • Spectral imaging • Digital subtraction • Heart rate control
High heart rate or arrhythmia	Blurring; stair-step or banding	• Advanced heart rate control • High temporal resolution • Widened exposure window • Optimal phase reconstruction • Multi-segment acquisition • Motion-correction software
Severe obesity	Excessive image noise	• Tube setting optimization • Increased contrast volume • Noise reduction software • Heart rate control

- The NICE report [4] lists six scenarios of difficult scan conditions (Table 7.1).
- In this chapter, we will discuss these challenging scan conditions and provide a practical approach for improving image quality.

7.2 Severe Coronary Artery Calcification

- Severe coronary artery calcification represents a common diagnostic challenge for CCTA, which can lead to miss-diagnosis, and unnecessary downstream testing (also see Chap. 9).
- Several studies reported that in patients with severe calcification, CCTA has reduced accuracy for the detection of obstructive disease (Fig. 7.1) [5, 6].
- Calcified plaques may cause blooming artifact on CCTA images caused by the partial volume effect in the setting of limited spatial resolution (Fig. 7.2).
- The partial volume effect results from disproportional consideration of highly attenuating structures in the image processing algorithm (overtaking the information in a given voxel) which leads to artificial enlargement of such high-density structures in the final image.
- The resultant "blooming" effect may lead to impaired visualization of the coronary artery lumen, resulting in overestimation of the severity of coronary artery stenosis [7, 8].
- High spatial resolution is the key remedy to reduce blooming artifacts but scanners providing ultra-high-resolution are not yet widely available.
- Use of noise reduction software, e.g., artificial intelligence/deep learning algorithms, is a promising approach to improve image quality in the setting of severe coronary artery calcification, particularly when used in combination with dedicated sharp convolution filters [9].
- Adjusting the window level settings and use of smallest available slice thickness along with a sharp convolution kernel is strongly recommended to help improving visualization of the artery lumen.
- Dual energy imaging has shown promise in this setting but this approach has not been realized in routine clinical practice.

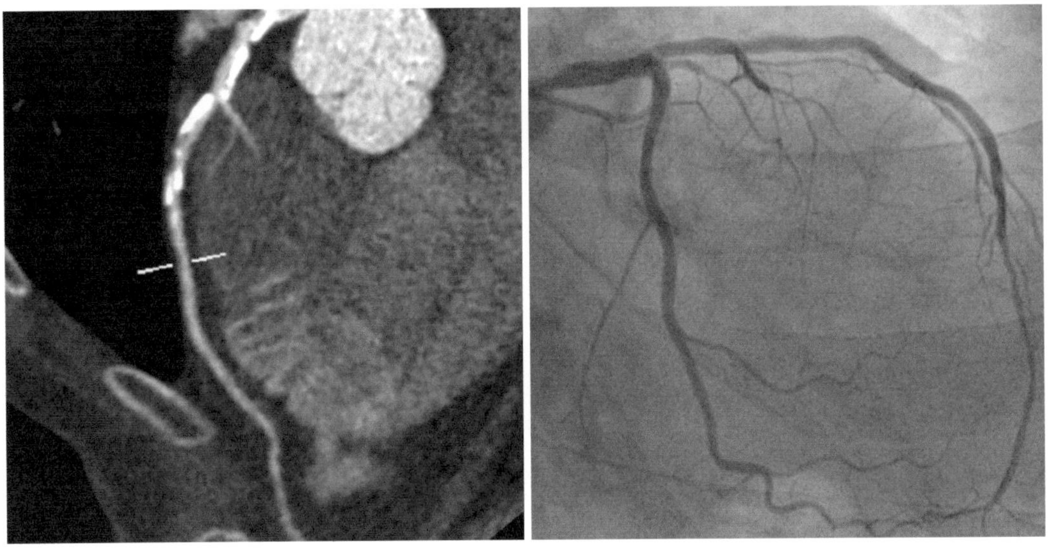

Fig. 7.1 Case example of a 65-year-old man presenting with chest pain. The left panel shows multiple calcified plaques in left anterior descending artery by CCTA. The right panel reveals no significant stenosis by invasive angiography

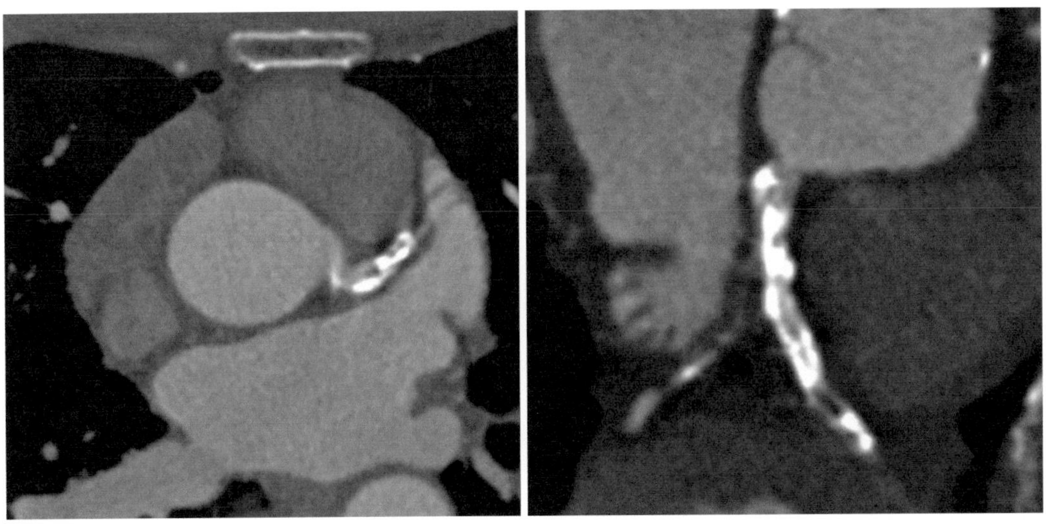

Fig. 7.2 Case example of a 72-year-old man with chest pain. CCTA images reveal densely calcified plaques obscuring the artery lumen

- Digital subtraction techniques require non-contrast scanning prior to CCTA and specific software, available with some vendors. Current results are not applicable to routine clinical practice, however.
- Optimal heart rate control does not affect spatial resolution but it eliminates blurring of coronary calcium, which further degrades image quality.

7.3 Presence of Coronary Artery Stents

- A dedicated chapter is provided to address this topic (please see Chap. 15).

7.4 Poor Heart Rate Control

- Motion and stair-step/slice misalignment artifacts due to high heart rate and heart rate variability may significantly reduce the CCTA diagnostic accuracy.
- Blurring occurs when the temporal resolution is insufficient to accurately register the moving structure. The right coronary artery is most commonly affected owing to its higher velocity and range of motion compared with other coronary segments (Fig. 7.3) [10].
- High temporal resolution, optimal cardiac phase selection, and good heart rate control may minimize or even eliminate image blurring from cardiac motion.
- Current generation CT scanners provide image acquisition with approximately 125–175 ms temporal resolution, which is generally adequate for coronary imaging with stable heart rates of 65 bpm and below.
- Volume scans with whole heart coverage are often able to provide good image quality in patients with high heart rates or even tachycardia due to ability to perform 2 or more full-coverage heart beat scans which facilitates multi-segmental image reconstruction with improved temporal resolution (see Chaps. 1 and 5).
- Wide-detector scanners are advantageous when the high heart rates are irregular (e.g., frequent ectopic beats, atrial fibrillation) because images may be acquired within one cardiac cycle only.
- Dual-source CT technology may have intrinsic a temporal resolution of 65–75 ms but image selection may be limited with rapid acquisition scan modes.
- Electrocardiogram (ECG)-gating techniques are necessary to identify optimal data for image reconstruction.
- Retrospective gating and full-cycle acquisition allow greater data selection but comes at the price of increased radiation dose (see Chap. 5 and 6).
- Intracycle motion-correction software may decrease coronary motion blurring in but results are variable (Fig. 7.4) [11–13].
- Generally, motion-free images are found in diastasis with lower heart rates (<65 beats/min) but less so with higher heart rates (>70 beats/min), in which case acquisition may include end-systole to identify images with little degradation due to motion [14].

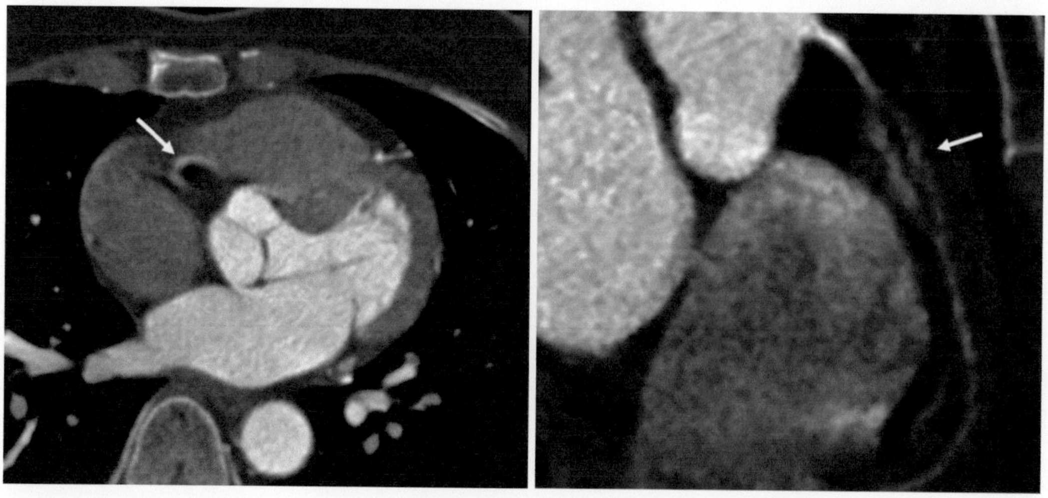

Fig. 7.3 Case example of a 62-year-old man with chest pain. CCTA images reveal blurring (arrows) in the proximal right coronary artery segment due to high heart rate (82 beats/min)

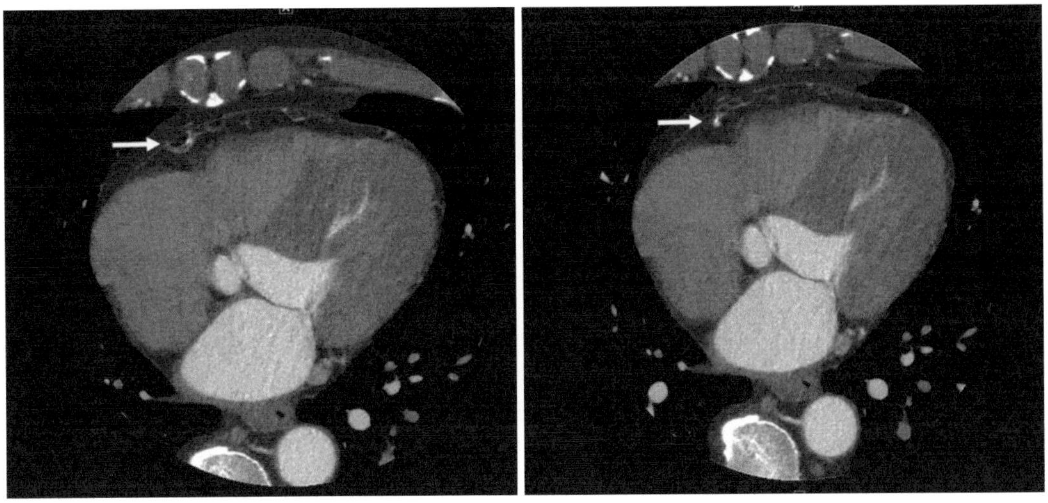

Fig. 7.4 Case example of a 52-year-old man with chest pain. The left panel shows blurring of the mid right coronary artery due to high heart rate (arrow). The right panel shows the same image after application of intracycle motion correction with improved results (arrow)

7.5 Cardiac Arrhythmia

- Cardiac arrhythmia, e.g., atrial fibrillation, premature atrial or ventricular contractions, during CCTA acquisition may cause artifacts or missing data, possibly rendering the scan as uninterpretable [15].
- If sufficient data were acquired, e.g., with retrospective gating, arrhythmia-induced artifacts may be corrected by reediting the reconstruction phases based on the continuous ECG registration during the acquisition (Fig. 7.5).
- Arrhythmia rejection modes are widely available and may switch acquisition modes when arrhythmia is detected, e.g., from prospective scan triggering to retrospective gating, but may result in excessive radiation doses.
- Optimal patient preparation and heart rate control are critical for achieving best scan results. The meticulous detail to patient preparation cannot be overstated.
- In patients with atrial fibrillation, selection of the best cardiac phase location is required for identifying optimal image reconstruction (Fig. 7.6).
- Cardiac phase selection using actual milliseconds past the R wave (e.g., 350–380 ms) may yield better results than selecting relative location of phases (e.g., 30–35%) to achieve optimal image quality, because location of systole during the cardiac cycle is relatively constant while the R-R interval substantially changes with the heart rate.

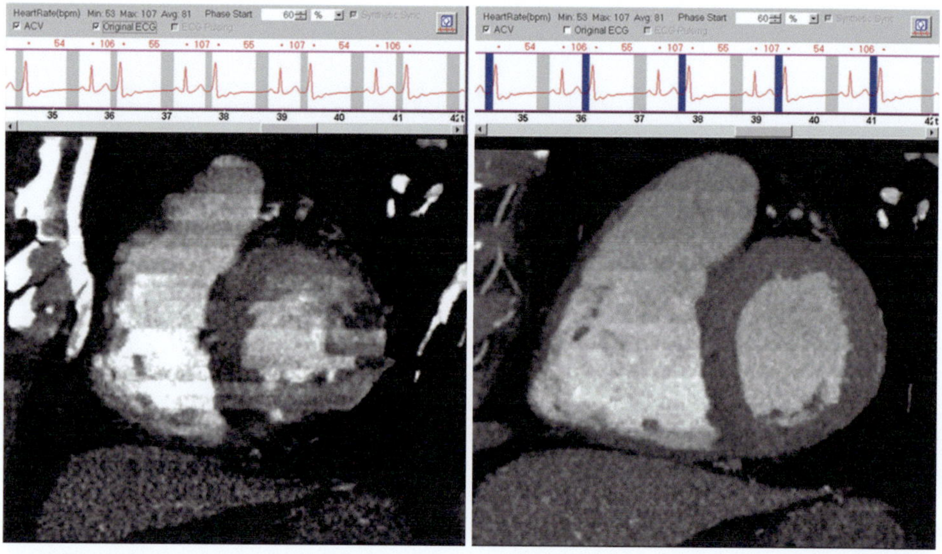

Fig. 7.5 Case example of a 62-year-old man with ventricular bigeminy. The left image shows multiple stair-step artifacts and resultant poor image quality. The right image shows the results of ECG editing and eliminating the signal from the ectopic beats (*dark blue line*) with markedly improved image quality

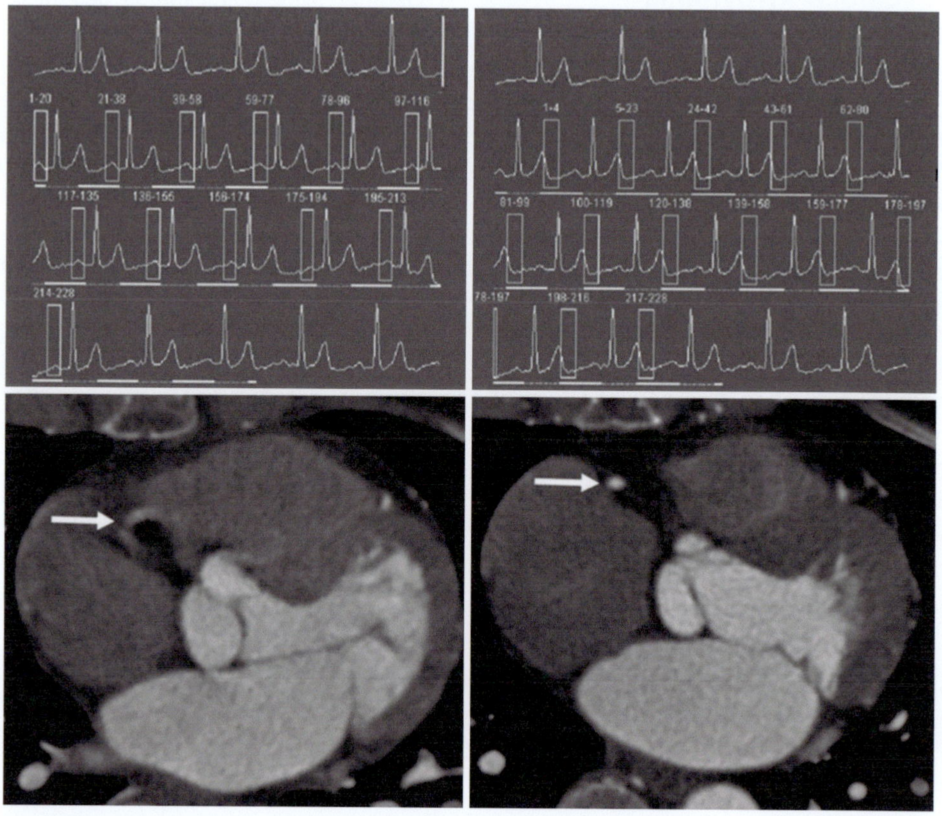

Fig. 7.6 Case example of a 57-year-old man with chest pain and heart rate of 78 bpm despite attempts of heart rate control. The left image was reconstructed from diastasis and displays blurring in the proximal right coronary (arrow). The right image was reconstructed from an end-systolic phase and shows markedly decreased motion artifact (arrow)

7.6 Excessive Image Noise in Obese Patients or Those with Implants/Devices

- Images in severely obese patients may be associated with low signal-to-noise ratio and excessive image noise as result of photon starvation in the setting of larger than typical attenuating tissue mass (Fig. 7.7).
- Scanner characteristics, e.g., tube power, may greatly affect the ability of acquiring diagnostic image quality in obese patients.
- In general, image quality is expected to be substantially impacted in patients with BMI >40 kg/m^2.
- X-ray tube settings typically need to be adjusted to offset high image noise [16].
- High peak tube voltage facilitates greater X-ray photon energy, stronger tissue penetration, and lower image noise at the expense of contrast [17, 18].
- Owing to decreasing contrast, increasing the kVp beyond 120 kVp (e.g., 130 kVp or 140 kVp) typically does *not* improve image quality while increasing radiation dose. For these reasons, use of 120 kVp is recommended even in morbidly obese patients.

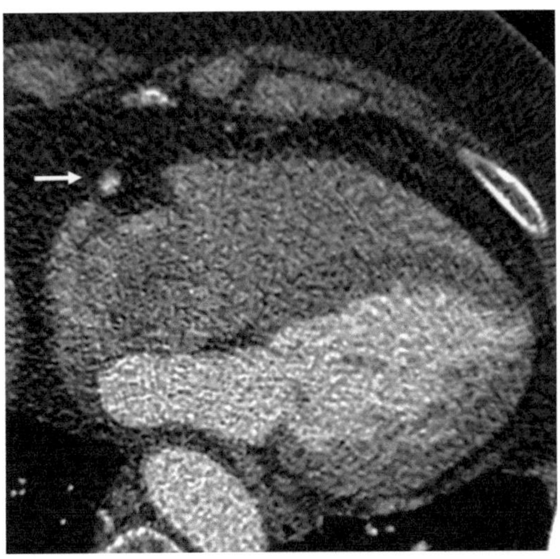

Fig. 7.7 Case example of a 69-year-old woman with a body mass index of 35 kg/m^2. Despite tube voltage setting of 120 kVp, excessive image noise was noted, affecting the interpretation of the right coronary artery (arrow)

- High tube current is helpful for generating more X-ray photons and increasing contrast. A powerful X-ray generator capable of delivering high tube currents (mA) is advantageous in the setting of severe obesity.
- Iterative or deep learning image reconstruction algorithms may improve image quality by reducing image noise [19].
- Postprocessing techniques reducing image noise include the use of thick slabs of maximum intensity projections and smooth reconstruction kernels (convolution filters).

7.7 Patients with Inability to Cooperate

- Breathing or patient motion during image acquisition may cause misregistration artifacts, which usually appear as shading or streaking in the reconstructed image (Fig. 7.8).
- The best approach to breathing artifacts is to prevent them with comprehensive breathing instructions and practice before contrast delivery (see Chap. 5).
- The use of positioning aids is sufficient to prevent voluntary movement in most patients. However, in some cases, it may be necessary to immobilize the patient by means of restraints and sedation.

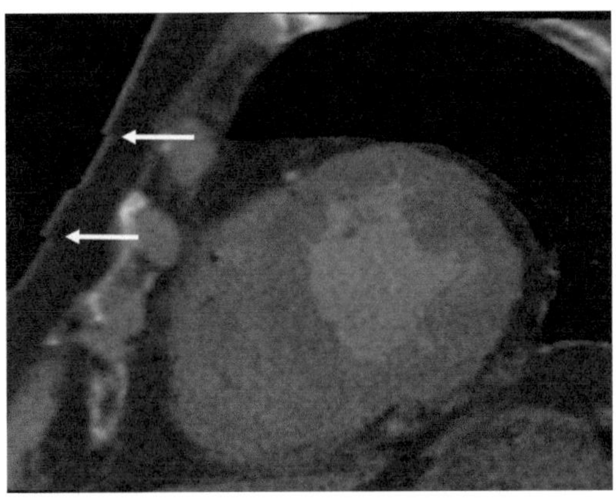

Fig. 7.8 Case example of a 71-year-old man with chest pain. The CCTA image reveals step artifacts throughout the heart and chest wall (arrows) from respiratory motion

- Using the shortest scan time possible helps minimize artifacts when scanning regions prone to movement.
- Single-beat acquisition decreases the risk of respiratory motion artifacts.
- A scan may need to be repeated if considerable motion artifacts render images nondiagnostic.

Key Points

- High image quality is the most important factor for rendering accurate diagnoses by CCTA.
- Patient preparation and meticulous attention to scan acquisition are key factors for obtaining diagnostic images [20].
- In clinical practice, we balance our goal for optimal image quality with the associated cost, i.e., toxicity from radiation and contrast volume, thus individualizing acquisition prescription for each patient.

References

1. Min JK, Shaw LJ, Berman DS. The present state of coronary computed tomography angiography a process in evolution. J Am Coll Cardiol. 2010;55(10):957–65.
2. Miller JM, Rochitte CE, Dewey M, Arbab-Zadeh A, Niinuma H, Gottlieb I, Paul N, Clouse ME, Shapiro EP, Hoe J, Lardo AC, Bush DE, de Roos A, Cox C, Brinker J, Lima JA. Diagnostic performance of coronary angiography by 64-row CT. N Engl J Med. 2008;359(22):2324–36.
3. Paech DC, Weston AR. A systematic review of the clinical effectiveness of 64-slice or higher computed tomography angiography as an alternative to invasive coronary angiography in the investigation of suspected coronary artery disease. BMC Cardiovasc Disord. 2011;11:32.
4. National Institute for health and care excellence (NICE). New generation cardiac CT scanners (Aquilion ONE, brilliance iCT, discovery CT750 HD and Somatom definition flash) for cardiac imaging in people with suspected or known coronary artery disease in whom imaging is difficult with earlier generation CT scanners. NICE diagnostics guidance [DG3]. 2012. http://www.nice.org.uk/guidance/DG3. Accessed 23 Jun 2016.
5. Park MJ, Jung JI, Choi YS, Ann SH, Youn HJ, Jeon GN, Choi HC. Coronary CT angiography in patients with high calcium score: evaluation of plaque characteristics and diagnostic accuracy. Int J Cardiovasc Imaging. 2011;27(Suppl 1):43–51.
6. den Dekker MA, de Smet K, de Bock GH, Tio RA, Oudkerk M, Vliegenthart R. Diagnostic performance of coronary CT angiography for stenosis detection according to calcium score: systematic review and meta-analysis. Eur Radiol. 2012;22(12):2688–98.
7. Vavere AL, Arbab-Zadeh A, Rochitte CE, Dewey M, Niinuma H, Gottlieb I, Clouse ME, Bush DE, Hoe JW, de Roos A, Cox C, Lima JA, Miller JM. Coronary artery stenoses: accuracy of 64-detector row CT angiography in segments with mild, moderate, or severe calcification—a subanalysis of the CORE-64 trial. Radiology. 2011;261(1):100–8.
8. Renker M, Nance JW Jr, Schoepf UJ, O'Brien TX, Zwerner PL, Meyer M, Kerl JM, Bauer RW, Fink C, Vogl TJ, Henzler T. Evaluation of heavily calcified vessels with coronary CT angiography: comparison of iterative and filtered back projection image reconstruction. Radiology. 2011;260(2):390–9.
9. Willemink MJ, de Jong PA, Leiner T, de Heer LM, Nievelstein RA, Budde RP, et al. Iterative reconstruction techniques for computed tomography part 1: technical principles. Eur Radiol. 2013;23:1623–31.
10. Kroft LJ, de Roos A, Geleijns J. Artifacts in ECG-synchronized MDCT coronary angiography. AJR Am J Roentgenol. 2007;189:581–91.
11. Fan L, Zhang J, Xu D, Dong Z, Li X, Zhang L. CCTA image quality improvement by using snapshot freeze technique under prospective and retrospective electrocardiographic gating. J Comput Assist Tomogr. 2015;39:202–6.
12. Lee H, Kim JA, Lee JS, et al. Impact of a vendor-specific motion-correction algorithm on image quality, interpretability, and diagnostic performance of daily routine coronary CT angiography: influence of heart rate on the effect of motion-correction. Int J Cardiovasc Imaging. 2014;30:1603–12.
13. Leipsic J, Labounty TM, Hague CJ, et al. Effect of a novel vendor-specific motion-correction algorithm on image quality and diagnostic accuracy in persons undergoing coronary CT angiography without rate-control medications. J Cardiovasc Comput Tomogr. 2012;6:164–71.
14. Abbara S, Arbab-Zadeh A, Callister TQ, et al. SCCT guidelines for performance of coronary computed tomographic angiography: a report of the society of cardiovascular computed tomography guidelines committee. J Cardiovasc Comput Tomogr. 2009;3:190–204.
15. Lesser JR, Flygenring BJ, Knickelbine T, Longe T, Schwartz RS. Practical approaches to overcoming artifacts in coronary CT angiography. J Cardiovasc Comput Tomogr. 2009;3:4–15.
16. Leschka S, Stinn B, Schmid F. Dual source CT coronary angiography in severely obese patients: trading off temporal resolution and image noise. Invest Radiol. 2009;44:720–7.
17. Sigal-Cinqualbre AB, Hennequin R, Abada HT. Low-kilovoltage multi-detector row chest CT in adults: fea-

sibility and effect on image quality and iodine dose. Radiology. 2004;231:169–74.
18. Leschka S, Stolzmann P, Schmid FT. Low kilovoltage cardiac dual-source CT: attenuation, noise, and radiation dose. Eur Radiol. 2008;18:1809–17.
19. Yang DH. Application of artificial intelligence to cardiovascular computed tomography. Korean J Radiol. 2021;22:1597–608.
20. Abbara S, Blanke P, Maroules CD, et al. SCCT guidelines for the performance and acquisition of coronary computed tomographic angiography: a report of the society of cardiovascular computed tomography guidelines committee: endorsed by the north American Society for Cardiovascular Imaging (NASCI). J Cardiovasc Comput Tomogr. 2016;10:435–49.

Recognizing and Addressing Artifacts in Cardiac CT

8

Jeannie Yu and James Iwaz

Abstract

This chapter reviews the most common artifacts that impact diagnostic coronary CT imaging and includes a concise description of the appearance, mechanisms, as well as potential preventive strategies and countermeasures. The artifacts discussed include several causes of motion artifact, partial volume averaging, metal or streak artifact, beam hardening, stair-step, banding and centerline pseudo-stenosis.

Keywords

Artifact · Partial volume · Streak · Metal
Beam hardening · Misregistration · Banding
Pseudo-stenosis

8.1 Introduction

- Recognizing and addressing artifacts is fundamental to learning cardiac CT, because they are common and may significantly impact the ability to obtain diagnostic quality images.
- The causes or mechanisms of common artifacts affecting coronary CT imaging are most frequently due to different kinds of motion, partial volume averaging, metal or streak, body habitus, contrast delivery, or technical issues related to acquisition, reconstruction, or post-processing [1, 2].
- Adequate patient preparation and thorough understanding of all aspects of scan acquisition are essential to avoid artifacts (also see Chaps. 1 and 5).
- Accuracy for detecting coronary stenoses is highly dependent on the absence of image artifacts with approximately 91–100% of cases of false positive and false negative interpretations being due to image artifacts [3]. Motion artifact alone accounts for 45% of non-diagnostic studies.
- Almost all CT image artifacts can be explained by limitations related to:
  - Temporal resolution.
  - Spatial resolution.
  - Image noise.
  - Reconstruction techniques.
- Artifacts can be observed even with the latest CT technology, and may be related to the following:
  - Scan technique.
  - Motion artifacts (coronary, cardiac and respiratory related).
  - X-ray tube settings.

J. Yu (✉) · J. Iwaz
University of California, Irvine, Irvine, CA, USA

Veterans Affairs Long Beach Healthcare System, Long Beach, CA, USA

Division of Cardiology, Tibor Rubin VA Medical Center, Long Beach, CA, USA
e-mail: James.Iwaz@va.gov

A. A. Zadeh, J. Hoe (eds.), *Practical Guide to Cardiac CT*,
https://doi.org/10.1007/978-981-97-6919-3_8

- Patient preparation (e.g., contraindications to nitroglycerin or beta blockers).
- Arrhythmia.
- Contrast volume/timing.
- Reconstruction and post-processing.
- Patient characteristics (e.g., severe obesity, metal implants, etc.)

8.2 Motion Artifacts

8.2.1 Coronary Artery Motion

- *Definition*: Blurring of the coronary artery due to coronary motion.
- *Appearance*: Artery will appear blurry with indistinct borders and can be described as star/seagull/boomerang in appearance. Most frequently impacts the right coronary artery because of its rapid motion in its mid segment during the cardiac cycle (Fig. 8.1).
- *Causes*:
  - Uncontrolled (high) or irregular heart rates, insufficient temporal resolution.
  - Coronary motion artifacts are accentuated in the setting of calcium or stents.
  - High heart rates may occur in the setting of contraindication to beta blockers or an unanticipated increase/change in heart rate during time of scan acquisition despite adequate pre-scan HR control, e.g., anxiety.
  - Using multi-segment reconstructions for high heart rates can result in motion artifact, particularly when more than two or three segments are used.
  - Suboptimal phase selection for reconstruction of vessel image, which can be relevant for both for low and high heart rates.
- *Solutions*:
  - *Prevention*: Tight heart rate control (see Chap. 5), sedation for anxious patients, clear patient instructions [4].
  - *Strategic Scanning and Reconstruction Protocols*:

    Diastolic imaging for the left anterior descending (LAD) and left circumflex (LCx) arteries and for heart rates <65 bpm (e.g., 75% phase or around 700 ms).

    Systolic imaging may be helpful for the right coronary artery (RCA), e.g., 45% phase.

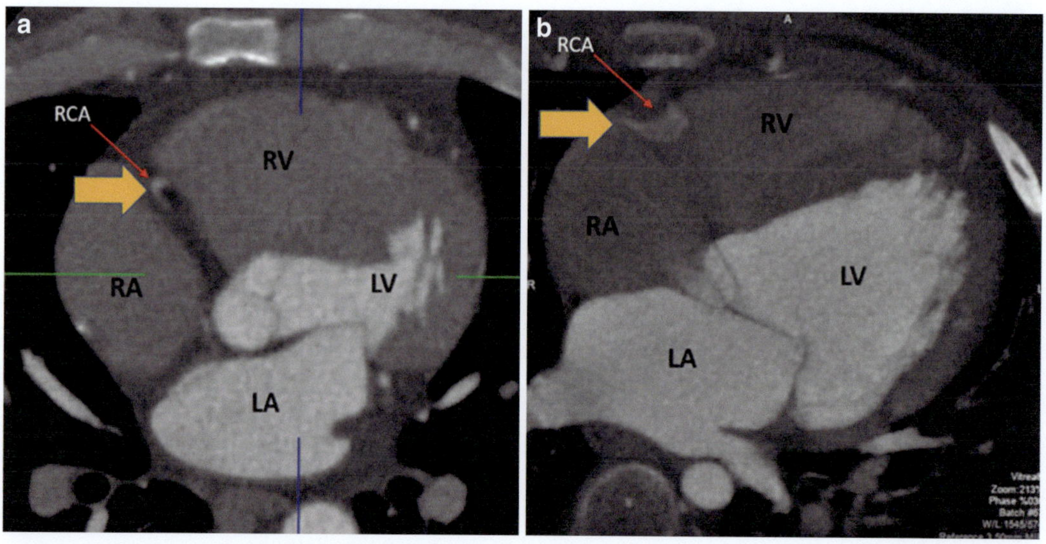

Fig. 8.1 Case example of coronary motion. Significant coronary motion noted in the right coronary artery which has a blurred, boomerang appearance, resulting in non-diagnostic image quality. In Panel **a**, there is a darker core which is commonly observed in coronary motion artifact. Given the severity of the artifact (Panel **b**), curved MPR and other reformatted images or post-processing techniques will be negatively impacted

Systolic imaging may also be helpful for patients with irregular rhythms (e.g., atrial fibrillation, ectopy) or higher heart rates above 65 bpm.

Consider avoiding multi-segment reconstruction protocols.

- *Post-processing*: ECG editing in post-processing for arrhythmias as well as motion correction and metal artifact reduction may be helpful if available.

8.2.2 Myocardial and Aortic Motion

- *Definition*: Blurring of the aorta or myocardium due to motion.
- *Appearance*: Motion of the aorta can manifest as indistinct borders or curvilinear artifact which may be mistaken for a dissection flap (Fig. 8.2). Aortic motion artifacts are typically more severe near the aortic root, due to translational motion from the heart. Cardiac motion can produce blurring and may even mimic perfusion defects when evaluating the myocardium.
- *Cause*: Cardiac or aortic motion due to insufficient temporal resolution.

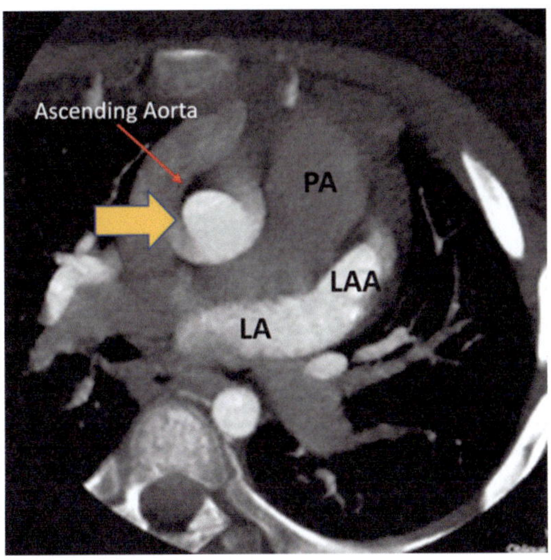

Fig. 8.2 Case example of aortic motion. Significant motion occurring during image acquisition resulted in a curvilinear artifact within the aorta. This artifact may mimic the appearance of a dissection flap

- *Solutions*:
  - Severe artifacts affecting the aortic root may require a repeat study with or without gating to rule out pathology, e.g., dissection.
  - Myocardial abnormalities that may be appear to be potential CT myocardial perfusion defects that do not follow a coronary territory are likely to be artifact.

8.2.3 Respiratory Motion

- *Definition*: Structures within the thorax demonstrate blurring due to breathing during scan acquisition.
- *Appearance*: Blurring, double images, or long-range streaking in the lung parenchyma, diaphragm, cardiac borders, and all other structures. The presence of steps in the ribcage or diaphragm are indicative of breathing (Fig. 8.3).
- *Cause*: Breathing or movements during breath holding during scan acquisition may result in motion related artifacts.

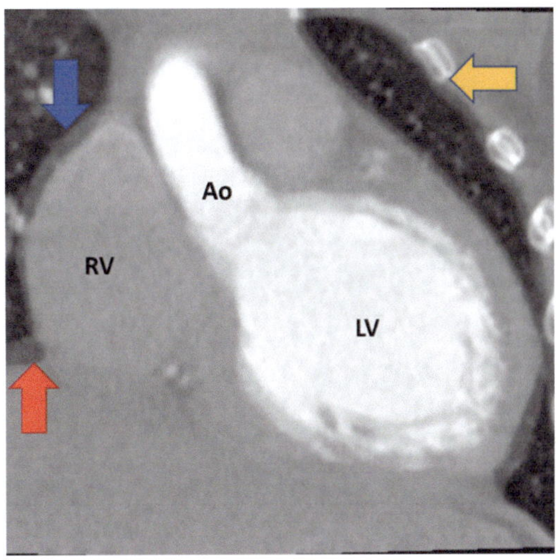

Fig. 8.3 Example of respiratory motion during scan acquisition. Respiratory artifact with blurring and double images is noted at the cardiac borders (blue arrow), diaphragm, and ribs. Involvement of the lung parenchyma, diaphragm (red arrow), and ribs (yellow arrow) differentiates breathing as the cause apart from cardiac motion

- *Solutions*:
  - Patient education and practice for appropriate breath holds, i.e., varying depths to identify most comfortable positing while avoiding Valsalva.
  - If the scan duration is too long, patients may have difficulty holding still—consider alternative, shorter scan acquisition.
  - Consider craniocaudal acquisition to avoid motion in the most important (i.e., proximal) vasculature.

8.3 Artifacts Related to Partial Volume Averaging

- *Definition*: Highly attenuating structures dominate the CT numbers for a given voxel, even if they represent only a small portion of the signal. For example, most of the voxel represents tissue next to a metallic clip with low attenuation. The small portion of the metallic clip with very high attenuation, however, will strongly skew the average Hounsfield unit toward a higher value—largely overriding the information of the low attenuating tissue next to the clip.
- *Appearance*: The borders of such highly attenuating structures may be blurred and appear "blooming," i.e., larger than they are.
- *Cause*: Limited spatial resolution resulting in larger voxel size with too much density averaging. The extent blooming will also depend on the density and shape of the objects (e.g., bulky calcifications, thick stent struts, Figs. 8.4 and 8.5).
- *Solutions*:
  - Use the thinnest possible slice thickness.
  - Consider ultra-high-resolution CT with less than 0.5 mm detector width.
  - Sharp convolution kernel (edge enhancement), which somewhat improves spatial resolution at the expense of image noise.
  - Window/Level adjustment (e.g., window 1500, level 400).
- *Caveats*: Do not increase MIP thickness (which worsens partial volume artifacts).

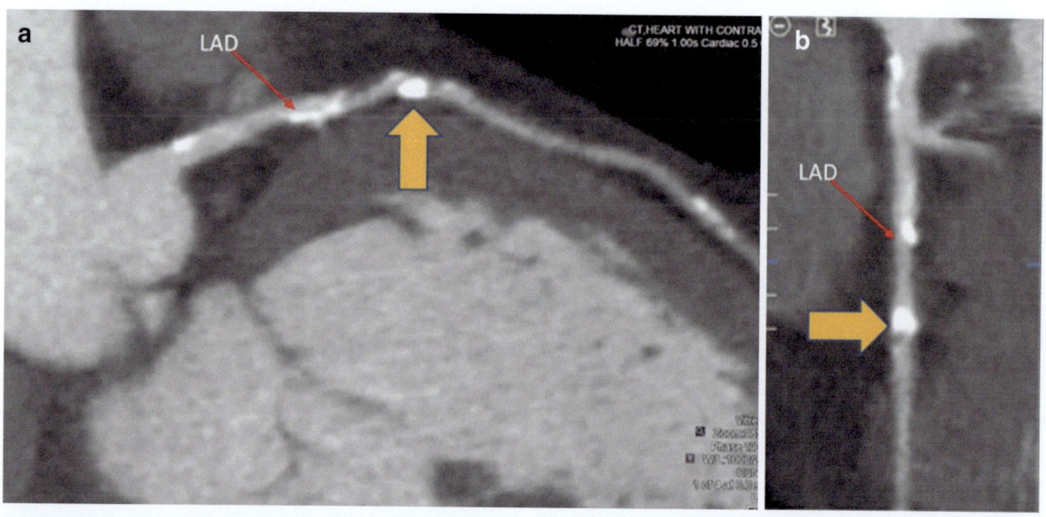

Fig. 8.4 Case example of "blooming" artifact from calcium due to partial volume averaging. Blooming can be noted in the larger, dense area of calcium in the mid-LAD. The blooming calcium obscures the lumen, hindering adequate assessment of lumen stenosis

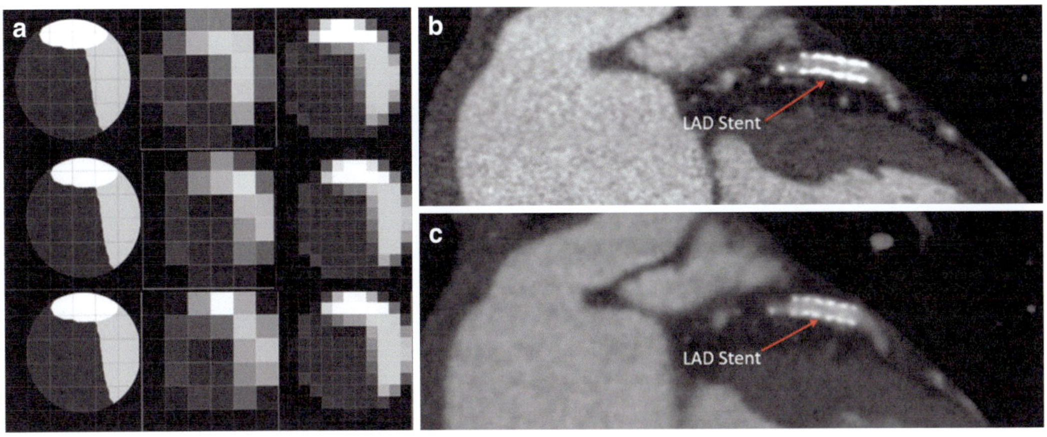

Fig. 8.5 Demonstration of the partial volume averaging effect along with a case example in a patient with a coronary stent. The impact of partial volume averaging can be particularly seen at interfaces between tissue or structures of largely different attenuation, resulting in indistinctness on the edges of the coronary lumen. In Panel **a**, spatial resolution is illustrated with the first column representing the histologic or real interface of three different tissue types. The second column and third column demonstrate the impact of lower and higher spatial resolution on the image representation of the actual structure. Partial volume averaging is more pronounced in the second column with larger voxels (lower spatial resolution). In Panels **b** and **c**, a coronary stent is shown using reconstructions at high and lower spatial resolution to demonstrate the impact on assessing highly attenuating structures

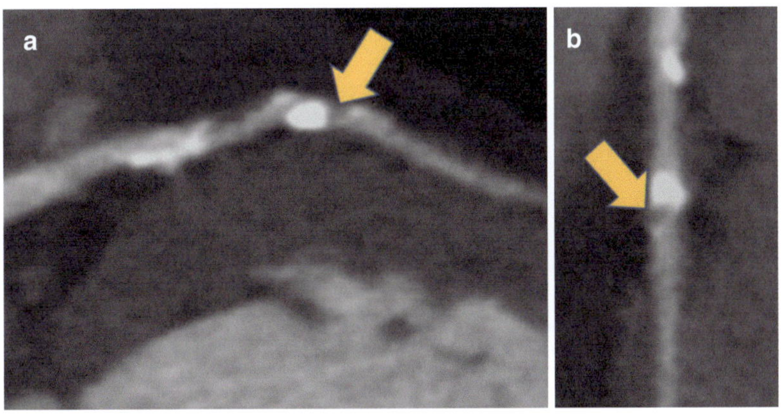

Fig. 8.6 Case example of beam hardening artifact. Beam hardening artifact is evident as the low attenuation areas adjacent to a calcified plaque. When present adjacent to stents or dense coronary calcifications, the beam hardening can be challenging to distinguish from noncalcified plaque or in-stent restenosis

8.4 Beam Hardening Artifacts

- *Definition*: X-rays beams of differing energies are being "filtered" by high-density structures, e.g., bone, metal, allowing only high energy X-rays to penetrate, thus leading to "hardening" of the beam.
- *Appearance*: Very low-density areas near high-density objects (e.g., calcification, metal, dense contrast) which may mimic thrombus or plaque or even perfusion defects (Fig. 8.6).
- *Cause*: Attenuation of low energy X-rays results in higher energy X-rays reaching the detector, which then are reconstructed with incorrectly assigned lower attenuation values near high attenuating objects.
- *Solutions*: Adjusting filters; reconstructing at a different phases; diluting contrast; virtual monoenergetic reconstructions. Beam hardening artifact near dense calcification or stent struts may be challenging to distinguish between true low-density plaque and artifact, but absolute densities may be helpful (low-density plaque is usually around 40–90 HU, whereas beam hardening will be similar to calcium or metal HU).

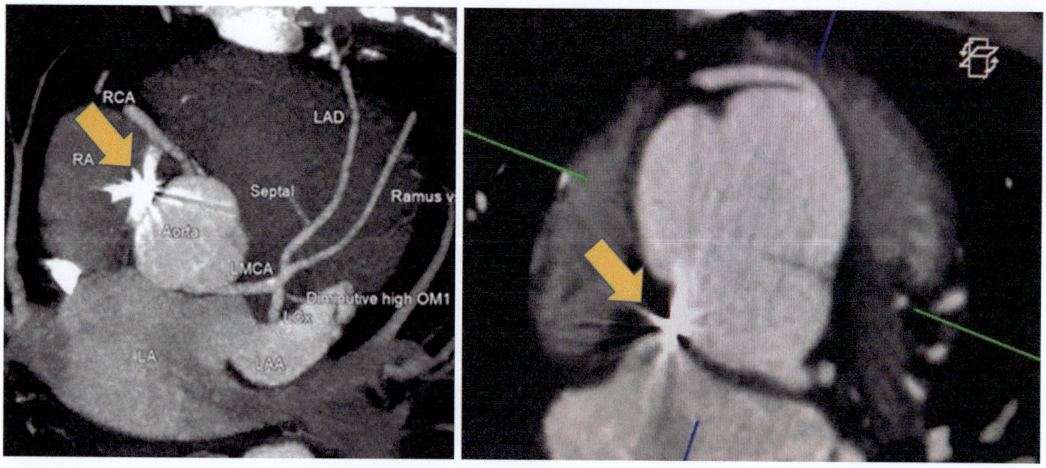

Fig. 8.7 Metal related streak artifact due to pacemaker leads. Metal streak artifact is noted in the right atrium at the level of the aortic valve, with the characteristic alternating bright and dark bands emanating from a high-density object such as a pacemaker lead. The bands can be prominent and sometimes obscure adjacent structures

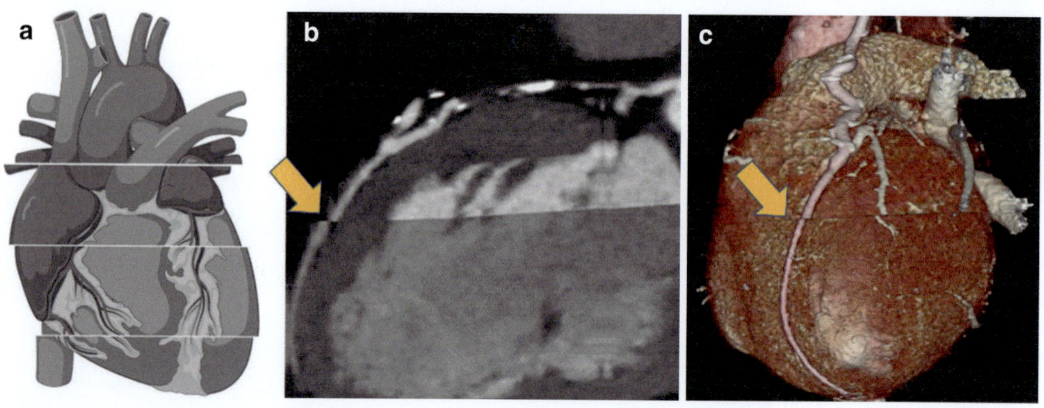

Fig. 8.8 Illustration of the misregistration artifact. Panel **a** illustrates the misregistration of acquired data volumes during a "step-and-shoot" acquisition due to arrhythmia. The misalignment of structures is demonstrated in curved MPR and volume rendering of the LAD (Panels **b**, **c**). (*Created with BioRender*)

8.5 Metal/Streak Artifacts

- *Definition*: Combination of beam hardening and partial volume averaging due to metal or other highly attenuating objects.
- *Appearance*: Light and dark bands originating from highly attenuating object (e.g., pacemaker lead, surgical clip) (Fig. 8.7).
- *Cause*: Combination of Sects. 8.3 (partial volume averaging) and 8.4 (beam hardening) with high attenuation objects—see above.
- *Solutions*: Increase tube potential and/or tube current. If RCA is affected, consider different phase reconstruction. Metal artifact reduction algorithms. For SVC related contrast artifacts, bi- or tri- phasic contrast injection protocols may be preferred (see Chap. 5).

8.6 Stair-Step or Misregistration

- *Definition*: The acquired slabs do not align perfectly. The related artifacts are also described as misregistration, misalignment, stair-step, interscan motion.
- *Appearance*: Linear artifacts are noted at the interface of different slabs that do not obey anatomic boundaries (Fig. 8.8).

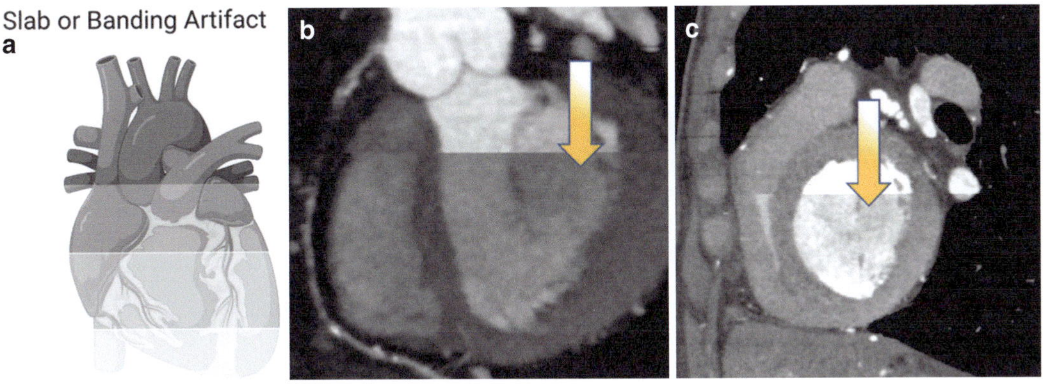

Fig. 8.9 Case example of slab/banding artifact. Slab or banding artifact as result of differences in contrast volume over time and throughout the scan. Panel **a** illustrates the sequential washout of contrast among acquired image slabs using a “step-and-shoot” acquisition. Panels **b** and **c** illustrate the effect in a clinical case example (arrows). (*Created with BioRender*)

- *Cause*: Heart rate variability/arrhythmia (e.g. ventricular or atrial ectopy) during sequential scanning.
- *Solutions*:
  - Beta blockers to achieve a regular heart rate.
  - Single-cycle acquisition, e.g., wide volume or high-pitch.
  - Arrhythmia rejection algorithms (see Chaps. 1 and 5).
- *Caveats*: Stair-step is NOT the same as banding artifact.

8.7 Slab or Banding Artifacts

- *Definition*: Slabs acquired do not have the same contrast enhancement. Gradation is noted across the full scan range.
- *Appearance*: Varying contrast enhancement among image slabs acquired with sequential, “step-and shoot” scanning (Fig. 8.9).
- *Cause*: Time delay between acquisition of image slabs in the setting of low contrast volume and/or long scan times.
- *Solutions*:
  - Single-cycle acquisition, e.g., wide volume or high-pitch.
  - Greater contrast volume.
  - Faster scan time.
  - Improve contrast timing.

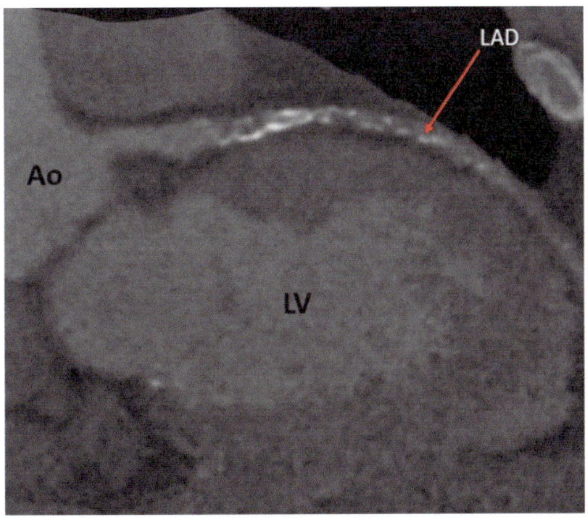

Fig. 8.10 Illustration of artifacts related to poor contrast opacification. Poor contrast enhancement of the coronary artery may challenge visualization of the lumen and differentiation to noncalcified plaque or thrombus

8.8 Poor Contrast Artifacts

- *Definition*: Artifacts due to inadequate contrast opacification of the blood vessels.
- *Appearance*: Mimicking of low attenuation plaque due to poor delineation of lumen/wall interface (Fig. 8.10).
- *Cause*: Insufficient contrast volume or poor contrast timing (e.g., slow contrast flow rate, long contrast transit time, low cardiac output,

improper timing, contrast extravasation, or technical error).

- *Solutions*:
  - Greater contrast volume and flow rate with a sufficiently large bore peripheral IV.
  - Troubleshoot the contrast timing which may include modifying the trigger location or HU threshold versus consideration of a timing bolus.
  - Test intravenous access.
  - Power injector trouble shooting.
  - Adjust post-processing (kernels, window leveling).

8.9 Ring Artifact

- *Definition*: Circular artifact due to hardware malfunction.
- *Appearance*: Clearly non-biological circular artifact within the CT dataset that does not obey anatomic boundaries.
- *Cause*: Detector element is mis-calibrated or malfunctioning, radius of the artifact is related to the position of the culprit detector element.
- *Solutions*:
  - Repair or replace the detector element.
  - Software recalibration.

8.10 Excessive Image Noise Related Artifacts

- *Definition*: Poor contrast and excessive image noise due to inadequate dose exposure factors (e.g., severe obesity, inadequate X-ray tube settings) [5].
- *Appearance*: Grainy appearance of structures with degraded spatial resolution (Fig. 8.11). The image noise may prevent assessment of the presence of noncalcified plaque.
- *Cause*: Inadequate dose prescription (too low tube voltage/tube current) in relation to patient size/body habitus.
- *Solutions*:
  - Patient selection.
  - Adjusting X-ray tube settings.
  - Noise reduction reconstruction algorithm.
  - Smooth convolution kernel.

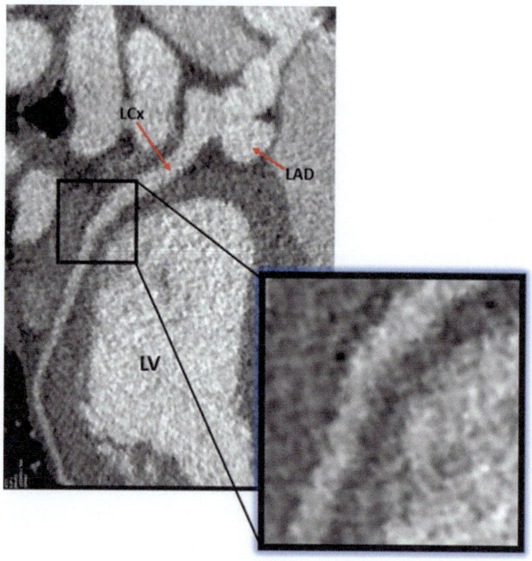

Fig. 8.11 Example of excessive image noise. Excessive image noise creates the artifactual appearance of noncalcified plaque at the lumen borders

8.11 Vessel Centerline Tracking Related Artifacts

- *Definition*: Interrupted lumen on curved multiplanar reformatted (MPR) images due to poor centerline tracking through the coronary lumen.
- *Appearance*: May appear like a typical coronary stenosis or as a full break in the coronary lumen (Fig. 8.12).
- *Cause*: Automated or manual centerline tracking failed to follow the true coronary lumen, which often occurs at branch points, bridging, tortuous segments or areas with significant noise or blooming. The reformatted images do not have contrast in the impacted areas and thus appear stenosed or interrupted.
- *Solutions*:
  - Validate centerline extraction and correct manually where the centerline exits the vessel.
  - Correlate any significant or suspicious stenoses with the axial data set.
  - Coronary stenosis evaluation should be done comprehensively with all tools available including walking the vessel manually.

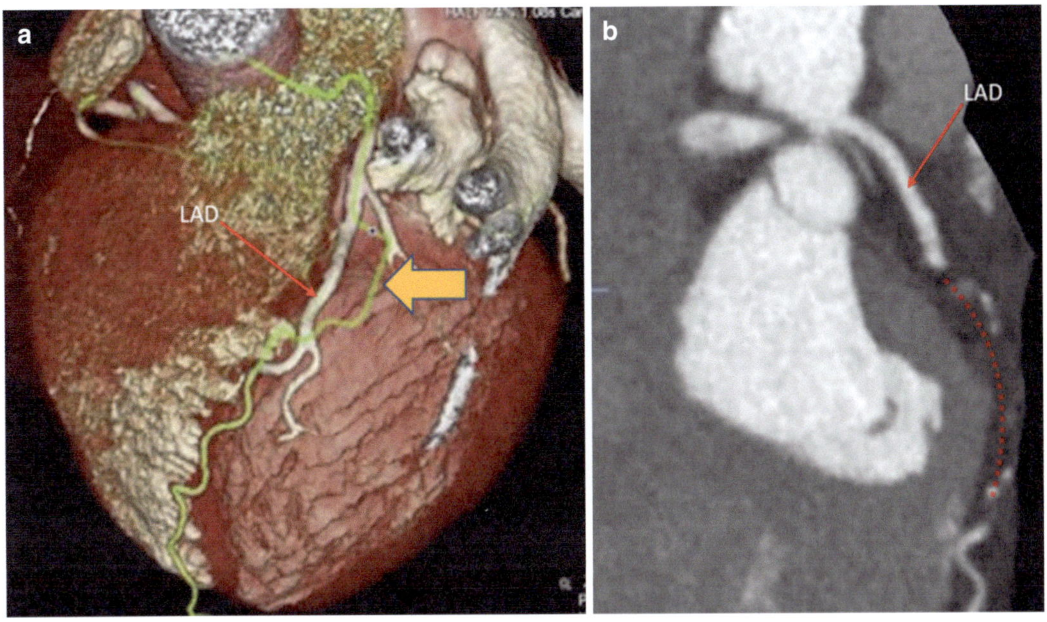

Fig. 8.12 Illustration of centerline errors. Inaccurate centerline tracking is noted in the left (Panel **a**), with the green line exiting the proximal LAD and coursing temporarily into the myocardium, then re-entering the lumen at the distal vessel, which leads to the curved multiplanar reformat of the LAD showing a long interruption in the contrast column that can mimic a long total occlusion (Panel **b**, red dotted line)

References

1. Abramson S. The complete guide to cardiac CT. 1st ed. Beijing: McGraw-Hill Education; 2012.
2. Abbara S, Achenbach S. CT and MR in cardiology. 1st ed. Toronto, ON: Elsevier; 2019.
3. Kroft LJ, de Roos A, Geleijns J. Artifacts in ECG-synchronized MDCT coronary angiography. AJR Am J Roentgenol. 2007;189(3):581–91. https://doi.org/10.2214/AJR.07.2138.
4. Kalisz K, Buethe J, Saboo SS, Abbara S, Halliburton S, Rajiah P. Artifacts at cardiac CT: physics and solutions. Radiographics. 2016;36(7):2064–83. Epub 2016 Oct 21. https://doi.org/10.1148/rg.2016160079.
5. Malagò R, et al. Artifacts in cardiac CT. In: Cademartiri F, Casolo G, Midiri M, editors. Clinical applications of cardiac CT. Milan: Springer; 2012. https://doi.org/10.1007/978-88-470-2522-6_27.

9 Calcium Scoring and Interpretation in Cardiac CT

Alexander C. Razavi, Carlo N. De Cecco, and Seamus P. Whelton

Abstract

Coronary artery calcium (CAC) is measured using non-contrast cardiac computed tomography. CAC scoring is simple to perform, low cost, and the associated radiation dose is generally low. Higher CAC scores are associated with an increasing risk of cardiovascular disease, while the absence of CAC (CAC = 0) is associated with a low 10-year risk for cardiovascular disease. CAC scores should be interpreted using the absolute value and the age, sex, race/ethnicity percentile value. CAC scoring significantly improves cardiovascular disease risk stratification beyond traditional risk factors, novel risk factors, and the Pooled Cohort Equations and can help to identify persons who may benefit from primary prevention therapies.

A. C. Razavi
Department of Medicine, Emory University School of Medicine, Atlanta, GA, USA

C. N. De Cecco
Department of Radiology, Emory University School of Medicine, Emory University, Atlanta, GA, USA

S. P. Whelton (✉)
Johns Hopkins Ciccarone Center for the Prevention of Cardiovascular Disease, Baltimore, MD, USA
e-mail: seamus.whelton@jhmi.edu

Keywords

Cardiac computed tomography · Coronary artery calcium · Cardiovascular disease · Risk prediction · Artificial intelligence

Abbreviations

ASCVD	Atherosclerotic cardiovascular disease
CAC	Coronary artery calcium
CACS	Coronary artery calcium score
CAD	Coronary artery disease
HU	Hounsfield unit
LAD	Left anterior descending artery
MESA	Multi-Ethnic Study of Atherosclerosis

9.1 Introduction and Basic Concepts

- Non-contrast cardiac computed tomography (CT) directly measures subclinical atherosclerosis in the form of coronary artery calcium deposits (CAC) [1].
- The Agatston score is the most commonly used method for quantifying CAC and was introduced by Arthur Agatston and colleagues in 1990 [2].
- CAC scoring significantly improves atherosclerotic cardiovascular disease (ASCVD) risk stratification beyond traditional risk factors [3].

A. A. Zadeh, J. Hoe (eds.), *Practical Guide to Cardiac CT*,
https://doi.org/10.1007/978-981-97-6919-3_9

- CAC = 0 is associated with a low 10-year risk for cardiovascular disease regardless of traditional risk factor burden [4].

9.2 Methods

9.2.1 Conventional CAC Data Acquisition and Scoring

9.2.1.1 Agatston Scoring Method

- The Agatston score was developed by Arthur Agatston and it remains the most commonly used method of reporting CAC [2].
- The method combines calcified plaque density and area into a numerical, continuous score, which facilitates ease of clinical interpretation (Fig. 9.1).
- Agatston CAC scores are commonly graded as zero, mild 1–99, moderate 100–399, and severe ≥400 (Fig. 9.2). Some grading differentiates mild CAC into very mild [1–10] and mild (11–99).
- Greater Agatston scores are associated with greater calcified atherosclerotic plaque burden but also correlate with overall, total atheroma volume.

9.2.1.2 CAC Volume, Mass, and Density Methods

- In addition to the Agatston score, the calcium volume, relative calcium mass, and calcium density scores [5] are also important approaches to quantify CAC, although these are less commonly used in clinical practice, largely because of fewer validation data for patient outcomes.
- The calcium volume score is calculated as the product of mean calcified voxels with at least 130 HU attenuation [6]. Unlike the Agatston score, it does not account for calcium density.
- Compared to the Agatston score, the calcium volume method is more vulnerable to the partial volume effect (see Chap. 13) and tends to both underestimate (lower density plaques) and overestimate (higher density plaques) volume.
- Mean calcium density performs better than peak calcium density for the prediction of ASCVD and coronary heart disease mortality when added to total calcium area burden in

Individual Plaque Score = Plaque Area x Density Weighting Factor
Total Score = Σ Individual Plaque Scores

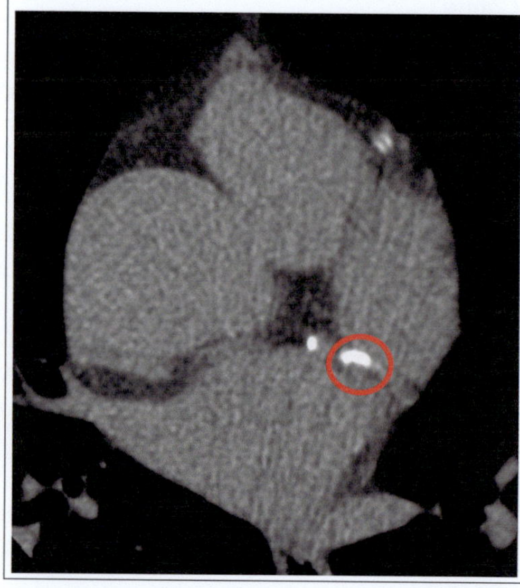

Density weighting factor	Hounsfield Units
1	130-199
2	200-299
3	300-399
4	≥400

Left Circumflex Plaque (circled)
Area = 35 mm^2
Peak Density = 709 HU
Plaque score = 35 * 4 = **140**

Fig. 9.1 Agatston CAC Scoring Methodology

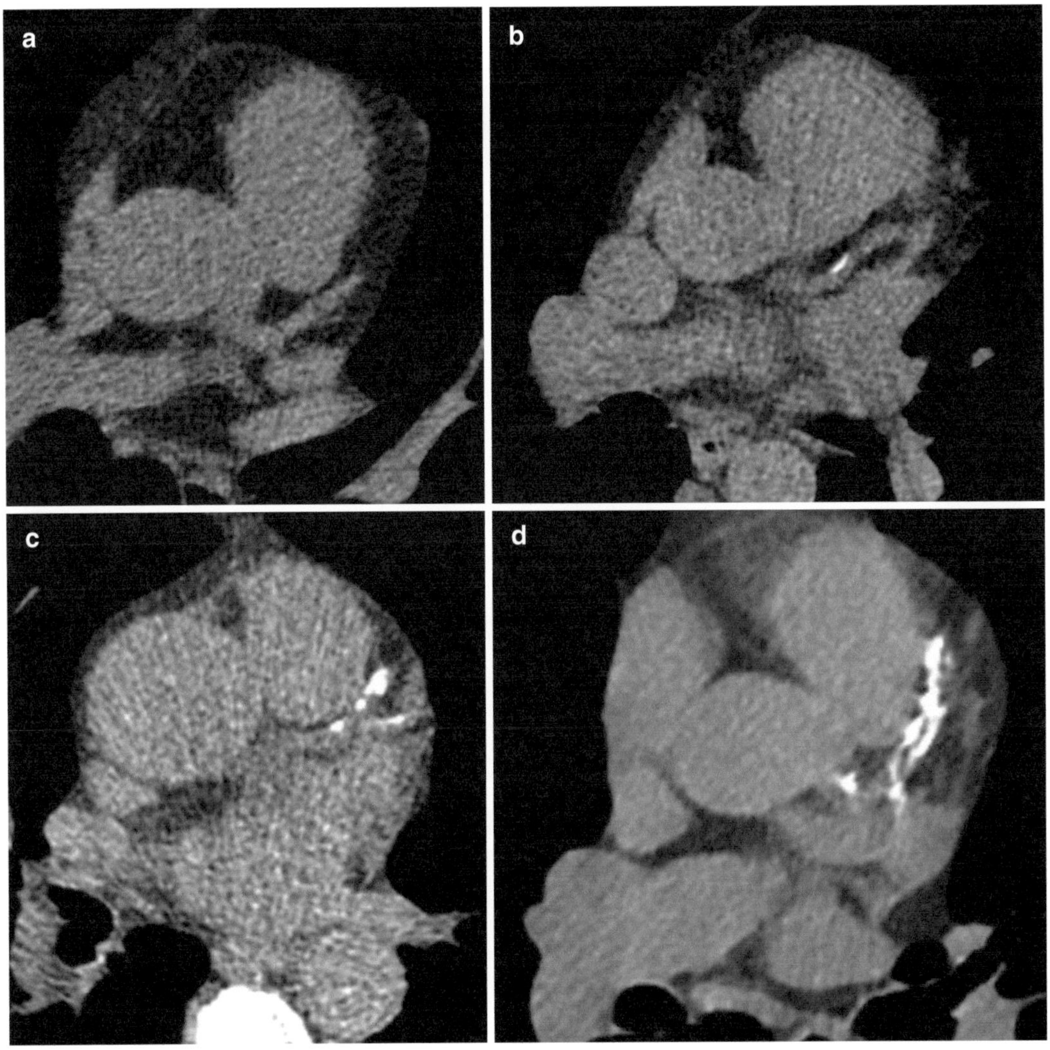

Fig. 9.2 CAC scan without calcification (**a**), mild LAD calcification (**b**), moderate LAD calcification (**c**), severe LAD calcification (**d**)

persons with prevalent CAC [7], but the net improvement in C-statistic is small.

- Dense plaques are thought to be more stable [8], while less dense plaques are generally considered less stable and more likely to result in an ASCVD event [9]. Calculating the CAC score using inversely weighted density categories provides a small improvement in ASCVD risk prediction [10].

9.2.1.3 Image Acquisition

- The traditional Agatston CAC protocol is an electrocardiogram-gated examination focusing on image acquisition at 75% of the R-R interval [11] (see also Chap. 5).
- CAC scans using the Agatston protocol are performed at 120 kV by convention to allow reproducibility among scanners and patients.
- Using parameters set forth by Agatston et al. [2], the image acquisition of calcium density on computed tomography is performed using a fixed slice thickness of 3 mm [11].
- CAC is identified/marked on each slice by the reader or software. As part of this process, the coronary artery containing plaque is located and the scores are calculated using automated software.

- Each plaque is scored based on area in mm^2, maximum calcium density in HU and CAC per vessel.
- The Agatston CAC score categorizes density into four groups with weighting factors of (1) 130–199 HU, (2) 200–299 HU, (3) 300–399 HU, and (4) ≥400 HU.
- Each individual plaque score is calculated as the plaque area times the density weighting factor.
- The total CAC score is calculated as the sum of each individual plaque scores (Fig. 9.1).
- CAC scores are reported as absolute scores on the integer scale but percentiles scoring based on age, sex, and race/ethnicity population percentiles should also be provided.
- We recommend using the percentile scores derived from the multi-ethnic study of atherosclerosis (MESA), as they were validated in individuals stratified by sex, age, and ethnicity [12] and can be easily obtained: https://www.mesa-nhlbi.org/Calcium/input.aspx
- The average effective radiation dose for CAC scans is approximately 1.0 mSv, typically ranging between 0.5 and 1.5 mSv [13, 14], depending on technology and patient characteristics.
- Such dose approximately corresponds to one third of the average annual dose from natural background radiation.

9.2.2 Unconventional CAC Scoring

- A fixed slice thickness of 3 mm reduces sensitivity in individuals with a low CAC burden and several studies have reported improved calcium detection using thinner sliced reconstructions [15–18].
- At the same time, individuals without CAC on 3 mm slice thickness generally have a low burden of CAC [18].
- While thinner slice (<3 mm) CACS increases sensitivity for the detection of CAC, categories (mild, moderate, and severe) across various slice reconstruction thickness protocols largely remain unchanged.
- Noncardiac, non-contrast CT scans (such as those performed for lung cancer screening) are commonly performed using 1 to 3 mm slice thickness. CAC scoring from these non-ECG gated CT chest scans yields similar results to those obtained using formal CAC scoring from ECG-gated cardiac CT scans [19].
- Noncardiac CT chest scans with intravenous contrast administration may also be used for gross identification of CAC, which may be reported as mild, moderate, or severe based on visual assessment. However, smaller and low-density calcified plaques may not be visible due to the presence of intravascular contrast.
- Although research efforts have shown promise for adequate adjustments, no clinically approved method is available and thus Agatston CAC scoring should not be performed using noncardiac CT chest scans with intravenous contrast administration.

9.3 Caveats

9.3.1 Motion Artifacts

- Cardiac motion is an important factor affecting the reproducibility of CAC scoring.
- While interscan variability of CAC scoring is low (mean difference of 17–24 Agatston units, 93–96% overall agreement [20], coronary artery motion artifact is the main contributing factor to interscan variation [21].
- There is no specific upper heart rate limit for CAC but in individuals with heart rate >90 bpm, considerations should be given to heart rate control if interscan variability (e.g., serial testing) is important.

9.3.2 Metallic Artifacts

- Metallic objects near or within the heart can cause artifacts that may interfere with CAC scoring.
- Pacemaker or ICD leads, particularly biventricular pacemaker leads in the coronary sinus,

can make interpretation of adjacent coronary arteries difficult, if not impossible.

- Metallic coronary stents should not be considered in the CAC score but coronary calcification within the stented segment may be missed.
- CAC scoring is of limited value in patients with known coronary artery disease, e.g., those with stents, although emerging data suggests that a CACS still may aid in risk prediction.

9.4 Automation and Artificial Intelligence in CAC Scoring

- Automation and artificial intelligence in CAC scoring (Fig. 9.3) holds promise for improving cardiac CT workflow across several areas, including enhancement of image quality, diagnostic classification, segmentation of struc-

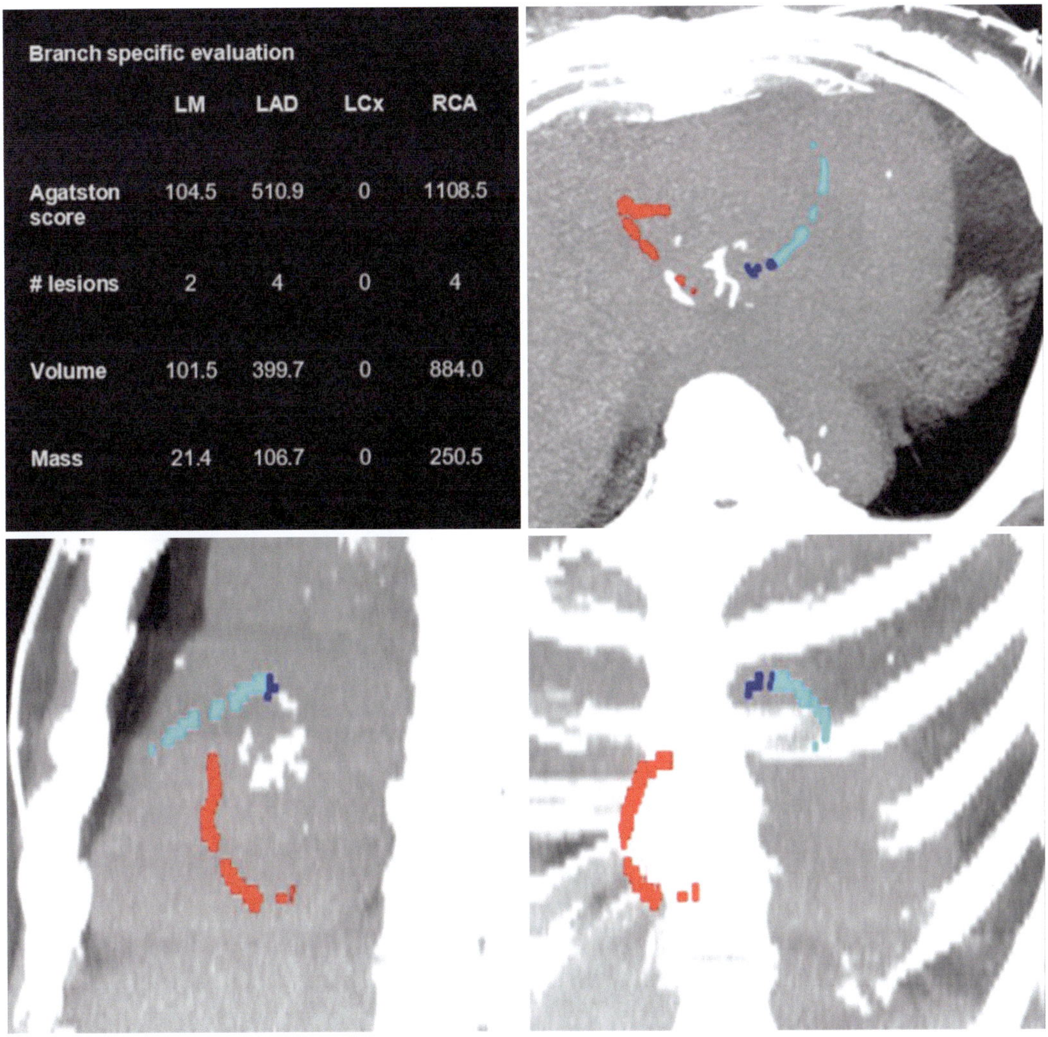

Fig. 9.3 Illustration of Automated CAC Quantification using Artificial Intelligence. Example of automated coronary artery calcium measurement from noncardiac chest CT using artificial intelligence convoluted neural network. Left main in blue, left anterior descending in teal, right coronary artery in red

tures, and facilitating unconventional CAC score, e.g., from noncardiac CT scans [22].
- It is likely that deep neural networks will be soon widely available for automatic detection and segmentation of, thoracic aortic calcium, and cardiac valve calcium, obtained from all CT scans of the thorax, including both ECG-gated and non-ECG studies [22].

9.5 Interpreting and Reporting CAC Scan Results

9.5.1 General Principles of Interpretation and ASCVD Risk Assessment

- Assessment of CAC has been studied predominantly in *asymptomatic* individuals for advanced risk stratification. Current data support the use of CACS particularly in persons at borderline or intermediate 10-year ASCVD risk (5–20%) to inform the decision whether to start statin or other lipid lowering therapy (IIa recommendation by ACC/AHA—see below).
- Recent evidence [23] and the 2021 multi-society chest pain guideline [24] now suggests a potential role for CACS also in patients with low-to-intermediate calculated 10-year ASCVD risk with stable angina, e.g., ruling out obstructive CAD with a zero score.
- Absolute CAC scores more strongly predict intermediate ASCVD risk compared to percentile scores [25]. However, percentile scores are better predictors of long-term or lifetime risk, especially among younger persons and groups in whom the prevalence of CAC >0 is low [26].
- Findings from the CAC Consortium [27] and MESA [28] demonstrated incremental predictive value of CACS beyond traditional risk factors and beyond the Pooled Cohort Eqs. 10-year ASCVD risk score (Fig. 9.4).
- CAC also provides superior risk assessment compared to novel ASCVD risk markers and the ACC/AHA risk-enhancing factors [29, 30].
- Subclinical atherosclerosis measured by CAC compares favorably to coronary stenosis evaluation for risk prediction [31, 32].

9.5.2 Influence of Sex and Ethnicity

- Women and persons who identify as Hispanic, African American, or Asian tend to have a lower CAC burden compared to age-adjusted Caucasian men [33, 34].
- CAC may be even more strongly predictive of ASCVD risk among women and non-white persons [33, 34].
- In addition to the absolute CAC burden, the development of plaque may also differ according to demographics. Observations suggest

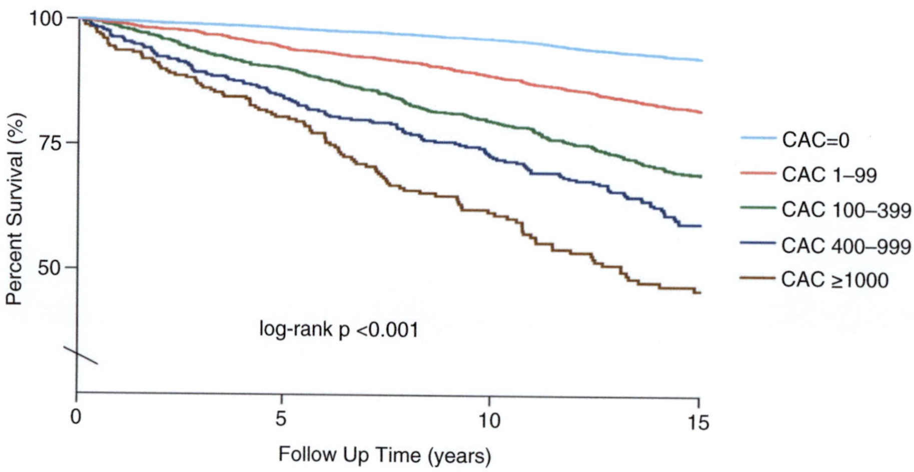

Fig. 9.4 CAC burden and survival free from ASCVD in MESA

that women tend to have a higher calcium density compared to men, but calcium density only significantly predicts ASCVD mortality in men and not in women after adjusting for traditional risk factors [33].

- South Asians may have a higher calcium density compared to Caucasians [35], but the implications of these findings remain unclear as South Asian ethnicity is a risk-enhancing factor while higher calcium density is believed to correlate with plaque stability.

9.5.3 Influence of Age

- In addition to sex and ethnicity, age is an important demographic variable to consider when interpreting CAC scores.
- Findings from the CAC Consortium demonstrated that approximately one in three at-risk young adults have evidence of CAC by age 49. Compared to younger adults with CAC = 0, individuals with CAC 1–99 and CAC ≥100 had 1.5- and 3.3-fold higher risk of ASCVD mortality, independent of traditional risk factors [36].
- The presence of ASCVD risk factors can inform the expected presence and extent of CAC and may inform the optimal time to screen for CAC in younger persons. Assuming a number needed to scan of 4 to detect CAC >0, the recommended age to for a potential first scan would be 37 in men and 50 years in women with diabetes, and 42 in men and 58 years in women without risk factors [37].
- CAC >0 in persons <40 years of age, even with very low CACS, is associated with a very high lifetime risk of clinical ASCVD [38].
- The utility of CAC scoring in persons >75 years of age is less clear given the very high prevalence of CACS >0. Nevertheless, CAC scoring in this age group is strongly associated with an increased risk for ASCVD events [39].
- While most major guidelines [40] recommend considering CAC scoring in persons as early as age 40 years with an intermediate 10-year ASCVD risk, few individuals fulfill these criteria for screening.
- CAC scoring in selected younger adults with risk factor(s) may be beneficial, especially diabetes, a strong family history of premature coronary heart disease, or those who have already accrued a significant exposure to risk factor(s).

9.5.4 Absence of CAC and the Warranty Period of CAC = 0

- The excellent prognosis of individuals with a CACS of zero has been largely consistent across studies despite presence of traditional risk factors, when considering population risk [41].
- The coined phrase "*the power of zero*" pertains to the very low absolute rate of ASCVD events in persons with CACS = 0, including in those conventionally considered high-risk based on traditional risk factors including, type 2 diabetes, metabolic syndrome, and those with low-density lipoprotein cholesterol ≥190 [42–44].
- Among eligible candidates, the number of persons with CACS of zero needed to treat with statins to prevent one event is up to 23-fold higher compared to those with CACS ≥100 [45].
- Approximately 40% of statin eligible persons without CAC at baseline maintain CACS = 0 over 15 years of follow-up with low associated ASCVD risk [46].
- Accordingly, the 2018 AHA/ACC Cholesterol Treatment [47] and 2019 ACC/AHA primary prevention guidelines issued a IIa recommendation for withholding statin therapy in intermediate risk adults with CACS = 0 [40].
- Even among persons in whom statin therapy is recommended regardless of ASCVD risk (type 2 diabetes and LDL-cholesterol ≥190), CACS = 0 is associated with a low 10-year risk [42, 43].
- Data from MESA suggest that the warranty period of a CAC score of 0 is at least 3–7 years [48].
- Older individuals with CACS = 0 are likely to have a shorter time for conversion to CACS >0 compared to younger persons [37], result-

Table 9.1 Recommended Rescan Interval for individuals with CAC = 0

Risk group	Recommended Rescan interval
Low 10-year ASCVD risk (<5%)	6–7 years
Borderline-intermediate 10-year ASCVD risk (5–20%)	3–5 years
High 10-year ASCVD risk (>20%)	3 years
Diabetes	3 years

Adapted from Dzaye et al. "Warranty Period of a Calcium Score of Zero: Comprehensive Analysis From the Multiethnic Study of Atherosclerosis" [3]
ASCVD atherosclerotic cardiovascular disease

ing in different recommended CAC rescan intervals depending on age/baseline ASCVD risk when the baseline CACS = 0 (Table 9.1).

9.5.5 Elevated CAC Burden

- Asymptomatic individuals with CACS ≥100 are likely to net benefit from aspirin therapy, whereas the risk of major bleeding outweighs ASCVD risk reduction for those with CACS <100 [49, 50].
- Similar findings have been observed regarding the intensity of blood pressure lowering, as CACS between 300 and 400 appears to signify an important threshold for further intensifying blood pressure lowering, according to the SPRINT trial [51, 52].
- Very high CACS (≥1000) has been reported in up to 4% of asymptomatic individuals undergoing screening [53], which is associated with similar ASCVD event risk compared to patients with stable, established ASCVD.
- Primary and secondary prevention is commonly defined by the history of a prior ASCVD event but individuals with very high CAC scores yet without prior ASCVD event have an ASCVD risk equivalent to persons with a prior ASCVD event [53].
- Compared to persons with CACS 0–100, there is a stepwise increase in the multivariable-adjusted risk for ASCVD events for individuals with CACS 101–399 (RR = 3.1, 95% CI: 1.2–7.9), CACS 400–999 (RR = 4.6, 95% CI: 1.8–8.8), and CACS ≥1000 (RR = 8.3, 95% CI: 3.3–22.1) [54].
- The trend toward increased ASCVD events in individuals with CACS ≥1000 compared to persons with CACS 400–999 is largely driven by the presence of angina, as opposed to hard outcomes, including resuscitated cardiac arrest, myocardial infarction, or cardiac death [55].
- CAC scores of 775–990 among primary prevention patients are associated with similar ASCVD mortality rates compared to those observed in the FOURIER trial (0.766 per 100 person-years), a modern secondary prevention cohort [56].
- Individuals with very high CACS also appear to have a high burden of extra-coronary calcification, including thoracic aortic and valvular calcification, which are associated with an increased risk of noncardiac ASCVD events [57].

9.5.6 Reporting

- CAC scores should be reported using a standardized format, including (1) absolute CAC score (Agatston score), (2) the age, sex, and race/ethnicity percentile, (3) the estimated probability of a non-zero calcium score, (4) extra-coronary calcification (e.g., aortic valve calcium, ascending/descending aortic calcium, etc.), and (5) and noncardiac findings.
- For further characterization, the presence and extent of CAC should be reported using the Coronary Artery Calcium Data and Reporting System (CAC-DRS), based on findings that persons with a greater total number of plaques, greater number of coronary vessels with CAC, and/or more diffuse distribution of CAC within the coronary arteries have an increased risk of ASCVD events.
- The Coronary Artery Calcium Data and Reporting System (CAC-DRS) takes into account the absolute calcium score (Agatston score), graded A0 (CACS = 0), A1 (mild CAC, 1–99), A2 (moderate CAC, 100–299), A3 (severe CAC, ≥300) and number of affected coronary arteries with CAC (N1–4 for involvement of left main, left anterior descending, left

circumflex, and right coronary artery) [58]. Example: A2/N1 for moderate CAC involving one coronary artery.

- The CAC-DRS represents a simple scoring system that can be used for dedicated cardiac CT and also for noncardiac chest CT. Visual inspection of CAC will be graded similar to the Agatston score: V0 (no calcium), V1 (mild CAC), V2 (moderate CAC), and V3 (severe CAC), along with the number of involved arteries (N1–4). For example, severe CAC noted on a chest CT, involving all 4 arteries, may be reported as V3/N4.
- An increased CAC-DRS has better ASCVD risk stratification than CAC score alone [59].

9.6 Conclusions

- The Agatston CAC score is the most widely used metric for effective ASCVD risk stratification in the modern era of Preventive Cardiology.
- CAC scoring improves ASCVD risk prediction beyond traditional risk factors, novel risk factors, and risk-enhancing factors.
- More detailed reporting of CAC burden, such as incorporating the CAC-DRS score, can improve CVD risk prediction.
- CAC = 0 is associated with a very low ASCVD risk regardless of traditional risk factors.
- CAC scores should be interpreted using both absolute and percentile results.
- CAC burden should be noted and reported on non-ECG gated noncardiac CT scans.
- Radiomics and artificial intelligence are likely to facilitate automated CAC scoring on all CT scans of the thorax in the near future.

References

1. Budoff MJ, Young R, Burke G, et al. Ten-year association of coronary artery calcium with atherosclerotic cardiovascular disease (ASCVD) events: the multi-ethnic study of atherosclerosis (MESA). Eur Heart J. 2018;39:2401–8.
2. Agatston AS, Janowitz WR, Hildner FJ, Zusmer NR, Viamonte M, Detrano R. Quantification of coronary artery calcium using ultrafast computed tomography. J Am Coll Cardiol. 1990;15:827–32.
3. Erbel R, Mhlenkamp S, Moebus S, et al. Coronary risk stratification, discrimination, and reclassification improvement based on quantification of subclinical coronary atherosclerosis: the Heinz Nixdorf recall study. J Am Coll Cardiol. 2010;56:1397.
4. Sarwar A, Shaw LJ, Shapiro MD, et al. Diagnostic and prognostic value of absence of coronary artery calcification. JACC Cardiovasc Imaging. 2009;2:675–88.
5. Alluri K, Joshi PH, Henry TS, Blumenthal RS, Nasir K, Blaha MJ. Scoring of coronary artery calcium scans: history, assumptions, current limitations, and future directions. Atherosclerosis. 2015;239:109.
6. Callister TQ, Cooil B, Raya SP, Lippolis NJ, Russo DJ, Raggi P. Coronary artery disease: improved reproducibility of calcium scoring with an electron-beam CT volumetric method. Radiology. 1998;208:807.
7. Dzaye O, Razavi AC, Dardari ZA, Berman DS, Budoff MJ, Miedema MD, Obisesan OH, Boakye E, Nasir K, Rozanski A, Rumberger JA, Shaw LJ, Mortensen MB, Seamus P, Whelto MJB. Mean versus peak coronary calcium density on non-contrast computed tomography: implications for calcium scoring and mortality risk prediction. JACC Cardiovasc Imaging. 2021;15:489.
8. Van Rosendael AR, Narula J, Lin FY, et al. Association of High-Density Calcified 1K plaque with risk of acute coronary syndrome. JAMA Cardiol. 2020;5:282.
9. Ehara S, Kobayashi Y, Yoshiyama M, et al. Spotty calcification typifies the culprit plaque in patients with acute myocardial infarction: an intravascular ultrasound study. Circulation. 2004;110:3424.
10. Criqui MH, Denenberg JO, Ix JH, et al. Calcium density of coronary artery plaque and risk of incident cardiovascular events. JAMA. 2014;311:271.
11. Agatston AS, Janowitz WR, Hildner FJ, Zusmer NR, Viamonte M, Detrano R. Quantification of coronary artery calcium using ultrafast computed tomography. J Am Coll Cardiol. 1990;15:827.
12. McClelland RL, Chung H, Detrano R, Post W, Kronmal RA. Distribution of coronary artery calcium by race, gender, and age. Circulation. 2006;113:30–7.
13. Messenger B, Li D, Nasir K, Carr JJ, Blankstein R, Budoff MJ. Coronary calcium scans and radiation exposure in the multi-ethnic study of atherosclerosis. Int J Cardiovasc Imaging. 2016;32:525.
14. Mettler FA, Huda W, Yoshizumi TT, Mahesh M. Effective doses in radiology and diagnostic nuclear medicine: a catalog. Radiology. 2008;248:254.
15. Mühlenbruch G, Klotz E, Wildberger JE, et al. The accuracy of 1- and 3-mm slices in coronary calcium scoring using multi-slice CT in vitro and in vivo. Eur Radiol. 2007;17:321.
16. Vliegenthart R, Song B, Hofman A, Witteman JCM, Oudkerk M. Coronary calcification at electron-beam CT: effect of section thickness on calcium scoring in vitro and in vivo. Radiology. 2003;229:520.

17. Groen JM, Greuter MJ, Schmidt B, Suess C, Vliegenthart R, Oudkerk M. The influence of heart rate, slice thickness, and calcification density on calcium scores using 64-slice multidetector computed tomography: a systematic phantom study. Invest Radiol. 2007;42:848.
18. Van Der Bijl N, De Bruin PW, Geleijns J, et al. Assessment of coronary artery calcium by using volumetric 320-row multi-detector computed tomography: comparison of 0.5 mm with 3.0 mm slice reconstructions. Int J Cardiovasc Imaging. 2010;26:473.
19. Christensen JL, Sharma E, Gorvitovskaia AY, et al. Impact of slice thickness on the predictive value of lung cancer screening computed tomography in the evaluation of coronary artery calcification. J Am Heart Assoc. 2019;8:e010110.
20. Budoff MJ, McClelland RL, Chung H, et al. Reproducibility of coronary artery calcified plaque with cardiac 64-MDCT: the multi-ethnic study of atherosclerosis. Am J Roentgenol. 2009;192:613.
21. Qanadli SD, Mesurolle B, Aegerter P, et al. Volumetric quantification of coronary artery calcifications using dual-slice spiral CT scanner: improved reproducibility of measurements with 180° linear interpolation algorithm. J Comput Assist Tomogr. 2001;25:278.
22. Singh G, Al'Aref SJ, Van Assen M, et al. Machine learning in cardiac CT: basic concepts and contemporary data. J Cardiovasc Comput Tomogr. 2018;12:192.
23. Grandhi GR, Mszar R, Cainzos-Achirica M, et al. Coronary calcium to rule out obstructive coronary artery disease in patients with acute chest pain. JACC Cardiovasc Imaging. 2021;15:271.
24. Gulati M, Levy PD, Mukherjee D, et al. AHA/ACC/ASE/CHEST/SAEM/SCCT/SCMR guideline for the evaluation and diagnosis of CHEST pain: a report of the American College of Cardiology/American Heart Association joint committee on clinical practice guidelines. Circulation. 2021;2021:144.
25. Budoff MJ, Nasir K, McClelland RL, et al. Coronary Calcium predicts events better with absolute Calcium scores than age-sex-race/ethnicity percentiles. MESA (multi-ethnic study of atherosclerosis). J Am Coll Cardiol. 2009;53:345–52.
26. McClelland RL, Chung H, Detrano R, Post W, Kronmal RA. Distribution of coronary artery calcium by race, gender, and age: results from the multi-ethnic study of atherosclerosis (MESA). Circulation. 2006;113:30–7.
27. Blaha MJ, Whelton SP, Al Rifai M, et al. Comparing risk scores in the prediction of coronary and cardiovascular deaths: coronary artery calcium consortium. JACC Cardiovasc Imaging. 2021;14:411.
28. Bild DE, Detrano R, Peterson D, et al. Ethnic differences in coronary calcification: the multi-ethnic study of atherosclerosis (MESA). Circulation. 2005;111:1313.
29. Yeboah J, McClelland RL, Polonsky TS, et al. Comparison of novel risk markers for improvement in cardiovascular risk assessment in intermediate-risk individuals. JAMA. 2012;308:788.
30. Patel J, Pallazola VA, Dudum R, et al. Assessment of coronary artery calcium scoring to guide statin therapy allocation according to risk-enhancing factors: the multi-ethnic study of atherosclerosis. JAMA Cardiol. 2021;6:1161.
31. Arbab-Zadeh A, Fuster V. from detecting the vulnerable plaque to managing the vulnerable patient: JACC state-of-the-art review. J Am Coll Cardiol. 2019;74:1582.
32. Mortensen MB, Dzaye O, Steffensen FH, et al. Impact of plaque burden versus stenosis on ischemic events in patients with coronary atherosclerosis. J Am Coll Cardiol. 2020;76:2803–13.
33. Shaw LJ, Min JK, Nasir K, et al. Sex differences in calcified plaque and long-term cardiovascular mortality: observations from the CAC consortium. Eur Heart J. 2018;39:3727–35.
34. Orimoloye OA, Budoff MJ, Dardari ZA, et al. Race/ethnicity and the prognostic implications of coronary artery calcium for all-cause and cardiovascular disease mortality: the coronary artery calcium consortium. J Am Heart Assoc. 2018;7:e010471.
35. Al Rifai M, Kanaya AM, Kandula NR, et al. Distribution of calcium volume, density, number, and type of coronary vessel with calcified plaque in south Asians in the US and other race/ethnic groups: the MASALA and MESA studies. Atherosclerosis. 2021;317:16.
36. Miedema MD, Dardari ZA, Nasir K, et al. Association of coronary artery calcium with long-term, cause-specific mortality among young adults. JAMA Netw Open. 2019;2:e197440. https://jamanetwork.com/journals/jamanetworkopen/fullarticle/2738350. Accessed 30 Sept 2019
37. Dzaye O, Razavi AC, Dardari ZA, et al. Modeling the recommended age for initiating coronary artery calcium testing among at-risk young adults. J Am Coll Cardiol. 2021;78:1573.
38. Miedema MD, Dardari ZA, Nasir K, et al. Association of coronary artery calcium with long-term, cause-specific mortality among young adults. JAMA Netw Open. 2019;2:e197440.
39. Wang FM, Rozanski A, Arnson Y, et al. Cardiovascular and all-cause mortality risk by coronary artery calcium scores and percentiles among older adult males and females. Am J Med. 2021;134:341.
40. Arnett DK, Blumenthal RS, Albert MA, et al. 2019 ACC/AHA guideline on the primary prevention of cardiovascular disease. J Am Coll Cardiol. 2019;74:e177–232.
41. Blaha M, Budoff MJ, Shaw LJ, et al. Absence of coronary artery calcification and all-cause mortality. JACC Cardiovasc Imaging. 2009;2:692–700.
42. Razavi AC, Wong N, Budoff M, et al. Predicting long-term absence of coronary artery Calcium in metabolic syndrome and diabetes. JACC Cardiovasc Imaging. 2020;14:219–29.
43. Sandesara PB, Mehta A, O'Neal WT, et al. Clinical significance of zero coronary artery calcium in individuals with LDL cholesterol ≥190 mg/dL: the

multi-ethnic study of atherosclerosis. Atherosclerosis. 2020;292:224.
44. Nasir K, Cainzos-Achirica M. Role of coronary artery calcium score in the primary prevention of cardiovascular disease. BMJ. 2021;373:n776.
45. Blaha MJ, Budoff MJ, Defilippis AP, et al. Associations between C-reactive protein, coronary artery calcium, and cardiovascular events: implications for the JUPITER population from MESA, a population-based cohort study. Lancet. 2011;378:684.
46. Razavi AC, Kelly TN, Budoff MJ, et al. Atherosclerotic cardiovascular disease events among statin eligible individuals with and without long-term healthy arterial aging. Atherosclerosis. 2021;326:56.
47. Sc S, Sperling L, Virani SS, Yeboah J. 2018 AHA/ACC/AACVPR/AAPA/ABC/ACPM/ADA/AGS/APhA/ASPC/NLA/PCNA guideline on the Management of Blood Cholesterol: a report of the American College of Cardiology/American Heart Association task force on clinical practice guidelines. J Am Coll Cardiol. 2019;73:e285–350.
48. Dzaye O, Dardari ZA, Cainzos-Achirica M, Blankstein R, Dzaye AO, Dardari ZA, Cainzos-Achirica M, Blankstein R, Agatston AS, Duebgen M, Yeboah J, Szklo M, Budoff MJ, Lima JAC, Blumenthal RS, Blaha MJ. Warranty period of a calcium score of zero: comprehensive analysis from the multiethnic study of atherosclerosis. JACC Cardiovasc Imaging. 2020;14:990–1002.
49. Cainzos-Achirica M, Miedema MD, McEvoy JW, et al. Coronary artery calcium for personalized allocation of aspirin in primary prevention of cardiovascular disease in 2019: The MESA study (multi-ethnic study of atherosclerosis). Circulation. 2020;141:1541.
50. Miedema MD, Duprez DA, Misialek JR, et al. Use of coronary artery calcium testing to guide aspirin utilization for primary prevention: estimates from the multi-ethnic study of atherosclerosis. Circ Cardiovasc Qual Outcomes. 2014;7:453.
51. Uddin SMI, Mirbolouk M, Kianoush S, et al. Role of coronary artery calcium for stratifying cardiovascular risk in adults with hypertension: the coronary artery calcium consortium. Hypertension. 2019;73:983.
52. McEvoy JW, Martin SS, Dardari ZA, et al. Coronary artery calcium to guide a personalized risk-based approach to initiation and intensification of antihypertensive therapy. Circulation. 2017;135:153.
53. Peng AW, Dardari ZA, Blumenthal RS, et al. Very high coronary artery Calcium (≥1000) and association with cardiovascular disease events, non-cardiovascular disease outcomes, and mortality: results from MESA. Circulation. 2021;143:1571–83.
54. Vliegenthart R, Oudkerk M, Hofman A, et al. Coronary calcification improves cardiovascular risk prediction in the elderly. Circulation. 2005;112:572.
55. Coylewright M, Rice K, Budoff MJ, et al. Differentiation of severe coronary artery calcification in the multi-ethnic study of atherosclerosis. Atherosclerosis. 2011;219:616.
56. Dzaye O, Razavi AC, Michos ED, et al. Coronary artery calcium scores indicating secondary prevention level risk: findings from the CAC consortium and FOURIER trial. Atherosclerosis. 2022;347:70.
57. Kianoush S, Al Rifai M, Cainzos-Achirica M, et al. Thoracic extra-coronary calcification for the prediction of stroke: the multi-ethnic study of atherosclerosis. Atherosclerosis. 2017;267:61.
58. Hecht HS, Blaha MJ, Kazerooni EA, et al. CAC-DRS: coronary artery Calcium data and reporting system. An expert consensus document of the Society of Cardiovascular Computed Tomography (SCCT). J Cardiovasc Comput Tomogr. 2018;12:185.
59. Dzaye O, Dudum R, Mirbolouk M, et al. Validation of the coronary artery Calcium data and reporting system (CAC-DRS): dual importance of CAC score and CAC distribution from the coronary artery Calcium (CAC) consortium. J Cardiovasc Comput Tomogr. 2020;14:12.

10 Coronary CT Anatomy

Jeannie Yu and James Iwaz

Abstract

This chapter reviews normal coronary and non-coronary cardiac structures that are of relevance in the interpretation of cardiac CT images, including typical coronary anatomy (origin, course, and branches), cardiac chambers, valves and subvalvular apparatus, pericardium, cardiac veins, and great vessels.

Keywords

Coronary arteries · Cardiac anatomy · Atrium Ventricle · Valve · Aorta · Pericardium · Cardiac veins

Abbreviations

ALCAPA	Anomalous origin of the left main from the pulmonary artery
Ao	Aorta
ASD	Atrial septum defect
CCTA	Coronary CT angiography
CRT	Cardiac resynchronization therapy
CS	Coronary sinus
CT	Crista terminalis or computed tomography
CTCA	CT coronary angiography
D	Diagonal branch(es)
IAS	Interatrial septum
IVS	Interventricular septum
LA	Left atrium
LAA	Left atrial appendage
LAD	Left anterior descending artery
LAO	Left anterior oblique
LCC	Left coronary cusp
LCx	Left circumflex coronary artery
LIMA	Left internal mammary artery
LM	Left main coronary artery
LMCA	Left main coronary artery
LV	Left ventricle
MIP	Maximum intensity projection
MPR	Multi-planar reformation
NCC	Noncoronary cusp
OM	Obtuse marginal branch(es)
PA	Pulmonary artery
PDA	Posterior descending artery
PFO	Patent foramen ovale
PV	Pulmonary vein
RAA	Right atrial appendage
RAO	Right anterior oblique
RCA	Right coronary artery
RCC	Right coronary cusp
RI	Ramus intermedius
RIMA	Right internal mammary artery
RPL	Right posterolateral

J. Yu (✉) · J. Iwaz
University of California, Irvine, Irvine, CA, USA

Veterans Affairs Long Beach Healthcare System, Long Beach, CA, USA

Division of Cardiology, Tibor Rubin VA Medical Center, Long Beach, CA, USA
e-mail: James.Iwaz@va.gov

A. A. Zadeh, J. Hoe (eds.), *Practical Guide to Cardiac CT*,
https://doi.org/10.1007/978-981-97-6919-3_10

RV	Right ventricle
SA	Sinoatrial
SCCT	Society of Cardiovascular Computed Tomography
SMT	Septomarginal trabeculation
VSD	Ventricular septum defect

10.1 Introduction

- This chapter reviews normal coronary and non-coronary cardiac anatomy as depicted by CT.
- Extra-cardiac findings are discussed elsewhere (Chap. 22).

10.2 Coronary Arterial Anatomy

- Knowledge of the coronary anatomy by CT is required to report CTCA scans and includes the following:
  - Segmental classification of coronary arteries (i.e., SCCT 18 segment model).
  - Coronary artery territories and corresponding myocardial segments.
  - Nomenclature and anatomical landmarks used with invasive angiography.
  - Anatomy relevant for percutaneous coronary and structural interventions.
- Typical anatomy consists of three major epicardial coronary arteries, which are the left anterior descending (LAD), left circumflex (LCx), and right coronary (RCA) arteries [1] (Fig. 10.1).
- The version referenced in this chapter is the SCCT coronary nomenclature which is comprised of 18 coronary artery segments [2]:

1	Proximal Right Coronary Artery (pRCA)	10	Second Diagonal Artery (D2)
2	Mid right coronary artery (mRCA)	11	Proximal left circumflex artery (pCx)
3	Distal right coronary artery (dRCA)	12	First obtuse marginal (OM1)
4	Right posterior descending artery (R-PDA)	13	Distal left circumflex artery (LCx)

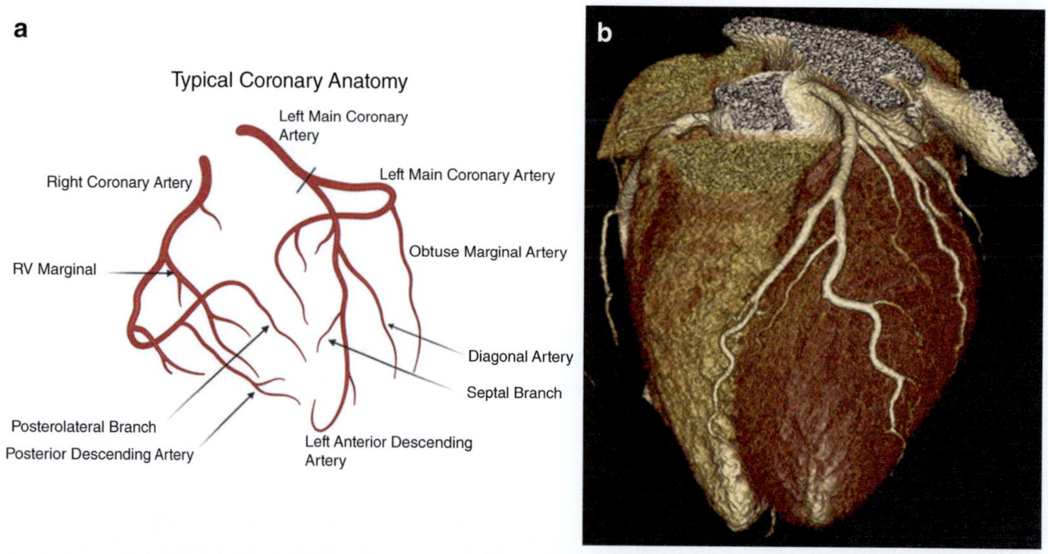

Fig. 10.1 Typical coronary anatomy. A schematic is on the left (**a**) which demonstrates the general course and relationship of the coronary arteries and is mirrored in the right panel (**b**) with volume rendered CT image demonstrating the location of coronary arteries in relation to the entire heart. The left main coronary artery gives rise to the left anterior descending artery and non-dominant left circumflex artery. The dominant right coronary artery originates from the right coronary cusp and supplies the posterior descending artery and posterolateral branch. (*Created with* BioRender.com)

5	Left Main coronary artery (LM)	14	Second obtuse marginal (OM2)
6	Proximal left anterior descending artery (pLAD)	15	Left posterior descending artery (L-PDA)
7	Mid left anterior descending artery (mLAD)	16	Right posterolateral branch (R-PLB)
8	Distal left anterior descending artery (dLAD)	17	Ramus intermedius (RI)
9	First diagonal artery (D1)	18	Left posterolateral branch (L-PLB)

- *Left Main Coronary Artery (LM or LMCA)* originates off the left coronary cusp within the aortic root and typically bifurcates into the left anterior descending artery and left circumflex artery (Figs. 10.2 and 10.3). Its length is defined from the ostium to the proximal aspect of the circumflex artery.
  - The LM arises typically at the 3–4 o'clock position in respect to the aorta as visualized on axial images.

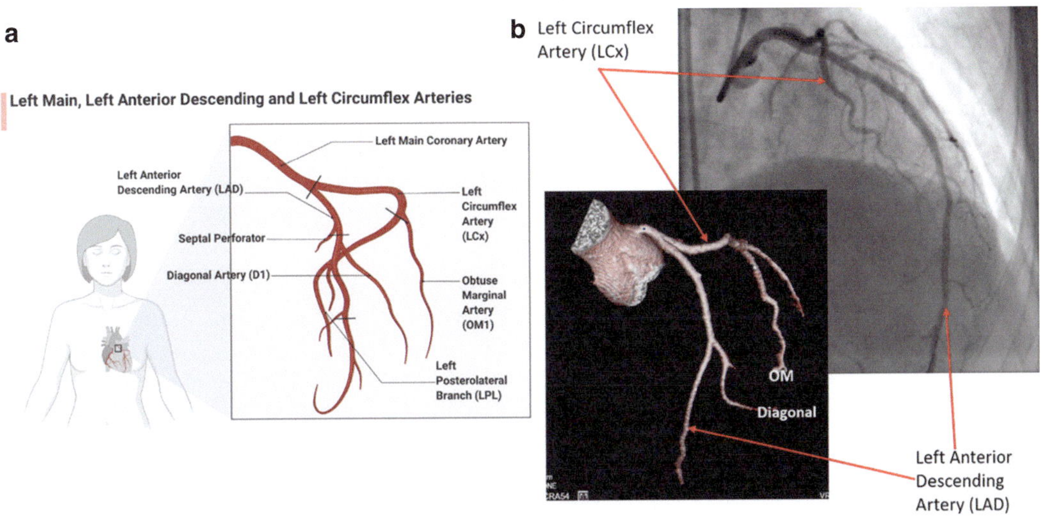

Fig. 10.2 The illustration in Panel **a** shows the left main coronary artery bifurcating into the left circumflex artery and left anterior descending artery. The LAD supplies both septal perforators to perfuse the majority of the interventricular septum as well as the diagonal branches which subtend the anterior left ventricle. Panel **b** shows a 3D volume rendering of the left coronary circulation and representative corresponding invasive angiogram with focus on the length of the LAD. Note that the circumflex is foreshortened on this image. (*Created with* BioRender.com)

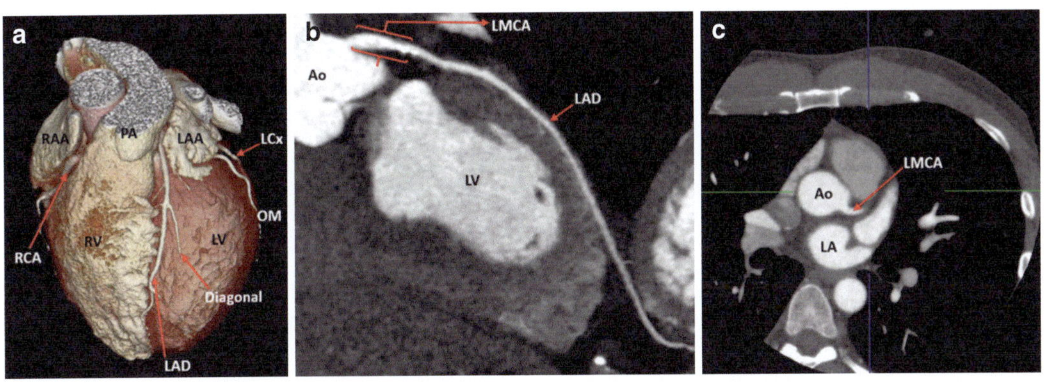

Fig. 10.3 CCTA representations of the LAD in 3D volume rendering of the anterior heart (Panel **a**), curved multiplanar reformation (MPR) of the LAD (Panel **b**), and axial view of the origin of the left main coronary artery arising from the left coronary cusp of the aortic root (Panel **c**)

  - If the LM arises at the 5–6 o'clock position (as seen with obesity and leftwards aortic root rotation), it can be more difficult to engage the ostium using standard catheters on invasive coronary angiography.
- *Left Anterior Descending (LAD) Artery* is the major epicardial branch from the left main coronary artery and courses down the anterior interventricular groove (Figs. 10.2 and 10.3).
  - *Septal branches* supply the interventricular septum (Figs. 10.4 and 10.5).
  - *Diagonal (D) branches* supply the anterior and anterolateral left ventricle.
  - *The proximal LAD* is demarked either by the first major septal perforator (used predominantly in North America) or the first major diagonal branch (used particularly in Europe).
  - The mid LAD is typically defined as half the distance from the end of the proximal segment to its distal end.
- *Left Circumflex (LCx) Artery* is the second major epicardial branch of the left main coronary artery and traverses the left atrioventricular groove and typically terminates within the groove or as a posterolateral branch (Figs. 10.6 and 10.7). It is divided into two segments: proximal (generally ostium to origin of obtuse marginal) and distal (beyond the obtuse marginal). A mid-segment may be defined for the region between the first and second obtuse marginal artery.
  - *Obtuse Marginal (OM)* are typically 1–3 branches that supply the lateral left ventricle.

    Note: Coronary artery bypass grafts usually connect to the obtuse marginal branches, as they are superficially

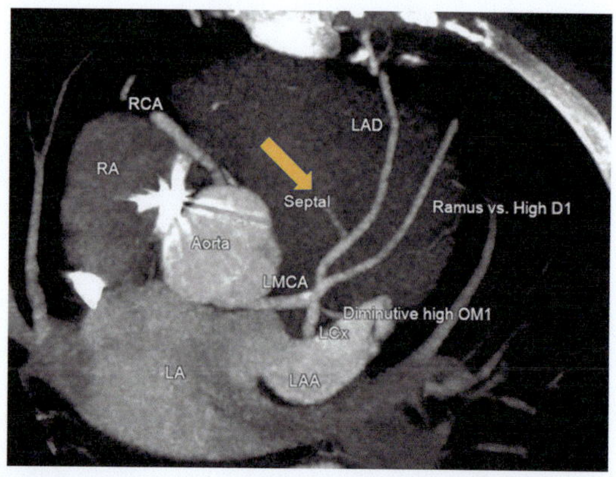

Fig. 10.4 Maximum intensity projection (MIP) MPR of the coronaries originating from the aortic root. The left main bifurcation is noted in this particular angulation reminiscent of a "spider view" (LAO Caudal) on invasive angiography. There is a branch that arises at the ostium of the left anterior descending artery, which likely represents a high first diagonal artery but could be labeled as a Ramus Intermedius in operative reports, given that this region is often obscured by the left atrial appendage

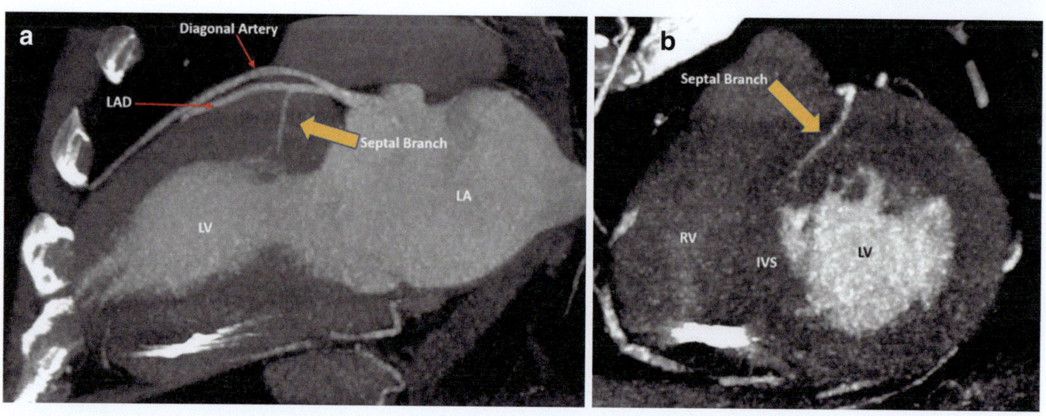

Fig. 10.5 The first septal perforator is accentuated in these projections including a 2 chamber (Panel **a**) and short axis (Panel **b**) MIP images. This case of hypertrophic cardiomyopathy demonstrated the use of CT imaging in pre-procedural planning for alcohol ablation versus surgical intervention

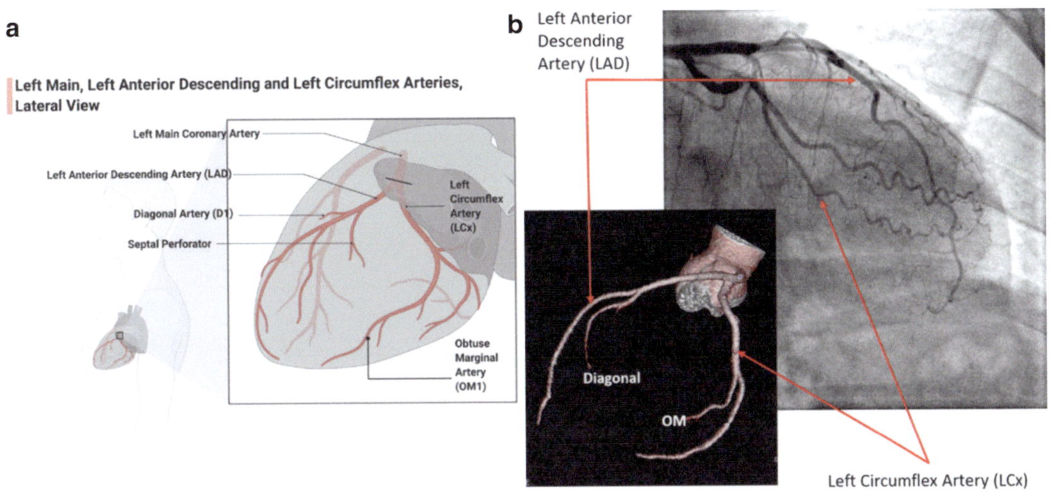

Fig. 10.6 The illustration on the left shows a lateral projection of the left coronary circulation with the left anterior descending coursing anteriorly and the left circumflex wrapping around the left atrioventricular groove (**a**). A representative corresponding invasive angiogram is shown in Panel **b** with the traditional orientation on invasive angiography (mirror image to the CCTA). (*Created with* BioRender.com)

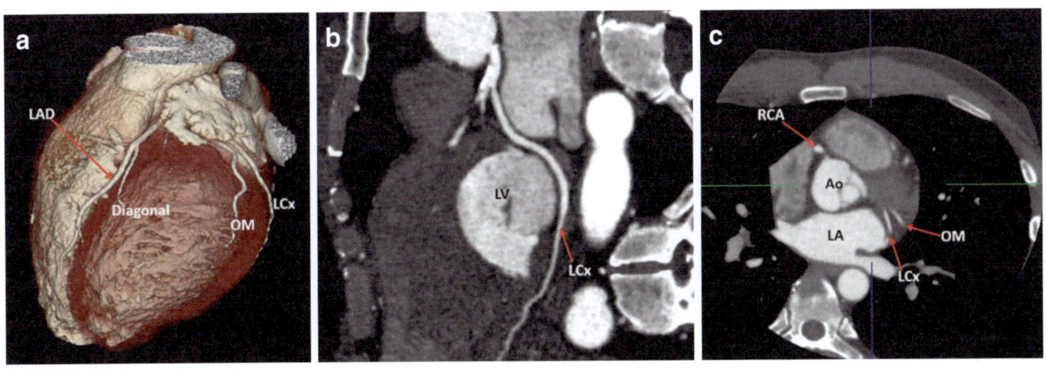

Fig. 10.7 The 3D volume rendered image (Panel **a**) provides an overview of the left coronary anatomy. The curved MPR of the left circumflex demonstrates the course of the vessel around the atrioventricular groove of the left ventricle (Panel **b**). Panel **c** shows on axial imaging the appearance of the circumflex and the orientation of the obtuse marginal branch which extends toward the left ventricular apex and subtends the anterolateral left ventricle

located, while the body of the LCx is more deeply situated in the left atrioventricular groove (Fig. 10.13) and generally unsuitable for grafting.

- *Posterolateral (LPL) branches* may arise from the distal LCx and supply the inferolateral left ventricle.
- Caliber tends to be smaller when non-dominant.
- Large posterolateral branches form the LCx may indicate co-dominant status of the LCx, particularly if RPL branches are absent.
- The LCx is considered dominant if it supplied the posterior descending artery.

- *Right Coronary Artery (RCA)* originates from the right coronary cusp and traverses the right atrioventricular groove and, in the majority of patients (approximately 80%), terminates as the PDA and RPL indicating right dominance (Figs. 10.8, 10.9, and 10.10). The RCA is divided into three segments: proximal, mid, and distal thirds which generally correspond with the first and second curvatures of the vessel.

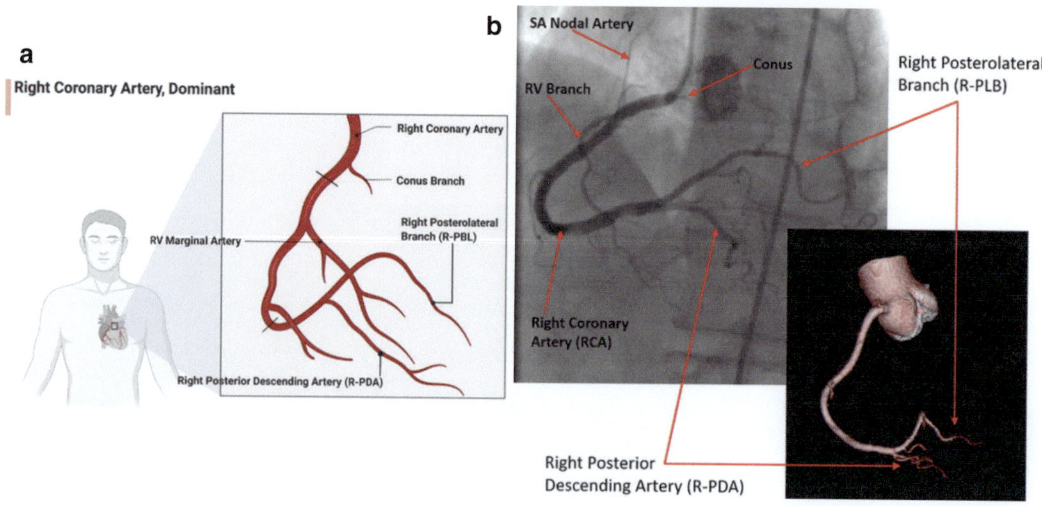

Fig. 10.8 The illustration on the left in Panel **a** shows the anatomy of a dominant right coronary artery, which is then represented in a volume rendering of the RCA and corresponding invasive angiogram with major branches, including the conus, SA nodal artery, RV or marginal branch, and terminating as the right posterior descending artery and right posterolateral branch (**b**). (*Created with* BioRender.com)

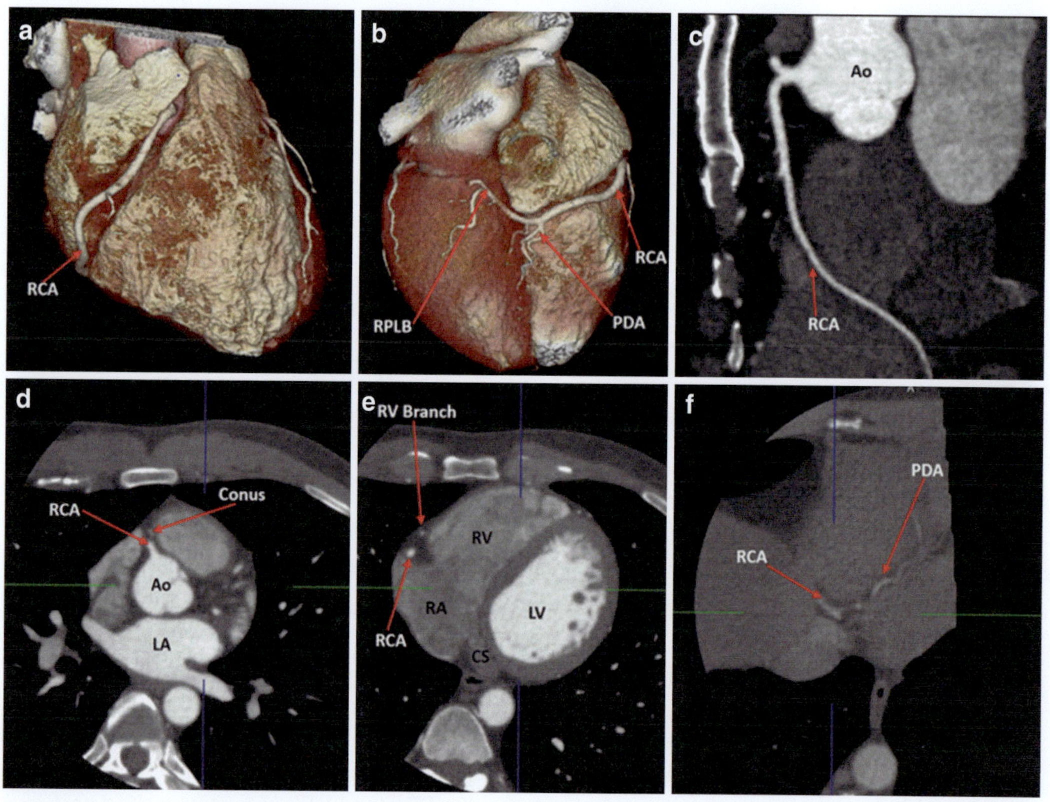

Fig. 10.9 The 3D volume rendering of the heart shown in right lateral and posterior views shows the relation and course of the right coronary artery and the visualized branches in relation to the cardiac structures (Panel **a**, **b**). A curved MPR of the right coronary artery (Panel **c**) shows the RCA wrapping around the right atrioventricular groove, surrounding the unopacified right ventricle. Axial views at three different levels (Panels **d**, **e**, and **f**) demonstrate the origin of the RCA from the right coronary cusp as well as the typical appearance of the conus, RV marginal, and posterior descending arteries

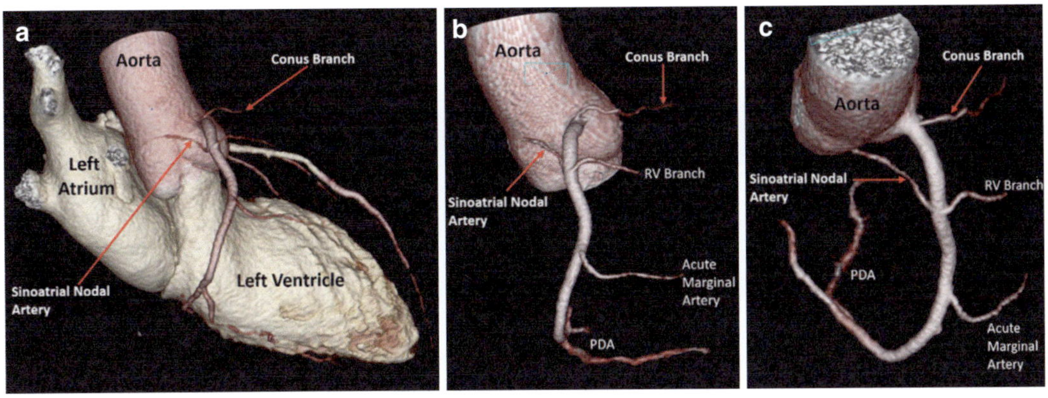

Fig. 10.10 The conus and sinoatrial nodal branches are demonstrated more explicitly on these projections. The conus extends anterior to subtend the muscular RV outflow tract, also known as the RV infundibulum. The SA nodal artery extends posteriorly to provide perfusion the SA node in the posterior left atrium

- *Conus Branch* supplies the right ventricular outflow tract known as the infundibulum and is the very first branch of the right coronary artery in 50–60% of cases (but can also arise from a separate ostium adjacent to the RCA).
- *Sinoatrial (SA) Nodal Artery* subtends the SA node and originates from the RCA in approximately 60% of cases (and LCx in the remaining 40%).
- *Right ventricular (RV) Branches* are more proximal branches that supply the lateral right ventricle.
- *Acute Marginal Branches (RV Marginals)* occur around the acute margin of the right ventricle, subtends the inferolateral aspects of the right ventricle.
- *Posterior Descending Artery (PDA)* begins at the crux of the heart and is the vessel that courses down the posterior interventricular groove, also often supplies the AV nodal branch.
- *Posterolateral (RPL) branches.*
- Caliber tends to be large when dominant.

• *Ramus Intermedius (RI)* is a branch that arises between LAD and LCx and represents a trifurcation of the left main coronary artery, subtending the anterolateral left ventricle.
  - This is a normal variant.
  - The RI may be small, of medium caliber, large, or arborizing.
  - Depending on its course, it may assume the typical course of an LAD/diagonal or an LCx/OM branch.

• *Coronary Dominance* can be categorized as right, left, or co-dominant, depending on the vessel from which the posterior descending artery (PDA) arises [3] (Fig. 10.9).
  - Co-dominance refers to the situation of both the RCA and LCx giving off a vessel that supplies the PDA territory or the LCx supplying all posterolateral branches.
  - Approximately 80% of patients are right dominant, and the remaining 20% will either be left dominant or co-dominant.
  - The dominant vessel will also typically supply the AV nodal artery.

• Correlation of Coronary Artery Anatomy by CCTA in the Cardiac Catheterization Laboratory.
  - It is important to understand how CCTA images correlate to invasive angiography images, both to communicate with interventional cardiologists as well as for procedure planning.
  - With invasive coronary angiography, one can adjust the projection in right and left directions as well as cranial and caudal directions.
  - Conventional angiography creates a 2D image of a 3D structure, so different views are necessary to adequately evaluate the coronary arteries. Each view provides a different perspective of the vessels.
  - The standard coronary angiography views are: right anterior oblique (RAO) cranial, RAO caudal, left anterior oblique (LAO) cranial, and LAO caudal (also known as the "spider shot") (Figs. 10.11 and 10.12).

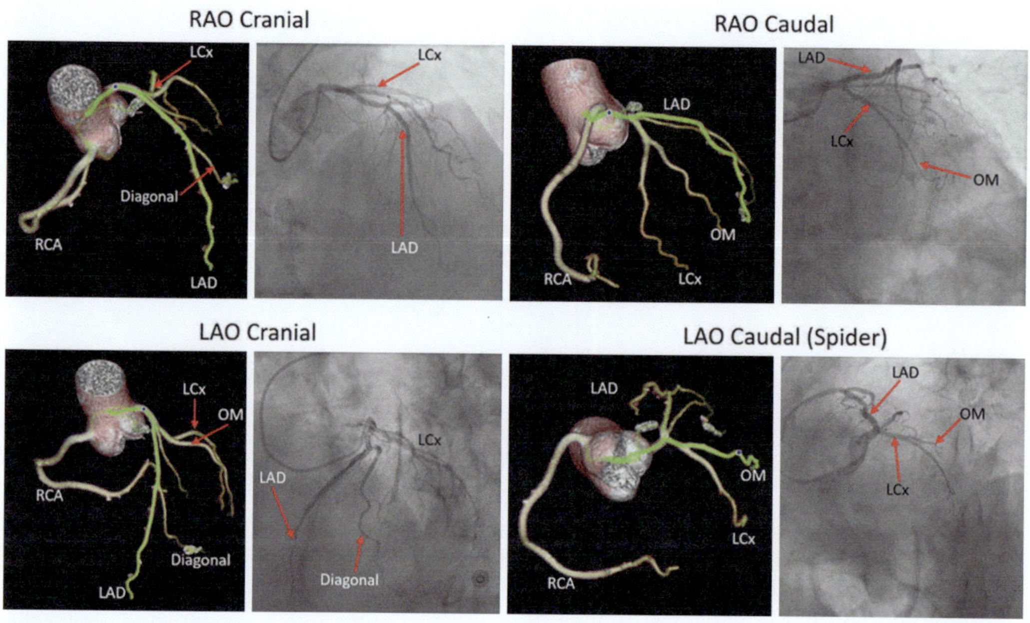

Fig. 10.11 Left coronary circulation with conventional angiography correlation. Common projections in the cardiac catheterization laboratory have been labeled with corresponding volume renderings of the coronary arteries on CCTA, including: RAO Cranial, RAO Caudal, LAO Cranial, and LAO Caudal (Spider) views

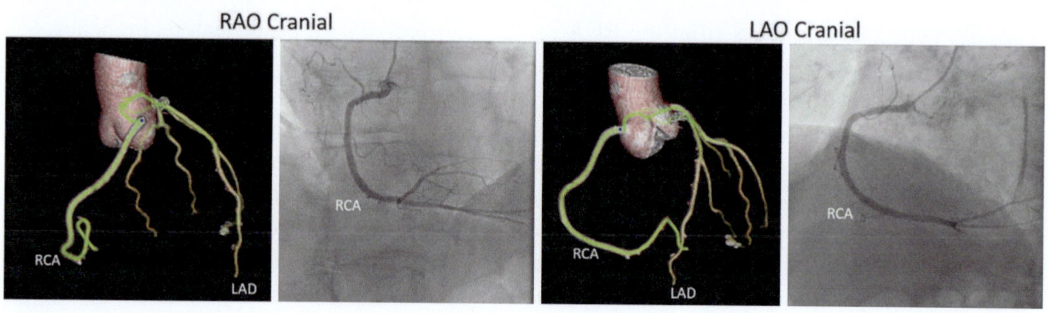

Fig. 10.12 Right coronary circulation with conventional angiography correlation. Common projections have been labeled with corresponding volume renderings of the coronary arteries on CCTA, including: RAO Cranial and LAO Cranial

10.3 Common Coronary Artery Bypass Anatomy (Fig. 10.13).

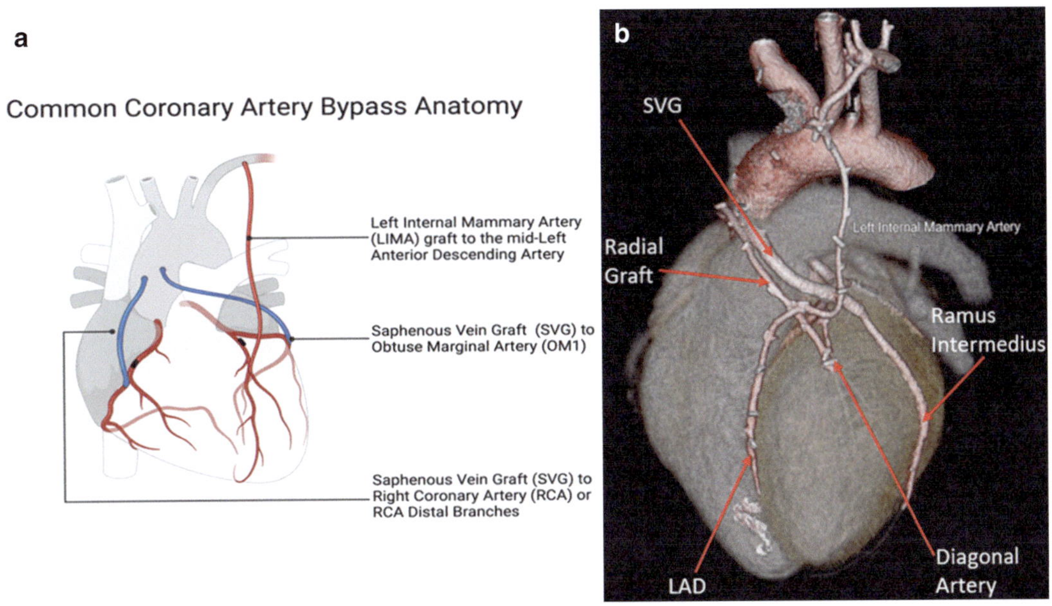

Fig. 10.13 Coronary artery bypass grafting on CCTA requires modification of the scan protocol, however, anatomy itself tends to follow common conventions. The left internal mammary artery (LIMA) is the most durable CABG graft, and is typically well-suited and used to bypass the left anterior descending artery. Reverse saphenous vein grafts are often used for the other vessels, though free radial and RIMA grafts are also common. For the LIMA/RIMA, it is imperative to image the origin of the vessel. Note that vein graft caliber is also noticeably larger than arterial grafts. Other configurations of bypass grafts beyond in situ grafts can include sequential/jump and composite T grafts. (*Created with* BioRender.com)

10.4 Cardiac Chambers and Non-Coronary Structures (Figs. 10.14 and 10.15)

- *Right Atrium (RA)* receives venous return from the body and heart, functioning as a reservoir, and transmits this blood to the right ventricle. The RA is notable on imaging for the following structures:
  - *Right Atrial Appendage (RAA)* is an outpouching off the anterolateral right atrium and is typically described as shallow with a large orifice, and RAA thrombus is thought to be uncommon though not well characterized.
  - *Crista Terminalis (CT)* is a smooth ridge of myocardium that extends vertically down the posterolateral aspect of the right atrium, and divides the smooth walled posterolateral right atrium (sinus venosus) and the pectinate muscles of the anterior RA and RAA (primitive right atrium) (Fig. 10.16):

    Can be mistaken for a right atrial mass. Important anatomic structure with relation to paroxysmal atrial fibrillation, atrial flutter, and other types of supraventricular tachycardia.
  - *Eustachian Valve* is a ridge of tissue that originates inferiorly at the insertion of the inferior vena cava and courses medially along the interatrial septum toward the fossa ovalis.
  - *Os of the Coronary Sinus* is located inferiorly and anteriorly to the Eustachian valve (Fig. 10.9, Panel e).
- *Right Ventricle (RV)* is the chamber that sends the venous, deoxygenated blood to the pulmonary vascular bed. The RV is characterized by an irregular crescent shape that is difficult to characterize with geometric assumptions (unlike the left ventricle), has prominent trabeculae in the apex, papillary muscles, tendons and in normal circumstances, a much thinner wall than the left ventricle (3–5 mm in end-diastole).

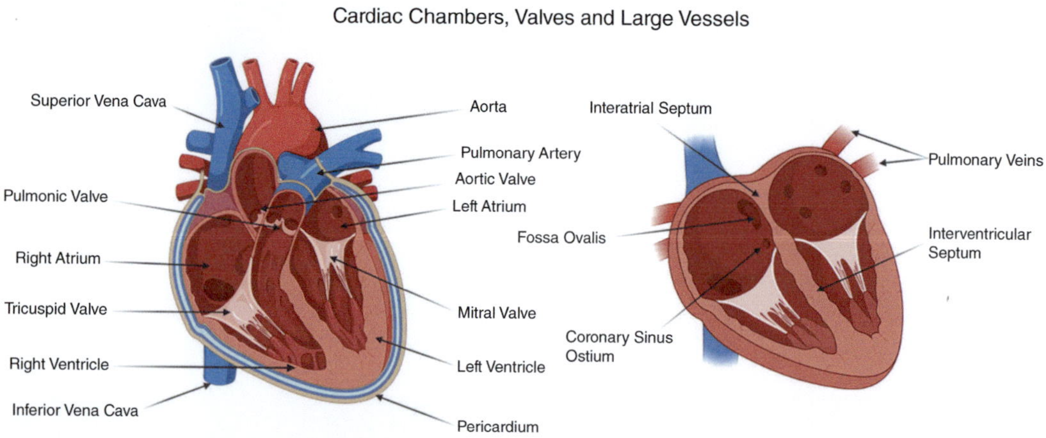

Fig. 10.14 Cardiac chambers, valves, and large vessels. Blood enters the right atrium from the superior and inferior vena cava as well as the coronary sinus, then is funneled through the tricuspid valve into the right ventricle, the right ventricular outflow track, past the pulmonic valve and out the main pulmonary artery to deliver the deoxygenated blood to the pulmonary vascular bed. The blood is oxygenated and then returned via the pulmonary veins to the left atrium, which sends the blood through the mitral valve to the left ventricle, the muscular pump that pushes the oxygenated blood to the system circulation through the left ventricular outflow tract, aortic valve, and into the aorta. (*Created with* BioRender.com)

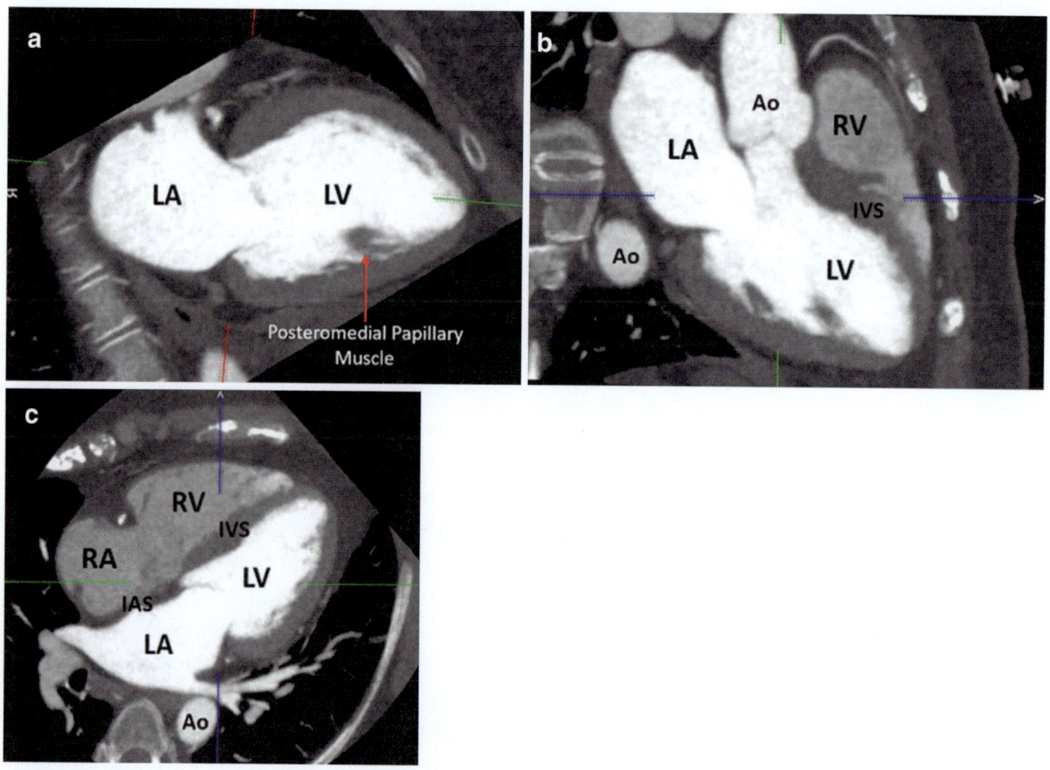

Fig. 10.15 Typical cardiac long axis views are recreated with multiplanar reformations (MPR). Panel **a** represents a 2-chamber view, with the left atrium and left ventricle. The valve plane visualizes the mitral valve. The anterior myocardial segments are visualized toward the top of the image, with the inferior segments toward the bottom of the image also notable for the posteromedial papillary muscle. Panel **b** shows a typical 3-chamber view, similar to the parasternal long axis window on echocardiography. The anteroseptal segments are noted (IVS), opposite to the inferolateral myocardial walls. Panel **c** illustrates the CT representation of a 4-chamber view

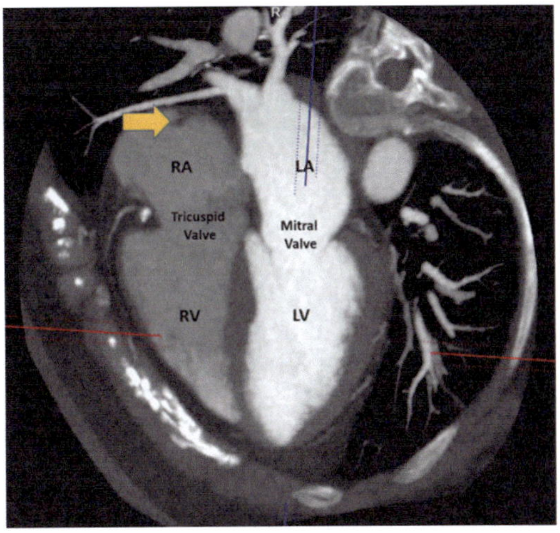

Fig. 10.16 This apical 4-chamber view with thick MIP is used to demonstrate the crista terminalis (yellow arrow) in the posterior right atrium which is a vertical ridge of tissue that is sometimes mistaken for a mass but is a normal structure

  - *Moderator Band* is a thick muscular tendon that is located in the RV apex and extends from the septum to the free wall (Fig. 10.17).
  - *Septomarginal Trabeculation (SMT) or Band* is another tendon toward the apex of the RV which typically bifurcates into two branches (posteriorly and anteriorly directed).
  - *RV Segments: The RV is generally divided into anterior, inferior, lateral, and RVOT wall segments* [4].
- *Left Atrium (LA)* is the receiving chamber of the oxygen-rich blood draining from the pulmonary vascular bed through the pulmonary veins and transmits blood to the left ventricle. The LA is notable for the following structures:
  - *Left Atrial Appendage (LAA)* is an outpouching off the lateral left atrium and is notable for the risk of thrombus formation in patients with atrial fibrillation, and can take on several different morphologies. Because the LAA has a narrow orifice and can have a shape that promotes stasis, particular attention must be made to distinguish filling defects from slow-flow versus thrombus. The inner surface of the LAA is notable for ridges of tissue called pectinate muscle (Fig. 10.18).

    Typical LAA Morphologies: Cactus, cauliflower, chicken wing, windsock; high, middle, and low.
  - *Coumadin Ridge (Eustachian Ridge)* is an invagination of tissue that projects into the left atrium from the lateral wall and is located between the os of the left atrial appendage and the left upper pulmonary vein. It is sometimes described as shaped like a "q-tip" (Fig. 10.18).
  - *Pulmonary Veins (PV)* drain into the posterior left atrium. Most commonly there are four pulmonary veins (left upper, left lower, right upper, right lower pulmonary veins). Significant variation can occur including common ostia, a right middle pulmonary vein and others (Fig. 10.19).
- *Interatrial Septum (IAS)* is the separation between the left and right atria and is formed by fusion of the septum primum and septum secundum. A central area of thinning in the IAS is known as the fossa ovalis and can be associated with either a potential structural defect (*patent foramen ovale, PFO*) or a fixed defect (*atrial septal defect, ASD*) with resultant shunting.
- *Left Ventricle (LV)* is a muscular chamber that serves as the pump to the systemic circulation and is described commonly as cone or bullet-shaped with two papillary muscles (posteromedial and anterolateral).
  - LV Myocardial Segments (See Figs. 10.20 and 10.21):

    Six Basal Segments: Basal anteroseptal, basal anterior, basal anterolateral, basal inferolateral, basal inferior, basal inferoseptal.

    S Mid Segments: Mid anteroseptal, mid anterior, mid anterolateral, mid inferolateral, mid inferior, mid inferoseptal.

    4 Apical Segments plus the apical cap: Apical anterior, apical lateral, apical inferior, apical septal, apical cap
- *Interventricular Septum* is the myocardium between the left and right ventricles and has two major components consisting of the thin membranous septum more proximally near the level of the atrioventricular valves and the thicker muscular septum. A defect in either of these areas would be consistent with a ventricular septal defect (VSD) (Fig. 10.21).

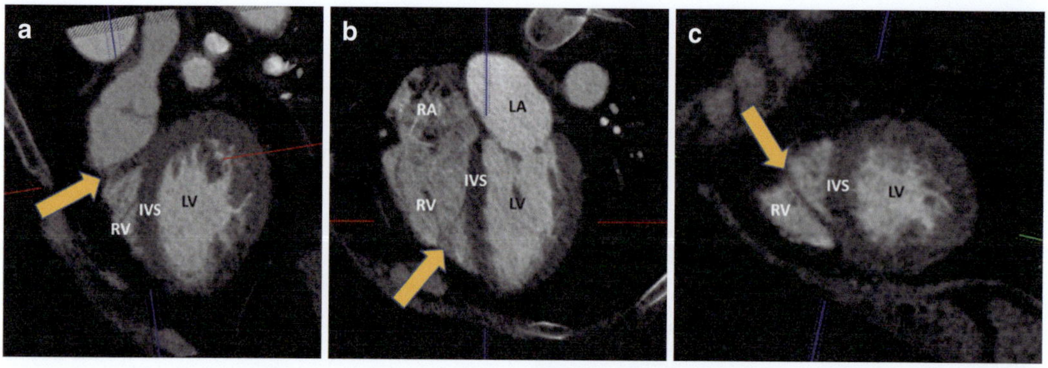

Fig. 10.17 Panel **a** demonstrates the septomarginal trabeculation near the right ventricular outflow tract and extending from the interventricular septum. Panels **b** and **c** show two different views of the moderator band in the RV apex

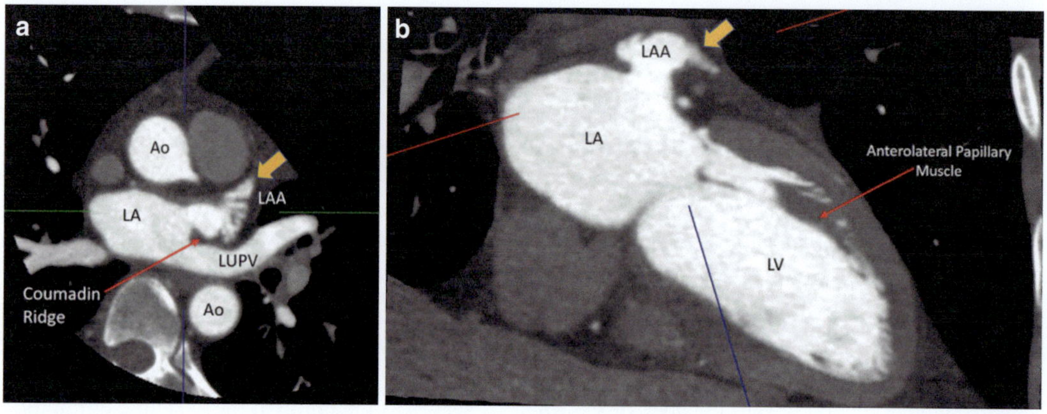

Fig. 10.18 The left atrial appendage (yellow arrow) is noted on axial imaging (Panel **a**) and the MPR of the 2-chamber view (Panel **b**) with numerous linear projections into the cavity representing pectinate muscle representing normal structure and should not be confused with thrombus or mass. The coumadin ridge, also known as the Eustachian Ridge is noted in Panel **a**, and represents an invagination of tissue or fold between the left atrial appendage and the left upper pulmonary vein

Fig. 10.19 The pulmonary veins are shown on the volume rendered posterior view of the left atrium. The typical configuration consists of four main pulmonary veins, including the left upper, left lower, right upper, and right lower pulmonary veins. It is common to also have common ostia as well as additional accessory veins, such as the right middle pulmonary vein

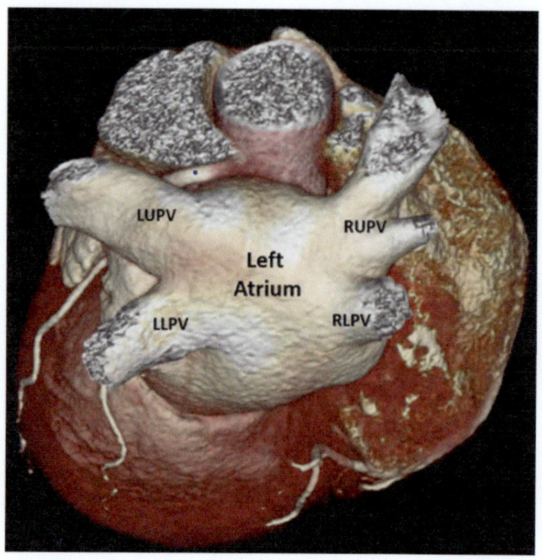

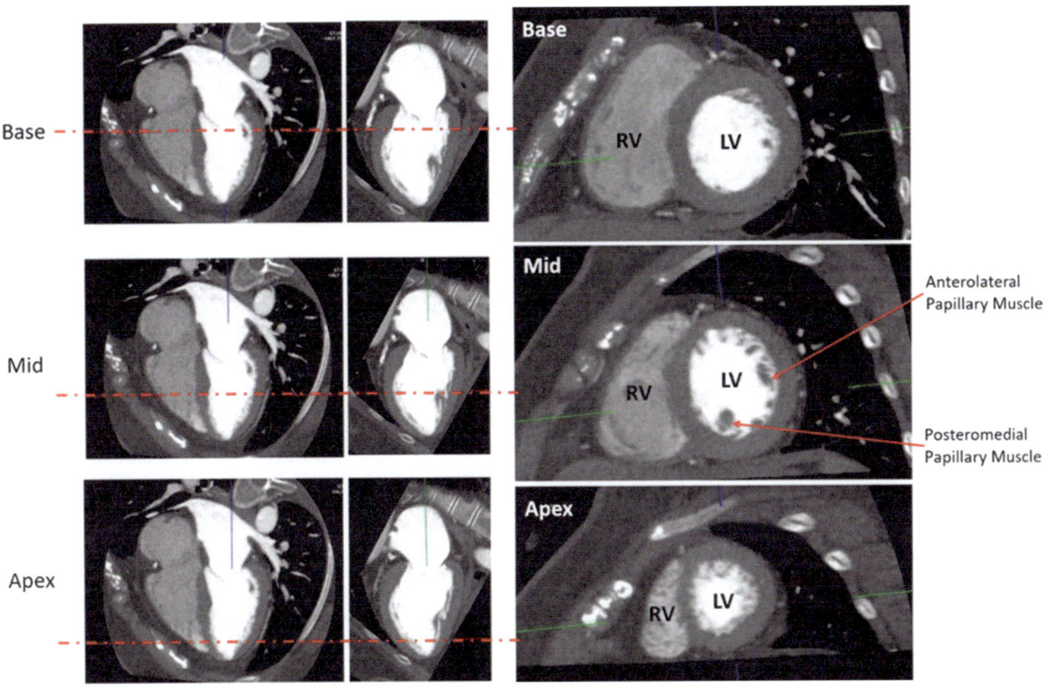

Fig. 10.20 The short axis levels of the myocardium classically used for perfusion diagrams have been recreated here with CCTA views. The corresponding 4-chamber and 2-chamber long axis views have also been included with a red-dotted line to indicate at what level the short axis was obtained for the traditional basal, mid, and apical levels

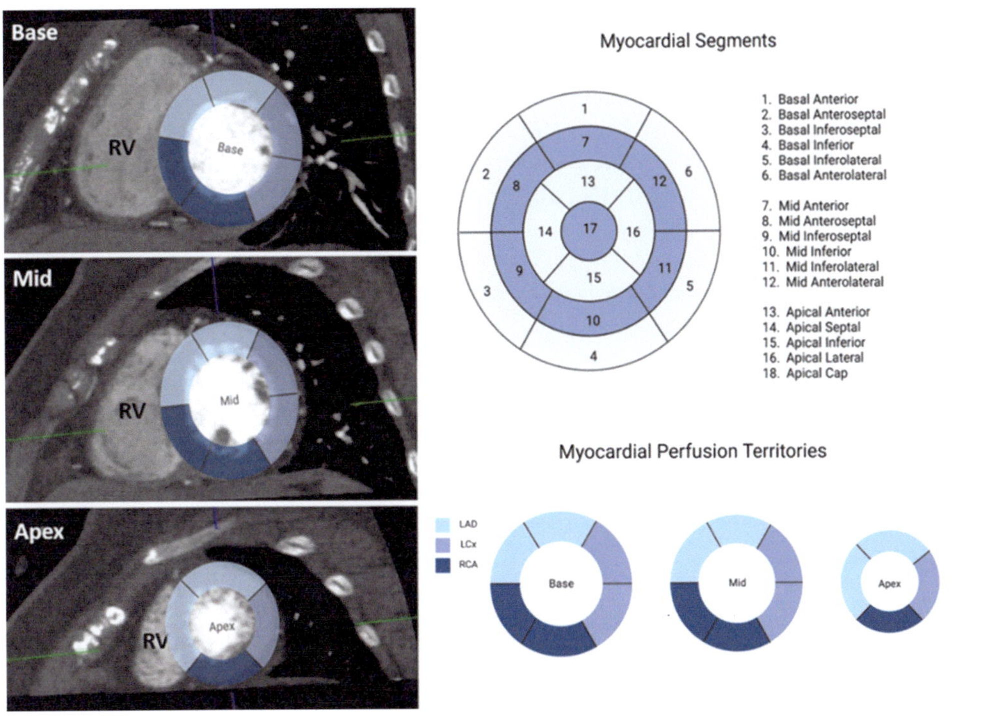

Fig. 10.21 Myocardial segments outlined in standard fashion with basal, mid, and apical levels. Common coronary perfusion territories are depicted (bottom right) with CT overlay by segment (left) at the basal, mid, and apical levels with alignment of the septal segments with the RV insertion points. (*Created with* BioRender.com)

10.5 Cardiac Valves and Subvalvular Apparatus

- *Tricuspid Valve* is located at the atrioventricular position between the right atrium and right ventricle and consists of three leaflets (anterior, posterior, and septal).
- *Pulmonic Valve* is a semilunar valve positioned between the right ventricular outflow tract and the main pulmonary artery and is characterized by three leaflets (anterior, right, and left).
- *Mitral Valve* is located at the atrioventricular position between the left atrium and left ventricle and consists of two leaflets (anterior and posterior) where the anterior leaflet is much more expansive than the posterior leaflet.
  - The mitral annulus is prone to develop calcification known as *mitral annular calcification.*
  - The posterior leaflet has three scallops (P1, P2, and P3) and the corresponding segments of the anterior leaflet are also assigned similarly (A1, A2, and A3) where A1/P1 are more laterally located and A3/P3 are more medially positioned.
- *Aortic Valve* is a semilunar valve positioned at the demarcation of the left ventricular outflow tract (LVOT) and the aortic root and is characterized by three cusps (right coronary, left coronary, and non-coronary cusps) (Fig. 10.22). When viewed in short axis or *en face*:
  - *Right Coronary Cusp* is adjacent to portions of the right atrium, tricuspid valve, right ventricle, and right ventricular outflow tract. The RCA arises from this cusp.
  - *Left Coronary Cusp* is the cusp from which the left main originates and is adjacent to either the left atrium and left atrial appendage (LAA) or the main pulmonary artery depending on the level and double-oblique angulation.
  - *Non-Coronary Cusp* is adjacent to the interatrial septum.
  - *Commissures* are the points at which the cusps insert into the aortic root and this space represent the cusp-to-cusp interface at these attachment sites to the aorta.
- *Papillary Muscles* and *Subvalvular Apparatus* are associated with the atrioventricular valves (i.e., tricuspid and mitral valves) and provide tethering to support normal valve opening and closure (Fig. 10.23).
  - Left-sided papillary muscles: Anterolateral and posteromedial (see Fig. 10.23).
  - Right-sided papillary muscles: Anterior, posterior, and septal.
  - Chordae tendinae are characterized as true (attaching to the valve leaflets) or false (attaching to anything else).
  - Both papillary muscles provide chordae tendinae to both leaflets.

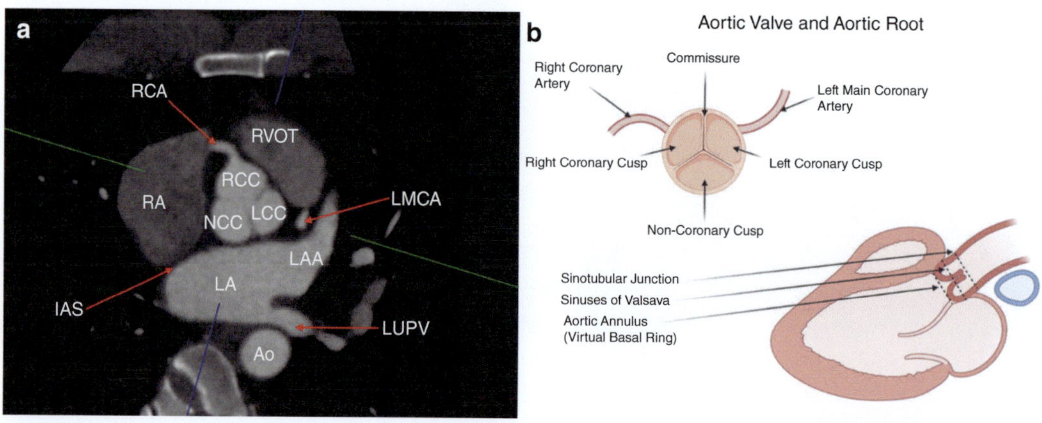

Fig. 10.22 Panel **a** shows the aortic root on axial imaging. The non-coronary cusp (NCC) is bisected by the interatrial septum (IAS). Aortic valve and common aortic root landmarks illustration. (*Created with* BioRender.com)

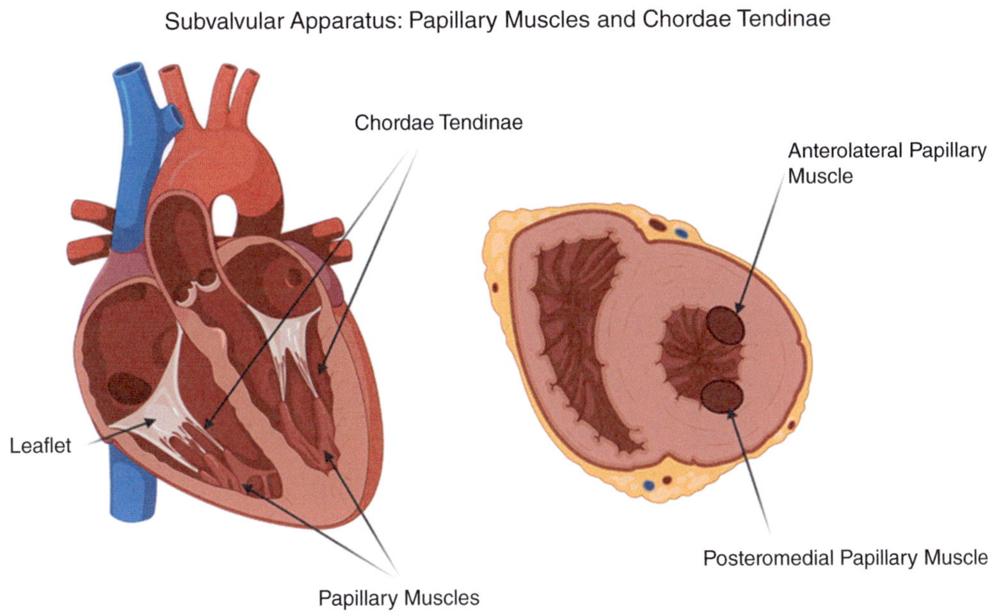

Fig. 10.23 The mitral and tricuspid valves are shown on the left with their associated subvalvular apparatus, including the chordae tendinae and papillary muscles. The right side shows the short axis location of the papillary muscles of the left ventricle: the posteromedial and anterolateral papillary muscles. (*Created with* BioRender.com)

10.6 Non-Coronary Vessels

- *Inferior Vena Cava (IVC)* is the large vein that drains into the inferior aspect of the right atrium (Fig. 10.14).
- *Superior Vena Cava (SVC)* is the large vein that drains into the superior aspect of the right atrium (Fig. 10.14).
- *Pulmonary Artery (PA)* is contiguous with the right ventricular outflow and is demarcated by the pulmonic valve, providing deoxygenated blood to the pulmonary vascular bed for oxygenation (Fig. 10.14).
- *Pulmonary Veins* drain the pulmonary vascular bed into the left atrium for pumping to the systemic circulation (Fig. 10.19).
- *Aorta (Ao)* is the large artery which is attached to the left ventricular outflow and is demarcated by the aortic valve, providing oxygenated blood to the systemic circulation. The aortic root is characterized by the following structures and landmarks (See Fig. 10.5):
  - *Sinuses of Valsalva are the most proximal portion of the aorta and are just distal to the aortic valve. There are three sinuses corresponding to the three aortic valve cusps.*
  - *Aortic Annulus or Virtual Basal Ring* is the junction between the Sinuses of Valsalva and the left ventricular outflow tract.
  - *Sinotubular Junction* is the junction between the Sinuses of Valsalva and the tubular ascending aorta.
  - *Ascending Thoracic Aorta.*
  - *Aortic Arch or Transverse Aorta* is the horizontal segment of the thoracic aorta and is the segment from which the following branches originate:
    - *Brachiocephalic Artery*, which then bifurcates into the right common carotid and right subclavian arteries.
    - *Left Common Carotid Artery.*
    - *Left Subclavian Artery.*
  - Descending Thoracic Aorta.

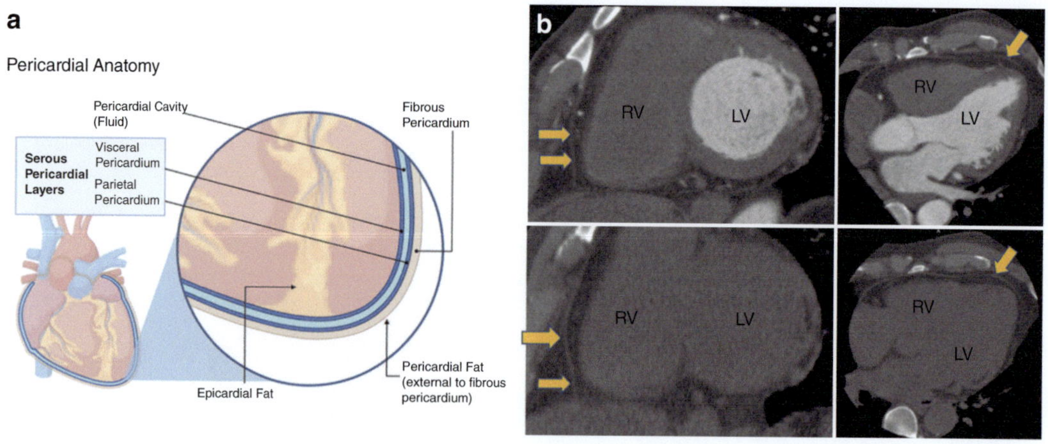

Fig. 10.24 Panel **a** illustrates the layers of the pericardium, with views of the pericardium on the right (Panel **b**)

10.7 Pericardium (Fig. 10.24)

- *Pericardium* consists of layers including the fibrous and serous pericardium. The serous pericardium includes the visceral pericardium (which is adjacent to the epicardial surface), a small amount of pericardial fluid, and the parietal pericardium. The nominal fluid at baseline allows lubrication for free cardiac movement within the pericardial sac. The pericardium can occasionally become calcified and thickened secondary to infection, inflammatory conditions, radiation, malignancy or other trauma.
- Normal pericardium thickness varies based on the region. On CT imaging, the width of the thinnest segments can range from 0.7 to 1.2 mm, but 2.0 mm is conventionally accepted as the upper limit of normal and a diameter of >4.0 mm in any area of the pericardium is considered abnormal.
- *Epicardial Fat* is the fat on the epicardial surface and often surrounds the coronary arteries.
- *Pericardial Fat* is the fat on the surface of the parietal pericardium.
- *Pericardial Effusion* represents fluid in the pericardial cavity, and can be serous, hemorrhagic or purulent. Attenuation values can help differentiate exudative (20–60 HU), transudative (<10 HU), or hemorrhagic effusions (>60 HU). When this fluid accumulates and develops pressure beyond the intracardiac filling pressures, hemodynamic compromise can result and this is called *cardiac tamponade*.

10.8 Cardiac Veins

The cardiac veins are not usually imaged on typical coronary CT protocols with arterial phase timing, but occasionally can be visualized or even obscure clear visualization of the coronaries depending on contrast timing (Fig. 10.25).

- *Great Cardiac Vein (GCV)* and courses around the left atrioventricular groove in a path adjacent to the Left Circumflex artery to usually terminate in the Coronary Sinus, drains the Anterior Interventricular Vein.
- *Posterior and Lateral Marginal Veins of the Left Ventricle* drain into the GCV or coronary sinus.
- *Anterior Interventricular Vein (AIV)* runs down the anterior interventricular groove parallel to the left anterior descending artery.
- *Middle Cardiac Vein (MCV)* runs down the posterior interventricular groove in the same distribution of the posterior descending artery and empties into the coronary sinus.
- *Small Cardiac Vein (SCV)* courses around the right atrioventricular groove and drains the right ventricular venous branches.
- *Coronary Sinus (CS)* receives the deoxygenated blood from all veins and returns this volume to the inferior right atrium (Fig. 10.9, Panel e).

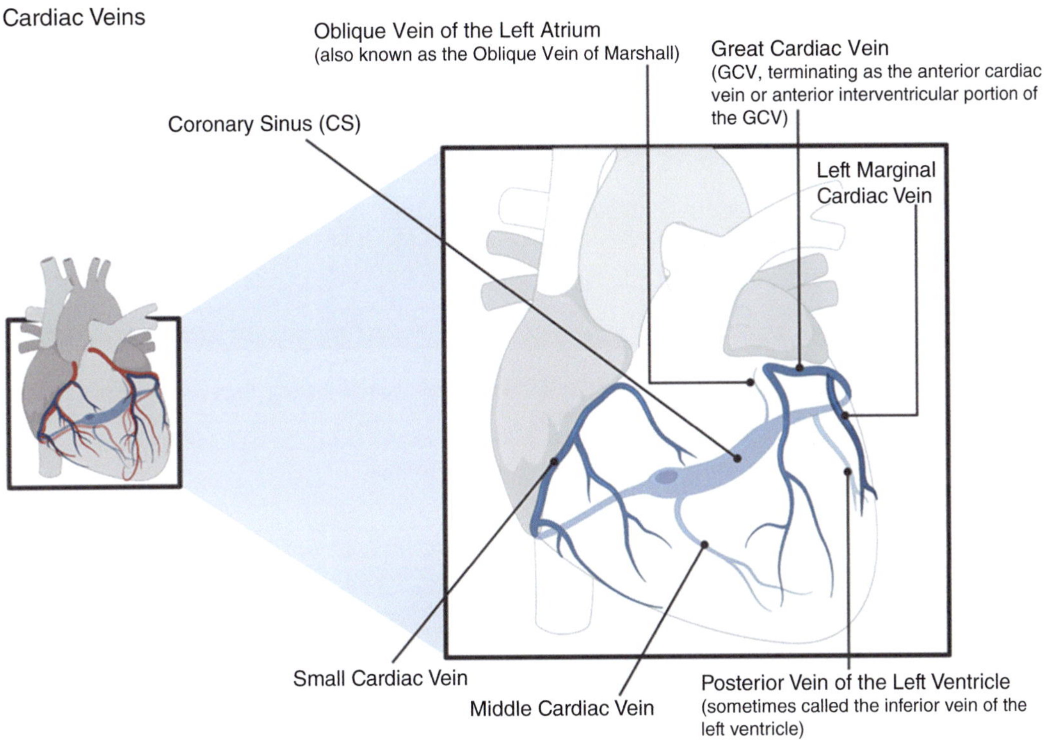

Fig. 10.25 The cardiac veins are illustrated along with the representation of the relationship of the veins to the coronary arteries. The anterior interventricular vein parallels the LAD, and along with the left marginal and posterior veins, drains into the great cardiac vein which then drains into the coronary sinus. The middle cardiac vein runs alongside the posterior descending artery, and along with the small cardiac vein, also drains into the coronary sinus

10.8.1 Cardiac Resynchronization Therapy (CRT) Considerations and CCTA

- Combined RV and LV pacing is performed in certain situations to improve cardiac function.
- Pacing of the LV is done by placing a lead in the great cardiac vein via the coronary sinus (generally posterolateral in location).
- The diameter and angle of the great cardiac vein can help in anticipating the degree of procedural difficulty.
- Vessel size is an important criterion for selecting the target vein.
- In order to visualize the venous anatomy, scanning is performed approximately 6–8 s after the peak enhancement in the descending aorta.

10.9 Coronary Artery Anomalies

- Normally, the left main originates the left coronary cusp and bifurcates into the LAD and left circumflex arteries. The RCA normally originated from the right coronary cusp.
- Coronary arteries that do not have a normal origin or course are considered anomalous.
- There is a range of severity of anomalies and the majority are not clinically significant.
- Scarce prospective data are available about the appropriate management of coronary artery anomalies and the benefit of interventions remains controversially discussed.
- Examples of coronary anomalies.
  - Separate ostia of the LAD and LCx with both arising from the left coronary

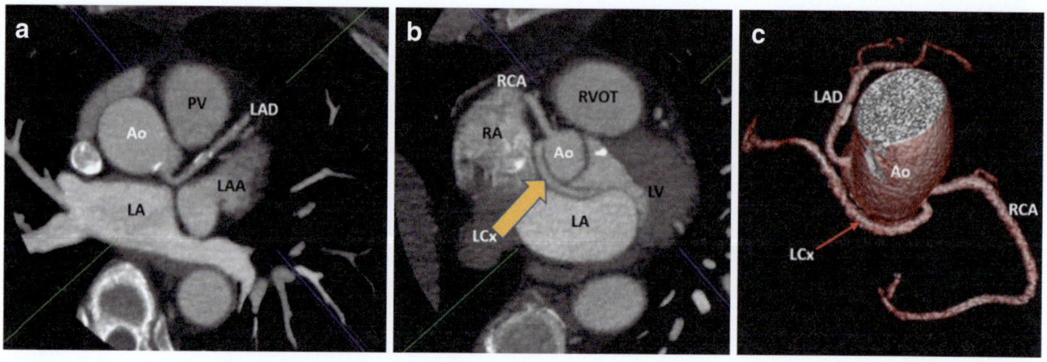

Fig. 10.26 A benign coronary anomaly is shown here. A long left main (Panel **a**) is the first indication of a potential coronary anomaly. Panel **b** and **c** demonstrate the non-dominant left circumflex artery originating just posterior to the right coronary artery from a separate and distinct ostium in the right coronary cusp, then taking a retro-aortic course to eventually subtend the typical anterolateral left ventricle

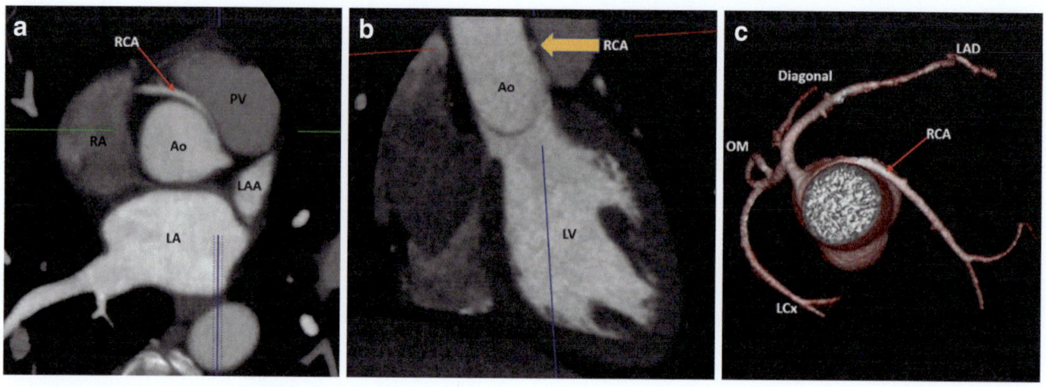

Fig. 10.27 Malignant anomalous right coronary artery originating from the (opposite) left coronary cusp. This vessel has several malignant features, including acute angle take off, inter-arterial course (between the aorta and pulmonary artery), slit-like orifice, and possible intramural component

cusp (Fig. 10.26). This anomaly is among the most common and considered benign.

- Another benign variant of separate ostial includes the LCx originating from the right coronary cusp with a retro-aortic course (Fig. 10.26).
- Anomalous origin of Left Main or RCA from the opposing coronary cusp.
  - Origin of the RCA from the left coronary cusp (Fig. 10.27).
  - Origin of the left main from the right coronary cusp.
  - These anomalies are considered not benign when the vessel traverses anteriorly between aortic root and pulmonary artery. If these anomalies are implicated in sudden cardiac death remains unclear, however.
  - *Some additional features are considered unfavorable*:
    - Acute take off angle (origin of vessel is acute).
    - Slit-like orifice.
    - Intramural course (vessel within the wall of the aorta).
- Anomalous origin from the pulmonary artery.
  - Most common form is anomalous origin of the left main from the pulmonary artery (ALCAPA).
  - Typically discovered in infants and may be associated with dyspnea and heart failure.

References

1. Libby P, Bonow RO, Mann DL, Tamaselli GF, Bhatt DL, Solomon SD. Braunwald's heart disease. 12th ed. Philadelphia, PA: Elsevier; 2022.
2. Cerqueira MD, Weissman NJ, Dilsizian V, Jacobs AK, Kaul S, Laskey WK, Pennell DJ, Rumberger JA, Ryan T, Verani MS, American Heart Association Writing Group on Myocardial Segmentation and Registration for Cardiac Imaging. Standardized myocardial segmentation and nomenclature for tomographic imaging of the heart. A statement for healthcare professionals from the Cardiac Imaging Committee of the Council on Clinical Cardiology of the American Heart Association. Circulation. 2002;105(4):539–42. PMID: 11815441. https://doi.org/10.1161/hc0402.102975.
3. Baim DS. Grossman's cardiac catheterization, angiography, & intervention. 7th ed. Philadelphia, PA: Lippincott Williams & Wilkins; 2021.
4. Rudski LG, Lai WW, Afilalo J, Hua L, Handschumacher MD, Chandrasekaran K, Solomon SD, Louie EK, Schiller NB. Guidelines for the echocardiographic assessment of the right heart in adults: a report from the American Society of Echocardiography endorsed by the European Association of Echocardiography, a registered branch of the European Society of Cardiology, and the Canadian Society of Echocardiography. J Am Soc Echocardiogr. 2010;23(7):685–713; quiz 786-8. PMID: 20620859. https://doi.org/10.1016/j.echo.2010.05.010.

11 Coronary Stenosis Assessment by CT

John Hoe

Abstract

Assessment for coronary artery disease by CCTA commonly includes estimation of coronary artery stenosis. This chapter describes systematic methods of how to visually estimate as well as to quantify diameter stenosis degree. Furthermore, the utility of area and area stenosis assessment is discussed as well as methods of detecting chronic total occlusions.

Keywords

Computed tomography angiography · Coronary artery disease · Atherosclerosis · Coronary stenosis

Abbreviations

3D-VR	3D volume rendered
CCTA	Coronary CTA
CPR	Curved planar reconstruction
CTO	Chronic total occlusion
DS	Diameter stenosis
ICA	Invasive coronary angiography
MIP	Maximum intensity projections
MLA	Minimal luminal diameter
MPR	Multiplanar reconstruction
NPV	Negative predictive value
PPV	Positive predictive value
QCTA	Quantitative coronary CTA
RD	Reference diameter
UHR-CT	Ultra-high-resolution CT

11.1 Pathophysiology of Coronary Arterial Lumen Narrowing

11.1.1 Introduction

- Coronary arterial lumen narrowing most commonly occurs as result of atherosclerotic disease. Rapid acceleration of lumen narrowing may occur after plaque disruption and healing or with associated vascular thrombosis.
- Lumen obstruction from vascular injury, e.g., dissection, is less common but critical to consider in the acute setting.
- Coronary lumen narrowing may occur as result of mechanical forces, e.g., myocardial bridging, which is rarely associated with adverse patient outcome.

J. Hoe (✉)
Department of Radiology, Mount Elizabeth Hospital, Singapore, Republic of Singapore

A. A. Zadeh, J. Hoe (eds.), *Practical Guide to Cardiac CT*,
https://doi.org/10.1007/978-981-97-6919-3_11

11.1.2 Brief Overview of Coronary Atherogenesis

- Typically, intimal hyperplasia of the coronary artery wall develops first with smooth muscle cell migration from the arterial wall media to the arterial wall intima.
- Due to endothelial dysfunction or injury, LDL cholesterol enters from the blood into the intima and is taken up by macrophages. These are loaded with lipid to form a lipid core. The lipid core accumulates and the external vascular wall remodels to accommodate the lipid rich core, also called positive remodeling. The size of the lumen of the artery does not at this stage change significantly (Fig. 11.1).
- As the lipid plaque accumulates, luminal narrowing may occur unless there is compensatory enlargement of the vessel, termed external (or positive) vascular remodeling.
- The lipid core may stabilize and undergo fibrocalcific changes as well as develop a thick fibrous cap.
- Erosion or rupture of the plaque may lead to healing or to vascular thrombosis which may cause an acute coronary syndrome [1].
- Further details on vulnerable/ high-risk plaque and plaque rupture are discussed in Chap. 13.

11.2 Diagnostic Accuracy of Coronary CTA (CCTA) for the Detection of Coronary Stenosis in Patients Presenting with Stable Symptoms

- Many studies and multicenter trials, mainly using 64 MSCT scanners, have been performed to assess the accuracy of CCTA to detect coronary stenosis ≥50% luminal diameter stenosis compared to invasive quantitative coronary angiography (QCA).
- The high sensitivity, usually >95% and high negative predictive value (NPV), usually >97%, suggests that CCTA can be used to reliably detect and exclude a coronary stenosis of ≥50% in selected populations, assuming adequate reader experience (Table 11.1).
- A negative CCTA scan result can reliably rule out the presence of severe CAD, especially in patients with low or intermediate risk of CAD.
- However, high pre-test probability of CAD (e.g., in populations with high disease prevalence) is associated with lower NPV [2].

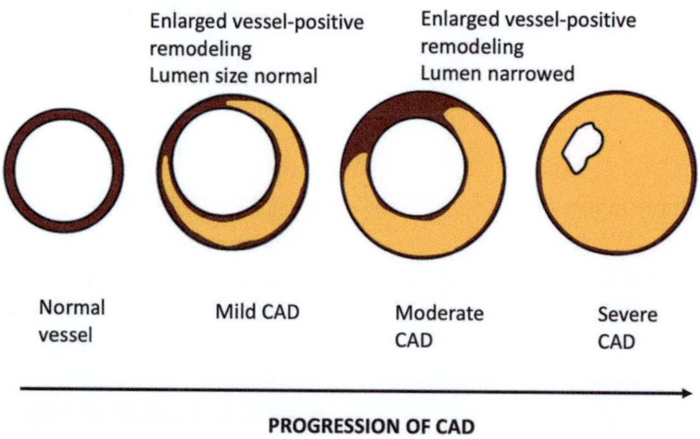

Fig. 11.1 Progression of coronary artery disease from normal artery wall and lumen to positive remodeling and lumen size unchanged to moderate and severe disease with lumen narrowing. (Diagram modified after Sandfort V, Lima JAC, Bluemke DA. Noninvasive Imaging of atherosclerotic plaque progession. https://doi.org/10.1161/CIRCIMAGING.115.003316 [1])

Table 11.1 Diagnostic performance of CCTA for detection of coronary diameter stenosis ≥50% by invasive angiography (per patient analysis) [2, 4–8]

Study	No of patients	Sensitivity	Specificity	PPV	NPV
Four multicenter studies (64 MSCT) (Stefani 2015)	1046	81%–99%	84%–93%	64%–92%	83%–99%
320 MDCT meta-analysis of 12 studies (Sun Z 2015)	1592	96% (mean)	86%(mean)	89% (mean)	93% (mean)
Dual source CT-first generation-meta-analysis (Jiang B 2014)	2047	97% (mean)	86% (mean)	85% (mean)	97% (mean)
256 MDCT single center (Petcherski 2013)	121	97%	97%	75%	100%
High-definition whole heart 256 MDCT single center (Mushtaq 2019)	100	98%	95%	88%	99%
Ultrahigh resolution 128MDCT single center (Takagi 2018)	38	100%	67%	94%	100%

- The positive predictive value (PPV) of CCTA is variable (~64–93%), depending on the disease prevalence in the study population. The low PPV means overestimation of ≥50% stenosis or false positive results.
- Particularly in low risk populations, false positive CCTA findings (stenosis ≥50%) may lead to unnecessary follow-up testing, including invasive coronary angiography (ICA).
- Among noninvasive tests for CAD (e.g., vs. exercise treadmill testing, stress echo, SPECT-MPI), CCTA is the most accurate modality for diagnosis and prognosis [3].

11.2.1 Limitations of Reported Diagnostic Accuracy Studies of CCTA Compared to ICA

- Limitations of diagnostic accuracy studies include:
  - Using a binary cut-off for diameter stenosis (DS) ≥50% stenosis.
  - Unlimited time to analyze the images.
  - Performance in expert academic centers or core laboratories.
  - Consensus reading of two expert readers.
  - Exclusion of segments with severe calcifications, artifacts, poor image quality.
- In clinical practice, patients cannot be excluded from analysis even if image quality is suboptimal, e.g., due to fast heart rates or high image noise.
- The presence of calcified plaques will also affect the PPV and NPV of the CCTA scan result.
- Therefore, results from clinical studies may not be achieved in many practices.
- Furthermore, more granular stenosis grading is often required in clinical practice than reported in studies.

11.3 Step-by-Step Approach of Stenosis Assessment

11.3.1 Visual Stenosis Evaluation

Step 1:

- Obtain an overview of the coronary tree by reviewing 3D-volume rendered (VR) images (Fig. 11.2).
- 3D-VR images may be helpful to avoid missing short stenoses as these can sometimes be missed on 2D viewing [9] (Fig. 11.3).
- Know the limitations of the 3D-VR images:
  - changing the thresholds can obscure or create a stenosis;

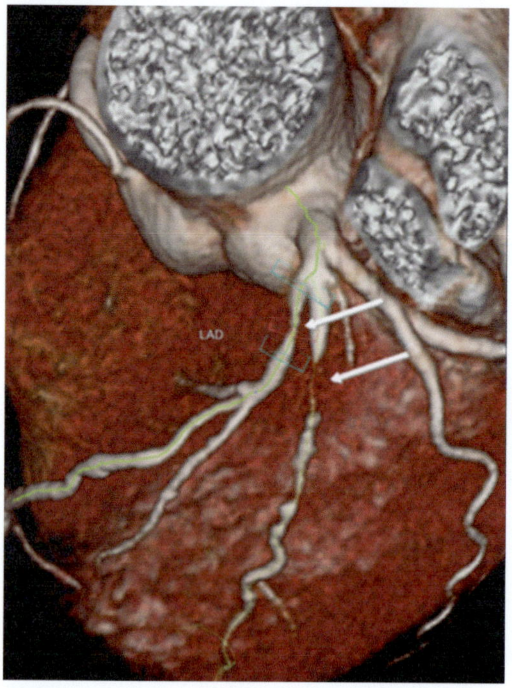

Fig. 11.2 3D-Volume Rendered (VR) image suggests a stenosis in the proximal left anterior descending artery (LAD) and ramus intermedius (RI) branch. Such finding should prompt further analysis of these segments

- 3D-VR images are not accurate for estimation of the degree of stenosis and are not useful if calcifications or stents are present.

- The SCCT guideline for interpretation and reporting of CCTA recommend review of axial, MPR, and MIP images while CPR image review is considered optional [10].

Step 2:

- The axial view images serve as the main source of coronary stenosis analysis because they require less postprocessing and thus contain less sources for errors.
- An initial overview is best achieved with thicker MIPs, e.g., 3 mm. Too thick MIPs may not disclose lesions.
- Lesions should then be interrogated with thin slab MIPs (e.g., 1 mm) or the source dataset (e.g., 0.25–0.625 mm depending on the minimum available detector width).
- Truly cross-sectional/axial images (i.e., without adjusting the plane) are rarely used for stenosis quantification because the minimum lesion diameters are typically not aligned in this plane, except for the mid-RCA.

Step 3:

- Oblique MPRs often provide the best option to obtain cross-sectional and long axis views in true orthogonal planes.
- Every stenosis should be assessed in at least two orthogonal views and/or cross-sectionally (Fig. 11.4) to account for irregular/eccentric lumen borders.
- Oblique MPRs were found to be most accurate for stenosis evaluation (superior to axial images, curved MPRs, MIPs, and 3D-VR images) [11] although we prefer cross-sectional assessment for luminal diameter stenosis (as discussed further below).

11.3.2 Quantification of Stenoses

Methods of quantifying stenoses by CCTA

- Emulating ICA, conventional assessment of stenosis degree by CCTA has rested on diameter measurements and calculating diameter stenosis (DS) in %.
- Other metrics for assessment of coronary stenosis, e.g., minimal luminal diameter (MLD in mm), minimal luminal area (MLA in mm^2), and area stenosis (AS in %) are less commonly used and are discussed further in Sect. 11.3.6.

11.3.3 Quantification of Diameter Stenosis

The three common methods of quantifying diameter stenosis by CCTA are:

11.3.3.1 Visual Estimation ("Eyeballing")

Visual estimates of diameter stenosis are typically provided with a range, thus representing a "semiquantitative" or qualitative approach, e.g.,

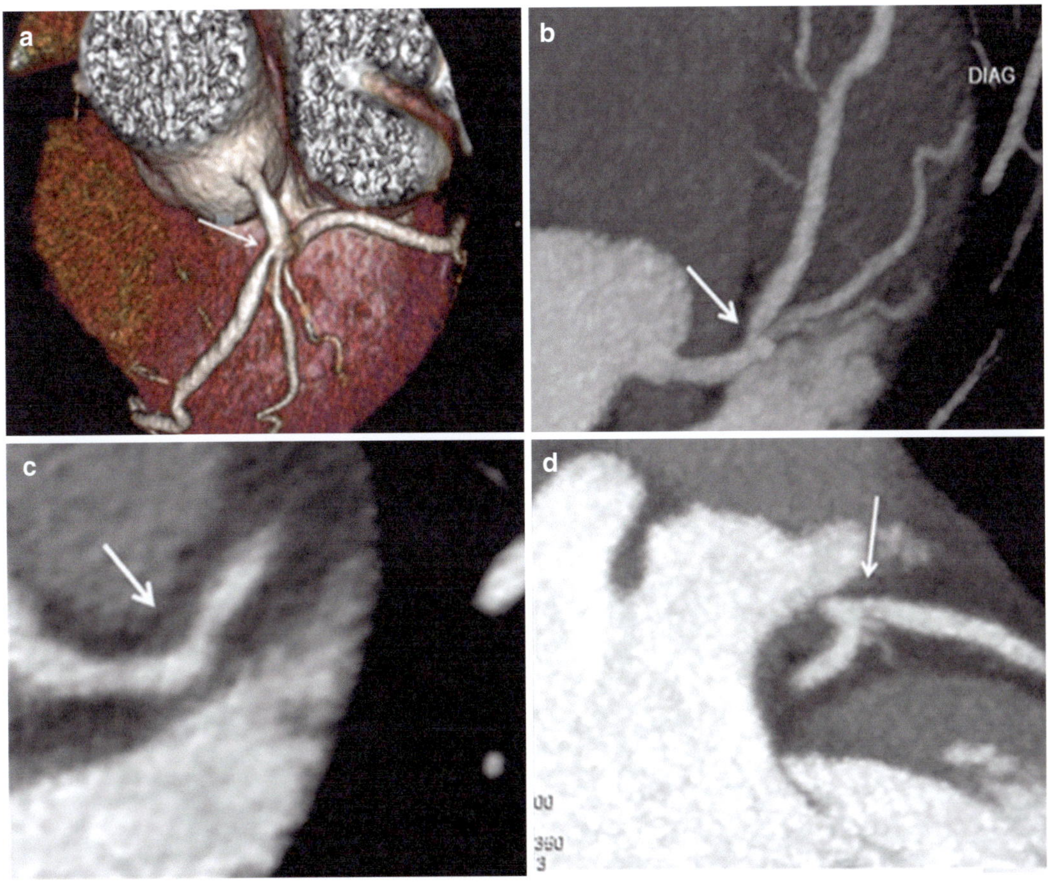

Fig. 11.3 Panels **a**–**d**. An ostial LAD stenosis of approximately 25%–50% can be well appreciated on the 3D-VR image (**a**) but may be missed on axial scans and Curved Planar Reformations (CPR) and thick slab maximum intensity projections (MIP) (panels **b**–**d**)

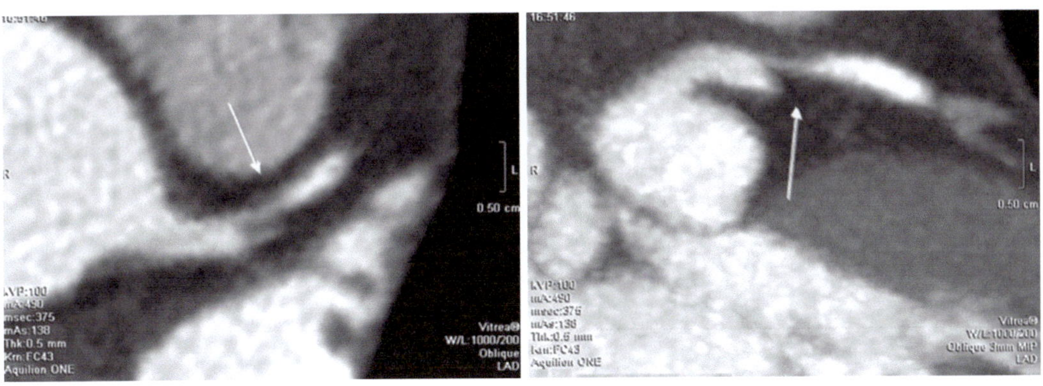

Fig. 11.4 A diameter stenosis of approximately 70–80% is seen in the proximal LAD on both axial and sagittal views

25–50%, etc. This method remains the predominant method of stenosis assessment in daily clinical practice despite the ease of aided contour detection.

- Visually estimate the DS% after comparing the contrast filled lumen at the site of maximal stenosis with the lumen of the normal reference site, this is usually expressed in as a percentage range of about 20–25% (Fig. 11.5).

Key Point
Selecting an appropriate reference site for comparing lumen diameter to the lesion site is critical and may greatly influence the stenosis degree. The reference site should be free of atherosclerosis and as close as possible to the lesion and not be affected by lumen tapering after large side branches. Ideally, the reference lumen diameter is derived from the average of a proximal and distal (in reference to the lesion) lumen diameter [12].

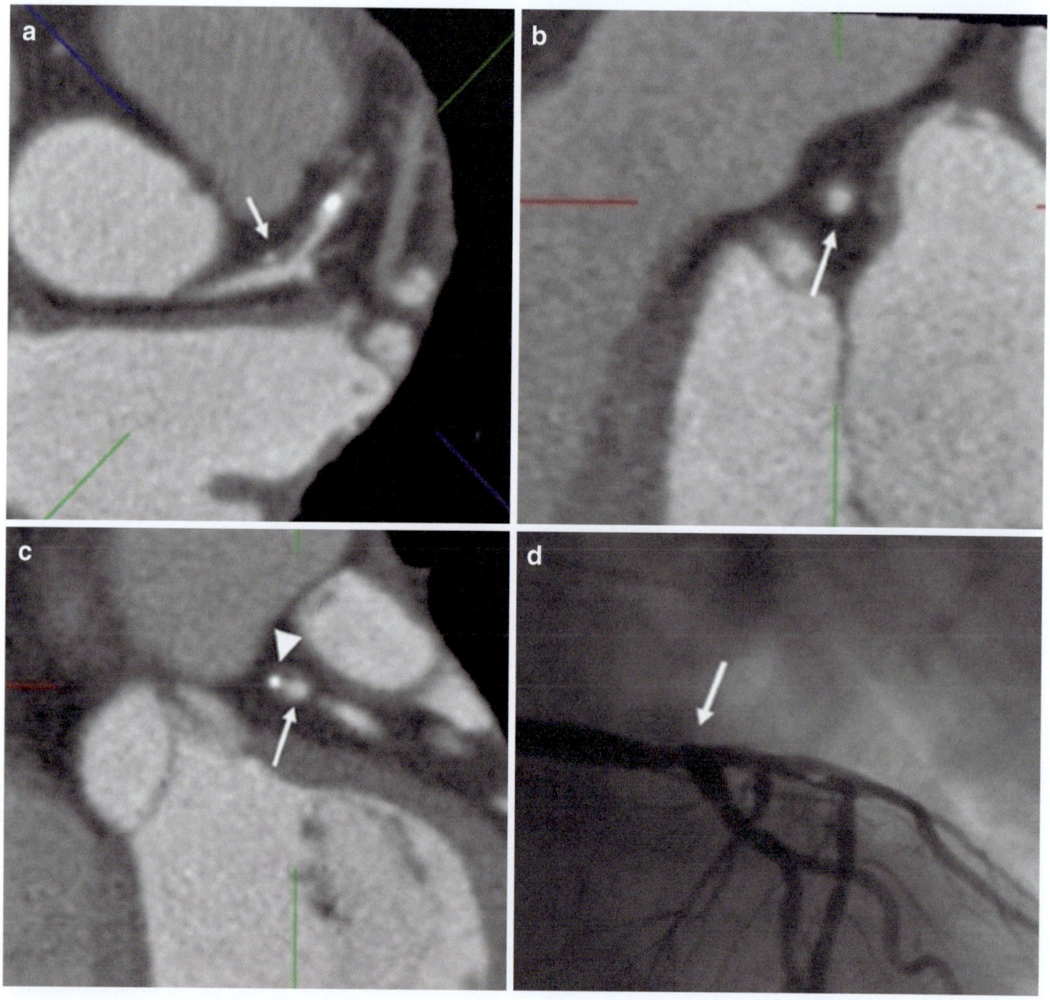

Fig. 11.5 (Panels **a–d**). Panel **a** shows a large eccentric plaque in the distal left main and ostial/proximal LAD with positive remodeling. If the reference diameter is selected in the distal left main, the LAD stenosis may be overestimated. Panel **b** provides a cross-sectional image of the mildly diseased left main proximal to the lesion. Panel **c** shows the site of maximum atheroma and lumen narrowing in the distal left main (arrow) which may be compared with the lumen dimensions in Panel **b** (a true, non-diseased reference site is not available). The resultant lumen narrowing is minimal, i.e., <25% DS. Note positive remodeling with noncalcified plaque and a speck of calcified plaque (arrowhead). Panel **d** reveals images from invasive coronary angiography (ICA), confirming only minimal narrowing of the distal left main. (Images: From Hoe J and Toh KH 2007 with permission of the publisher. Copyright ©2007, Springer)

11.3.3.2 Direct, Manual Measurement of Lumen Stenosis

- This entails using measurement tools, e.g., calliper, ruler, and determining the minimal lumen diameter (MLD, mm) at the site of most severe lumen narrowing in relation to appropriate reference diameters (Fig. 11.6) [12].
- Ideally, the MLD is determined from cross-sectional images perpendicular to the centerline of the vessel.
- The stenosis degree (DS%) is determined by this formula: (RD − MLD/RD] × 100. Alternatively: (1 − [MLD/RD]) × 100 (Fig. 11.7).
- Another method of manually measuring the MLD is to create a long axis view of the stenosis (angio like view) parallel to the long axis of the vessel and comparing the luminal diameter at the stenosis with a normal reference site proximal or distal to the stenosis (average of proximal and distal normal reference diameter without interrupting side branches) (Fig. 11.8).

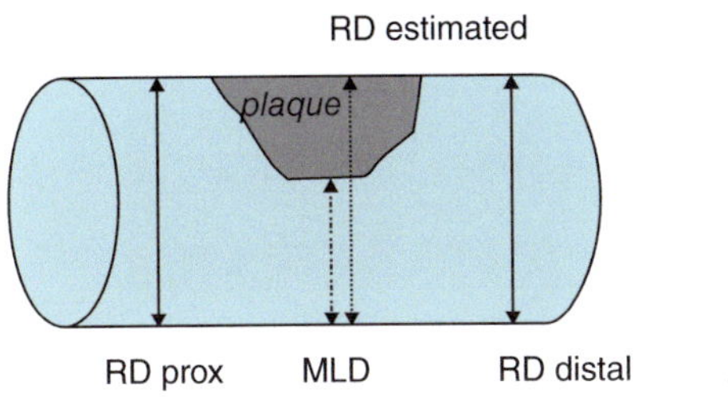

Fig. 11.6 The smallest diameter at the lesion site should be compared to the average normal reference diameters proximal or distal to the stenosis (RD prox and RD distal)

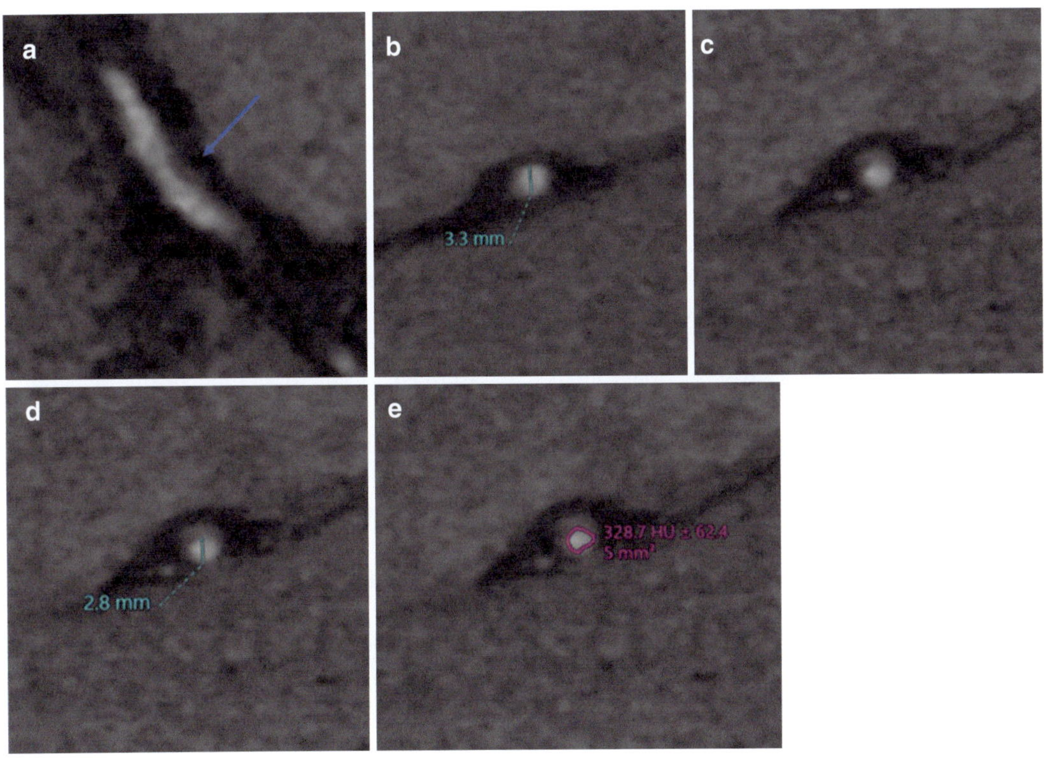

Fig. 11.7 (Panels **a**–**e**) An example of performing manual MLD measurements at the site of maximal stenosis and at the nearest normal reference site. The panels reveal: (**a**) Axial view of a distal RCA stenosis (arrow) on a 2.0-mm MIP image. (**b**) Cross-section view on an MPR image of the normal proximal reference site with manual measurement of the minimal luminal diameter (MLD) in mm. (**c**) Cross-section view of the site of maximal stenosis in the distal RCA without measurements. (**d**) Cross-section view of the site of maximal stenosis with manual measurements of MLD in mm. (**e**) Cross-section view of the site of maximal stenosis with manual measurement of minimal luminal area (MLA) in mm^2 (See Sect. 11.3.5)

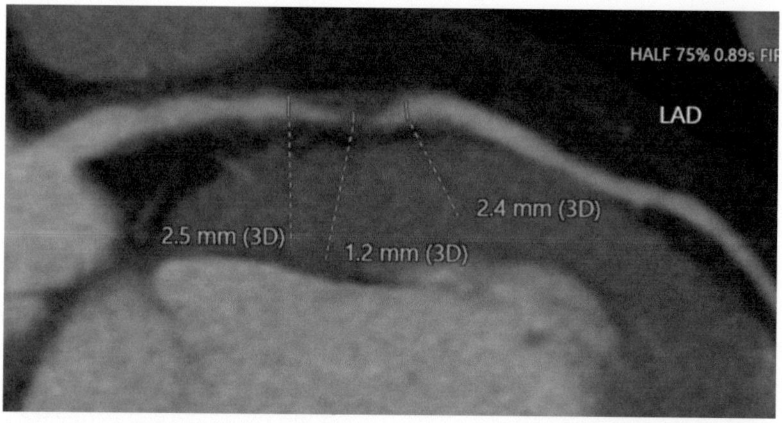

Fig. 11.8 A long axis CPR view of the mid-LAD is shown revealing a stenosis with minimum diameter of 1.2 mm compared to the normal proximal and distal reference sites of 2.5 mm and 2.4 mm. The resultant DS = [(2.5 mm–1.2 mm)/2.5 mm] × 100 = 52%. By visual estimation, the stenosis is more severe, i.e., >70% DS, demonstrating the known tendency to visually overestimate stenoses compared to quantification

- *MPR vs. MIP for Stenosis Quantification*
  - MIP images may obscure stenoses because pixels containing high density contrast in the lumen of the coronary artery are retained while low density plaque pixels are less well represented. Thus, the MIP images may lead to underestimating stenoses (Fig. 11.9).
  - Using the source MPR datasets (e.g., 0.5, 0.625 mm) or thin slice 1–2 mm MIPs rather than >3–5 mm thick slice MIP images is likely to improve stenosis evaluation, especially for cross-sectional image analysis.
  - If the MIPs images are too thick, the stenosis may be underestimated due to partial volume averaging artifacts, particularly related to calcified plaques.

> **Key Point**
> Stenosis assessment using MIP thickness of greater than the vessel size (e.g., >2–3 mm) may lead to underestimating lumen narrowing or even to missing visualization of plaque altogether.

11.3.3.3 Automated or Semiautomated Lumen Contour Analysis (QCTA)

- Most dedicated CT analysis workstations offer QCTA and several commercially available software analysis packages exist (online or offline).
- The software typically either automatedly or semiautomatedly (requires prompting) tracks the contrast filled vessel lumen and identifies the outer vessel wall. The space between vessel wall and lumen borders is typically ascribed to atherosclerotic plaque and often are color coded for easy identification.
- Plaque characterization is commonly available based on the attenuation values of plaque components, e.g., fatty plaque with low density characteristics.
- While contour detection has been improved over the past years, challenges remain particularly with suboptimal image quality and severe calcification.
- Centerline tracking likewise has much improved but manual corrections may be required with suboptimal image quality.

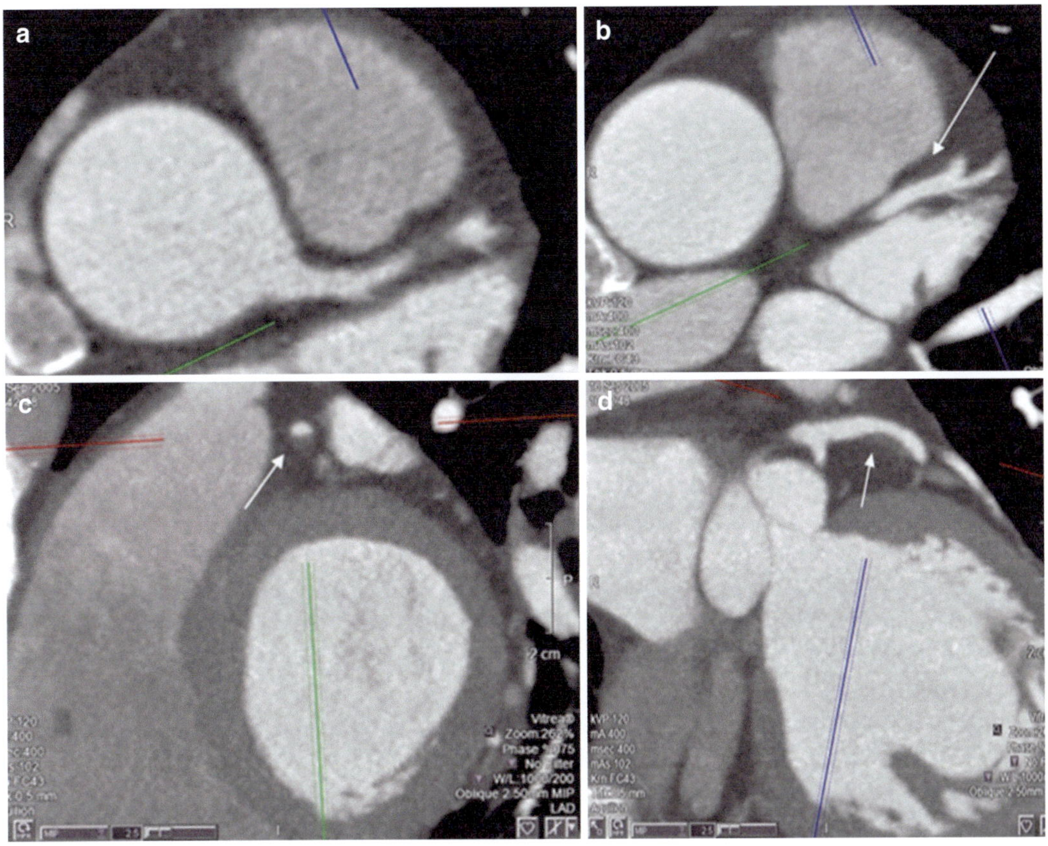

Fig. 11.9 (Panels **a–d**) Atherosclerotic plaque in the proximal LAD can be seen on axial 0.5-mm images (Panel **a**) but not on 3-mm axial MIP images (Panel **b**). Orthogonal views (Panels **c** and **d**) confirm the presence of plaque in the proximal LAD with a diameter stenosis of 25–49%. (From Hoe J and Toh KH 2007 with permission of the publisher. Copyright ©2007, Springer)

- Side-branch detection varies by software and some require user input.
- Software stenosis assessment may occur with or without direction to specific sites or vessels. Similarly, there are various options for automated vs. manual reference site determination.
- In general, software packages focus on determining diameter stenosis, minimum lumen diameter, and minimal lumen area.
- Using a standardized post-processing method, quantitative has been shown to be reproducible but results are less reliable with suboptimal image quality [13].
- Compared to expert analysis, current generation QCTA is associated with adequate sensitivity but low specificity [14], i.e., a tendency for QCTA to overestimate the degree of stenosis [15].
- With continued improvements, QCTA may become the standard of lumen and vessel analysis but validation studies and a consensus on methodology and derived metrics are still lacking.
- QCTA currently does not seem to improve the accuracy of visual estimation but is still useful as an additional tool for quantification of coronary stenosis, e.g.,:
  - To confirm initial visual estimation in difficult situations—such as near an ostium when no normal nearby reference site is available.
  - When large calcified plaques are present.

- For use of MLA mm^2 or area stenosis % (discussed below).
- When coronary plaque analysis is simultaneously assessed with total atheroma volume and plaque characteristics [16].

Key Point

Stenosis assessment using current generation CCTA varies by ±20–25% degrees vs. invasive angiography but recently introduced UHR-CT may overcome CCTA's limitation regarding its spatial resolution.

11.3.4 Quantifying Stenoses in Clinical Practice

- Although CCTA diagnostic accuracy for detecting patients with coronary artery disease is high, there is considerable variability for the degree of stenosis determined by CCTA vs. ICA. The reasons for this discrepancy are numerous, including reader variability for both CCTA and ICA, limits of spatial resolution of CCTA, and limits of displaying complex anatomy accurately by ICA [12].
- Clinical studies with 64-slice CT scanners have shown stenosis degrees varying by ±25%, (within 95% probability range/±2 standard deviations) compared to QCA [17].
- Wide detector scanners, e.g., using 256 or 320-slice CT, have not shown an improvement for stenosis quantification over 64-slice technology (which is unsurprising as spatial resolution is similar) [18].
- Preliminary results from studies using ultra-high-resolution CT (UHR-CT) are promising for improved diagnostic accuracy with detector width of <0.5 mm, even in the presence of severe calcifications [19].
- UHR-CT using photon-counting technology is now commercially available, with through-plane spatial resolution of 0.2 mm and 0.4 mm. Preliminary results indicate high diagnostic accuracy including in patients with severe coronary calcifications and prior stent placement [20].
- Unaided, visual CCTA estimates of stenoses using a 5-point grading system was no worse than manual semiquantitative assessment in one study [21].
- Given the wide limits of agreement, current practice remains focused on visual, multi-tiered grading with broad stenosis ranges to evaluate coronary stenoses.

11.3.5 Use a 5-Point Grading Scale to Report CCTA Stenosis

- The 5-point grading scale has been adopted for clinical practice and is the method currently recommended by the SCCT to report CCTA stenosis [22].
- Examples of standardized reporting of CCTA stenosis shown below [22] (Fig. 11.10).
- Details on reporting Cardiac CT are discussed in Chap. 25.

SCCT Grading system for stenosis severity: degree of luminal diameter stenosis DS%	Terminology	CAD-RADS category
0%	No plaque or visible stenosis	CAD-RADS 0
1–24%	Minimal stenosis	CAD-RADS 1
25–49%	Mild stenosis	CAD-RADS 2
50–69%	Moderate stenosis	CAD-RADS 3
70–99%	Severe stenosis	CAD-RADS 4
100%	Occluded	CAD-RADS 5

11.3.6 Other Metrics Than Diameter Stenosis Assessment for Quantifying Stenosis

- Diameter stenosis assessment has significant limitations for stenosis assessment when the lumen is non-circular; yet it remains the standard metric because of its routine use in the cardiac catheterization laboratory and in clinical studies.

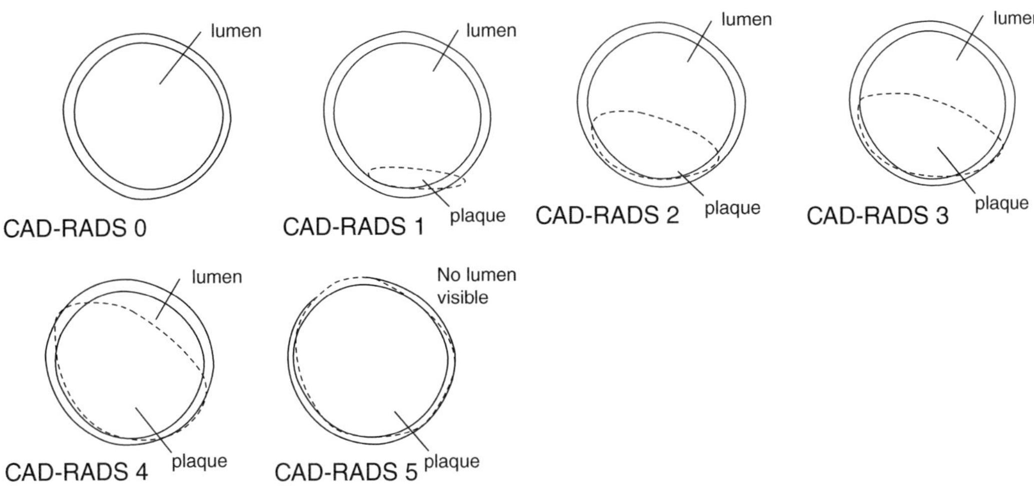

Fig. 11.10 Stenosis Grading. (Modified after: Cury R. CAD-RADS Coronary Artery Disease-Reporting and Data system. JCCT 2022: 16;536 [22])

- Appropriate use criteria statements for PCI [23] defined a physiological significant stenosis by ICA as:
  - ≥70% luminal diameter narrowing by visual assessment measured in the worst view projection (≥50% for a left main stenosis).
  - 40%–70% luminal narrowing by visual assessment associated with an abnormal FFR ≤0.80.
- Other common methods to quantify stenosis include:
  - Minimal luminal diameter (MLD).

    The advantage of MLD alone, given in mm, is that it does not require a reference measurement and thus reduces one source of variability. It can be measured in the long axis view but is best obtained on cross-sectional images as they allow to easily to identify the true MLD.

    The MLD as a metric of stenosis degree is uncommonly used in clinical practice.

    Examples for significant thresholds identified for invasive angiography (Appropriate Use Criteria for PCI) [23] are:

      <2.8 mm for the left main coronary artery.

      <2 mm for the proximal LAD.
  - Minimal luminal area (MLA).

    MLA measurements, given in mm^2, may be used as a metric for quantifying stenosis, often as a supplementary tool in addition to DS%.

    The measurements may be obtained manually or by QCTA software, using true cross-sectional views of the vessel, similar to the use by intravascular ultrasound (IVUS) (Fig. 11.7e).

    Thresholds for significant lumen narrowing have been established by IVUS and may vary according to vessel size [23–25]:

      <6 mm^2 for the left main coronary artery.

        a smaller cut-off may be more appropriate for Asian patients (4.5–4.8 mm^2) [25].

        If MLA of the LM ≥6.0 to 7.5 mm, PCI may be deferred.

      <4 mm^2 for proximal coronary artery segments.

      <3 mm^2 for mid-segments.

    The 2021 Appropriate Use Criteria for PCI [25] state that MLA assessment by IVUS is particularly useful for indeterminate left main disease by ICA, because of IVUS' greater spatial resolution and cross-sectional analysis.

- Area stenosis (AS).

  Percent area stenosis (AS%) may be obtained manually or via QCTA. It is uncommonly used in clinical practice although there are conceptual advantages over diameter stenosis as AS% by QCTA performs similarly to IVUS.

  For computing AS%, MLA is compared to a normal reference area, similar to DS% assessment. Alternatively, MLA is compared to the vessel area of the same cross-section. This approach, often used in histopathology and with IVUS imaging, neglects the concept of external vascular remodeling, however, and thus may poorly correlate to other metrics of stenosis assessment.

  QCTA tends to overestimate MLA mm^2 compared to IVUS but AS% assessment correlates well with IVUS [13].

  Assuming circular lumen geometry, a 50% DS corresponds to a 75% AS, while 75% DS corresponds to a 94% AS [26] (Fig. 11.11).

  Like MLA, AS% may be used mainly to determine how PCI should be performed to guide stent implantation, especially for the left main coronary artery and complex lesions [25].

Key Points (Table 11.2)

- Visual estimates remain default approach to quantify diameter stenosis (DS) in %, commonly using a 5-point grading scale of 0%, 1–24%, 25–49%, 50–69%, 70–99%, 100%.
- Manual measurements of MLD and MLA are not often performed because of the advances of QCTA.
- QCTA software may provide MLA (mm^2), AS (%), as well as DS (%) but performance varies, particularly with less than optimal image quality. QCTA may be useful when no appropriate normal reference site is identified, for stenosis near an ostium or bifurcation of an artery, or if calcified plaques are present obscuring visualization of the lumen, especially when diffuse disease is present.
- Key thresholds for significant stenoses by CCTA are:
  - MLA—For left main <6 mm^2, for proximal non-left main artery <4 mm^2.
  - AS%—For any artery >90% AS usually corresponds to >70% DS.

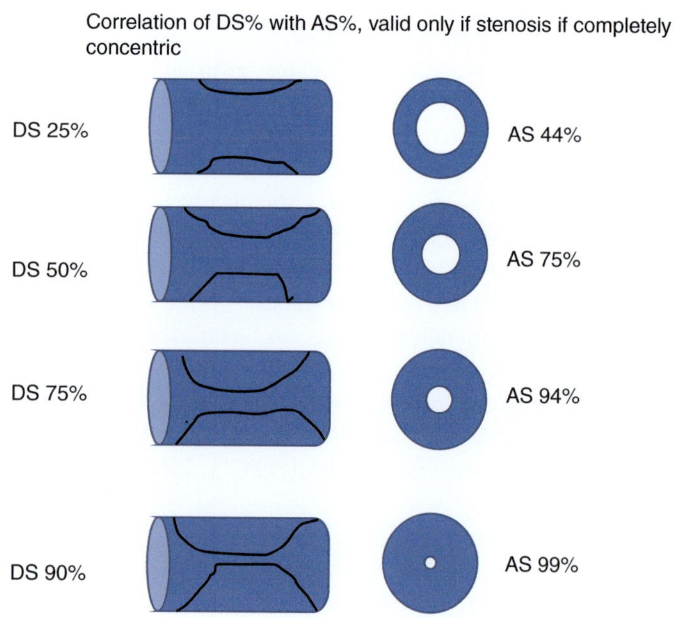

Fig. 11.11 Correlation of diameter stenosis DS% and area stenosis AS%

Table 11.2 Comparison of different methods of quantification of coronary stenosis

	Visual estimation	Manual or semiautomated measurement	Automated software QCTA
Uses and advantages	• Easy application and default method for clinical quantification of stenosis • Accurate vs. ICA by ±20–25%	• Occasionally use; especially when calcified plaques present, at bifurcations or ostia	• Largely research tool at present • Faster processing than manual evaluation
Disadvantages	• Subjective/reader dependent • Variability for reference site selection	• Time consuming • Variability for reference site selection	• Performance varies based on software and image quality • No standards for reporting
Diameter stenosis (DS%) as quantification metric	Default metric used as it is similar to what is used at ICA	Can be calculated if lumen diameter at normal reference site also measured	Readily calculated by software but nearest normal reference site /s needs to be manually selected and determining reference site varies and remains challenging Use CAD-RADS 5 -point grading scale for reporting and not the DS% result generated by QCTA
Minimal luminal diameter (mm)	Cannot be visually estimated	Can be calculated from long axis or cross-sectional views	• Readily calculated by software • Accuracy varies by software and image quality • Generally <2.8 mm for LM or <2 mm for proximal LAD indicate significant stenosis
MLA in mm^2	Cannot be visually estimated	Can be calculated by software after manual contouring	• Readily calculated by software • Niche application for LMD: <6 mm^2 for LM (<4.8 mm^2 in Asians)
Area stenosis AS in %	Cannot be visually estimated	Can be calculated by software after manual contouring	• Readily calculated by software • AS>90% is significant and is ≥70% DS

11.4 Limitations of ICA as the Reference Standard

- Discrepancies between CCTA quantification of stenosis versus ICA or QCA are commonly seen in clinical practice. Reasons may include:
  - ICA has superior spatial resolution to common CT technology.
  - ICA reader variability may be ±20%, especially for 40%–70% stenoses.
  - Compared with QCA, visual assessment at ICA tends to overestimate lesion severity and the difference between visual estimation and QCA is ±10–20% [26].
  - Reference site selection may differ between CT vs. ICA with large impact on resultant diameter stenosis. QCA may employ algorithms for interpolating a reference diameter at lesion site while CT based algorithms either use single or dual reference sites) (Fig. 11.7).
- In clinical practice, it helps educating patients and referring providers regarding the variability of stenosis assessment by CCTA as well as ICA and the challenges in the setting of suboptimal image quality.

Summary (Fig. 11.12)

- DS% is most commonly used as the metric to report coronary stenosis by CCTA and ICA. (Both are typically based on visual estimation).
- Supplementary tools for automated assessment are helpful if contours are adequately traced.
- Fully automated contour detection for stenosis assessment has not been approved for clinical use.

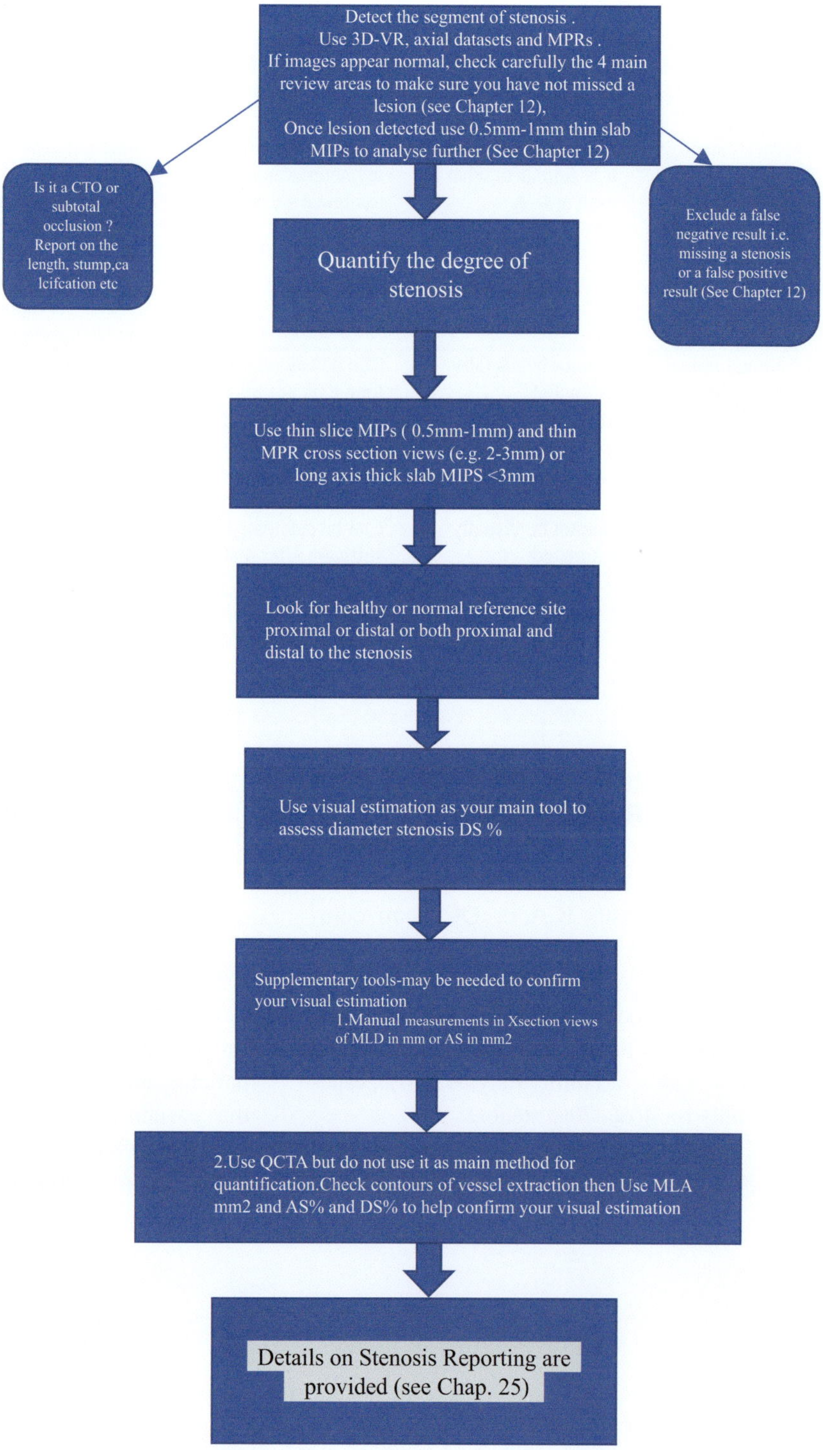

Fig. 11.12 Overview and flow chart of how to read a CCTA scan for stenosis evaluation

- There is considerable variability of stenosis assessment by both CCTA and ICA leading to ±20–25% differences.
- In general, CCTA stenosis estimates tend to be higher compared to ICA (<50% DS by CCTA is unlikely to be found to be significant by ICA).
- For the less experienced CCTA reader, follow-up and correlation with the ICA findings is strongly recommended to allow calibration and improvement of agreement.

11.5 Diagnosis of a Chronic Total Occlusion (CTO) on CCTA

- The presence of a CTO may be missed by less experienced readers or misinterpreted as severe stenosis of >70% DS which may have implications for management (Fig. 11.13).
- Recognizing a CTO on the CCTA scan may help planning of revascularization.
- Key to recognize CTO is to identify soft tissue density material in the lumen with no contrast—usually best seen on cross-sectional views. Complete absence of contrast suggests a total occlusion at that level.
- As there may be contrast seen in the lumen distal to the occluded artery, a less experienced reader may report a severe stenosis (>70–90%) rather than a total occlusion (100%).
- The contrast material distal to the occlusion often is due to retrograde flow from collaterals (Fig. 11.14).
- At ICA, the lumen of the artery distal to the CTO is often not visualized by direct injection of contrast into the artery, but collaterals may be visualized after injection of contrast into the contralateral artery.
- It can be very difficult to differentiate between a CTO (100%) and subtotal occlusion (99%) on CCTA (Fig. 11.15).
- A CTO tends to show longer occlusion length ≥15 mm and is more often associated with other features such as more frequent side branches and calcification at the stump [28].
- A CTO is usually easily recognized on a 3D-VR image (Fig. 11.16).
- Certain features may be helpful to the interventional cardiologist in planning the management of a CTO:
  - Length of stenosis—short or long, e.g., >2 cm.
  - Presence of multiple occlusions separated by contrast filled segments.
  - Shape of stump—tapered or blunt.
  - Presence of calcification at the stump of the occlusion or within the segment of occlusion (more than 50% of the cross-sectional area of calcium is considered severe).
  - Presence of collaterals—although these are not usually by CCTA.
  - Tortuosity of the artery proximal or distal to the CTO-bending of the vessel >45%.
  - Track and position of the opacified distal vessel [28].
- Consider scoring systems to aid PCI for CTOs based on CCTA findings such as J-CTO score (Multicentre CTO Registry of Japan) and CT-RECTOR score (Computed Tomography Registry of Chronic Total Occlusion Revascularization) [29].
- Pre-PCI CCTA may improve PCI success rates and outcomes [30, 31].

Summary of Key Points

- CTO may be difficult to differentiate from a subtotal occlusion, especially for stenosis length <15 mm.
- Consider reporting CCTA features such as length of the CTO, presence of calcium at the stump, >45 bending of the artery proximal or distal to CTO, etc.
- The correct diagnosis on CCTA may facilitate proper planning of revascularization.

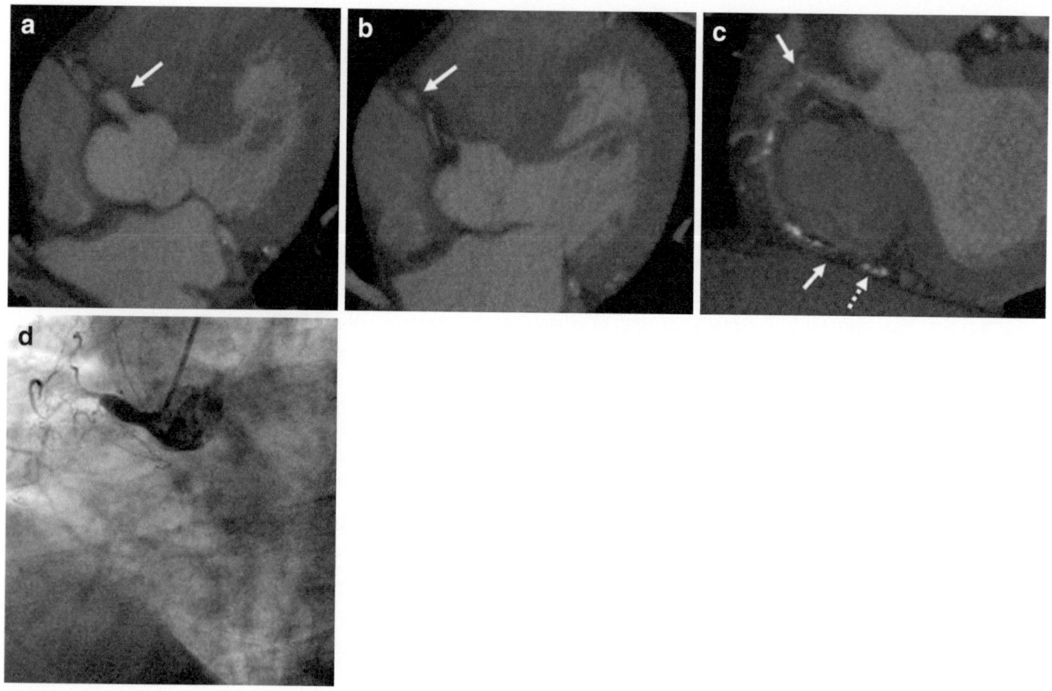

Fig. 11.13 (Panels **a**–**d**) Long CTO ranging from the proximal to distal RCA. Note the abrupt change of contrast in the proximal RCA (Panel **a**) and no contrast in the lumen of the mid-RCA (Panel **b**). The length of the CTO is indicated between arrows. Faint opacification of distal RCA (dashed arrow, Panel **c**) may indicate collateral flow. ICA shows CTO of RCA with no opacification of mid- or distal-RCA without an option to estimate the length of CTO (Panel **d**)

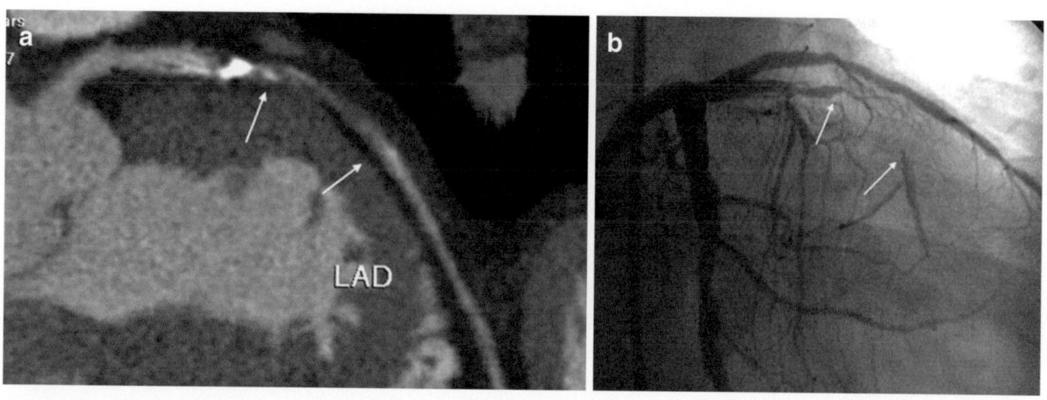

Fig. 11.14 (Panels **a** and **b**) Panel **a** reveals a CTO of the mid-LAD by CCTA with a segment of non-opacified lumen with reconstitution of contrast in the distal LAD (by collaterals, not seen here). Panel **b** confirms findings by ICA (arrows). Note presence of large calcified plaque at the stump of the occlusion

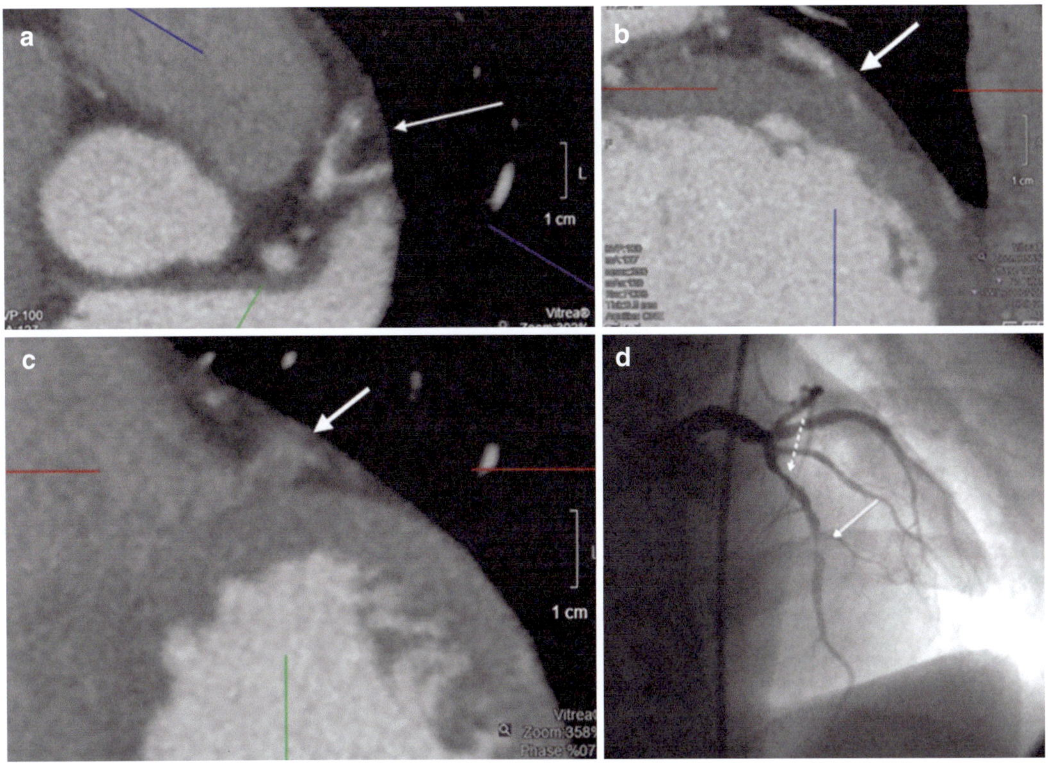

Fig. 11.15 (Panels **a**–**d**) Axial images (**a**) show a short segment of disease in mid-LAD which on the longitudinal images and cross-sectional images reveal no contrast in the lumen (**b** and **c**). This is likely a CTO or a subtotal occlusion (STO) due to its short length. ICA reveals a STO (arrow). There is also a segment of stenosis in the proximal LAD (dotted arrow) but CT images not shown here

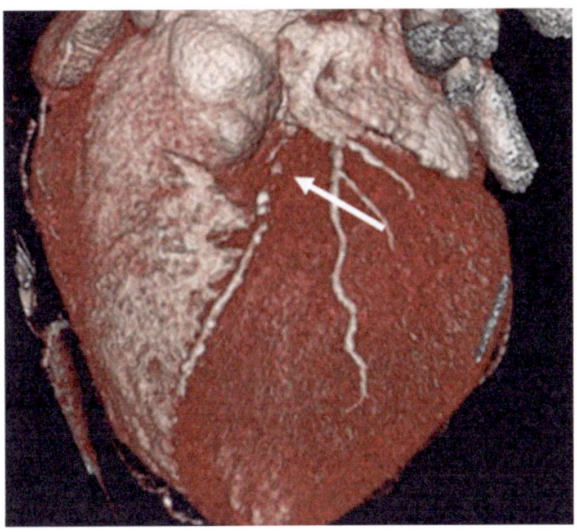

Fig. 11.16 A CTO of the proximal LAD seen on a 3D-VR image and confirmed by ICA (not shown here)

11.6 Stenosis Due to Coronary Artery Dissection

- Stenoses may be nonatherosclerotic in nature. Particularly, in younger, female patients presenting with acute chest pain.
- The stenosis in this setting is due to intramural hematoma with separation of the layers of the coronary artery and may or may not be associated with an intimal tear.
- Many patients will present as ACS and emergently go to the cardiac catheterization laboratory.
- CCTA is increasingly being used for detecting spontaneous coronary artery dissection (SCAD) as well as for follow-up imaging.

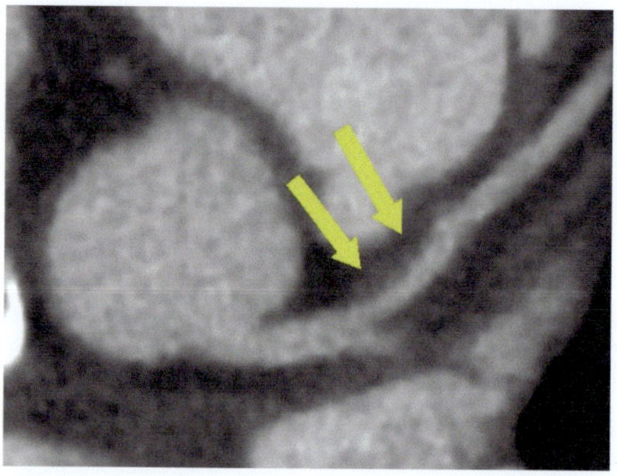

Fig. 11.17 A 30-year-old healthy woman presented to the emergency department after hours of emesis, a few weeks after delivery of her third child. Her troponin levels were elevated and CCTA reveals mild lumen narrowing in the proximal LAD due to a thickened vessel wall, filled with low density tissue. Her history suggests coronary artery dissection rather than noncalcified atherosclerosis. She underwent ICA which confirmed the findings (images not shown)

- Typical findings of CCTA are presence of an intramural hematoma visualized as a sleeve like thickening of the vessel wall and presence of a dissection seen as a low density or dark linear structure between the contrast filled false and true lumen.
- The findings are typically difficult to differentiate from noncalcified atherosclerosis (Fig. 11.17).
- The associated lumen narrowing largely varies as well as its shape.
- Calcium is typically not present and the vessel wall thickening is rather homogenous.
- Note that findings can be subtle on CCTA and easily missed especially in distal vessels [32–34].

11.7 Stenosis Due to Myocardial Bridging

- Myocardial bridging (MB) is a common anatomical variant and is defined as an intramyocardial segment of a coronary artery, which would normally have an epicardial course but is encased by myocardium.
- This is most commonly seen involving the mid-LAD and is generally considered benign.
- Associations with angina, myocardial ischemia or infarction and ventricular arrythmias have been reported but a causal link remains controversial [35], except for extreme cases.
- The prevalence of MB detected on CCTA is higher than on angiographic series as the bridging is more readily detected on CCTA, ranging from 3.5% to 38.3%, with an average of 21% [36, 37].
- Atherosclerotic disease tends to spare the tunneled segment of the artery but can be seen proximally.

Myocardial bridging can be classified into three anatomic patterns (Fig. 11.18):

- Superficial and incomplete
- The artery is in direct contact with myocardium and is partially encased by muscle.
- Superficial and complete
  - The artery is fully encased by muscle for depth of <7 mm.
- Deep
  - The artery is fully encased by muscle for depth of >7 mm [37].
- Myocardial bridging may be clinically significant when it is associated with ventricular compression, seen by ICA as "milking effect" when a short segment of stenosis is seen at the end systolic phase with normal lumen size during the end diastolic phase.
- 97.5% of cases of MB with dynamic compression at ICA were associated with full deep encasement of the artery [36]. Dynamic compression was also associated with longer segments of MB.
- The diagnosis of MB at CCTA is made when soft tissue with the same density as the adjacent myocardium, and not the lower density of noncalcified plaque, is seen covering the coronary artery segment, typically located in the mid LAD.
- The presence of dynamic compression of the segment of MB can be seen on CCTA during the systolic and diastolic phase images. However, most CCTA scans are only acquired

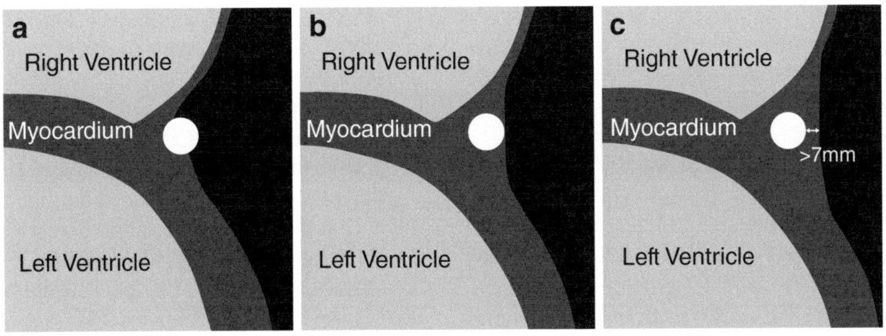

Fig. 11.18 Anatomic Patterns of MB shown in short axis view (after Kim PJ et al. Circulation 2009) [36]. Panels **a–c** show: Panel **a**: Superficial and partially encased artery in direct contact with the myocardium (see Fig. 11.19a). Panel **b**: Superficial and fully encased artery (<7 mm) (see Fig. 11.19b). Panel **c**: Deep and fully encased artery (>7 mm) (see Fig. 11.19c)

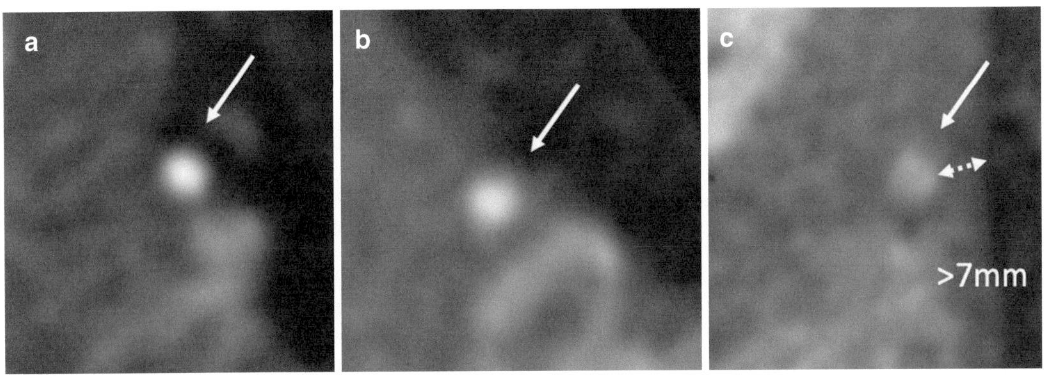

Fig. 11.19 Examples of anatomical patterns of MB. Lumen of artery is white. (**a**) Superficial MB with incomplete encasement. (**b**) Superficial MB with complete encasement, <7 mm in thickness. (**c**) Deep MB with complete encasement, >7 mm in thickness

during diastole in patients with low heart rates, to reduce radiation dose, and so the systolic datasets are typically not available for analysis.

Key features of MB by CCTA:

- Length and type, i.e., superficial (partially or fully encased) or deep (>7 mm).
- Systolic compression (if available).
- Further evaluation by ICA may include the use of dobutamine infusion; nitroglycerine, and IVUS may be helpful based on clinical findings or presence of ischemia on functional testing [38].

References

1. Sandfort V, Lima JAC, Bluemke DA. Noninvasive imaging of atherosclerotic plaque progession. Status of coronary computed tomography angiography. Circ Cardiovasc Imaging. 2015;8:e003316. https://doi.org/10.1161/CIRCIMAGING.115.003316.
2. Stefani GG, Windecker S. Can coronary computed tomography angiography replace invasive angiography? Circulation. 2015;131:418–26. https://doi.org/10.1161/CIRCULATIONAHA.114.008148.
3. Arbab-Zadeh A. Stress testing and non-invasive coronary angiography in patients with suspected coronary artery disease: time for a new paradigm. Heart Int. 2012;7:e2. https://doi.org/10.4081/hi.2012.e2.

4. Sun ZH, Lin CH. Diagnostic value of 320-slice coronary CT angiography in coronary artery disease: a systematic review and meta-analysis. Curr Med Imaging. 2014;10:272–80. https://doi.org/10.2174/1573405610041501211408336.
5. Jiang B, Wang J, Lu X, Cai W. Dual source CT versus single source 64 section CT angiography for coronary artery disease. A meta-analysis. Clin Radiol. 2014;69:861–9. https://doi.org/10.1016/j.crad.2014.03.023.
6. Petcherski O, Gaspar T, Halon DA, Peled N, Jaffe R, Molnar R, et al. Diagnostic accuracy of 256-row computed tomographic angiography for detection of obstructive coronary artery disease using invasive quantitative coronary angiography as reference standard. Am J Cardiol. 2013;111:510–5. https://doi.org/10.1016/j.amjcard.2012.10.036.
7. Mushtaq S, Conte E, Pontone G, Pompilio G, et al. Interpretability of coronary CT angiography performed with a novel whole heart coverage high-definition CT scanner in 300 consecutive patients with coronary artery bypass grafts. JCCT. 2020;14:137–43. https://doi.org/10.1016/j.jcct.2019.08.004.
8. Takagi H, Tanaka R, Nagata K, Ninomiya R, Arakita K, Schuijf JD, et al. Diagnostic performance of coronary CT angiography with ultra-high-resolution CT: comparison with invasive coronary angiography. Eur J Radiol. 2018;101:30–7. https://doi.org/10.1016/j.ejrad.2018.01.030.
9. Hoe J, Toh KH. A practical guide to reading CT coronary angiograms-how to avoid mistakes when assessing for coronary stenosis. Int J Cardiovasc Imaging. 2007;23:617–33. https://doi.org/10.1007/s10554-006-9173-9.
10. Leipsic JL, Abbara S, Achenbach S, Cury R, et al. SCCT guidelines for the interpretation and reporting of coronary CT angiography: a report of the Society of Cardiovascular Computed Tomography Guidelines Committee. JCCT. 2014;8:342–58. https://doi.org/10.1016/j.jcct.2014.07.003G.
11. Ferencik M, Ropers D. Abbara S et al diagnostic accuracy of image postprocessing methods for the detection of coronary artery stenoses by using multidetector CT. Radiology. 2007;243:696–702. https://doi.org/10.1148/radiol.2433060080.
12. Arbab-Zadeh A, Hoe J. Quantification of coronary arterial Stenoses by multidetector CT angiography in comparison with conventional angiography: methods, caveats and implications. J Am Coll Cardiovasc Imaging. 2011;4:191–202. https://doi.org/10.1016/j.jcmg.2010.10.011.
13. Reinhart S, Vazquez G, Qian Z, Murrieta L, et al. Quantitative measurements of coronary arterial stenosis, plaque geometry and composition are highly reproducible with a standardized coronary arterial computed tomographic approach in high quality CT datasets. JCCT. 2011;5:35–43. https://doi.org/10.1016/j.jcct.2010.09.006.
14. Anders K, Achenbach S, Petit I, Daniel WG. Accuracy of automated software guided detection of significant coronary artery stenosis by CT angiography: comparison with invasive catherization. Eur Radiol. 2013;23:1218–25. https://doi.org/10.1007/s00330-012-2717-6.
15. Min HJ, Mim SM, Lee SY, Choi JH, et al. Diagnostic performance of algorithm for computer-assisted detection of significant coronary artery disease in patients with acute chest pain: comparison with invasive coronary angiography. Am J Roentgenol. 2014;202:730–7. https://doi.org/10.2214/AJR.13.11419.
16. Meah M, Singh Williams MC, Dweck MR, et al. Reproducibility of quantitative plaque measurement in advanced coronary artery disease. JCCT. 2021;15:333–8. https://doi.org/10.1016/j.jcct.2020.12.008.
17. Raff GL, Gallagher MJ, O'Neill WW, Goldstein JA. Diagnostic accuracy of non-invasive coronary angiography using 64-slice spiral computed tomography. J Am Coll Cardiol. 2005;46:552–7. https://doi.org/10.1016/j.jacc.2005.05.056.
18. Korosoglou G, Mueller D, Lehrke S, Steen H, et al. Quantitative assessment of stenosis and atherosclerotic plaque composition using 256-slice computed tomography. Eur Radiol. 2010;20:1841–50. https://doi.org/10.1007/s00330-010-1753-3.
19. Latina J, Shabani M, Kapoor K, Whelton SP, et al. Ultra-high-resolution coronary CT angiography for assessment of patients with severe coronary calcifications: initial experience. Radiol Cardiothorac Imaging. 2021;3:e210053. https://doi.org/10.1148/ryct.2021210053.
20. Hagar TB, Sochynski MS, Saffer R, Rau A, Taron J, Weiss J, et al. Accuracy of ultrahigh -resolution photon-counting CT for detecting coronary artery disease in a high-risk population. Radiology. 2023;307(5):e223305. https://doi.org/10.1148/radiol.223305.
21. Cheng V, Gutstein A, Wolak A, Suzuki Y, et al. Moving beyond binary grading of coronary arterial stenoses on coronary computed tomographic angiography: insights for the imager and referring clinician. J Am Coll Cardiol Imaging. 2008;1:460–71. https://doi.org/10.1016/j.jcmg.2008.05.006.
22. Cury R, Leipsic J, Abbara S, Achenbach S, Berman D, et al. CAD-RADS 2.0-2022 coronary artery disease-reporting and data system. An expert consensus document of the Society of Cardiovascular Computed Tomography (SCCT), The American College of Cardiology (ACC) the American College of Radiology (ACR) and the north American Society for Cardiovascular Imaging (NASCI). JCCT. 2022;16:536. https://doi.org/10.1016/j.jcct.2022.07.002.
23. Patel MR, Calhoon JH, Dehmer GJ, Grantham JA, et al. ACC/AATS/AHA/ASE/ASNC/SCAI/SCCT/STS 2017. Appropriate use criteria for coronary revascularisation in patients with stable ischemic heart disease. J Am Coll Cardiol. 2017;69:2212–41. https://doi.org/10.1016/j.jacc.2017.02.001.
24. Hecht H, Roubin G. Usefulness of computed tomographic angiography guided percutaneous coronary

intervention. Am J Cardiol. 2007;99:871–5. https://doi.org/10.1016/j.amjcard.2006.10.049.
25. Lawton SJ, Tamis-Holland JE, Bangalore S, Bates ER, et al. 2021 ACC/AHA/SCAI Guideline for Coronary Artery Revascularization: Executive Summary: A Report of the American College of Cardiology/American Heart Association Joint Committee on Clinical Practice Guidelines. Circulation. 2022;145:e4–e17. Online ahead of print. https://doi.org/10.1161/CIR.0000000000001039.
26. Ota H, Takase K, Hiroya R, Tsuboi T, et al. Quantitative vascular measurements in arterial occlusive disease. Radiographics. 2005;25:1141–58. https://doi.org/10.1148/rg.255055014.
27. Nallamothu BK, Spertus JA, Lanksy AJ, Cohen DJ, et al. Comparison of clinical interpretation with visual assessment and quantitative coronary angiography in patients undergoing percutaneous coronary intervention in contemporary practice. Circulation. 2013;127:1793–800. https://doi.org/10.1161/CIRCULATIONAHA.113.001952.
28. Choi JH, Kim EK, Kim SM, Kim HY, et al. Non-invasive discrimination of chronic total occlusion and subtotal occlusion by coronary computed tomography angiography. J Am Coll Cardiol Intv. 2015;8:1143–53. https://doi.org/10.1016/j.jcin.2015.03.042.
29. Opolski MP, Achenbach S, Schuhback A, Rolf A, et al. Coronary computed tomographic prediction rule for time-efficient guidewire crossing though chronic total occlusion: insights from the CT-RECTOR Multicenter Registry (Computed Tomography Registry of Chronic Total Occlusion Revascularization). JACC Cardiovasc Interventions. 2015;8:257. https://doi.org/10.1016/j.jcin.2014.07.031.
30. Hoe J. CT coronary angiography of chronic total occlusions of the coronary arteries: how to recognize and evaluate and usefulness for planning percutaneous coronary interventions. Int J Cardiovasc Imaging. 2009;25:43–54. https://doi.org/10.1007/s10554-009-9424-7.
31. Hong SJ, Kim BK, Cho I, Kim HY, et al. Effect of coronary CTA on chronic total occlusion percutaneous coronary intervention: a randomised trial. J Am Coll Cardiol Img. 2021;14:1993–2004. https://doi.org/10.1016/j.jcmg.2021.04.013.
32. Aslam A, Stojanovska J, Khokhor US, Weinberg RL, et al. Spontaneous coronary artery dissection: an underdiagnosed clinical entity—a primer for cardiac imagers. Radiographics. 2021;41:1897–915. https://doi.org/10.1148/rg.2021210062.
33. Hayes SH, Tweet MS, Adlam D, Kim ESH, et al. Spontaneous coronary artery dissection. J Am Coll Cardiol. 2020;76:961–84. https://doi.org/10.1016/j.jacc.2020.05.084.
34. Ufuk F, Kilic ID. Spontaneous coronary artery dissection. Radiology. 2022;302:25. https://doi.org/10.1148/radiol.2021211385.
35. Ko SM. An overview of myocardial bridging with a focus on multidetector CT coronary angiographic findings. Korean Circ J. 2008;38:583–9. https://doi.org/10.4070/kcj.2008.38.11.583.
36. Kim PJ, Gham H, Kim SY, Namgung J, et al. Frequency of myocardial bridges and dynamic compression of Epicardial coronary arteries. A comparison between computed tomography and invasive coronary angiography. Circulation. 2009;119:1408–16. https://doi.org/10.1161/CIRCULATIONAHA.108.788901.
37. Konen E, Goitein OG, Sternik L, Eshet Y, et al. The prevalence and anatomical patterns of intramuscular coronary arteries: a coronary computed tomographic angiographic study. J Am Coll Cardiol. 2007;49:587–93. https://doi.org/10.1016/j.jacc.2006.09.039.
38. Corban MT, Hung OY, Eshtehardi P, Rasoul-Arzrumly E, et al. Myocardial bridging. Contemporary understanding of pathophysiology with implications for diagnosis and therapeutic strategies. J Am Coll Cardiol. 2014;63:2346–55. https://doi.org/10.1016/j.jacc.2014.01.049.

Further Reading

Karl CA, Leschka S, Stolzmann P, Glaser-Gallion N, Wildermuth S, Alkadhi H. A systematic approach for analysis, interpretation, and reporting of coronary CTA studies. Insights Imaging. 2012;3:215–28. https://doi.org/10.1007/s13244-012-0167-y.
Sundaram B, Patel S, Agarwal P, Kazerooni EA. Anatomy and terminology for the interpretation and reporting of cardiac MDCT: part 2, CT angiography, cardiac function assessment and noncoronary and extracardiac findings. AJR Am J Roentgenol. 2009;192:584–98. https://doi.org/10.2214/AJR.08.1178.
Zimmerman S, Fishman E, editors. Pearls and pitfalls in cardiovascular imaging: pseudolesions, artifacts, and other difficult diagnoses. Cambridge: Cambridge University Press; 2015. https://doi.org/10.1017/CBO9781139152228.

12 Pitfalls in Coronary CTA Interpretation

John Hoe

Abstract

This chapter discusses the causes of stenosis misinterpretation and how to avoid it. False positive results of CCTA, which are overestimating the severity of coronary stenosis compared to the standard of invasive angiography, are more common than a false negative diagnosis (missing the presence of plaque or a significant stenosis) but the latter has a more serious impact on patient outcomes and management. This chapter outlines how to recognize plaque in challenging locations, such as at ostia, bifurcations, or are affected by degraded image quality. Heavily calcified plaques represent a particular challenge, and are generally associated with false positive results, though less commonly also with underappreciation of stenosis severity. Methods of approaching calcified plaques are being provided.

Keywords

Computed tomography angiography · Coronary artery disease · Atherosclerosis · Coronary stenosis

J. Hoe (✉)
Department of Radiology, Mount Elizabeth Hospital, Singapore, Republic of Singapore

A. A. Zadeh, J. Hoe (eds.), *Practical Guide to Cardiac CT*,
https://doi.org/10.1007/978-981-97-6919-3_12

Abbreviations

3D-VR	3D volume rendered
CCTA	Coronary CTA
CPR	Curved planar reconstruction
CTO	Chronic total occlusion
DS	Diameter stenosis
ICA	Invasive coronary angiography
MRP	Multiplanar reconstruction
NPV	Negative predictive value

12.1 Introduction

- The diagnostic accuracy of coronary CTA compared with invasive coronary angiography (ICA) using QCA for the detection of coronary artery stenosis of ≥50% diameter stenosis (DS) is well known and has been documented in many single center and multicenter studies (See Chap. 11).
- The high sensitivity and high negative predictive value (NPV) in symptomatic patients with no known CAD suggest that coronary CTA may be used to detect and exclude obstructive stenosis. It also means CCTA is less likely to underreport a stenosis of ≥50% DS.
- A false positive finding means that a "significant" stenosis reported by CCTA was not confirmed by invasive angiography (ICA), i.e., was found to be of less severe lumen narrowing. A false positive result may lead to unnec-

essary testing, including ICA, but it is a potentially less serious error than missing significant stenoses.

- A false negative result indicates underestimating the degree of stenosis or missing a significant or severe stenosis altogether. This may have a serious impact on patient prognosis and management. Even missing presence of nonobstructive plaque may have prognostic and treatment implications for the patient.
- False positive results are about three times more common than false negative results [1, 2].
- The most common causes of stenosis misinterpretation are motion artifacts, excessive image noise, and severe plaque calcification. Small vessels (e.g., <2 mm in diameter) are often not optimally assessable and contained stenoses may be missed.
- If a repeat scan is required e.g., due to respiratory artifact or poor contrast injection, early recognition, i.e., before the patient is taken off the scanner table, facilitates patient management.

12.2 How to Avoid False Positive CCTA Scan Results

12.2.1 Calcified Plaques Are the Most Common Cause of False Positive Results

1. Calcified plaques cause two types of artifacts on CCTA: "blooming" and "beam hardening" (see Chap. 8).
2. Methods to reduce effect of these artifacts and improve image quality in clinical practice are:
   (a) Scanning with a higher tube current −120 kVp instead of using 100 kVp or 80 kVp. Note that there is no image improvement when using higher tube voltages of 130 kVp or higher.
   (b) Scanning with a higher tube current mAs, e.g., overriding the automated low dose settings.
   (c) Post-processing images using a high convolution filters—these are CT vendor specific, e.g., B46f, FC05.
   (d) Widening window width and window level—1500/300 or extremely widened WW/WL 2700/900 for heavy calcifications.
   (e) Assessing calcium size as a proportion of the contrast lumen size on cross-sectional images to estimate the likelihood of a severe stenosis (if there is severe calcification with no residual contrast filled lumen visible, there is a 80% probability of a severe stenosis) [3]. A suggested method of reading the scan if visualization of the contrast filled lumen is obscured by the calcified plaque (Fig. 12.1).
   (f) Novel and new software and hardware technologies are being used to improve visualization of the lumen in the presence of calcified plaques from CCTA images:
      - Using different kV energies to scan.
      - Spectral CT scanner using multi-energy acquisition.
      - Calcium image subtraction using calcium score scan as mask.
      - Ultra-high-resolution CT.

12.2.2 Motion Artifacts

- Motion artifacts may mimic a stenosis and may occur even with low heart rates (e.g., <65 per minute [bpm]), especially if there is considerable heart rate variability or ectopy.
- The mid-RCA is most prone to false positive stenoses because of its excessive motion during the cardiac cycle (Fig. 12.2).
- To reduce misinterpretations due to motion artifacts, we recommend to routinely reconstruct at least two different sets of data (in milliseconds or percentages), preferably far apart (e.g., for a 70–80% RR interval acquisition one should use 70%, 75%, and 80%).

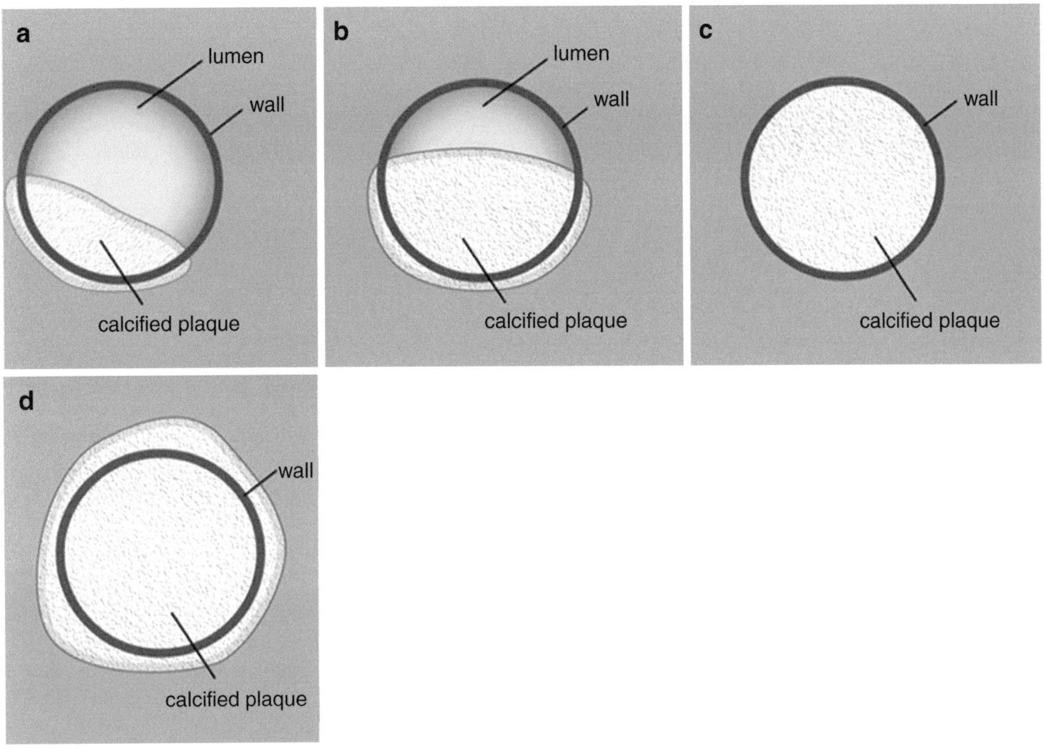

Fig. 12.1 (Panels **a**–**d**) Panel **a** shows a calcified plaque (white) obscuring <50% of the contrast filled lumen (gray), thus unlikely to be associated with a significant stenosis (>50% DS). Panel **b** depicts a calcified plaque obscuring>50% of the lumen rendering it impossible to determine if a significant stenosis present and further evaluation is recommended. Panels **c** and **d** show the lumen completely obscured (100%) by calcified plaque or >100% with presence of positive remodeling. The likelihood of a significant stenosis is high in this setting. (*Ref Makmur & Hoe2015. Copyright approval obtained from Springer*)

- If there is a lesion on one phase but not on others, the finding is likely related to motion artifact. If a stenosis is seen on multiple phases, it is likely to be a "real" lesion and not due to motion artifact [4].
- A "real" stenosis typically reveals evidence of atherosclerotic plaque, best seen on cross-sectional images [4].

12.2.3 Step Artifacts

- They can be difficult to recognize especially if they are parallel to imaging plane, e.g., distal RCA, PDA.
- They may occur due to breathing or motion artifacts or due to scanning mode.
- Step artifacts are frequently encountered with the sequential (step and shoot) scanning mode.
- Use of wide-volume scanners (e.g., 256/320 scanners) reduces the risk of step artifacts.

12.2.4 Coronary Artery Vasospasm

- Spasm may cause an apparent stenosis, especially if no nitroglycerine is used or is contraindicated (Fig. 12.3).
- If there is an apparent stenosis by CCTA but not by ICA, intracoronary administration of ergonovine may be used to provoke a spasm and demonstrate a possible cause of angina [5].

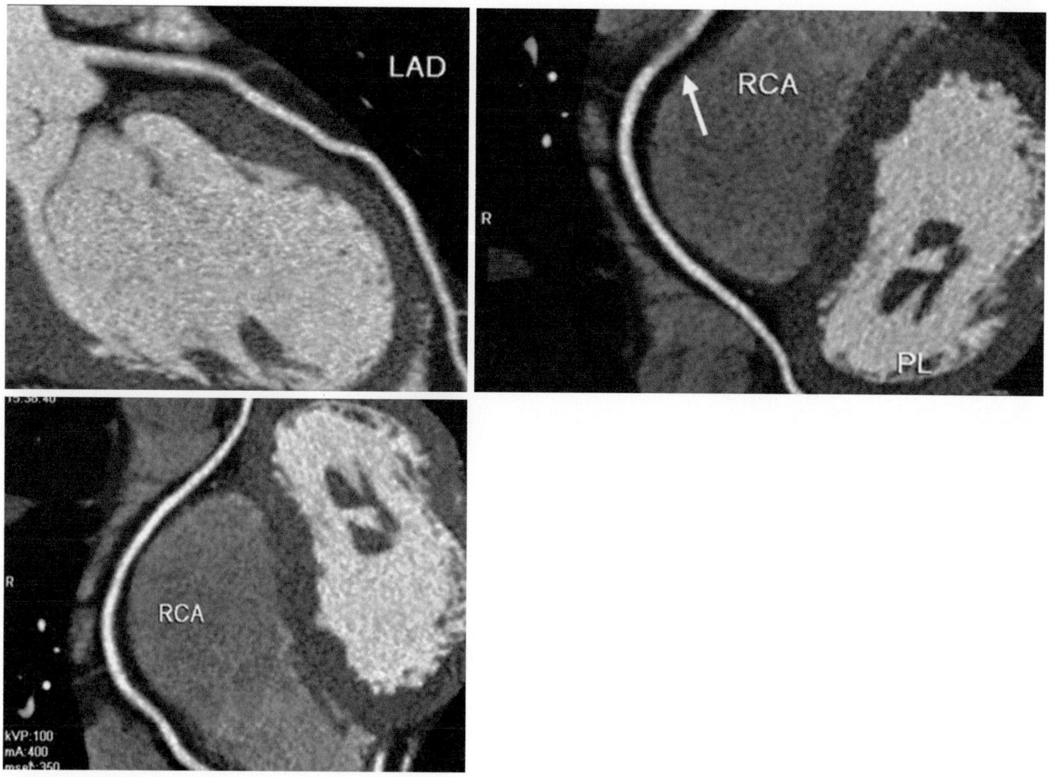

Fig. 12.2 This patient had a low but variable heart rate (56–63 bpm) during scan acquisition. A potential stenosis is seen in the mid-RCA (arrow) when reconstructed at 75% phase but no lesion is noted when images were reconstructed at 752 ms after the R wave

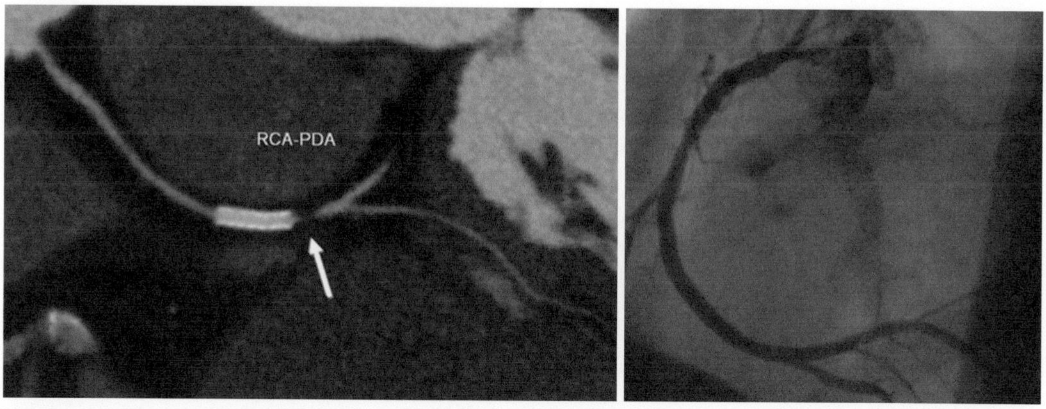

Fig. 12.3 A 51-year-old woman with prior PCI and stent placement presented with recurrent chest pain. CCTA shows a segment of stenosis in the RCA distal to the stent. Nitroglycerine was not used because the patient became hypotensive after use of betablocker to lower her heart rate. At ICA, no stenosis seen in the RCA

12.2.5 False Positive Related to Poor Contrast Filling of Distal Vessels

- This may occur as result of inadequate contrast injection rates or volume, poor venous access, high heart rate (and rapid contrast dilution), or lack of nitroglycerine use (and small vessel size).
- The resultant finding is a small vessel with poor contrast opacification (Fig. 12.4).

Summary
How to avoid false positive CCTA scans

- Large calcified plaques are the most common cause of misdiagnosis, which may be avoided using higher kVp (but no more than 120 kVp), sharp kernels, and appropriate WW/WL settings.
- At least two datasets of acquired scan data should be reconstructed, at different phase % or milliseconds, preferably wide apart, to verify consistency of lesion.
- In patients with high heart rates, image reconstruction in both systole and diastole, is recommended.
- Knowledge on how to recognize step artifacts will reduce the risk of misdiagnosis.
- If nitroglycerine is not given during scan acquisition, the possibility of coronary artery spasm or underfilled distal artery as a cause of false positive results should be considered.

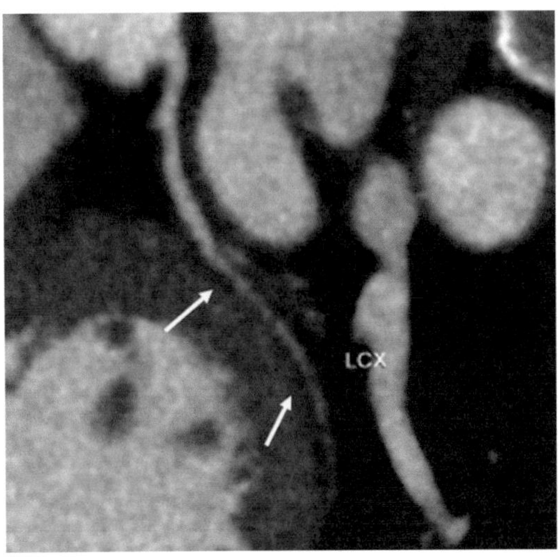

Fig. 12.4 A 64-year-old woman with good heart rate control (51 bpm). Adequate opacification is seen in the proximal LCx but contrast and visualization of the distal LCx is poor, possibly indicating severe lumen narrowing. Subsequent ICA (image not included here) revealed normal LCx. The false positive finding likely is due to insufficient radiation dose and associated image noise as well as small vessel size

12.3 Causes and Remedies of False Negative CCTA Results

False negative typically refers to missing "significant" stenoses as defined by ICA but may also relate to underreporting *any* coronary atherosclerotic disease. The following steps are recommended to reduce the risk of underreporting disease.

12.3.1 Use 3D-VR Images for an Overview of the Coronary Arteries

This helps to detect a segment of stenosis that may not be obvious or is easily seen on the axial data sets (see also Chap. 11, Figs. 11.2 and 11.3).

The limitations of the 3D VR images need to be considered:

- changing the window leveling may obscure or create a stenosis,
- 3D images generally are not accurate for estimating stenosis degree,
- calcifications or stents render interpretation even less accurate.

12.3.2 Use Oblique MPRs Routinely and Systematically Along the Longitudinal Plane of the Artery

Begin reading the scans in detail using the axial views as the datasets are the least post processed

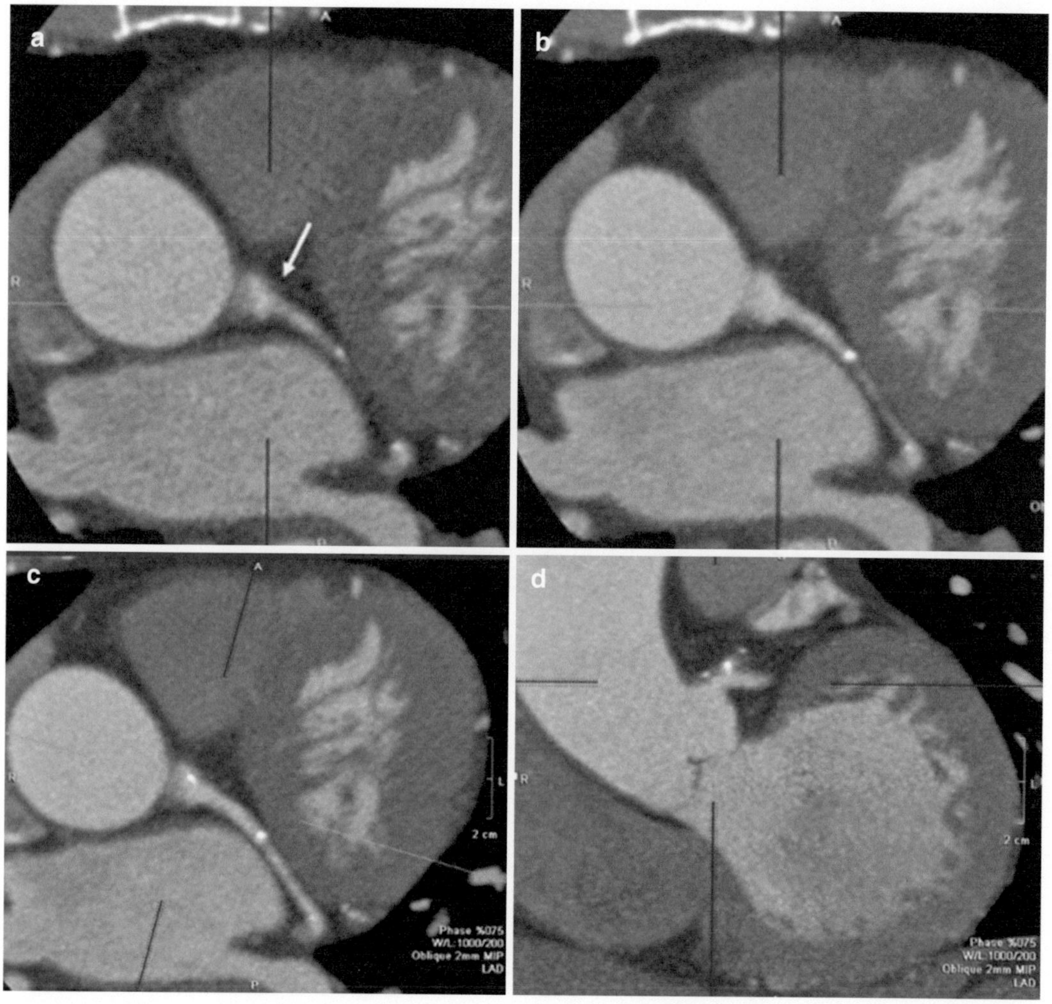

Fig. 12.5 (Panels **a**–**d**) Ostial left main disease which may be missed. Panels **a** and **b**: Normal appearing left main LM (arrow) viewed on axial image at 0.5-mm slice thickness (**a**) or using 3-mm MIP (**b**). Panel **c** shows the crosshairs of the MPR tool placed along the long axis of the LM and the orthogonal image. Panel **d** reveals ostial LM mixed, non-calcified and calcified, atherosclerotic plaque

- Oblique MPR image plans may allow detecting ostial or bifurcation disease, which may otherwise be missed.
- This is particularly important for left main or ostial LAD disease (Figs. 12.5 and 12.6, [3]).
- Missing a significant bifurcation lesion by CCTA has implications for planned PCI which becomes more complex in that setting (Type B lesion), often requiring two guide wires and special techniques for stent placement.

Key Points

- Start reading images by scrolling through the axial image set. Each vessel should be interrogated using the workstation's MPR tool, viewed in its long axis using oblique MPR views and on the corresponding orthogonal planes, with special emphasis on the ostia of the left main and LAD, and on major bifurcations [4].

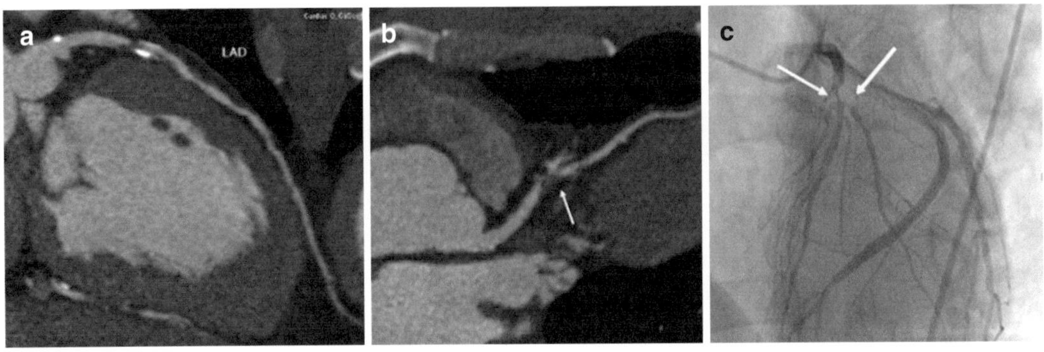

Fig. 12.6 (Panels **a**–**c**) Panel **a** shows a CPR image of the LAD showing a short segment of severe stenosis in proximal segment. Panel **b**: CPR image of diagonal branch showing a severe ostial stenosis of the diagonal branch. This stenosis was also easily seen on the 3D-VR images as well as MPR images (not shown here). Panel **c**: ICA images confirming the two stenoses

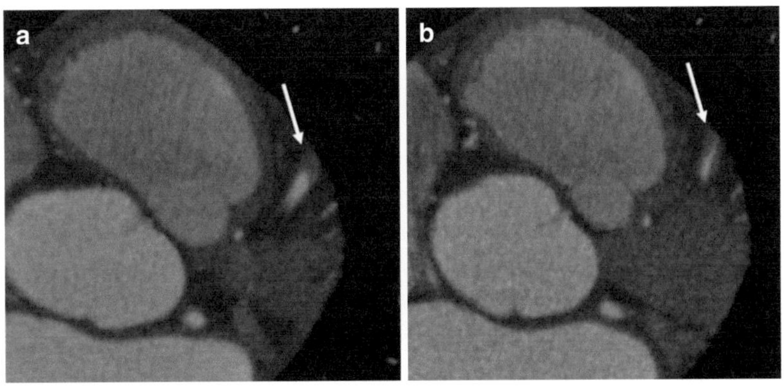

Fig. 12.7 An area of dark density (black lumen sign) in the mid-LAD abruptly appears while scrolling through the axial datasets (Panel **a**). The following axial image (Panel **b**) reveals non-calcified plaque with associated lumen stenosis, which could be easily missed

- CPR images are helpful but disease may be missed at the edge of an artery if there are errors with centerline tracking (less common with contemporary software).
- MPR images with thickness greater than the size of the artery (e.g., >3 mm) should be avoided for stenosis assessment.

12.3.3 Use the "Black Lumen" Sign to Help in Detecting Non-Calcified Disease

- If the bright lumen on axial dataset images suddenly becomes dark, often at its margins, interrogate the vessel by using oblique MPRs to look for non-calcified atherosclerotic disease.
- A brief, sudden change of the lumen contrast density may be easily missed, as it may only be seen on a few mouse clicks and thus it is better to avoid using the mouse scroll button as it may lead to skipping the stenosis (Fig. 12.7).

12.3.4 Check Three Key Areas Where Stenosis May be Missed Before Reporting a Normal Scan

These areas are notorious for missing disease due to challenging viewing planes:

- Mid-LAD and ostium of D1 and D2 branches.
- Proximal or distal circumflex or OM branch (Fig. 12.8).
- Distal RCA and PDA [4].

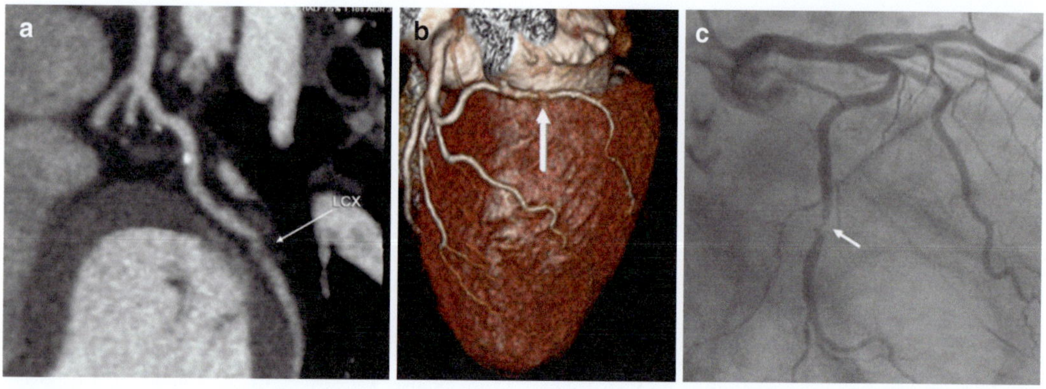

Fig. 12.8 (Panels **a**–**c**) Panel **a** shows a CPR image of left circumflex with a short segment of severe lumen narrowing that was missed on the initial read of the axial image datasets but was confirmed on oblique MPR images (not shown). Panel **b** shows a 3D-VR image suggesting a short stenosis which was confirmed by ICA (Panel **c**)

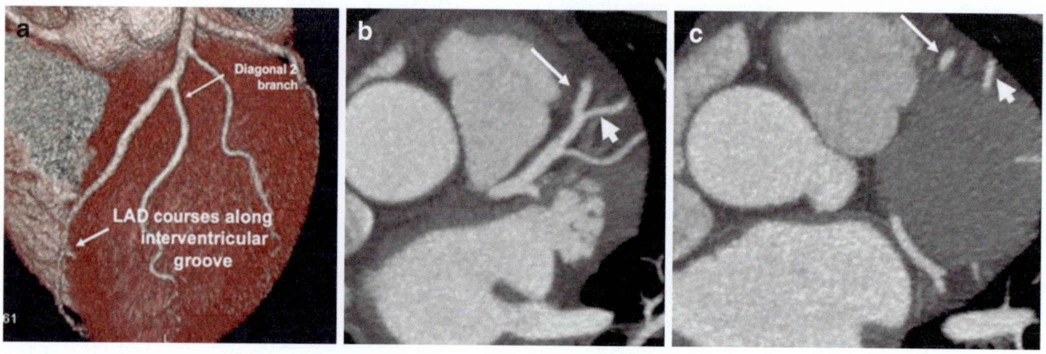

Fig. 12.9 (Panels **a**–**c**) Panel **a**—Normal expected course of the LAD in the interventricular groove with second diagonal traveling laterally (short arrow). Panels **b** and **c**: Distal images are shown for the LAD (thin arrow) and second diagonal branch (short arrow)

12.3.5 Know the Normal Course of the LAD to Avoid Missing a CTO

- In Chap. 11, the possibility to falsely report a CTO as severe stenosis was discussed.
- Knowledge of the typical course of the LAD on CCTA images helps in avoiding this mistake and facilitates detecting CTO of the mid or distal LAD.
- Missing a CTO diagnosis has implications for the planning of PCI because, as a Type C lesion, it requires considerably more time and preprocedural planning.

The LAD typically travels along the interventricular groove to the left ventricular apex (Fig. 12.9), best seen on axial images and 3D-VR (for confirmation). Vessels lateral to the interventricular groove are generally diagonal branches. With a CTO of the mid or distal LAD, the diagonal may be mistaken for the LAD as it may be the only contrast-filled vessel traveling distally (Fig. 12.10).

12.3.6 False Negative Reporting Due to Presence of Small, Calcified Plaques

- While calcified plaques are typically associated with false positive reports, eccentric, small calcified plaques partially obscuring lumen may falsely lead to the assumptions

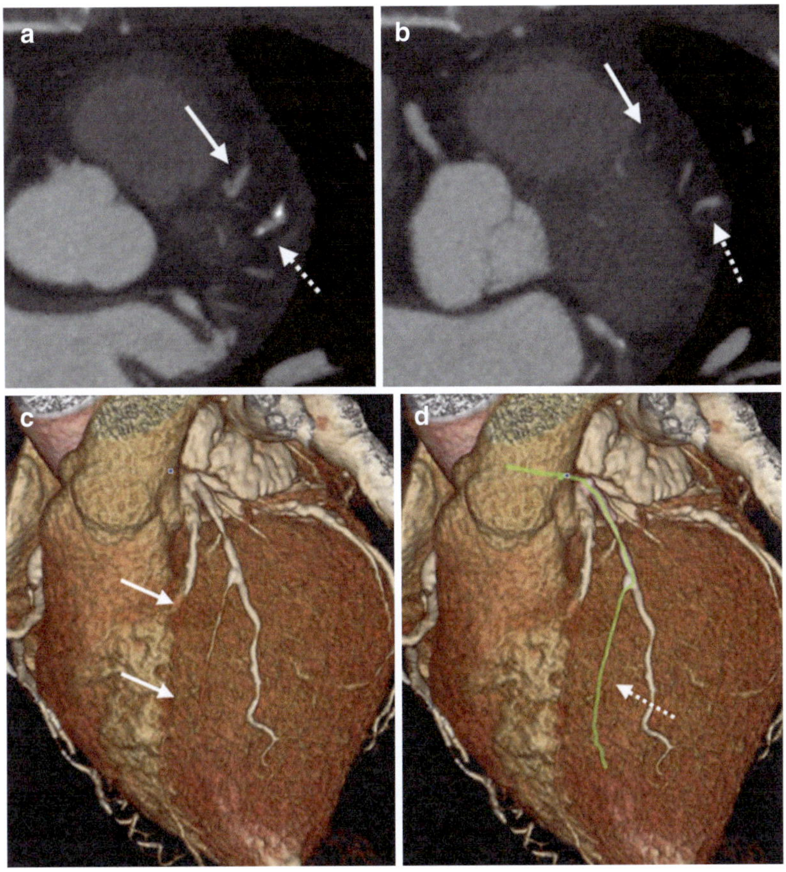

Fig. 12.10 (Panels **a–d**) Panel **a**: Mid-LAD is opacified (arrow), as is the diagonal branch (dotted arrow). Panel **b**: The distal LAD is poorly opacified and hard to visualize (arrow). This is a CTO of the distal LAD while the diagonal branch (dotted arrow) remains opacified and could be mistaken for the distal LAD. Panel **c**: VR image showing lack of contrast filled vessel lumen at the expected positions of the mid and distal LAD segments (arrows) suggesting CTO (ICA images confirmed, not shown). Panel **d**: 3D-VR image demonstrates how the software tool mistakenly tracked the diagonal branch and labeled it "LAD"

that missed detail is due to partial volume effect and not to plaque.

- This may be particularly misleading in the setting of small, spotty calcifications opposite to each other (Fig. 12.11) [6].

Key Point

- The clinical history and symptoms should weigh heavily when reviewing the CCTA images and further testing, e.g., ICA, should be considered in cases of a mismatch between reporting and symptomatology [7].

12.3.7 Small Vessel Size Can be a Cause of a False Negative Result

With an artery diameter of less than 2 mm, it may be difficult to appreciate lumen stenoses—a limitation related to the spatial resolution of current CT scanners.

Locations where stenoses are prone to be missed:

- Distal LAD.
- Distal diagonal branches.
- Distal Left circumflex.
- Distal OM branch.
- PDA.

12.3.8 Excessive Image Noise May Result in False Negative Findings

Excessive image noise may result in poor image quality such that the contrast filled lumen may not be well visualized. The most common causes of excessive image noise are:

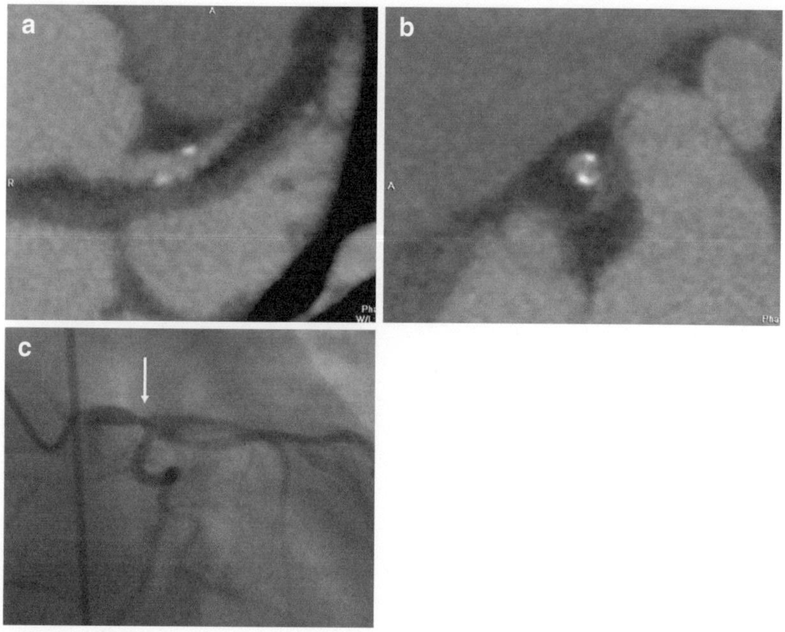

Fig. 12.11 (Panels **a**–**c**) A case of a 44-year-old man presenting with chest pain. Panels **a** and **b** show two small, spotty calcifications opposite each other in distal LM without obvious significant stenosis. Panel **c** reveals a stenosis of >50% in the distal LM by ICA which was prompted by persistent symptoms. (*Images reprinted from Ref Makmur & Hoe 2015. Copyright approval obtained from Springer*)

- Underpenetration/ low radiation dose settings. Inappropriately low tube current settings lower radiation dose at the expense of image noise and risk of false negative findings [8].
  - Appropriate use of iterative reconstruction (IR) or deep learning algorithms may reduce image noise and may allow lower tube current—within limits. This choice of choosing different IR algorithms to reduce noise in images is CT vendor specific.
  - Avoid acquiring scans with ultralow radiation doses but inadequate image quality.
- Very obese patients. Although maximum tube current output may be sufficient to acquire CCTA, in severely obese patients, image noise may be inadequate for accurate diagnosis due to photon starvation and associated image noise.

12.3.9 Coronary Motion Artifacts

Motion artifacts is a less common cause of false negative scan result but frequently found to be the culprit of false positive findings. The mid-RCA is particularly affected. Good heart rate control is the remedy.

12.3.10 Combination of factors leading to poor image quality.

Even when individual factors are not grave, a combination of suboptimal heart rate control (e.g., contraindication to use of beta blockers), inadequate contrast opacification of the artery (e.g., i.v., access problems), poor vasodilation (e.g., contraindication to use of nitroglycerine) may sum up to poor overall image quality and possible false negative findings.

Summary

How to avoid a false negative result (i.e., missing presence of plaque or a significant stenosis)

- Use of 3D-VR images for an overview and verifying the coronary anatomy.
- Routine use of oblique MPRs of the arterial long axis along with orthogonal planes, with particular emphasis on ostial and bifurcation lesions (LM!).
- Use of MPR slabs not be thicker than 2–3 mm.
- CPR images in support of above with attention to correct centerline tracking.

- Use of the "dark lumen" sign to help you detecting non-calcified plaques.
- Review of three problem areas before reporting normal results.
- Knowledge of the typical LAD anatomy to detect distal CTO.
- Consideration of small, eccentric calcified plaques, especially those opposite each other, as cause of missing a significant short, stenosis.
- Optimizing image quality in each patient and awareness of artifacts related to inadequate heart rate control, excessive image noise, and poor vasodilation.

References

1. Meijer AB, Ying LO, Gelejins J, Kroft LJM. Meta-analysis of 40 and 64 MDCT angiography for assessing coronary artery stenosis. AJR. 2008;191:1667–75. https://doi.org/10.2214/AJR.07.4022.
2. Yan RT, Miller JM, Rochitte C, Dewey M, et al. Predictors of inaccurate coronary arterial stenosis assessment by CT angiography. JACC Cardiovasc Imaging. 2013;6:963–72. https://doi.org/10.1016/j.jcmg.2013.02.011.
3. Cerci R, Vavere AL, Miller JM, Yoneyama K, Rochitte CE, Dewey M, et al. Patterns of coronary arterial lesion calcification by a novel, cross-sectional CT angiographic assessment. Int J Cardiovasc Imaging. 2013;29(7):1619–27. PMID: 23702949; PubMed Central PMCID: PMC3796157. https://doi.org/10.1007/s10554-013-0240-8.
4. Hoe J, Toh KH. A practical guide to reading CT coronary angiograms—how to avoid mistakes when assessing for coronary stenosis. Int J Cardiovasc Imaging. 2007;23:617–33. https://doi.org/10.1007/s10554-006-9173-9.
5. Kang KM, Choi SI, Chun EJ, Kim JA, et al. Coronary vasospastic angina: assessment by multidetector CT coronary angiography. Korean J Radiol. 2012;13(1):27–33. https://doi.org/10.3348/kjr.2012.13.1.27.
6. Makmur A, Hoe J. The challenge of coronary calcium on coronary computed tomographic angiography (CCTA) scans: effect on interpretation and possible solutions. Int J Cardiovasc Imaging. 2015;31:145–57. https://doi.org/10.1007/s10554-015-0773-0.
7. Patel MR, Bailey SR, Bonow RO, Chambers CE, Chan PS, et al. ACCF/SCAI/AATS/AHA/ASE/ASNC/HFSA/HRS/SCCM/SCCT/SCMR/STS 2012 appropriate use criteria for diagnostic catheterization: a report of the American College of Cardiology Foundation Appropriate Use Criteria Task Force, Society for Cardiovascular Angiography and Interventions, American Association for Thoracic Surgery, American Heart Association, American Society of Echocardiography, American Society of Nuclear Cardiology, Heart Failure Society of America, Heart Rhythm Society, Society of Critical Care Medicine, Society of Cardiovascular Computed Tomography, Society for Cardiovascular Magnetic Resonance, and Society of Thoracic Surgeons. J Am Coll Cardiol. 2012;59(22):1995–2027. https://doi.org/10.1016/j.jacc.2012.03.003.
8. van der Bijl N, Joemai RMS, Mertens BJA, de Roos A, et al. Effect of dose reduction on image quality and diagnostic performance in coronary computed tomography angiography. Int J Cardiovasc Imaging. 2013;29:453–61. https://doi.org/10.1007/s10554-012-0096-3.

Advanced Plaque Evaluation by CT 13

Armin Arbab Zadeh

Abstract

Assessment of the presence and extent of coronary atherosclerotic disease is central to the evaluation of patients with suspected coronary heart disease. Risk of myocardial infarction or cardiovascular death is strongly related to the total coronary atheroma burden. While coronary calcium scanning allows an estimate of calcified coronary atheroma burden, it cannot account for noncalcified atherosclerosis. Automated arterial contour detection enables rapid assessment of total coronary atheroma burden which is predictive of patient outcome. However, standards for assessment and reporting have not been established and inter-scan reproducibility is modest at this time. Data supporting automated plaque detection over visual estimates for clinical practice are lacking. Similarly, there are no data demonstrating improved patient outcome informed by advanced coronary atherosclerotic plaque characterization vs. conventional methods. The field is rapidly evolving, however, and it is likely that automated coronary atheroma assessment will eventually be the mainstay of coronary artery disease evaluation.

Keywords

Coronary atherosclerosis · Plaque · Atheroma · Plaque burden · Vulnerable plaque · High-risk plaque

Abbreviations

AHA	American Heart Association
MPR	Multi-planar reformation
PAV	Percent atheroma volume
SCCT	Society of Cardiovascular Computed Tomography
TAV	Total atheroma volume

13.1 Background

- Most acute coronary events are the results of coronary atherosclerotic plaque rupture or erosion and associated vascular thrombosis [1]. Certain plaque features, e.g., thin fibrous cap and large lipid pool, have been associated with plaque ruptures and thus generated immense interest for early detection by imaging for possible prevention [1].
- Although many studies suggested a predictive value of various plaque features by CT, the concept of single "vulnerable" plaques remains controversial [2].

A. A. Zadeh (✉)
Department of Medicine, Johns Hopkins University, Baltimore, MD, USA
e-mail: arminzadeh@jhu.edu

A. A. Zadeh, J. Hoe (eds.), *Practical Guide to Cardiac CT*,
https://doi.org/10.1007/978-981-97-6919-3_13

- Criticism relates to (1) methodological flaws of studies claiming predictive value, (2) evidence that most plaque ruptures occur clinically silently, and (3) failure of interventional treatment of "vulnerable" plaques to reduce acute coronary events [3].
- "High-risk" plaque is a more recently used term which may relate to single plaques (and hence is associated with the same limitations discussed above) [4] or to plaque *volume*. The latter has different implications than the single plaque concept because it builds on the proven concept that atheroma burden is linearly correlated with adverse patient outcome [5].
- Whether "high-risk" plaque volume adds to the assessment of total atheroma volume remains controversial. A recent analysis of the ISCHEMIA trial found little value over conventional coronary artery disease grading [6].
- Assessment of plaque calcification has been associated with predictive value for PCI success [7].

> **Key Points**
> Despite considerable interest in coronary atherosclerotic plaque characterization, adequate supporting evidence for its clinical value is lacking with the possible exception of informing proceduralists of densely calcified lesions considered for percutaneous coronary intervention.

13.2 Methods for Advanced Plaque Characterization by CCTA

- Baseline plaque assessment consists of describing the presence of calcified, noncalcified, or mixed atherosclerotic disease based on visual detection of calcium within the plaque.
- Advanced plaque assessment considers additional features which have been associated with "high-risk" of adverse patient outcome:
  - External vascular remodeling.
  - Spotty calcification.
  - "Napkin ring" sign
  - Low density plaque.
- Note that neither a causal relationship between such plaque characteristics and adverse patient outcome nor clinical value of these assessments has been established.

External (also known as positive) vascular remodeling

- Remodeling status is determined by comparing the vessel dimension at lesion site, e.g., diameter or area, to an appropriate reference site.
- The *remodeling index* is commonly defined by:
- *Lesion Vessel Dimension/Reference Vessel Dimension* (Fig. 13.1).
- While any remodeling index >1 indicates external remodeling, most publications use a threshold of 1.1 or greater to indicate external remodeling.
- The clinical significance of determining remodeling status remains doubtful. While several studies claim value for risk prediction, an adjustment for disease burden was often not performed. The PROSPECT study using intravascular ultrasound found no predictive value of external remodeling.

Spotty Calcification

- Spotty calcification is characterized by chunks of calcium within otherwise noncalcified plaque.
- Extrapolating from histology findings that focal calcification may increase the risk of plaque rupture, spotty calcification detected by CCTA has been considered a "high-risk" feature.
- Data in support of "high-risk" status have been inconsistent, however, and there is doubtful value of detecting spotty calcification for clinical care.
- Detection of spotty calcification by CCTA requires the identification of calcium components within noncalcified plaque which is typically straightforward due to high X-ray attenuation of calcium (Fig. 13.2).

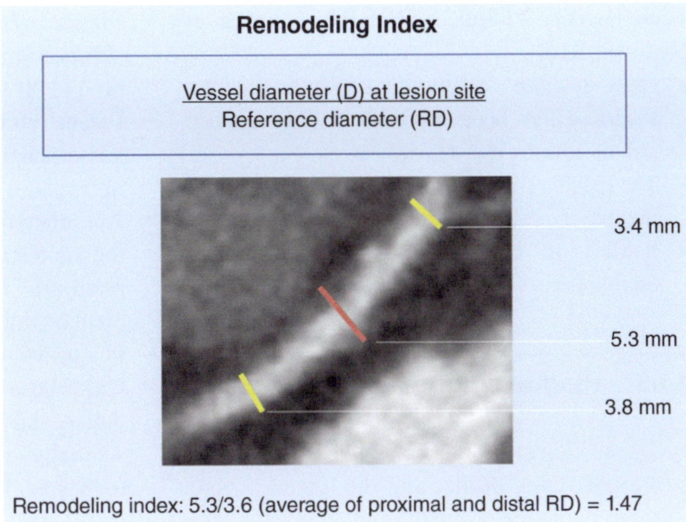

Fig. 13.1 The Remodeling Index

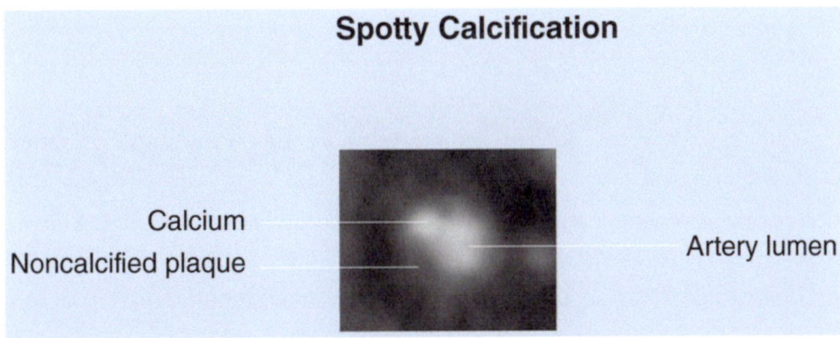

Fig. 13.2 Spotty Calcification

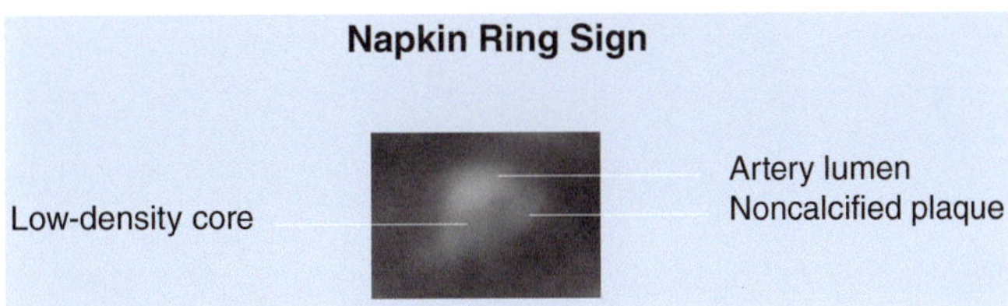

Fig. 13.3 The Napkin Ring Sign

Napkin Ring Sign

- Noncalcified plaque wrapping a very low density circular center within a plaque gives the appearance of a napkin ring (Fig. 13.3).
- Comparison with histopathology suggests that the low density area corresponds to the necrotic core within a plaque.
- Given the similarities with features of a "vulnerable" plaque, e.g., large lipid or necrotic core surrounded by a thin cap, the napkin ring sign has been associated with "vulnerability."
- Positive predictive value for ACS is exceedingly low, however, and there is doubtful value of detecting these plaques for clinical care.

Low Density Plaque

- Low density (AKA low attenuation) plaque is commonly defined as plaque with less than 30 HU density.
- It has been associated with necrotic or lipid plaque components detected by histopathology.
- Several studies suggest predictive value of low density plaque for adverse events though most did not adjust for overall disease burden.
- The largest, most rigorous study on the predictive value of low density plaque found no increased risk after adjustment [6].
- Value for clinical care has not been established.

High Density Plaque as Possible Marker of Reduced Risk

- High calcium density on coronary calcium scanning has been associated with reduced risk of adverse events [8].
- The mechanisms remain unclear and this finding may be related to survival bias.
- Value for clinical care has not been established.

13.3 Plaque Volume Assessment

- Tissue detected by CT between the outer arterial vessel border and the lumen is considered plaque even though it negates the thickness of the adventitia (average of 0.2 mm) [9].
- Plaque area is commonly computed by subtracting the lumen area from the vessel area [10]
- Plaque volume integrates plaque area over vessel length with interpolating measurement intervals, e.g., 0.25 or 0.5 mm. [10]
- Automated and semi-automated arterial contour detection software available on various platforms allows rapid determination of plaque volumes (Fig. 13.4).
- Plaque volumes by CT correlate overall well with those by intravascular imaging techniques and histopathology, but they may substantially overestimate atheroma burden due to the inability to differentiate between normal vessel wall volume and early disease stages, particularly in the setting of increased image noise [11].

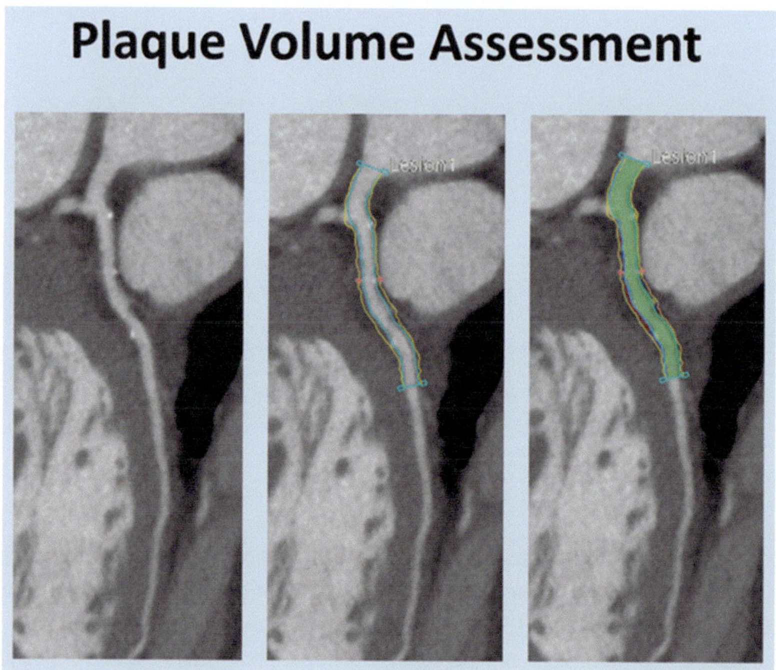

Fig. 13.4 Plaque Volume Assessment. The left panel shows the left main and left anterior descending coronary artery in a curved MPR view revealing evidence of partially calcified atherosclerosis. The mid panel shows the same image after semi-automated contour detection of the lumen and vessel borders. The software provides the plaque volume within the proximal and distal borders of the selected segments. Vessel and segment selection for analysis may occur manually or automatedly. The contours detected by the software may be manually edited according to the observer's visual assessment. The right panel shows the same image after plaque characterization according to tissue attenuation. The software provides several plaque categories which may be individualized, e.g., targeting low attenuation plaque associated with lipid-rich plaque vs. fibrous vs. calcified plaque. The software provides individual plaque proportions and volumes along with color coding for improved visualization

- Atheroma volume is strongly predictive of patient outcome. If, however, atheroma volume quantification provides superior risk prediction compared to a simple, semi-quantitative assessment, e.g., no, mild, moderate, severe by visual assessment, has not been demonstrated.
- There is interest in serial assessment of atheroma volume to determine plaque progression, but lack of standardization and considerable inter-scan variability remain major hurdles for widespread adoption [12].
- Atheroma volume can be further characterized according to its attenuation characteristics, which has been associated with common plaque tissue types, e.g., fibrous, calcified, lipid-rich, etc. [9].
- The accuracy of determining plaque types by CT is limited and description is best restricted to noncalcified, calcified, or partially calcified plaque.

13.4 Common Plaque Volume Metrics Derived from Arterial Contour Tracing

- There is no consensus on the desirable metrics obtained by plaque volume assessment.
- Common plaque volume metrics reported in the literature are displayed in Table 13.1.

13.5 Limitations of Plaque Volume Assessment and Outlook

- Several software packages are commercially available for coronary arterial lumen and vessel contour detection with variable validation data vs. intravascular imaging and/or histology.
- No standards have been established for measuring, computing and reporting plaque volume metrics though the SCCT issued a consensus statement for some guidance [13].
- Unless plaque volume is normalized for normal wall volume, "plaque" volume derived by subtracting lumen from vessel volume overestimates true plaque volume.
- No reference values have been established for reliable correlation with conventional coronary artery disease severity or with risk of adverse events.
- Inter-reader (limits of agreement +40 to −50%) and inter-scan reproducibility (+24 to −25%) is modest for plaque volume determination, limiting assessment of plaque progression at this time [12].
- Software algorithms are improving and their reliability and accuracy are expected to improve considerably over the next few years.
- Processing times also have markedly decreased and it is expected that standard,

Table 13.1 Common plaque volume metrics

Metric	Definition	Common range
Total Atheroma Volume (TAV)	Cumulative atheroma volume across analyzed segments per person	0–5000 mm^3
TAV normalized to total analyzed vessel length	Total atheroma volume/total vessel length (m)	0–10 mm^3/m
Percent Atheroma Volume (PAV)	(Total atheroma volume/total vessel volume)*100	0–70
Population normalized PAV	(Total atheroma volume/total vessel length)* average total vessel length analyzed in population	0–5000 mm^3

Note that values for TAV and PAV are highly dependent on software performance and image characteristics, and may be lower by a factor of 10 when normalized to visually absent atherosclerosis [8] commercially available image workstations will be routinely equipped with contour detection software for rapid assessment of atheroma burden, plaque characterization, lumen narrowing, and estimated hemodynamic impact in the near future.

- Numerous validation studies are underway investigating the utility of automated plaque and lumen volume as well as stenosis assessment, increasingly using artificial intelligence algorithms, to further augment performance.
- It is likely that automated atheroma, lumen, and stenosis assessment will evolve into the primary mode of coronary artery disease assessment for guiding patient management.

References

1. Arbab-Zadeh A, Nakano M, Virmani R, Fuster V. Acute coronary events. Circulation. 2012;125(9):1147–56.
2. Arbab-Zadeh A, Fuster V. The myth of the vulnerable plaque—transitioning from a focus on individual lesions to atherosclerotic disease burden for coronary artery disease risk assessment. J Am Coll Cardiol. 2015;65(8):846–55. https://doi.org/10.1016/j.jacc.2014.11.041.
3. Arbab-Zadeh A, Fuster V. The risk continuum of atherosclerosis and its implications for defining CHD by coronary angiography. J Am Coll Cardiol. 2016;68(22):2467–78.
4. van Rosendael AR, Bax JJ, Arbab-Zadeh A. Noninvasive assessment of coronary atherosclerosis by cardiac computed tomography for risk stratifying patients with suspected coronary heart disease. J Cardiovasc Comput Tomogr. 2019;13(5):235–41. https://doi.org/10.1016/j.jcct.2019.08.009.
5. Arbab-Zadeh A. Does "vulnerable" atherosclerotic plaque modify coronary blood flow?: how myths perpetuate. JACC Cardiovasc Imaging. 2020;13(3):757–9. https://doi.org/10.1016/j.jcmg.2019.07.011.
6. Nurmohamed NS, Min JK, et al. Atherosclerosis quantification and cardiovascular risk: the ISCHEMIA trial. Eur Heart J. 2024; ehae471. https://doi.org/10.1093/eurheartj/ehae471.
7. Tzimas G, Gulsin GS, Takagi H, et al. Coronary CT angiography to guide percutaneous coronary intervention. Radiol Cardiothorac Imaging. 2022;4(1):e210171.
8. Criqui MH, Denenberg JO, Ix JH, et al. Calcium density of coronary artery plaque and risk of incident cardiovascular events. JAMA. 2014;311(3):271–8. https://doi.org/10.1001/jama.2013.282535.
9. Bakhshi H, Meyghani Z, Kishi S, et al. Comparative effectiveness of CT-derived atherosclerotic plaque metrics for predicting myocardial ischemia. JACC Cardiovasc Imaging. 2018;12:1367.
10. Kishi S, Magalhaes T, Cerci R, et al. Semi-automatedly derived total atherosclerotic plaque burden by CT angiography for predicting clinically driven coronary artery revascularization: a comparison with expert stenosis assessment in the CORE320 study. Circulation. 2013;128:A9822.
11. Conte E, Mushtaq S, Pontone G, et al. Plaque quantification by coronary computed tomography angiography using intravascular ultrasound as a reference standard: a comparison between standard and last generation computed tomography scanners. Eur Heart J Cardiovasc Imaging. 2020;21(2):191–201. https://doi.org/10.1093/ehjci/jez089.
12. Meah MN, Singh T, Williams MC, et al. Reproducibility of quantitative plaque measurement in advanced coronary artery disease. J Cardiovasc Comput Tomogr. 2021;15(4):333–8. https://doi.org/10.1016/j.jcct.2020.12.008.
13. Nieman K, Garcia-Garcia HM, et al. Standards for Quantitative Coronary Computed Tomography Angiography (CCTA): An expert consensus statement by the society of cardiovascular computed tomography (SCCT). J Cardiovasc Comput Tomogr. 2024:S1934–5925(24)00341-1. https://doi.org/10.1016/j.jcct.2024.05.232. Online ahead of print.

14 Functional CT Assessment of Coronary Stenoses

Richard J. Bloomingdale and Kavitha M. Chinnaiyan

Abstract

Determining the hemodynamic impact of coronary artery stenoses has implications for patient management but conventional tools, e.g., diameter stenosis, are only modestly predictive. Fractional flow reserve (FFR) has been the gold standard adjudicator of hemodynamically significant coronary stenosis in the cardiac catheterization laboratory. Software algorithms utilizing models of computational flow dynamics have enabled FFR estimations obtained from static coronary CT angiography (CCTA) images. Optimal scan parameters including achieving an appropriate heart rate, vasodilation with nitroglycerin, and minimizing image noise and motion are necessary to ensure sufficient image quality for CT-derived FFR (CT-CT-FFR). CT-FFR must be interpreted in conjunction with CTA findings with attention to individual anatomic considerations. Lesion-specific values of <0.75 are considered hemodynamically significant, and values >0.8 are considered non-flow limiting, while values in the 0.75–0.80 range are intermediate, requiring further consideration of clinical and imaging factors. This chapter discusses concepts of functional assessment of coronary artery stenoses with CCTA as well as guidance for acquisition and interpretation.

Keywords

Coronary stenoses · CT-FFR · Hemodynamics · Lumen narrowing

Abbreviations

AU	Agatston units
CFR	Coronary flow reserve
CMR	Cardiac magnetic resonance
CPP	Coronary perfusion pressure
FFR	Fractional flow reserve
ICA	Invasive coronary angiography
MMAR	Myocardial mass at risk
MPI	Myocardial perfusion imaging
MVD	Microvascular disease
PET	Positron emission tomography
SPECT	Single-photon-emission computed tomography

14.1 Basic Concepts of Coronary Blood Flow Regulation

- Myocardial perfusion occurs with the delivery of oxygenated blood via the epicardial coro-

R. J. Bloomingdale
Corewell Health, Royal Oak, MI, USA
e-mail: richard.bloomingdale@corewellhealth.org

K. M. Chinnaiyan (✉)
Oakland University William Beaumont University, Corewell Health, Royal Oak, MI, USA
e-mail: kavitha.chinnaiyan@beaumont.edu

A. A. Zadeh, J. Hoe (eds.), *Practical Guide to Cardiac CT*,
https://doi.org/10.1007/978-981-97-6919-3_14

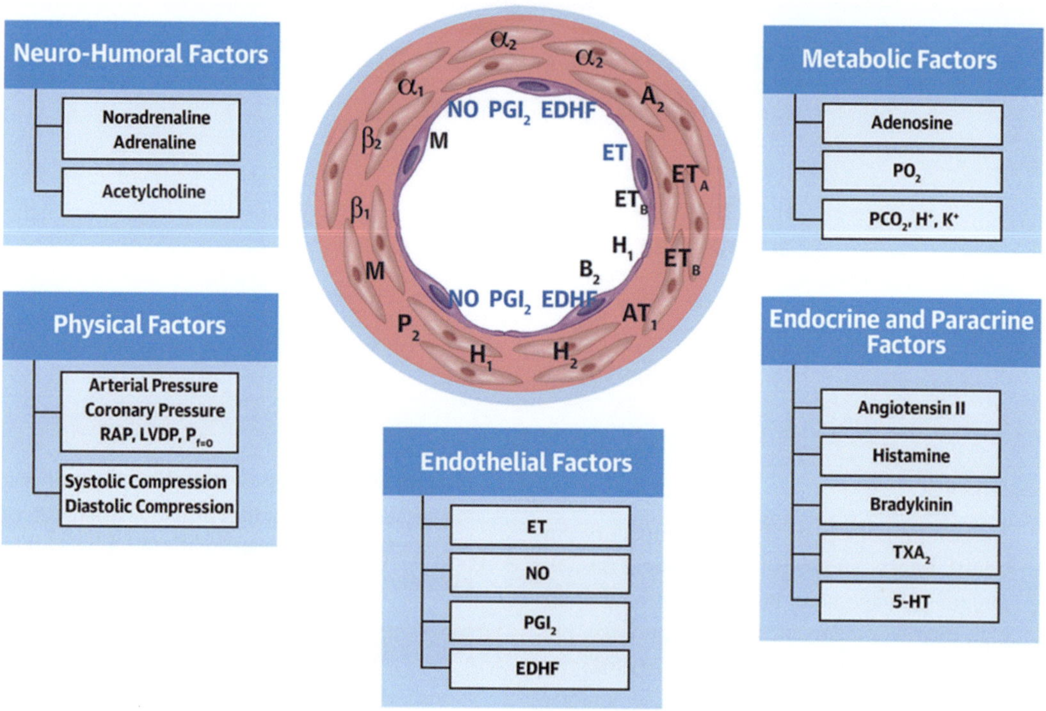

Fig. 14.1 Autoregulatory mechanisms of coronary artery blood flow. (*Reprinted with permission* [1])

nary vessels and is affected by tightly regulated local and systemic factors.

- While the aortic diastolic pressure drives blood flow into the myocardium toward the subepicardium, left ventricular diastolic pressure resists this flow at the subendocardium; the difference between these two pressures is *coronary perfusion pressure* (*CPP*).
- Muscular compression of the intramyocardial vessels in systole coupled with an increase in the intracavitary pressure reduces coronary flow; myocardial relaxation during diastole restores it.
- Numerous other factors affect regulation of coronary flow including neural, hormonal, endothelial, and metabolic processes (Fig. 14.1) [1].

14.2 Coronary Flow Reserve

- Coronary flow in the resting heart remains relatively constant due to autoregulation driven by vasodilatory mechanisms (See Fig. 14.2, red line). Coronary flow typically does not drop until CPP is <40 mmHg. Pharmacologic induction of vasodilation can increase blood flow in normal arteries four to fivefold (See Fig. 14.2, blue line) [2].
- Abnormalities in blood flow can result due to focal stenosis, diffuse disease, or small-vessel disease [3]. Absolute coronary flow can be determined invasively with a flow wire or non-invasively with quantification techniques with CT, PET, SPECT, and other modalities (as milliliters per minute). However, clinical applicability of absolute flow measurement is limited because coronary flow varies widely between patients and arteries [4]. Absolute flow reserve is a physiologic measure that compares hyperemic flow to resting flow and is influenced by loading conditions, heart rate, and other factors [5]. Relative flow reserve compares maximal coronary flow in a diseased region of an artery to the flow in the normal segment of the same artery but can only be utilized when this normal segment exists. CFR can be assessed with invasive flow meters, dynamic CT (see Chap. 18), PET, SPECT, CMR, or myocardial contrast echocardiography [6].

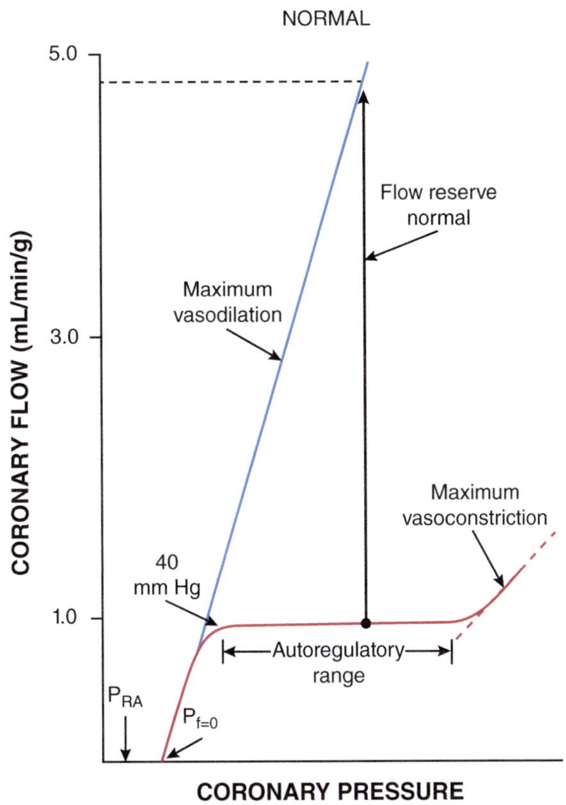

Fig. 14.2 Coronary flow is maintained at a constant level across a wide range of coronary perfusion pressures in the normal artery (red line). In the absence of a coronary stenosis, flow can increase four to fivefold with pharmacologic vasodilation (blue line). (*Adapted with permission* [2])

- *Fractional flow reserve* is the ratio of post-stenotic coronary pressure to the aortic pressure during maximal vasodilation and reflects what the maximum flow in the artery would be if it were not diseased [2] (see details below).

14.3 Determinants of Myocardial Ischemia

- The rate-pressure product (heart rate × systolic blood pressure) partly determines the myocardial workload, which influences the high oxygen-demand myocyte metabolism [7].
- CFR decreases with an *increase* in heart rate (because the diastolic time available for perfusion decreases), an *increase* in preload or radial wall stress, an *increase* in resting flow (increased systolic pressure or contractility), a decrease in arterial oxygen supply (anemia or hypoxia), or due to microvascular dysfunction resulting in abnormal vasodilation (see Fig. 14.3) [2].

Normal myocardial perfusion is sustained up to the lowest pressure at which there is maximal dilation of the resistance vessels.

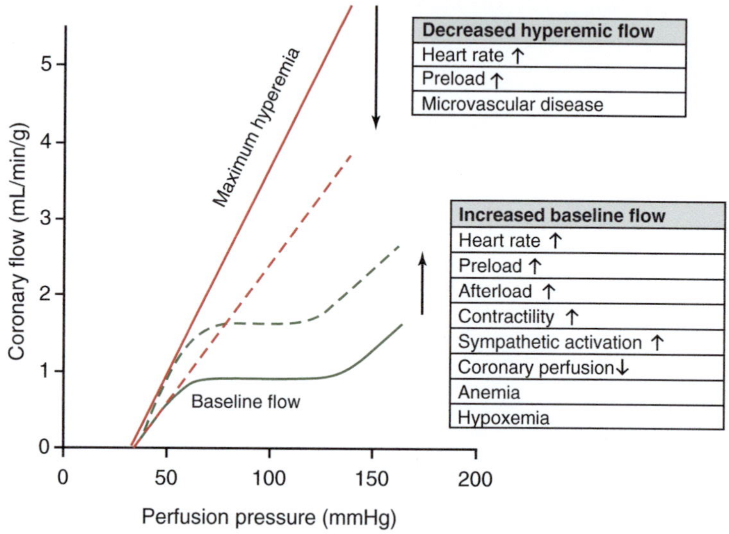

Fig. 14.3 Myocardial ischemia results from oxygen supply mismatch from increased baseline flow or decreased hyperemic flow, each of which are influenced by multiple factors. (*Reprinted with permission* [6])

14.4 The Concept of Fractional Flow Reserve

- Fractional flow reserve (FFR) compares flow distal to a stenotic area to a normal segment of a maximally vasodilated coronary artery; approximating maximal blood flow that would be achievable under normal conditions. FFR is calculated by dividing the downstream pressure in a stenotic coronary by the pressure in the aorta [4].
- Since FFR is derived under maximal hyperemic conditions, it represents the *fraction* of maximal coronary or myocardial blood flow that is preserved in the context of the stenotic lesion [1].
- An FFR value of ≤0.80 derived during invasive coronary angiography (ICA) with a pressure wire has excellent diagnostic accuracy (>90%) for identifying coronary stenoses resulting in myocardial ischemia [8].
- The FAME (FFR vs. angiography for multivessel evaluation) study demonstrated decreased MACE in FFR vs. angiographically guided percutaneous coronary intervention (PCI) patients, though largely driven by fewer periprocedural events as result of deferred interventions. Nevertheless, the concept of FFR guided PCI was widely adopted [9, 10].

14.5 Conventional vs. Functional Assessment of Coronary Stenoses

- Conventionally, coronary stenosis on CTA can be assessed quantitatively or semi-quantitatively for severity of stenoses, with greater than 70% diameter lumen narrowing by visual assessment (approximately 50% by quantification) commonly associated with hemodynamic significance.
- Images can be assessed on a per-segment basis for the number and severity of lesions, and on a per-lesion basis for diameter stenosis, minimal lumen diameter (MLD) and minimal lumen area (MLA) lumen, plaque or atheroma volume and composition, the presence of the so-called high-risk plaque features including positive remodeling, spotty calcification, napkin ring sign, and low attenuation plaque (see also Chap. 11).
- In one study of 210 patients undergoing CTA and ICA, MLA ≤1.8 mm^2 and MLD ≤1.2 mm were the most accurate cut-offs for the prediction of hemodynamically significant stenosis on ICA, with a higher accuracy than relative percent stenosis [11]. However, vessel size should be considered.

- It is possible to derive the myocardial mass at risk (MMAR) from CTA images. In a study of 111 patients, there was a significant correlation between an invasive FFR ≤ 0.8 and MMAR/MLD [12].
- Machine learning techniques have recently examined the utility of advanced plaque quantification. In addition to total plaque volume, the type of plaque such as calcified, noncalcified, low attenuation or fibrofatty results in superior prognostication for downstream major adverse cardiac events beyond stenosis severity alone. The multicenter, prospective CAPIRE study included 544 patients and demonstrated that quantitative plaque volume measurement outperformed not only traditional risk factors, clinical risk algorithms and biomarkers but also stenosis on CTA, qualitative assessment of high-risk plaques for predicting MACE over 5 years. Noncalcified plaque was associated with the highest risk for MACE [13]. However, there were very low event rates in this study due to exclusion of higher risk patients.
- In the DeFACTO trial of 252 patients, plaque volume and high-risk features of low attenuation and positive remodeling on CTA were predictive of reduced FFR even in nonobstructive lesions that would be considered nonsevere on angiography [14].
- An analysis from the NXT study of 484 coronary vessels demonstrated that large, low attenuation plaques were the strongest predictors of lesion-specific ischemia by invasive FFR [15].
- The importance of volumetric plaque analysis was further demonstrated in the multicenter, prospective, diagnostic derivation-validation CREDENCE study in which enrolled patients underwent CTA and myocardial perfusion imaging (MPI) followed by ICA and FFR. Compared to the presence of ischemia on MPI, stenosis severity and plaque burden on CTA including noncalcified atheroma volume and the number of lesions with high-risk plaque were more strongly associated with a vessel-specific FFR ≤0.80 [16]. In addition to re-demonstrating the association between stenosis and FFR, this study was hypothesis-generating for that of diffuse atherosclerosis resulting in a smaller vessel lumen, which can only be determined by evaluating the whole vessel rather than focusing on individual areas of stenoses.
- Other emerging technologies for evaluation of coronary disease on CTA include wall shear stress and axial plaque stress, which improve identification of high-risk plaque and plaque rupture.
- Wall shear stress is tangential force per unit area acting on and parallel to the luminal surface of the endothelium, whereas axial plaque stress is the force on the plaque due to pressure gradient that increases axial tension on the upstream segment of the plaque and decreased stress on the downstream end of the plaque.
- In one analysis of the DeFacto study of 100 patients, high wall shear stress was associated with stenosis severity, low attenuation plaque and positive remodeling. Wall shear stress was inversely associated with invasive FFR [17].
- The EMERALD study examined various hemodynamic indices including wall shear stress, axial plaque stress, CT-FFR and ΔCT-FFR in identification of high-risk plaques associated with acute coronary syndromes in 72 patients who had undergone CTA within the preceding 2 years. Compared to non-culprit lesions, culprit lesions demonstrated significantly lower CT-FFR, greater ΔCT-FFR, wall shear stress and axial plaque stress [18].
- Transluminal attenuation gradient (TAG) is a novel process that can assess the severity of coronary stenosis, which is a change in Hounsfield Units (HU) per 10-mm length of the coronary artery, defined as the linear regression coefficient between luminal attenuation (in HU) and length from the ostium (mm), which can determine the hemodynamic significance of a stenotic lesion. TAG has been shown to correlate with the degree of diameter stenosis, with the ability to discriminate between nonobstructive and obstructive coronary arteries [19]. However, TAG has not been studied extensively, especially in comparison with FFR.

14.6 CT-Derived FFR (CT-FFR)

- CT-Derived FFR (CT-FFR or CT-FFR) utilizes data from coronary CT angiography (CTA) at rest to generate CT-Derived FFR (CT-FFR or CT-FFR) utilizes data from coronary CT angiography (CTA) at rest to generate a mathematical model of coronary flow, pressure, and resistance (see Fig. 14.4) [20].
- The CT-FFR mathematical modeling is dependent on the following assumptions (see Fig. 14.5):
  - Total coronary blood flow in resting conditions is directly proportional to the overall myocardial mass.
  - Coronary microvascular resistance at rest is inversely proportional to the size of the epicardial coronary arteries.
  - The hyperemic response derived on invasive angiography is predictable enough to replicate in a computational model. This principle can be mimicked by decreasing the microvascular resistance by a factor of 0.21. In coronary CTA, this reduction is achieved by the administration of nitroglycerin, which is necessary for CT-FFR assessment.
  - Flow and pressure in the coronary system can be calculated with the Navier–Stokes equation [21].
- The above-mentioned mathematical assumptions require a supercomputer, which generates a three-dimensional model of the coronary tree using segmented coronary CTA data.
- Analysis may be performed on-site or remote. In the latter scenario, coronary CTA data are transferred to a remote location via secure networks and patient-specific CT-FFR data are received after analysis (see Fig. 14.5).
- Onsite computational fluid analysis-based algorithms may incorporate machine learning or deep learning for faster processing.
- Alternative models predicting hemodynamically significant stenoses bases on plaque characteristics, e.g., plasticity, have been recently introduced and may represent another option for CT-based functional assessment of coronary artery stenoses.
- Myocardial perfusion imaging for assessment of myocardial ischemia is discussed in Chap. 18.

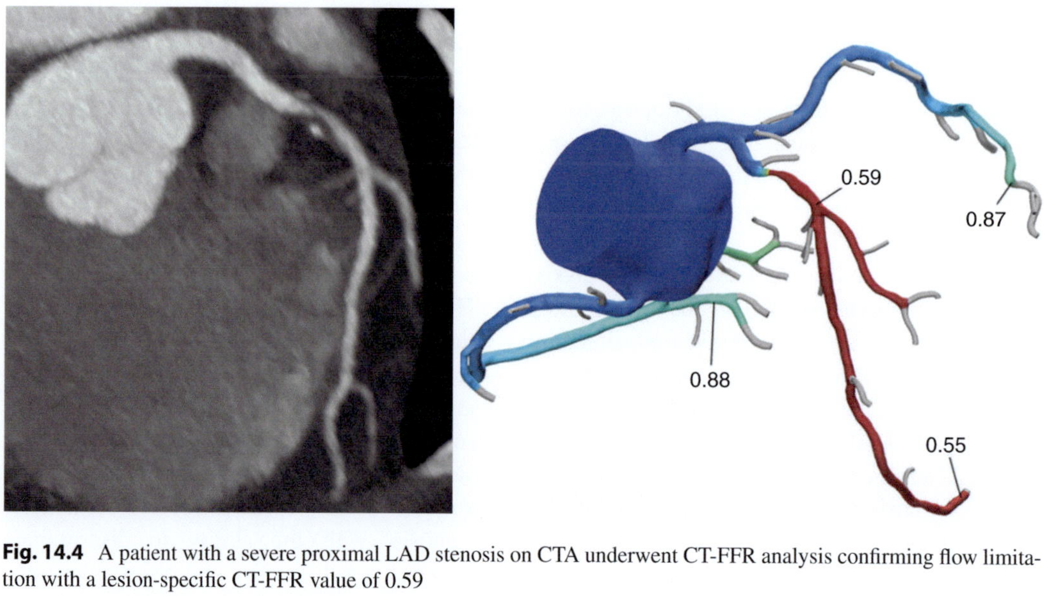

Fig. 14.4 A patient with a severe proximal LAD stenosis on CTA underwent CT-FFR analysis confirming flow limitation with a lesion-specific CT-FFR value of 0.59

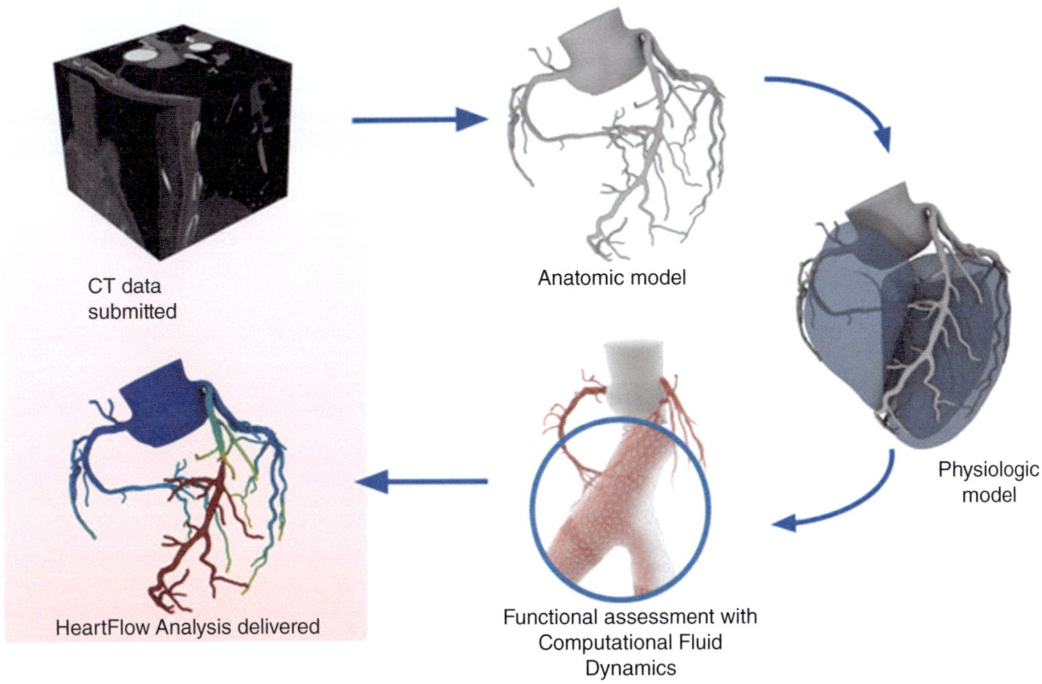

Fig. 14.5 Anatomical data combined with key assumptions about mass, resistance, and hyperemia are used to calculate a coronary flow model utilizing computational fluid dynamics. (*Reprinted with permission* [10])

14.7 Interpreting CT-FFR

- CT-FFR data are received as continuous values that are derived along the coronary arteries and are color-coded for at-a-glance interpretation.
- CT-FFR results must be interpreted along with the coronary CTA findings (see Fig. 14.6), specifically the location of stenosis.
- Interpretation of CT-FFR must include careful review of the CTA images since even minor artifacts or poor image quality can impact data output leading to false positive or negative values (see Sect. 14.13).
- CT-FFR values should be evaluated in the following ways:
  - Specific to the lesion, where the information from the coronary CTA is correlated with the location of the CT-FFR value. Typically, this is 2 cm distal to the lesion and is demonstrated to be more accurate and clinically valuable than a single value obtained at the distal vessel [22, 23].
  - Distal coronary value, which is of particular interest when there is diffuse disease in the corresponding coronary artery and when positive, may represent ischemia related to the overall atherosclerotic burden. Distal positivity in the absence of significant disease is of uncertain clinical significance and may represent a discordance between the coronary volume and myocardial mass (volume/mass ratio, or V/M), such as in the presence of left ventricular hypertrophy, small coronary arteries or microvascular disease (MVD). The significance of a positive CT-FFR value at the distal vessel in the absence of significant coronary disease is unclear and needs to be studied further.
- CT-FFR values for clinical interpretation are similar to those derived on invasive angiography. A value of >0.8 is considered non-significant for ischemia, whereas a value of <0.75 is indicative of a hemodynamically significant coronary stenosis. CT-FFR values of 0.75–0.8 are indeterminate and require further investigation for ischemia.

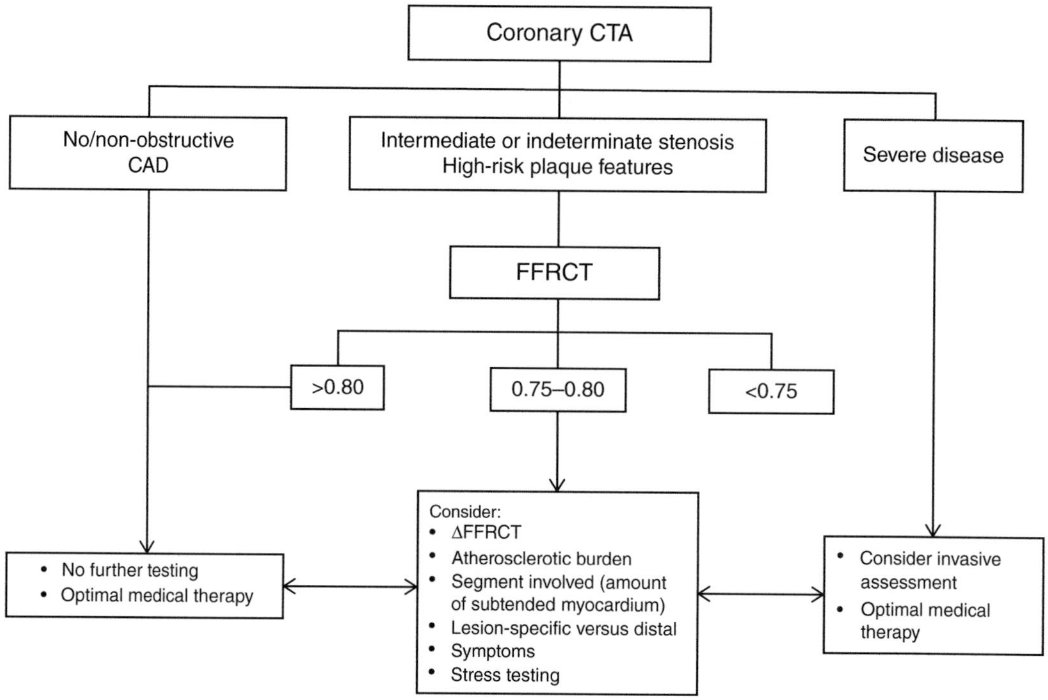

Fig. 14.6 Suggested algorithm for CT-FFR interpretation. A CT-FFR value of 0.80 or greater, in general, warrants no further testing, whereas patients with a value of <0.75 may benefit from invasive coronary evaluation in the adequate clinical context. In patients with intermediate values (0.75–0.80), additional factors should be considered, e.g., symptoms, atherosclerotic burden, lesion location. Emerging data suggest that ΔCT-FFR, lesion length on coronary CTA, and the amount of subtended myocardium may provide incremental data on patient management and prognosis

- It is important to remember that while cut-off values are useful, CT-FFR is better viewed as a continuum, and interpretation by the physician caring for the patient should consider clinical factors such as the presence of symptoms, atherosclerotic burden, and data from other ischemia testing, such as stress testing.
- Furthermore, the evaluation of translesional FFR flow gradient or ΔCT-FFR can be of incremental use in patients with positive CT-FFR. In such patients, a ΔCT-FFR >0.13 can further adjudicate those that would benefit from revascularization [24].

14.8 Workflow of Remote CT-FFR Assessment

Establishing the Workflow

- For a remote analysis setup, establishing an efficient workflow is important to ensure appropriate indications, good quality, and timely interpretation, which influence clinical outcomes as well as cost-effectiveness.
- Offsite image analysis requires establishing workflows that are collaborative between CTA requesting and interpreting physicians, use of electronic medical records, well-trained CT technologists, adequate patient preparation to ensure the best image quality, and timely reporting of results.
- Since the beginning of its widespread clinical availability, the turnaround time of remote CT-FFR has decreased considerably. However, the turnaround time must be considered when utilizing CT-FFR particularly in patients with acute chest pain [25]. The current turnaround time is 2–4 h in outpatients or in those with stable symptoms, and 1–2 h in those with acute symptoms. Further reductions are anticipated.

- CT-FFR in all patients undergoing CTA is neither needed nor cost-effective, since at present, there is an additional cost for the FFR analysis through commercially available vendors. The 2021 multi-society guidelines for chest pain evaluation recommend considering CT-FFR evaluation in patients with intermediate stenosis on CTA (40–70%). Consensus among the institution's interpreting physicians is helpful to determine which patients may benefit the most from CT-FFR (such as intermediate stenoses, high-risk plaque features, indeterminate stenosis due to calcification).
- The most important factor in CT-FFR acquisition is good image quality, which cannot be overemphasized.

14.9 CT-FFR Ordering and Report Integration

- If CT-FFR analysis is determined to be indicated at the time of the interpretation of the coronary CTA, the reader should ideally include an addendum at the end of the fully dictated report detailing the coronary segments of concern for which CT-FFR is being requested including the stenosis severity, presence of obscuring calcification, and/or high-risk plaque features (Fig. 14.7).
- A screenshot of the vessel segment in the body of the report can be helpful for the ordering physician as well as a second CT reader who may be reporting the CT-FFR findings at a later time.
- The initial CT reader should ensure a CT-FFR order is in the system (typically placed as an optional add-on by the original ordering physician).
- The images are then uploaded to the third-party vendor servers via a secure DICOM transfer.
- Email notification alerts the CT team that CT-FFR results are completed and available online through the vendor website.
- The CT-FFR results are then interpreted either with the interactive 3D model or the static PDF results with pins highlighting the CT-FFR values 1–2 cm after each stenosis.

CT-FFR ORDER ADDENDUM

The abnormal results of the Cardiac CT warrant CT-FFR Coronary Analysis (HeartFlow, Inc*) to define the extent of lesion-specific ischemia in the proximal left anterior descending, distal left circumflex, and mid right coronary arteries. Results will be available in 12–24 hours if technical quality is sufficient for analysis (Emergency Department Ct-FFR study results will be available in 2–3 hours).

Indication for request of CT-FFR analysis (check all that apply):

- [ ] Mild coronary artery stenosis (26–50% stenosis) in selected patients who may benefit from CT-FFR
- [ ] Moderate coronary artery stenosis (51–70% stenosis)
- [ ] Severe coronary artery stenosis (>70% stenosis) of uncertain significance
- [x] Uncertain stenosis severity due to calcified plaque in the coronary artery
- [ ] Presence of high risk plaque features
- [ ] Other

Coronary CT Angiography Image:

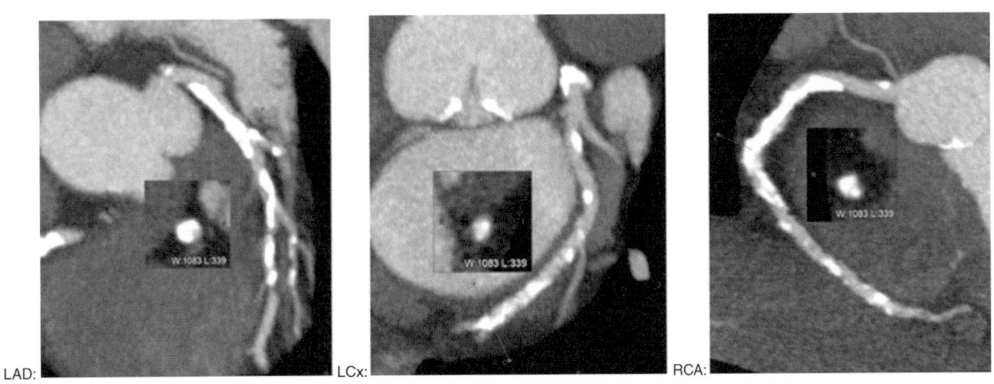

* CT-FFR is an FDA-approved noninvasive technique for defining lesion-specific ischemia that correlates with invasive FFR. The overall assessment requires integration of the CTA findings, CT-FFR model and clinical correlation.

Fig. 14.7 Sample report addendum of a study being sent for CT-FFR analysis including the indication for the request and images of the vessel segments in question

CT-FFR CORONARY ANALYSIS

CT-FFR values were evaluated corresponding to CTA identified lesions, as illustrated below in original CTA report (see "Indication for request for FFRCT analysis").

Interpretation:

1. The uninterpretable stenosis in the **proximal LAD coronary artery** (due to heavy calcification) has a **low likelihood of lesion-specific ischemia** with a CT-FFR value of **0.86**
2. The uninterpretable stenosis in the **mid LAD coronary artery** (due to heavy calcification) has an **high likelihood of lesion-specific ischemia** with a CT-FFR value of **0.79**
3. The uninterpretable stenosis in the **distal circumflex coronary artery** (due to heavy calcification) has a **high likelihood of lesion-specific ischemia** with a CT-FFR value of **0.74**
4. The uninterpretable stenosis in the **proximal right coronary artery** (due to heavy calcification) has a **high likelihood of lesion-specific ischemia** with a CT-FFR value of **0.70**

FFRCT IMAGE INSERT

(Include FFRCT values distal to all segments with stenosis >50% or stenosis >25% in the left main, proximal LAD or when high risk plaque features present)

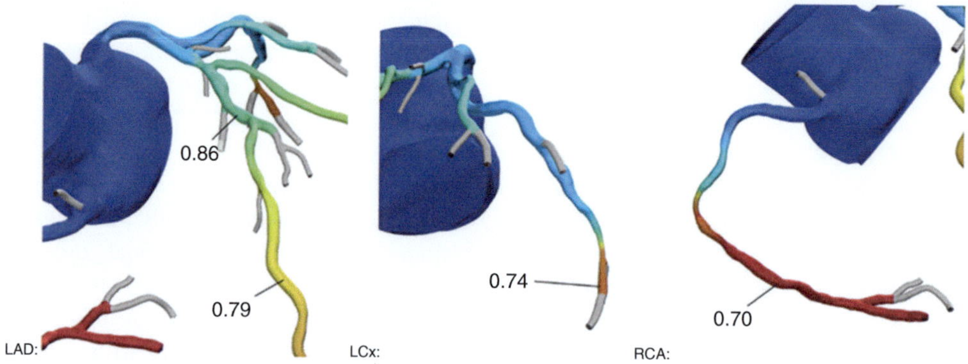

Interpreting Physician: @ME@ **Date/Time: @NOW@**

Summary of CT-FFR Values
a. >0.80 (distal to the stenosis): Low likelihood of lesion-specific ischemia
b. ≤0.80 (distal to the stenosis): High likelihood of lesion-specific ischemia
c. Assessment of lesion-specific ischemia by CT-FFR should rely on CT-FFR values measured approximately 10–15 mm distal to the lesion of interest, rather than from the terminal vessel. FFRCT values <0.80 measured from the terminal vessel do not necessarily indicate lesion-specific ischemia, particularly if there is only mild disease in the more proximal segments of the vessel.

Fig. 14.8 Example of a CT-FFR result addendum

- If a different reader is interpreting the CT-FFR results, the source CT images should be re-evaluated to ensure accurate interpretation.
- The report is then addended with the CT-FFR results including screenshots of the coronary tree model and CT-FFR value pins (if possible). See Fig. 14.8.
- Integration of the static PDF report may allow treatment team members to see the CT-FFR results in systems where images cannot be included in the body of the report (Fig. 14.9).
- A schematic of the workflow for interpretation of a CTA and CT-FFR in a multi-reader setting is detailed in Fig. 14.10.

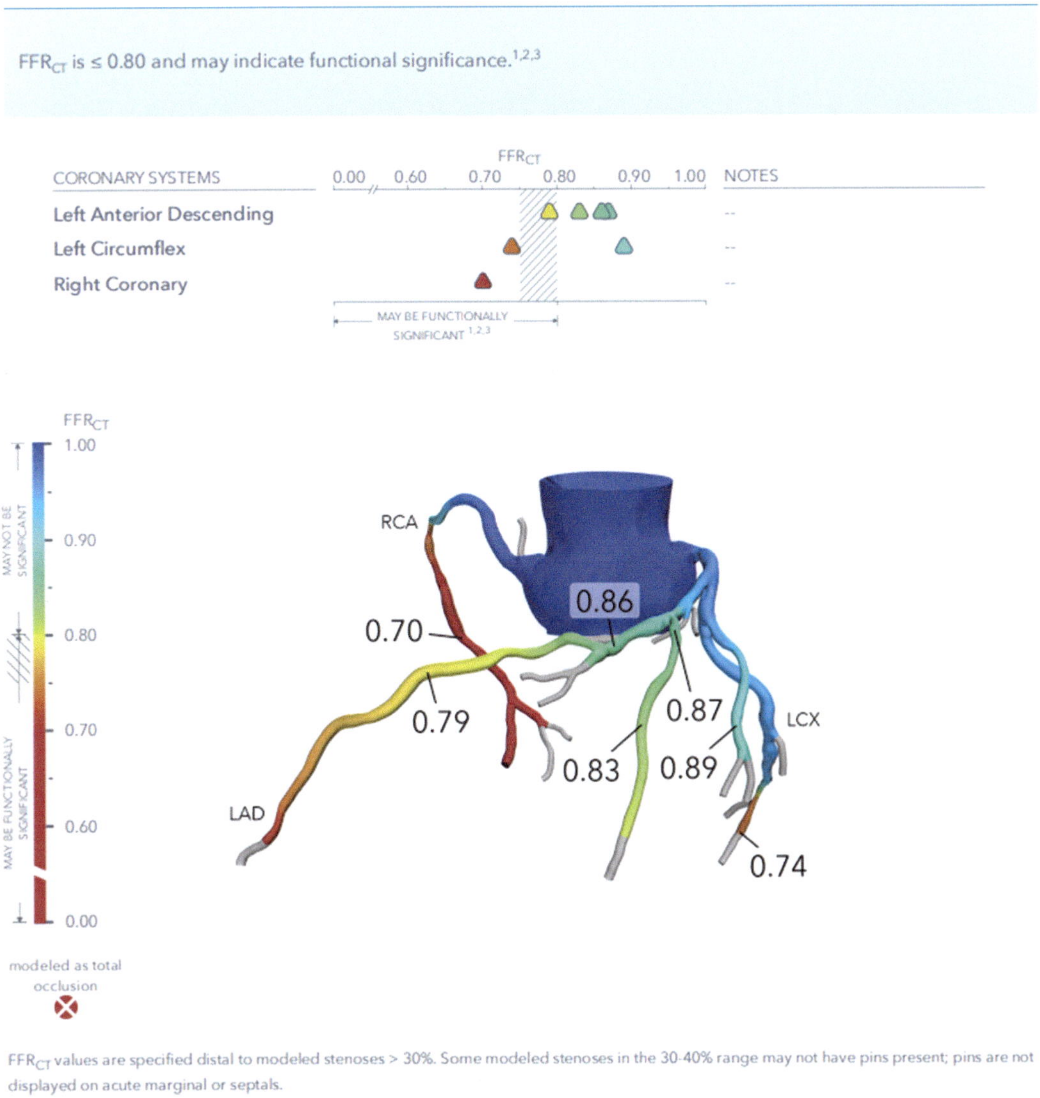

Fig. 14.9 Example of a static PDF report

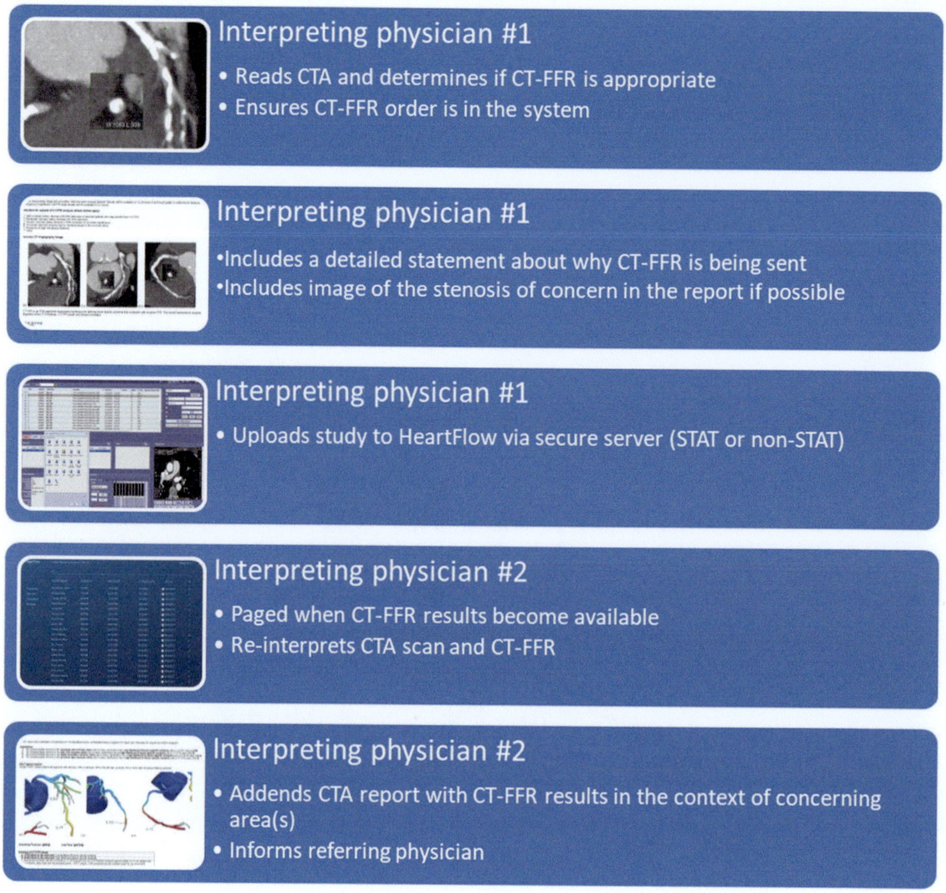

Fig. 14.10 Workflow for CTA and CT-FFR ordering, interpretation, and report integration

14.10 Most Studied Clinical Use of CT-FFR

- CT-FFR may be useful in patients with intermediate degrees of stenosis (variously described as 40–90%) on CTA, where adjudication of its physiologic importance is needed for clinical decision-making regarding revascularization.
- The 2021 Multi-society Chest Pain Guideline gives a Class 2a recommendation for add-on CT-FFR analysis in patients who undergo coronary CTA for acute or stable chest pain with 40–90% stenosis in a proximal or mid vessel unless they have high-risk coronary artery disease or frequent angina, in which case invasive angiography has a Class 1 recommendation [26].
- Numerous studies have demonstrated that in patients with intermediate degrees of coronary stenoses on CTA, a negative CT-FFR (value of >c0.80) can be used to avoid invasive angiography and revascularization (see Fig. 14.11) [27, 28].
- The diagnostic accuracy of coronary CTA improves incrementally with addition of plaque feature assessment as well as CT-FFR, and together outperform the accuracy of stress MPI as detailed in the CREDENCE trial [16].
- CT-FFR evaluation may also be useful in patients with calcified coronary lesions where the adjudication of stenosis and their significance is limited. Preliminary studies demonstrate an inverse relationship between coronary artery calcium scores (CACS, in Agatston units) and CT-FFR values (see Fig. 14.12) [29].

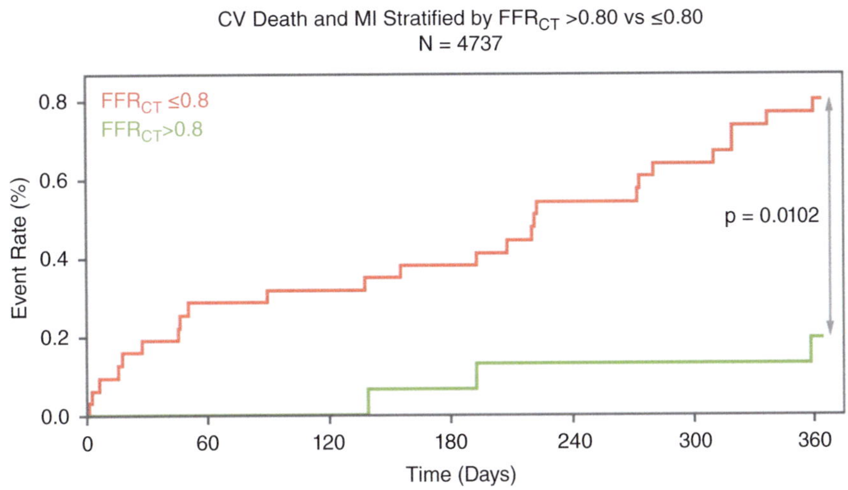

Fig. 14.11 Patients with CT-FFR > 0.8 have lower CV Death and MI compared to those with CT-FFR <0.8 at 1 year. (*Reprinted with permission* [28])

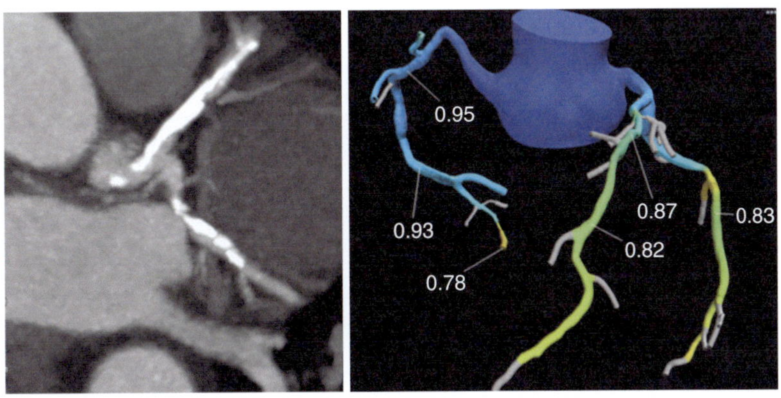

Fig. 14.12 A patient with heavily calcified left anterior descending and left circumflex arteries which can be assessed with CT-FFR

- Blooming artifact of heavy calcification can overestimate the degree of coronary stenosis.
- Elevated CACS has no significant impact on CT-FFR performance even with CACS >400 AU, however, very high scores, e.g., CACS >1000, are associated with reduced specificity [30].
- Extensive calcification that obscures the coronary lumen precludes assessment of CT-FFR.

14.11 Myocardial Volume/Mass in CT-FFR

- CT-FFR may be useful in the evaluation of MVD, where the V/M ratio is expected to be lower. Small studies have suggested the utility of CT-FFR in patients with MVD [31]. Larger studies with robust correlations with other modalities such as cardiac PET or MRI are needed.
- Volume and mass data can be derived from standard CTA images through specialized algorithms without the employment of CT-FFR.
- Of particular value in emerging studies is the concept of subtended myocardial mass at risk. Early studies suggest that in addition to stenosis severity, the myocardial territory as assessed on coronary CTA is independently affected by invasive FFR, which should be considered when interpreting CT-FFR [32]. Subtended myocardial mass evaluation does not require CT-FFR analysis and can be derived independently from standard CTA images with specific tools and algorithms.

14.12 CT-FFR and Lesion Length

- In addition to the degree of stenosis, lesion length may have a significant effect on ischemia, particularly related to intermediate stenoses on invasive angiography. In invasive angiography studies, a lesion length > 16 mm was shown to predict an FFR value <0.80 in intermediate lesions [33]. CT-FFR studies are needed to examine the correlation between lesion length and CT-FFR values.

14.13 Limitations of CT-FFR

- Good image quality is critical for adequate CT-FFR analysis and interpretation.
- Image noise affecting the coronary vessels affects the ability to identify lumen boundaries, may reduce the accuracy of the CT-FFR analysis, and if significant may result in the inability to analyze the study (see Fig. 14.13).
- Scanners with narrow detector coverage are susceptible to misalignment artifact which can result in pseudostenosis.
- Blending algorithms should be turned off on data sets sent for CT-FFR analysis to prevent false positive results (see Fig. 14.14).
- Nitroglycerin administration is necessary to induce the coronary vasodilation (see above) since CT-FFR calculations depend on the assumption of hyperemia.
- A dose of 0.8 μg is recommended over a 0.4 μg dose due to increased coronary vasodilation and fewer false positive CT-FFR results (see Fig. 14.15) [34].

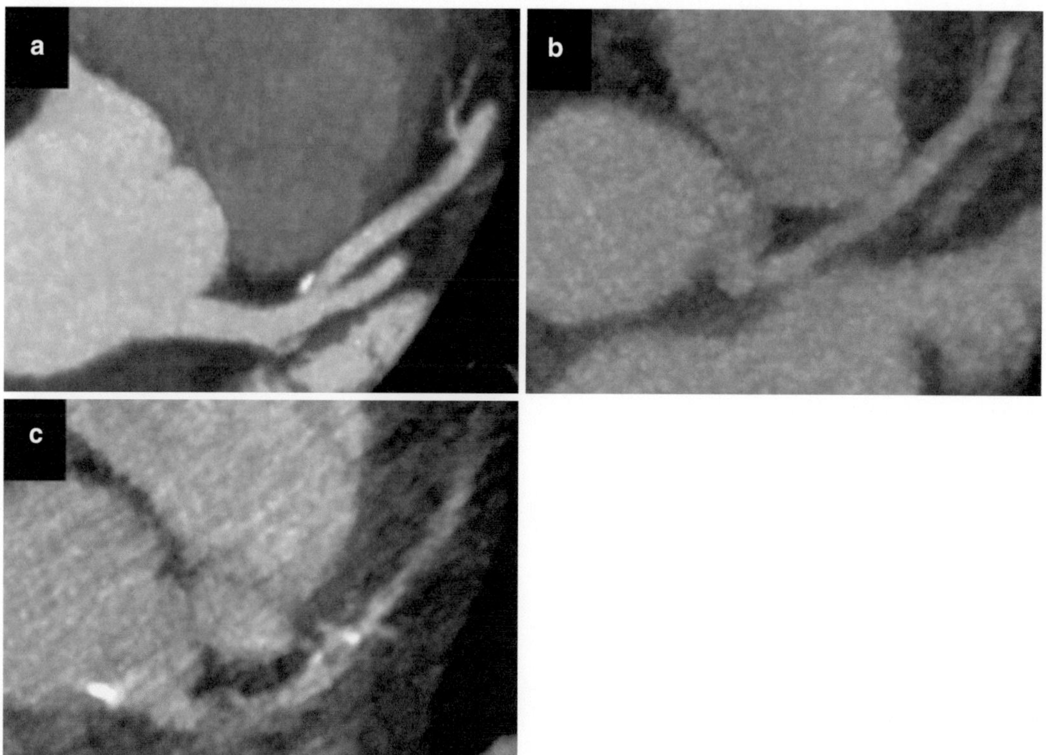

Fig. 14.13 Image noise degrades coronary lumen assessment and may preclude accurate boundary identification. Panel **a** shows excellent contrast-to-noise (CNR). Panel **b** has marginal CNR. Panel **c** has poor CNR precluding CT-FFR analysis

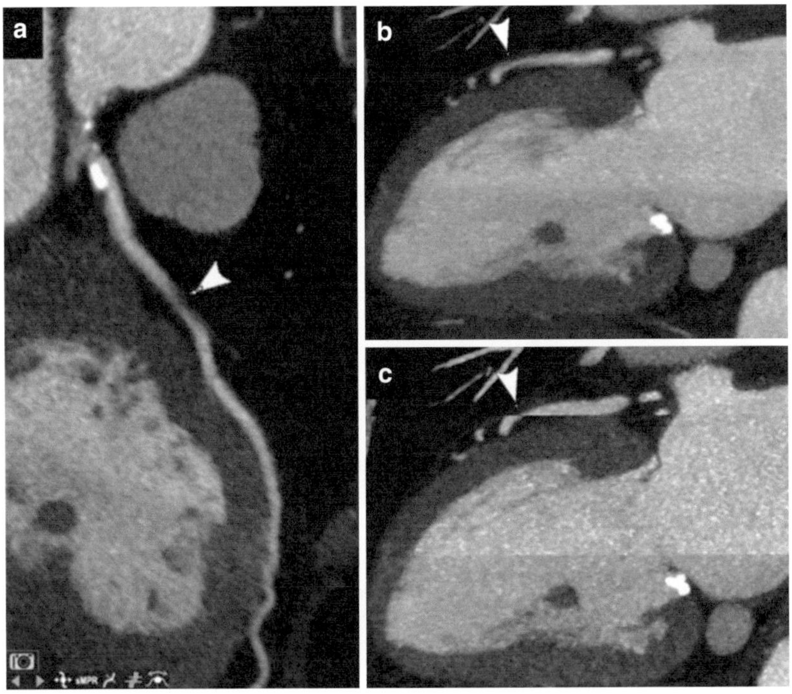

Fig. 14.14 Luminal narrowing due to pseudostenosis is seen in the LAD on a CPR reconstruction in panel **a**. Panel **b** shows the sagittal oblique view of the stenosis. Panel **c** demonstrates the same sagittal oblique view with blending algorithms turned off, and a misalignment artifact is seen causing a pseudostenosis

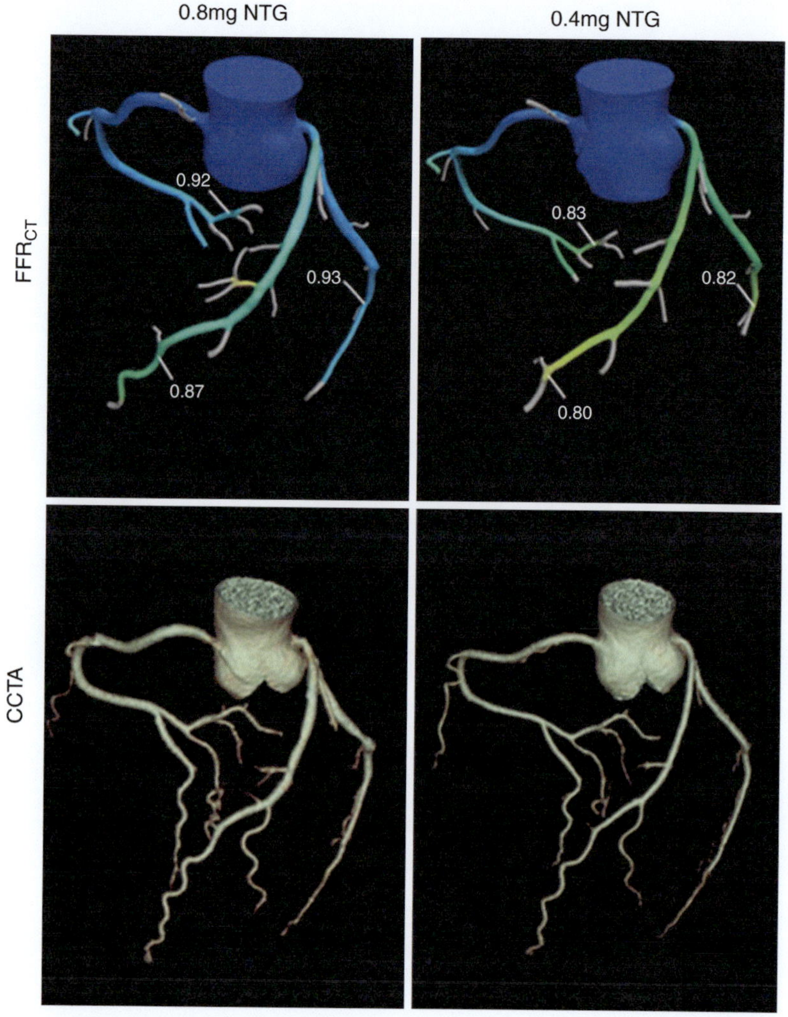

Fig. 14.15 The same patient was imaged with a dose of 0.4 and 0.8 mg of nitroglycerin. The lower dose resulted in less vasodilation and lower corresponding CT-FFR values. (*Reprinted with permission* [34])

14.14 Conclusions

- CT-derived FFR provides an assessment of the hemodynamic significance of coronary stenoses based on static CCTA images.
- While the concept is appealing, CT-FFR adds costs and time to CCTA assessment.
- CT-FFR may be useful in coronary lesions of intermediate stenosis, where their hemodynamic significance is uncertain and requires adjudication.
- Ensuring image quality is of paramount importance in ensuring clinical meaningful CT-FFR.
- Interpretation of CT-FFR is nuanced and requires incorporating coronary CTA findings.
- CT-FFR values represent a continuum and thresholds should not be regarded as absolute.
- Further refinements of CT-FFR may ease its application and may help facilitating real-time diagnosis of hemodynamically significant coronary artery disease.

References

1. Johnson NP, Gould KL, De Bruyne B. Autoregulation of coronary blood supply in response to demand: JACC review topic of the week. J Am Coll Cardiol. 2021;77(18):2335–45.

2. Duncker DJ, et al. Regulation of coronary blood flow in health and ischemic heart disease. Prog Cardiovasc Dis. 2015;57(5):409–22.
3. Taqueti VR, Di Carli MF. Clinical significance of noninvasive coronary flow reserve assessment in patients with ischemic heart disease. Curr Opin Cardiol. 2016;31(6):662–9.
4. Pijls NH, et al. Fractional flow reserve. A useful index to evaluate the influence of an epicardial coronary stenosis on myocardial blood flow. Circulation. 1995;92(11):3183–93.
5. Gould KL, Kirkeeide RL, Buchi M. Coronary flow reserve as a physiologic measure of stenosis severity. J Am Coll Cardiol. 1990;15(2):459–74.
6. Feher A, Sinusas AJ. Quantitative assessment of coronary microvascular function: dynamic single-photon emission computed tomography, positron emission tomography, ultrasound, computed tomography, and magnetic resonance imaging. Circ Cardiovasc Imaging. 2017;10(8):e006427.
7. Goodwill AG, et al. Regulation of coronary blood flow. Compr Physiol. 2017;7:321–82.
8. Tonino PA, et al. Fractional flow reserve versus angiography for guiding percutaneous coronary intervention. N Engl J Med. 2009;360(3):213–24.
9. De Bruyne B, et al. Fractional flow reserve-guided PCI versus medical therapy in stable coronary disease. N Engl J Med. 2012;367(11):991–1001.
10. Taylor C, Petersen K, Xiao N, Sinclair M, Bai Y, Lynch SR, Updepac A, Schaap M. Patient-specific modeling of blood flow in the coronary arteries. Comput Methods Appl Mech Eng. 2023;417:116414.
11. Plank F, et al. Quantitative coronary CT angiography: absolute lumen sizing rather than %stenosis predicts hemodynamically relevant stenosis. Eur Radiol. 2016;26(11):3781–9.
12. Sadamatsu K, et al. The functional severity assessment of coronary stenosis using coronary computed tomography angiography-based myocardial mass at risk and minimal lumen diameter. Cardiovasc Ther. 2020;2020:6716130.
13. Andreini D, et al. Coronary plaque features on CTA can identify patients at increased risk of cardiovascular events. JACC Cardiovasc Imaging. 2020;13(8):1704–17.
14. Park HB, et al. Atherosclerotic plaque characteristics by CT angiography identify coronary lesions that cause ischemia: a direct comparison to fractional flow reserve. JACC Cardiovasc Imaging. 2015;8(1):1–10.
15. Gaur S, et al. Coronary plaque quantification and fractional flow reserve by coronary computed tomography angiography identify ischaemia-causing lesions. Eur Heart J. 2016;37(15):1220–7.
16. Stuijfzand WJ, et al. Stress myocardial perfusion imaging vs coronary computed tomographic angiography for diagnosis of invasive vessel-specific coronary physiology: predictive modeling results from the computed tomographic evaluation of atherosclerotic determinants of myocardial ischemia (CREDENCE) trial. JAMA Cardiol. 2020;5(12):1338–48.
17. Han D, et al. Relationship between Endothelial Wall shear stress and high-risk atherosclerotic plaque characteristics for identification of coronary lesions that cause ischemia: a direct comparison with fractional flow reserve. J Am Heart Assoc. 2016;5(12):e004186.
18. Lee JM, et al. Identification of high-risk plaques destined to cause acute coronary syndrome using coronary computed tomographic angiography and computational fluid dynamics. JACC Cardiovasc Imaging. 2019;12(6):1032–43.
19. Steigner ML, et al. Iodinated contrast opacification gradients in normal coronary arteries imaged with prospectively ECG-gated single heart beat 320-detector row computed tomography. Circ Cardiovasc Imaging. 2010;3(2):179–86.
20. Tanabe Y, et al. Combined assessment of subtended myocardial volume and myocardial blood flow for diagnosis of obstructive coronary artery disease using cardiac computed tomography: a feasibility study. J Cardiol. 2020;76(3):259–65.
21. Koo BK, et al. Diagnosis of ischemia-causing coronary stenoses by noninvasive fractional flow reserve computed from coronary computed tomographic angiograms. Results from the prospective multicenter DISCOVER-FLOW (diagnosis of ischemia-causing Stenoses obtained via noninvasive fractional flow reserve) study. J Am Coll Cardiol. 2011;58(19):1989–97.
22. Cami E, et al. Importance of measurement site on assessment of lesion-specific ischemia and diagnostic performance by coronary computed tomography angiography-derived fractional flow reserve. J Cardiovasc Comput Tomogr. 2021;15(2):114–20.
23. Omori H, et al. Determination of the optimal measurement point for fractional flow reserve derived from CTA using pressure wire assessment as reference. AJR Am J Roentgenol. 2021;216(6):1492–9.
24. Takagi H, et al. Trans-lesional fractional flow reserve gradient as derived from coronary CT improves patient management: ADVANCE registry. J Cardiovasc Comput Tomogr. 2022;16(1):19–26.
25. Chinnaiyan KM, et al. Clinical use of CT-derived fractional flow Reserve in the Emergency Department. JACC Cardiovasc Imaging. 2020;13(2 Pt 1):452–61.
26. Gulati M, et al. 2021 AHA/ACC/ASE/CHEST/SAEM/SCCT/SCMR guideline for the evaluation and diagnosis of CHEST pain: a report of the American College of Cardiology/American Heart Association joint committee on clinical practice guidelines. Circulation. 2021;144(22):e368–454.
27. Fairbairn TA, et al. Real-world clinical utility and impact on clinical decision-making of coronary computed tomography angiography-derived fractional flow reserve: lessons from the ADVANCE registry. Eur Heart J. 2018;39(41):3701–11.
28. Patel MR, et al. 1-year impact on medical practice and clinical outcomes of FFRCT: the ADVANCE registry. JACC Cardiovasc Imaging. 2020;13(1 Pt 1):97–105.
29. Norgaard BL, et al. Clinical outcomes following real-world computed tomography angiography-derived

fractional flow reserve testing in chronic coronary syndrome patients with calcification. Eur Heart J Cardiovasc Imaging. 2021;22(10):1182–9.
30. Zhao N, et al. Effect of coronary calcification severity on measurements and diagnostic performance of CT-FFR with computational fluid dynamics: results from CT-FFR China trial. Front Cardiovasc Med. 2021;8:810625.
31. Grover R, et al. Coronary lumen volume to myocardial mass ratio in primary microvascular angina. J Cardiovasc Comput Tomogr. 2017;11(6):423–8.
32. Yang DH, et al. Incremental value of subtended myocardial mass for identifying FFR-verified ischemia using quantitative CT angiography: comparison with quantitative coronary angiography and CT-FFR. JACC Cardiovasc Imaging. 2019;12(4):707–17.
33. Iguchi T, et al. Impact of lesion length on functional significance in intermediate coronary lesions. Clin Cardiol. 2013;36(3):172–7.
34. Holmes KR, et al. Impact of sublingual nitroglycerin dosage on FFRCT assessment and coronary luminal volume-to-myocardial mass ratio. Eur Radiol. 2019;29(12):6829–36.

Coronary Stent CT Imaging and Interpretation

15

Edward P. Shapiro

Abstract

Coronary stenting is a common form of coronary artery revascularization, and the evaluation of symptoms in patients who have had stent placement is a frequent clinical problem in cardiology. Unfortunately, artifacts including blooming and beam hardening make the visualization of the lumen within a stent difficult, and stent assessment using conventional CT scanners is often problematic. Later generation stents and those with large diameters, e.g., of 3.5 mm or greater, can usually be well seen. Avoidance of reduced X-ray tube voltage and use of a sharp kernel during reconstruction may be helpful. New technological developments, such as ultra-high-resolution CT, hold promise in improving stent assessment.

Keywords

Stent · PCI · Stent restenosis · Stent thrombosis · Blooming · Beam hardening

E. P. Shapiro (✉)
Division of cardiology, John Hopkins University, Baltimore, MD, USA
e-mail: eshapiro@jhmi.edu

Abbreviations

BMS	Bare metal stent
DES	Drug-eluting stent
EID	Energy integrating detector
MPR	Multi-planar reformation
PCCT	Photon-counting computed tomography

15.1 Background

- In the 1980s, balloon angioplasty, the original percutaneous technique for restoring coronary patency was largely supplanted by placement of bare metal stents (BMS), which reduced the risk of abrupt vessel closure. Neointimal hyperplasia and in-stent restenosis was common until stents were coated with anti-proliferative agents (drug-eluting stents [DES]), which reduced restenosis rates to about 5–10% but also increased the risk of acute thrombosis, necessitating the administration of dual antiplatelet therapy. Bare metal stents are still placed in some patients, particularly those who are poor candidates for prolonged treatment with dual antiplatelet agents.
- Acute thrombosis in DES usually results in clear evidence for myocardial infarction and urgent invasive angiography, so there is generally not a role for CT in its evaluation. In contrast, the occurrence of less dramatic chest

A. A. Zadeh, J. Hoe (eds.), *Practical Guide to Cardiac CT*,
https://doi.org/10.1007/978-981-97-6919-3_15

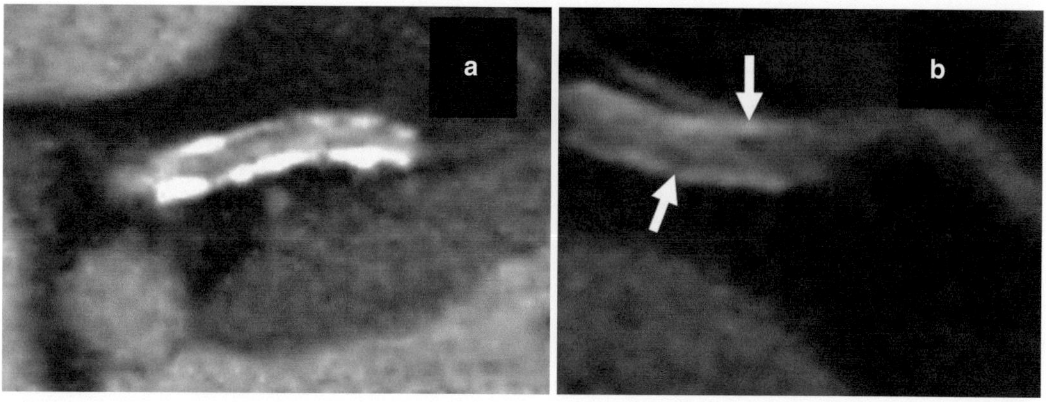

Fig. 15.1 Panels A and B. In-stent restenosis is difficult to assess in the setting of "blooming" of the stent borders (**a**) and beam hardening artifacts (**b**, arrows)

pain syndromes that may be due to restenosis is a frequent clinical problem in which the use of CCTA would reduce the need for invasive angiography.

- Assessment of restenosis by current generation CT technology is hindered by the phenomenon of "blooming," that is, very dense structures like metal and calcium appear to occupy more space than they do in reality. Blooming results in the obscuring of the part of the lumen adjacent to the stent, which is where in-stent stenosis begins, and in less contrast attenuation within the lumen (Fig. 15.1a). Difficulty also arises in distinguishing beam hardening artifacts adjacent to the dense metal, from lesions. (Fig. 15.1b).
- As a consequence, appropriate use guidelines for coronary CT angiography consider assessment of stent patency in symptomatic patients as inappropriate if the stent diameter is <3 mm or unknown, and uncertain if the stent diameter is ≥3 mm. An exception is the assessment of stents in the left main coronary artery, assuming the stent diameter is at least 3 mm.
- While many single center studies report acceptable accuracy of detecting in-stent restenosis by CT [1], sensitivity and specificity substantially varies. In the multicenter international Core64 study, the overall sensitivity, specificity, positive predictive value, and negative predictive value to detect 50% in-stent stenosis were 33.3%, 91.7%, 57.1%, and 80.5%, respectively, with a modest overall accuracy of 77.1% for the 64% of stents that were assessable [2]. In another study, the diagnostic accuracy for detecting in-stent stenosis was 66.7% [3]. In contrast, in another, where 87% of patients were assessable, CTA was 96% sensitive and 72% specific with a positive predictive valve of 79% and negative predictive value of 99% [4]. Many CT experts recommend against using CT if the main reason for performing the evaluation is stent assessment, unless the stent size is >3.5 mm (see "stent size," below).

15.2 Factors Influencing Adequacy of Visualization

- Scanner type
  - Scanners with ≥64 slices fare much better than those with less than 64 slices.
  - Ultra-high-resolution CT, using 0.25 mm detector width, results in larger measured lumen sizes, smaller measured strut thickness, higher visual scoring, and better differentiation of plaque vs. lumen [5].
  - Compared to energy integrating detectors (EID), photon-counting CT (PCCT) systems improve spatial resolution and reduce noise, blooming artifacts, and radiation dose and early evidence suggests that these scanners will be superior for stent assessment [6].

- Some CT systems allow image reconstruction that simulate monoenergetic sources either by using dual sources each with a different kV setting or by using layered detectors that achieve spectral separation at the detector level. These "virtual" monoenergetic images at low kV can increase the contrast-to-noise ratio, and at high kV can reduce beam hardening artifacts, effects that are potentially useful for evaluation of stents [7].
- Some wide detector systems acquire non-contrast and contrast images within a single breath-hold, to derive a subtraction image that removes the stent [8]. However, neither of these techniques have been widely adopted.

- Stent size
  - Stent diameter is the most important factor influencing the accuracy of assessing for in-stent restenosis. While only 50% of the true lumen is visible with stents of diameter 2.25 mm, at least 80% is visible if the stent diameter is 4.0 mm (Fig. 15.2). In general, stents of 3.5 mm or greater can be well assessed [9], and those less than 3.0 mm are usually not well seen. Those sized 3.0 mm are well seen 60–80% of the time [10].

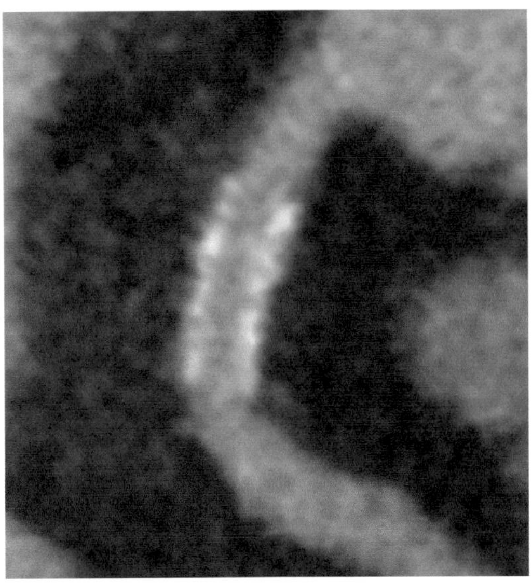

Fig. 15.2 Example of a large (4.0 mm diameter) stent in the proximal right coronary artery disease with adequate visualization of the stent lumen, revealing no evidence of in-stent restenosis

- Stent type
  - Stents with struts thicker than 100 μm are often un-assessable. Early-generation drug-eluting stents (DES) used a stainless-steel platform with a strut thickness of 130–150 μm (for example Cypher 140 μm, Taxus 132 μm) while current generation DES usually have stent struts measuring 50–90 μm (for example XienceV is 81 μm) [11]. The newer stents are therefore more easily evaluated by CT.
  - The use of bioabsorbable stents would largely solve the problem of stent "blooming," but the first generation bioabsorbable stent was clinically inferior to available DES, and at this time their use outside research protocols awaits further development.
- Scan parameters
  - Use of a higher X-ray tube voltage improves stent visualization but may result in unacceptable radiation exposure [12]. In general, when scanning a patient with stents, the tube voltage should remain at the current CT standard of 120 kV.
  - All of the usual parameters that affect image quality are important to optimize in-stent imaging (see Chapters I, II, V). That is, the heart rate should be effectively managed, nitroglycerin should be given, spatial and temporal resolution should be optimized, and the contrast bolus should be adequate, with well-timed images. Iterative reconstruction should be used.
- Reconstruction kernel
  - A kernel is a set of filters used during reconstruction of CT images (see Chapters I, II). A kernel described as "sharp" will improve edge detection but will also increase image noise. A kernel described as smooth will blur the edges and reduce image noise (Fig. 15.3). Stents are best evaluated using the sharpest kernel available. For example, using a series of one manufacturer's four available kernels from smooth to sharp allowed 53.3%, 58.3%, 69.4%, and 73.9% of the true lumen size to be seen.

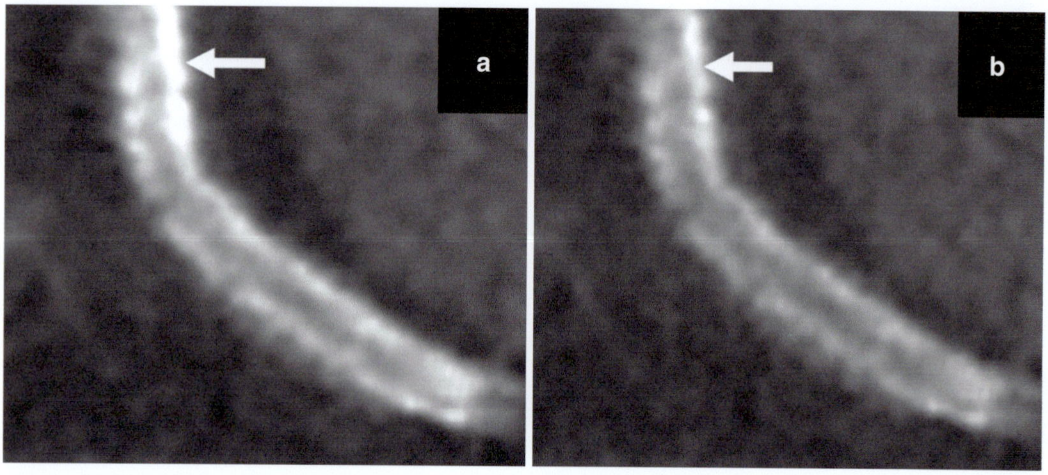

Fig. 15.3 Stent visualization with a smooth (**a**) vs. sharp convolution kernel (**b**)

- Stent angle
  - The angle that the stent direction makes with respect to the gantry may have an effect on stent visualization, especially if the in-plane resolution is not exactly the same as the through plane resolution (that is, voxels are not perfectly isotropic) [5].

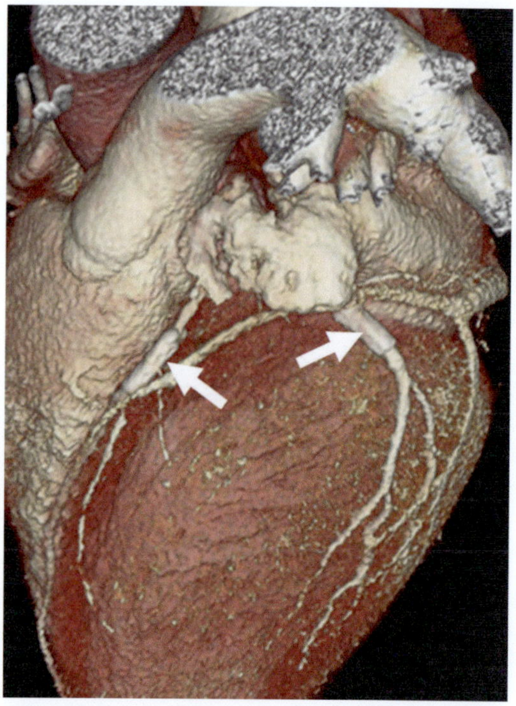

Fig. 15.4 Stents (arrows) in the left anterior descending and circumflex arteries visualized on 3D images

15.3 Study Interpretation on the Workstation

- 3D views
  - Proximal stents may be obscured by outer structures such as the pulmonary artery and the left atrial appendage. More distal stents may appear to be wrapped around the outside of the artery rather than being within the lumen on the 3D images (Fig. 15.4). This, of course, is due to the fact that only the lumen and not the wall is seen on the 3D image, plus the blooming of bright structures.
- Axial views
  - In axial views, stents are usually displayed in planes oblique to their orientation, and thus are difficult to interpret.
- Curved MPR views
  - These are useful for stent visualization but may require increasing the window width and level to best visualize the stent edge and distinguish it from the contrast filled lumen. Automatic lesion quantification software may be of little use because of the difficulty of tracing the lumen within the highly attenuating metal.
- MPR
  - Planes are adjusted to obtain longitudinal and cross-sectional images. The slices

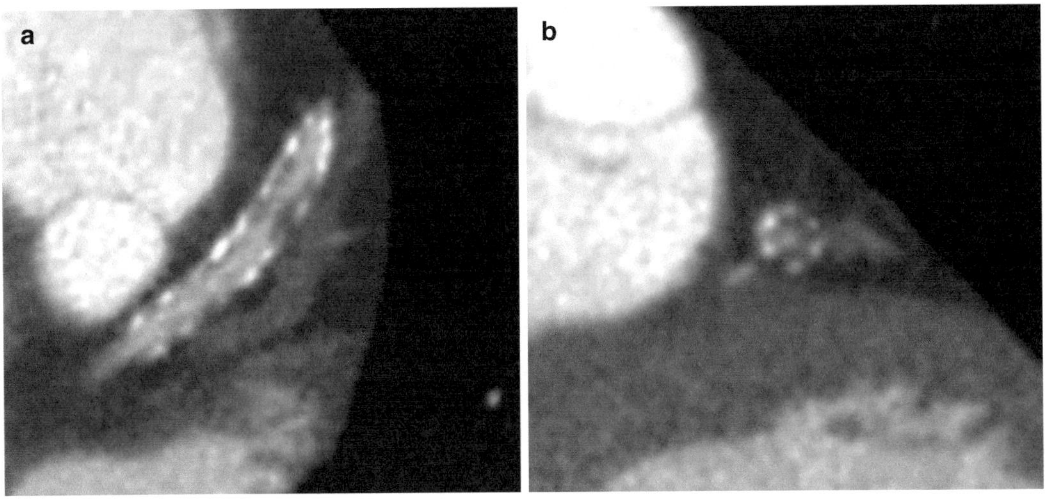

Fig. 15.5 Example of in-stent restenosis in longitudinal (**a**) or cross-sectional display (**b**)

should be as thin as possible to minimize the "blooming" artifact.

- The window width and level will usually have to be increased above what is used for native coronary segments.
- Lesions are due to endothelial proliferation rather than atherosclerosis, and usually appear in longitudinal images as gray or black lines adjacent to the bright metal (Fig. 15.5a). In cross-sectional images, they may be circumferential (Fig. 15.5b).
- It may be difficult to estimate the "percent stenosis" of these lesions, as a reference segment may be difficult to identify and measure. The reference segment may be estimated as the distance between the midpoints of the apparent strut thickness on opposite sides of the stent.
- Where multiple stents were placed in a long segment of atherosclerosis, the overlap can usually be identified.
- Strut fractures can sometimes be seen as a gap in the metal structure of the stent. These may form a nidus for the development of restenosis.
- Acute stent thrombosis usually causes obvious clinical evidence of infarction that requires urgent invasive angiography and re-stenting. Occasionally the thrombus is not fully occlusive, and infarction may not be obvious. In this situation, CCTA may be helpful as these thrombi are often easily visualized (Fig. 15.6).

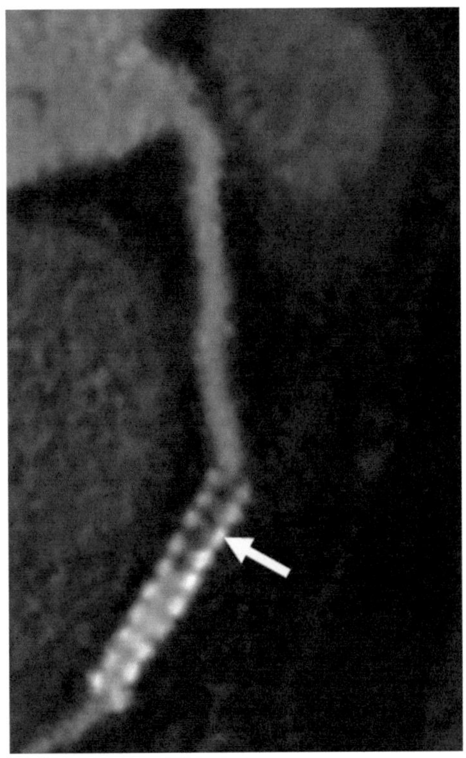

Fig. 15.6 An example of acute, partial stent thrombosis (arrow)

15.4 Summary

- Stent evaluation by current generation CCTA technology remains challenging and practice guidelines do not endorse the use of CCTA in this setting except for assessment of left main stents.
- Stent evaluation is often adequate in the setting of optimal image quality and stent diameter of at least 3.5 mm.
- Accuracy of detecting in-stent restenosis decreases with smaller stent sizes and less than optimal image quality.
- Optimization of acquisition and postprocessing are critical for adequate stent evaluation and use of 120 kV tube voltage and sharp reconstruction kernels are standard.
- Alternative imaging should be strongly considered if scan conditions are not optimal.

References

1. Kumbhani DJ, Ingelmo CP, Schoenhagen P, Curtin RJ, Flamm SD, Desai MY. Meta-analysis of diagnostic efficacy of 64-slice computed tomography in the evaluation of coronary in-stent restenosis. Am J Cardiol. 2009;103(12):1675–81.
2. Wykrzykowska JJ, Arbab-Zadeh A, Godoy G, Miller JM, Lin S, Vavere A, Paul N, Niinuma H, Hoe J, Brinker J, Khosa F, Sarwar S, Lima J, Clouse ME. Assessment of in-stent restenosis using 64-MDCT: analysis of the CORE-64 multicenter international trial. Am J Roentgenol. 2010;194(1):85–92.
3. Dowsley TF, Chepelev L, McArdle B, Alam M, Dwivedi G, Chow BJW. Improved diagnostic accuracy when combining computed tomography angiography and corrected coronary opacification in patients with coronary stents. Acta Cardiol. 2017;72(1): 53–60.
4. Eckert J, Renczes-Janetzko P, Schmidt M, Magedanz A, Voigtländer T, Schmermund A. Coronary CT angiography (CCTA) using third-generation dual-source CT for ruling out in-stent restenosis. Clin Res Cardiol. 2019;108(4):402–10.
5. Nishii T, Funama Y, Kato S, Iwasawa T, Yasuda N, Ota Y, Kawagoe H, Oda S, Tsutsumi T. Daisuke Utsunomiya; comparison of visibility of in-stent restenosis between conventional-and ultra-high spatial resolution computed tomography: coronary arterial phantom study. Jpn J Radiol. 2021;40:279.
6. Petritsch B, Petri N, Weng AM, Petersilka M, Allmendinger T, Bley TA, Gassenmaier T. Photon-counting computed tomography for coronary stent imaging: in vitro evaluation of 28 coronary stents. Investig Radiol. 2021;56(10):653–60.
7. Gupta A, Kikano EG, Bera K, Baruah D, Saboo SS, Lennartz S, Hokamp NG, Gholamrezanezhad A, Gilkeson RC, Laukamp KR. Dual energy imaging in cardiothoracic pathologies: a primer for radiologists and clinicians. Eur J Radiol Open. 2021;8:100324.
8. Yamaguchi T, Ichikawa K, Takahashi D, Sugaya T, Furuya J, Igarashi K. A new contrast enhancement protocol for subtraction coronary computed tomography requiring a short breath-holding time. Acad Radiol. 2017;24:38–44.
9. Sheth T, Dodd JD, Hoffmann U, Abbara S, Finn A, Gold HK, Brady TJ, Cury RC. Coronary stent assessability by 64 slice multi-detector computed tomography. Catheter Cardiovasc Interv. 2007;69(7):933–8.
10. Rixe J, Achenbach S, Ropers D, Baum U, Kuettner A, Ropers U, Bautz W, Daniel WG, Anders K. Assessment of coronary artery stent restenosis by 64-slice multi-detector computed tomography. Eur Heart J. 2006;27(21):2567–72.
11. Udrişte AS, Niculescu A-G, Grumezescu AM, Bădilăl E. Cardiovascular stents: a review of past, current, and emerging devices. Materials (Basel). 2021;14(10):2498.
12. Esposito A, Colantoni C, De Cobelli F, Del Vecchio A, Palmisano A, Calandrino R, Del Maschio A. Multidetector computed tomography for coronary stents imaging: high-voltage (140-kVp) prospective ECG-triggered versus standard-voltage (120-kVp) retrospective ECG-gated helical scanning. J Comput Assist Tomogr. 2013;37(3):395–401.

16 Coronary Artery Bypass Graft CT Imaging and Interpretation

Edward P. Shapiro

Abstract

Cardiac CT angiography is an appropriate tool for the assessment of recurrent symptoms in patients who have undergone coronary artery bypass grafting. Multiple studies have shown high accuracy for determining whether arterial and venous grafts are occluded, and good accuracy in detecting stenosis without occlusion. Image acquisition is best obtained using a prospectively triggered scan protocol, and should span a long z-axis, from the lung apices to the diaphragm. Analysis should include evaluation of patency and presence of narrowing or obstruction of both grafts and native coronary arteries distal to the grafts. Three-dimensional representation and the generation of curved MPR images are of value in image analysis. Visualizing the site of anastomosis requires special attention. Occluded saphenous grafts usually display a residual "nubbin" that can easily be seen on axial images. Unusual grafts, and surgical errors or complications, may occasionally be observed.

Keywords

CABG · LIMA · RIMA · Saphenous vein · Revascularization · Conduit · Nubbin · Anastomosis

Abbreviations

CABG	Coronary artery bypass grafting
LAD	Left anterior descending artery
LCx	Left circumflex coronary artery
LIMA	Left internal mammary artery
MIP	Maximum intensity projection
MPR	Multi-planar reformation
PCI	Percutaneous coronary intervention
RCA	Right coronary artery
RIMA	Right internal mammary artery
SVG	Saphenous vein graft

16.1 Background

- Coronary artery bypass grafting (CABG) is the most commonly performed cardiac surgery procedure worldwide, with annual volumes exceeding 300,000 in the USA.
- The left internal mammary artery (LIMA) is the preferred conduit for grafting the left anterior descending artery (LAD), the most important vascular bed, and its use is the key to the survival benefit of CABG over medical ther-

E. P. Shapiro (✉)
Division of Cardiology, John Hopkins University, Baltimore, MD, USA
e-mail: eshapiro@jhmi.edu

A. A. Zadeh, J. Hoe (eds.), *Practical Guide to Cardiac CT*,
https://doi.org/10.1007/978-981-97-6919-3_16

apy in patients with severe 3-vessel coronary disease and reduced left ventricular function.

- The 10-year graft patency rate for LIMA to LAD is about 95% [1]. The right internal mammary artery (RIMA) can be used to graft the LAD if the LIMA is unusable, or the RIMA can be used in conjunction with the LIMA (bi-internal mammary artery grafting). The free radial artery is the currently recommended conduit for the next most important vascular bed, as long as the native vessel lesion is severe enough to assure that competitive flow will not occur. The gastroepiploic artery may be used as a conduit, but this is uncommon as its implantation requires surgical access to both the chest and the abdomen.
- Venous grafts are the next in preference but their follow-up patency rate is lower than that of arterial conduits. Early disease of saphenous vein grafts (SVG) is caused by thrombosis. Twelve to 25% of SVGs occlude within 6 months of grafting [2]. Additional processes contribute to deterioration of venous grafts; intimal hyperplasia occurs between 1 and 12 months, and atherosclerosis causes late graft disease starting as early as 1 year after CABG [3].
- Chest pain in patients who have undergone CABG is a frequent clinical problem that is traditionally investigated with functional testing or invasive catheterization, but the use of CCTA for this purpose is appropriate [4] and increasing. Assessing grafts by CCTA is easier than evaluating native arteries because of grafts' relative immobility (thus less motion artifacts), wider luminal diameter, and lower rate of severe calcifications.
- CCTA also enables the assessment of native coronary vessels distal to the anastomoses, as well as of surgical complications.

16.2 Use of CTA Prior to CABG

- In patients who have had previous CABG in whom re-do CABG or other chest surgery is necessary, cardiac CTA is useful in defining the location of still-functioning grafts with respect to the sternum, so that these can be avoided when opening the chest. This application was considered appropriate in the 2010 appropriate use guidelines [4].
- In patients with anomalous coronary arteries who need CABG because of concomitant coronary disease or other unusual situations, cardiac CT is the preferred tool to define the course of the arteries and plan the procedure. Surgery for anomalous coronary origin usually consists of a coronary "unroofing" procedure rather than CABG.

16.3 Use of CTA for Graft Assessment

- The first report of the use of CT for evaluating grafts appeared in 1980, using an early generation scanner, before the introduction of cardiac gating, multi-slice CT, or arterial conduits [5], and reported a sensitivity and specificity of both 95% in determining SVG patency. With gating, and 16 and then 64 slice scanning SVG's could be characterized in much more detail, and the sensitivity and specificity for occlusion reached 99% and 96%, respectively [5].
- Many years later, a study using 16-slice technology reported a high sensitivity of 100% and specificity of 98% for detecting graft occlusion, however, only moderate sensitivity and specificity (82% and 88%) was observed in the detection of bypass stenosis [6].
- Accuracy continued to improve with the advances of CCTA, and a sensitivity of 98.3% and specificity of 97.4% for stenosis were reported and using a 320 detector scanner, [7] with a meta-analysis suggesting a pooled sensitivity and specificity of 96.1% and 96.3% [8].

16.4 Study Acquisition for Graft Assessment

- Assessment of grafts requires a scan of the full chest, starting at the apexes of the lungs to include the subclavian arteries, and ending at the diaphragmatic surface of the heart.

- Prospective scan triggering is strongly preferred over retrospective gating to minimize radiation exposure; this is especially important considering the long scan length in the Z-axis which adds to the radiation burden.
- The best acquisition protocol to use depends on the capabilities of the scanner. The use of CCTA with less than 64 slices is usually not practical in view of the long breath hold that would be needed to cover the whole chest. Scans may be:
  - Prospective helical, with low pitch similar to that used in retrospective studies;
  - Prospective axial ("step and shoot") where slabs of a thickness determined by the collimation (e.g., 64 slices × 0.5 mm thickness per slice yields 32 mm thick slabs) obtained from a series of heart beats are stacked together without overlap;
  - Prospective high pitch helical acquisition using a dual source system.
  - Scanners with wide array detectors covering up to 16 cm can ordinarily image the whole heart in a single beat, but cannot cover the entire chest, generally requiring two very thick axial slabs obtained from two heart beats to be combined.
- Some scanners have the ability to gate only a portion of the Z-axis during helical scanning, enabling the superior portion of the image, which does not require cardiac gating, to be acquired more rapidly.

16.4.1 Possible Use of Cardiac CTA in Conjunction with Invasive Angiography

- Invasive angiography in a patient with history of CABG may involve prolonged searching in the ascending aorta for ostia of grafts that may not easily be found. Since any vessel occlusion must be confirmed, the searching for grafts may involve excessive catheter manipulation in the aorta with the associated risk of athero-emboli. Some angiographers prefer to have data from CT prior to invasive angiography to obtain non-invasive evidence of graft occlusion if it is suspected.

16.4.2 Study Interpretation on the Workstation

- If available, the operative report is useful to define where grafts were originally placed.
- 3D views
  - The three-dimensional shaded surface display of the heart and vasculature is especially helpful in assessing bypass grafts, since the occlusion of SVGs can be easily appreciated and the small remaining nubbins on the aortic wall are clearly visible (Fig. 16.1).
  - These displays are generally reconstructed with software that removes non-cardiac structures from the image. Since the LIMA and RIMA are somewhat distant from the heart during the proximal 2/3 of their course, they are often automatically

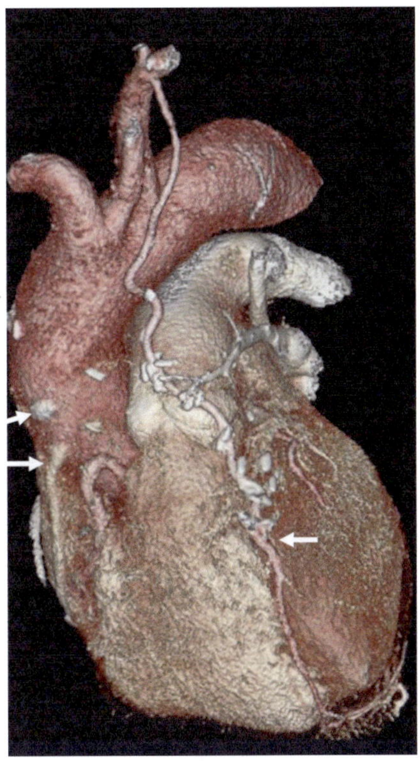

Fig. 16.1 A 3-D volume reconstruction is shown from a patient who had CABG: LIMA to LAD, SVG to LCx, and SVG to RCA. The SVG to LCx occluded at its origin with a nubbin seen (left-most arrow). The SVG to RCA (middle arrow) is patent. The LIMA is also patent with the anastomosis visible (right-most arrow)

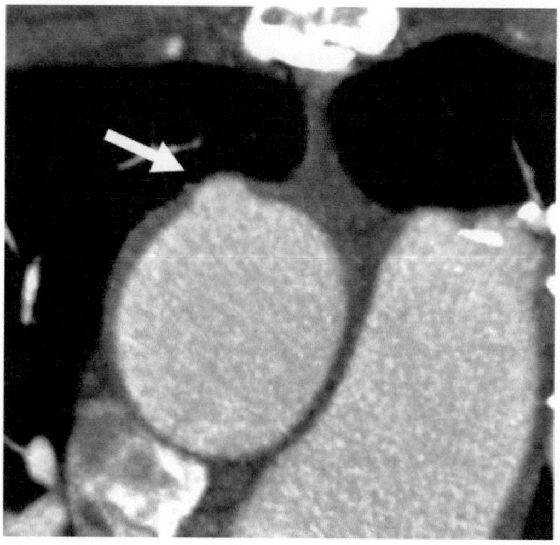

Fig. 16.2 An axial image of a nubbin remaining after SVG occlusion (arrow) is shown

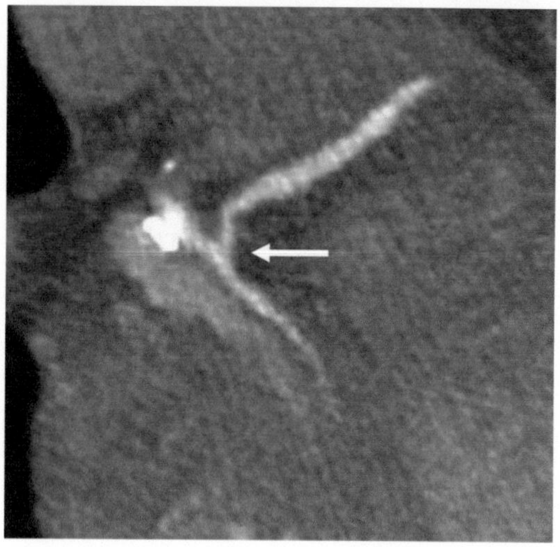

Fig. 16.3 Formation of a "Y" shape with patent anastomosis of SVG (on left) joining with native posterior descending artery (on right)

removed from the 3D image. The various workstations have mechanisms for restoring the 3D image of these vessels.
  - The LIMA and RIMA, if used, often contain multiple metal clips placed to stop bleeding from the many small intrathoracic arteries that emerge from the IMAs.
- Axial images
  - Viewing the axial plane, moving from superior to inferior, further defines the anatomy. Axial images of the aorta may display characteristic nubbins, the remnants of occluded grafts (Fig. 16.2).
- Coronal images
  - The grafted LIMA usually runs near the junction of the mediastinum and the left lung and can easily be followed from the subclavian artery to the anastomosis in the coronal plane.
- cMPR images
  - cMPR views are very useful for visualizing the full extent of the graft, including the proximal anastomosis to the aorta (or origin from the subclavian artery), the body of the graft, and the distal anastomosis. The distal anastomosis may be visualized by rotating the "virtual" image plane such that a "Y" shaped structure is seen, with the top limbs of the "Y" representing the native vessel and the end-to-side graft anastomosis, and the bottom stem representing the receiving native artery (Fig. 16.3). Lumen narrowing at the anastomosis is difficult to quantify given the artifacts from metallic clips.
  - Venous grafts often vary in caliber throughout their course. Narrow portions not containing atherosclerotic plaque probably do not represent significant stenoses unless they are narrower than the receiving artery.
  - While a clump of clips can create artifacts and obscure a small location of the mammary artery, this usually does not create a clinical problem since very focal lesions are not expected in this artery, which is extremely resistant to atherosclerosis. An exception is at the anastomotic site, where a localized obstruction can indeed occur (Fig. 16.4).
  - When the body of a mammary graft narrows, which can be caused by competitive flow, a long segment is usually involved.
  - While cMPR are often helpful, they may fail to correctly follow a vessel, giving a false appearance of stenosis. Similarly, a

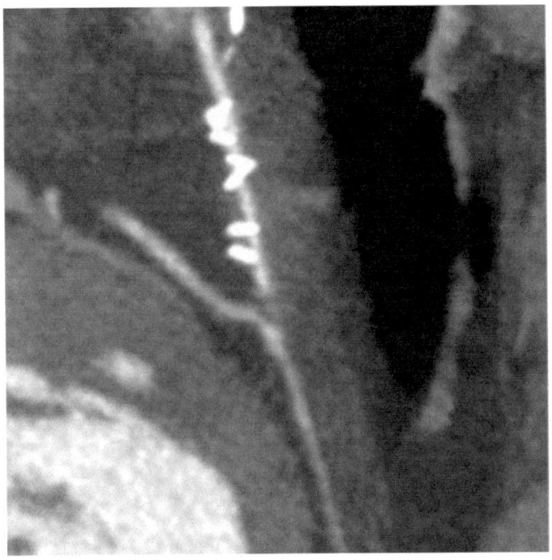

Fig. 16.4 Stenosis at the anastomosis of LIMA to LAD

cMPR may track correctly until it reaches the anastomosis and then follow the native vessel proximally rather than distally, causing the reader to miss a distal native vessel stenosis.
    - An additional format, sometimes called angio-MIP, allows the cMPR to be displayed in a view simulating an invasive angiogram, which is useful in some cases.
- Oblique planes manipulated such that longitudinal and cross-sectional sections of the grafts can be seen
    - As discussed above under "cMPR," the proximal anastomosis (or origin), body, and distal anastomosis of the graft should be assessed in all cases. In rare scenarios, subclavian artery stenosis can cause angina in a patient with a mammary graft, so that vessel should be also viewed, if possible.
    - The portion of the native artery proximal to the insertion of the graft undergoes shear stress changes and often shows extensive progression of atherosclerosis, including severe calcification. This portion of the native vessel may be difficult to assess, often containing severe lumen obstruction which necessitated the bypass.

16.5 Summary

16.5.1 Common Post-CABG Findings on CCTA

- Nubbin sign—A dimple in the aorta representing a remnant of an occluded graft (Fig. 16.2).
- String sign—Diffuse narrowing of a segment of a mammary graft, or the entire vessel.
- Clips without contrast between them—The mammary is occluded/atretic but the clips reveal where it runs (Fig. 16.5).
- Tented native arteries—A graft that is too short may pull on a native coronary artery resulting in a tented appearance. These grafts may occlude (Fig. 16.6).

16.5.2 Uncommon Post-CABG Findings on CCTA

- Patent LIMA branch causing poor graft flow—An unnoticed branch of a LIMA, which was not ligated during surgery, may steal coronary flow from the grafted portion resulting in inadequate perfusion (Fig. 16.7).

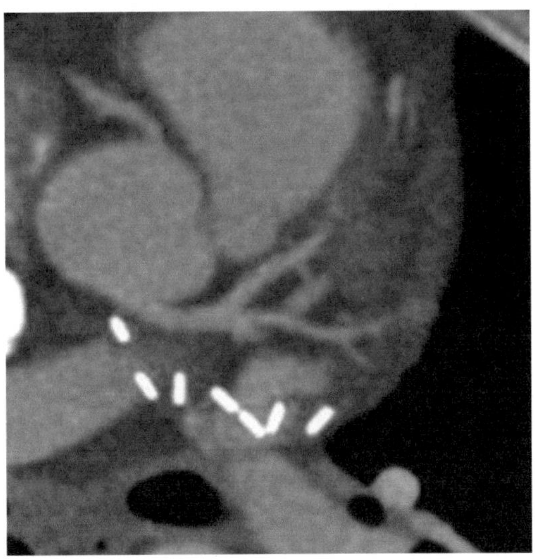

Fig. 16.5 A case of an occluded RIMA graft to LCX, revealing only a series of clips. The surgeon had used the transverse sinus as the shortest pathway between the right and left sides of the heart

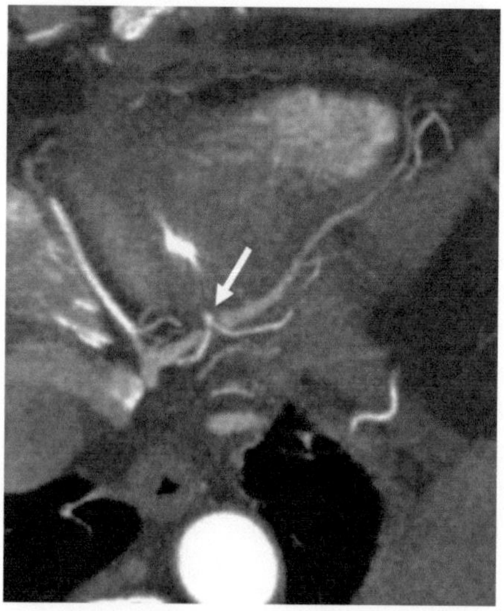

Fig. 16.6 A tented posterior descending artery (arrow), remaining after occlusion of an SVG graft that was too short

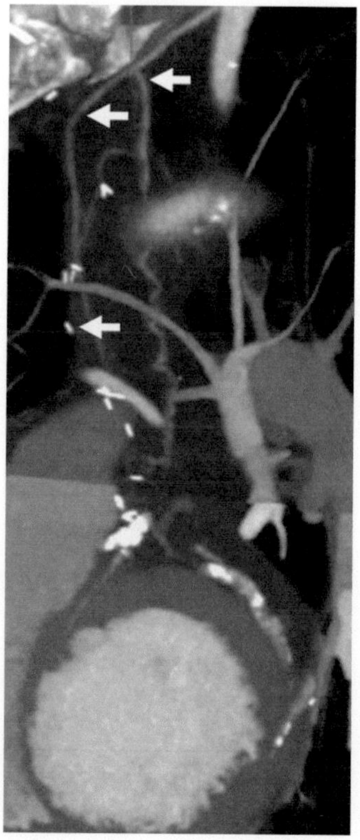

Fig. 16.7 LIMA with multiple patent branches (arrows) of which one was used to bypass the LAD, with poor results due to competitive flow

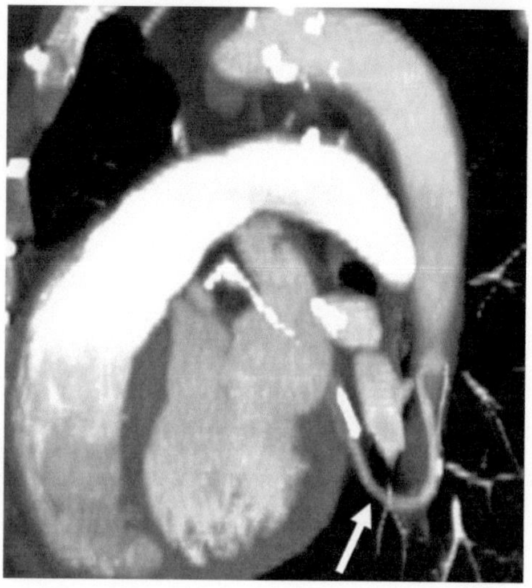

Fig. 16.8 SVG from the descending aorta to the LCx. This patient had undergone a re-do CABG to graft the LCx and the operative report was not available. At invasive angiography, injection of the native left coronary showed competitive flow into the LCx, but the graft could not be found despite an extensive search in the aorta

- Coronary graft pseudoaneurysms—These may develop at the anastomosis sites.
- Unique graft locations—Rarely, a graft may originate from the descending aorta (Fig. 16.8).
- Surgical errors—Rarely, a graft may be anastomosed to the wrong vessel (Fig. 16.9).

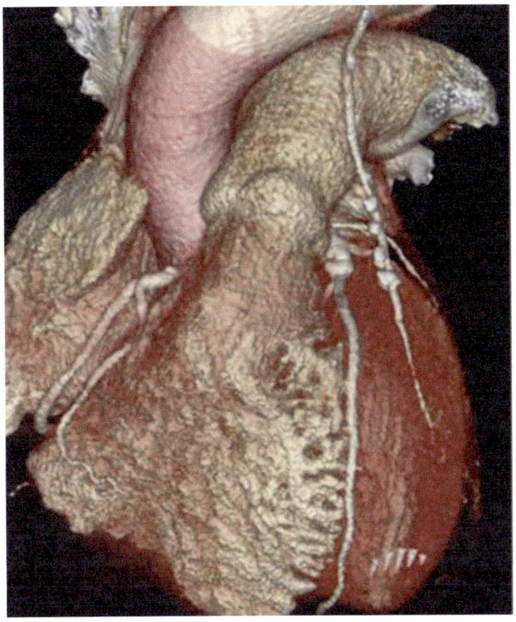

Fig. 16.9 A case of a LIMA graft attached to the wrong target vessel. The patient had a severe stenosis at the ostium of the LAD and underwent a minimally invasive single vessel CABG. The diagonal was grafted instead of the LAD. He subsequently had PCI of the LAD

References

1. Tatoulis J, Buxton BF, Fuller JA. The right internal thoracic artery: the forgotten conduit – 5766 patients and 991 angiograms. Ann Thorac Surg. 2011;92:9–15.
2. Fitzgibbon GM, Kafka HP, Leach AJ, et al. Coronary bypass graft fate and patient outcome: angiographic follow-up of 5065 grafts related to survival and reoperation in 1388 patients during 25 years. J Am Coll Cardiol. 1996;28:616–26.
3. Kim FY, Marhefka G, Ruggiero NJ, et al. Saphenous vein graft disease: review of pathophysiology, prevention, and treatment. Cardiol Rev. 2013;21:101–9.
4. Taylor AJ, Cerqueira M, Hodgson JMCB, Mark D, Min J, O'Gara P, Rubin GD. ACCF/SCCT/ACR/AHA/ASE/ASNC/NASCI/SCAI/SCMR 2010 appropriate use criteria for cardiac computed tomography. Circulation. 2010;122(21):e525–e55.
5. Brundage BH, Lipton MJ, Herfkens RJ, Berninger WH, Redington RW, Chatterjee K, Carlsson E. Detection of patent coronary bypass grafts by computed tomography: a preliminary report. Circulation. 1980;61:826–31.
6. Anders K, Baum U, Schmid M, Ropers D, Schmid A, Pohle K. Coronary artery bypass graft (CABG) patency: assessment with high-resolution submillimeter 16-slice multidetector-row computed tomography (MDCT) versus coronary angiography. Eur J Radiol. 2006;57:336–44.
7. Mushtaq S, Conte E, Pontone G. Interpretability of coronary CT angiography performed with a novel whole-heart coverage high-definition CT scanner in 300 consecutive patients with coronary artery bypass grafts. J Cardiovasc Comput Tomogr. 2020;14(2):137–43.
8. Chan M, Ridley L, Dunn DJ, Tian DH, Liou K, Ozdirik J, Cheruvu C, Cao C. A systematic review and meta-analysis of multidetector computed tomography in the assessment of coronary artery bypass grafts. Int J Cardiol. 2016;221:898–905.

LV and RV Evaluation by CT

17

Eun-Ju Kang and Jongmin John Lee

Abstract

This chapter summarizes the technical issues associated with the assessment of the cardiac ventricular chambers and the myocardium. Furthermore, practical applications for clinical cardiothoracic imaging are also suggested.

Keywords

Computed tomography · Myocardium · Left ventricle · Right ventricle

Abbreviations

ARVC	Arrhythmogenic right ventricular cardiomyopathy
CAD	Coronary artery disease
CMR	Cardiac magnetic resonance imaging
DCMP	Dilated cardiomyopathy
ECG	Electrocardiogram
EF	Ejection fraction
HCMP	Hypertrophic cardiomyopathy
LA	Left atrium
LAD	Left anterior descending artery
LV	Left ventricle
LVID	LV end-diastolic internal dimension
MBF	Myocardial blood flow
MPR	Multiplanar reformation
PET	Positron emission tomography
PWT	Posterior wall thickness
RA	Right atrium
RCA	Right coronary artery
RV	Right ventricle
SPECT	Single photon emission computed tomography
SVC	Superior vena cava
SWT	Septal wall thickness

17.1 Introduction

- Cardiac CT provides detailed three-dimensional volumetric information of the cardiac chambers. Using automated contour detection algorithms, ventricular volumes and mass are readily available. When images are obtained throughout the cardiac cycle, the assessment of cardiac function and wall motion can be obtained [1, 2].
- Echocardiography remains the primary imaging modality for cardiac structure and function assessment but operator dependency and

E.-J. Kang (✉)
Department of Radiology, College of Medicine, Dong-A University, Busan, Republic of Korea
e-mail: medcarrot@dau.ac.kr

J. J. Lee
Department of Radiology, School of Medicine, Kyungpook National University, Daegu, Republic of Korea
e-mail: jonglee@knu.ac.kr

A. A. Zadeh, J. Hoe (eds.), *Practical Guide to Cardiac CT*,
https://doi.org/10.1007/978-981-97-6919-3_17

limited use of 3-dimensional techniques may lead to variable results.

- Cardiac magnetic resonance imaging (CMR) is considered the gold standard for assessing cardiac structure and function, but its use is limited by the relatively high cost, long scan times, and its incompatibility for patients with claustrophobia or ferromagnetic metal devices.
- Therefore, cardiac CT is valid alternative method for cardiac chamber assessment, particularly with a simultaneous evaluation of the coronary arteries.

17.2 Scanning Methods

- Principally, acquisition for chamber assessment can be obtained by either retrospective electrocardiography (ECG)-gated scanning method or prospective scan triggering.
- With retrospective ECG-gated scanning, CT images are being obtained during the whole cardiac cycle (one RR interval) and reconstructed through multiple phases (10-phase or 20-phase).
- The derived metrics, e.g., LV end-diastolic wall thickness, volume, and wall motion abnormalities compared well to CMR two-dimensional echocardiography in terms of accuracy and reproducibility [3, 4].
- In prospective ECG-triggered scanning, CT images are acquired for selected phases of the cardiac cycle, usually during the mid-diastole or end-systole phase, which are often adequate for coronary assessment but less useful for the evaluation of myocardial thickness or chamber size. However, data are available to adjust mid-diastolic ventricular dimensions for estimation of end-diastolic data.
- A triphasic contrast injection protocol is preferred to reduce streak artifacts in the right atrium (RA) or superior vena cava (SVC): Start with pure contrast injected at 4–6 mL/s, followed by a contrast/saline mix (5:5–8:2) chased with a small bolus of saline. The total volume of contrast media is dependent on the CT machine, scanning protocol or patient body habitus (body weight, body surface area, etc.), and usually ranges between 50 and 120 mL.
- For the accurate evaluation of left ventricular (LV) myocardial thickness and volumes, end-diastolic should be selected.
- Largest chamber volumes in end-diastole may be selected by visual assessment or by the result from contour tracing (accuracy of tracing should be verified).

17.3 Recommended Reconstruction and Viewing Techniques

- The thickness of the myocardium is commonly measured at the interventricular septum on the short-axis multiplanar reformation (MPR) view.
- For clinical use, 4-chamber view, 2-chamber view, and LV outflow tract view (or 3-chamber view) images are commonly reformed, which provide easy comparisons with echocardiography, CMR, cardiac SPECT, or PET (Fig. 17.1).
- MPR images of cardiac chambers are automatically generated by commercial software, and LV volumes are automatically calculated by thresholding the Hounsfield units in the volumetric dataset for one cardiac cycle (RR interval, with increments of 10 or 20 phase) of reconstructed images. The software also automatically indicates the LV epicardial and endocardial contours, and if necessary, further features may be added (Fig. 17.2).
- Using the mid-diastole phase CT images (which are typically selected for coronary artery evaluation) for assessment of chamber size is likely to results in underestimation, because volume increases in end-diastole. Formulas for correcting mid-diastolic volumes have been developed.
- LV thickness, on the other hand, may be overestimated in mid- vs. end-diastole [5] (Fig. 17.3).

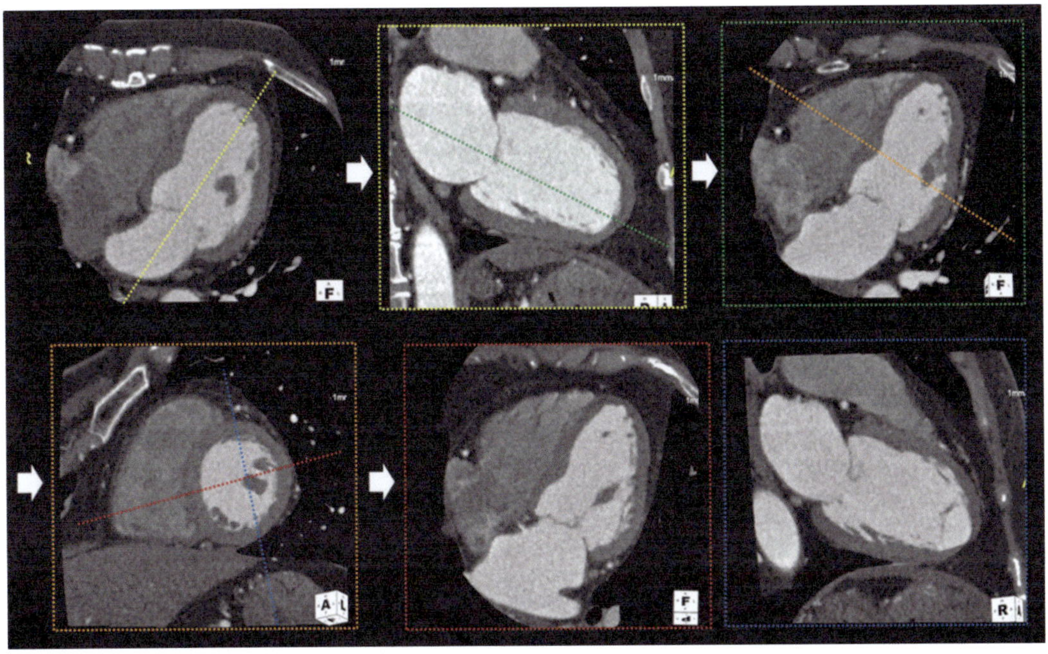

Fig. 17.1 Reformation technique for major cardiac image planes (bottom images; short axis, 4-chamber, and 2-chamber images) from a transaxial image (left upper) using MPR on 3D-softwere. Step 1—On the transaxial image, place oblique MPR line (yellow line) through mitral valve and apex, which can produce vertical long axis plane (upper middle). Step 2—then place MPR line (green line) gones through mitral valve and apex to produce horizontal long axis plane (upper right). Step 3—the short-axis view is obtained from a orthogonal MPR (orange line) to vertical long axis of left ventricle. Step 4—the 4-chamber and 2-chamber images can obtained from the horizontal plane that connect cardiophrenic angle to LV (red line) chamber, and a line perpendicular to it (blue line)

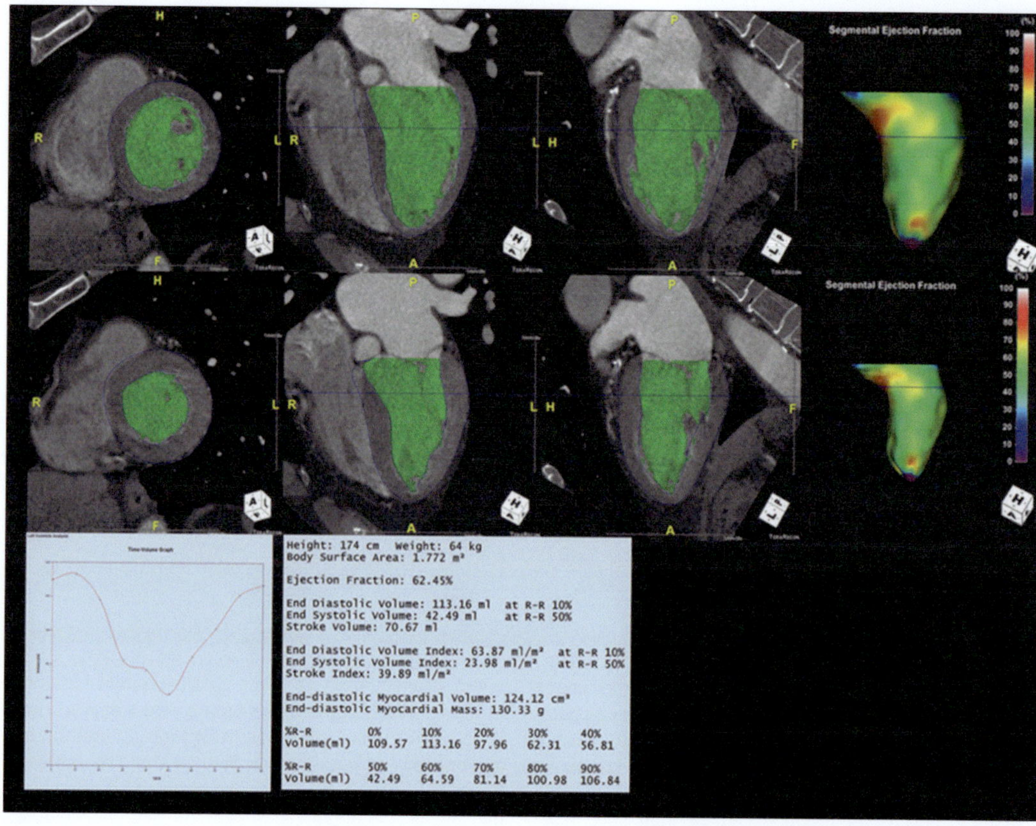

Fig. 17.2 Semiautomatic measurements for LV volume, mass and functional parameters using the cardiac specific 3D software tool

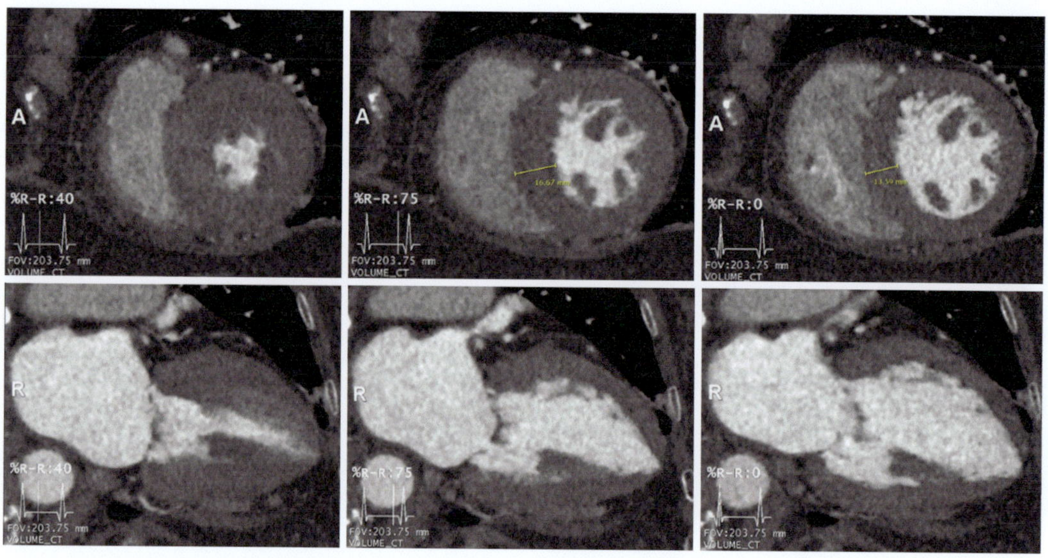

Fig. 17.3 LV myocardial change according to the cardiac phase. Note that the LV systolic phase (left) reveals a maximum thickness of the myocardium, and the difference of LV thickness is significant between the mid-diastolic (middle) and end-diastolic (right) phases

17.4 Measurements and Normal Reference Values

- Normal reference values for LV dimensions (volume, mass, and functional parameters) vary in the literature due to study population characteristics (sex, age, race, etc.) and the type of imaging modality used (echocardiography, MRI, CT) used.
- By echocardiography, the reference range of LV wall thickness in end-diastole phase is 6–10 mm, thus LV hypertrophy is usually defined by septal or posterior wall thickness ≥ 11 mm in end-diastole.
- The thickness of the LV myocardium is commonly measured by means of the interventricular septum (septal wall thickness, SWT) and posterior wall thickness (PWT) on the short-axis MPR at the chorda level. Normally the SWT is slightly thicker than the PWT. Normal reference values are provided in Table 17.1.
- The LV end-diastolic internal dimension (LVID) is usually measured at the mid-ventricle level on 4-chamber MPR on cardiac CT. Normal reference values are given in Table 17.1.
- In general, compared with CMR, the value of the LV mass is larger, and the LV volume is smaller on cardiac CT, due to the difference in the modality and measurement method, such as the exclusion or inclusion of the papillary muscles in the cardiac chamber. The comparison of previously published data for reference values for LV parameters is summarized in Table 17.1 [1, 6, 7], (Fig. 17.4).

Table 17.1 Normal LV dimension, volumes, and functional parameters

	Kang et al. 2017	Stolzmann et al. 2008	Kawel-Boehm et al. 2020
Image modality	CT	CT	MR
Country/subject number	Korea/172	United States/120	Meta-analysis
Men			
LV ID (cm)	4.8 ± 0.5	4.5 ± 0.5	5.2 ± 0.5
SWT(cm)	1.1 ± 0.2	0.9 ± 0.2	0.8 ± 0.1
PWT (cm)	0.9 ± 0.2	0.9 ± 0.2	0.7 ± 0.1
LV EDV (mL)	113 ± 26	144 ± 38	155 ± 30
LV EDVI (mL/m^2)	62 ± 14	–	79 ± 15
LV ESV (mL)	42 ± 15	47 ± 19	55 ± 15
LV ESVI (mL/m^2)	23 ± 8	–	29 ± 9
LV mass (g)	145 ± 29	167 ± 38	121 ± 28
LV MI (g/m^2)	80 ± 14	86 ± 18	62 ± 11
SV(mL)	71 ± 18	95 ± 29	103 ± 21
EF (%)	63 ± 8	66 ± 9	64 ± 8
Women			
LV ID (cm)	4.8 ± 0.6	4.4 ± 0.5	4.9 ± 0.5
SWT(cm)	0.9 ± 0.2	0.8 ± 0.1	0.7 ± 0.1
PWT (cm)	0.8 ± 0.1	0.8 ± 0.2	0.6 ± 0.1
LV EDV (mL)	98 ± 21	115 ± 7	123 ± 22
LV EDVI (mL/m^2)	60 ± 11	–	73 ± 12
LV ESV (mL)	34 ± 12	40 ± 12	43 ± 11
LV ESVI (mL/m^2)	21 ± 8	–	25 ± 7
LV mass (g)	108 ± 20	129 ± 29	83 ± 21
LV MI (g/m^2)	66 ± 11	68 ± 13	49 ± 10
SV(mL)	65 ± 15	76 ± 18	83 ± 16
EF (%)	66 ± 8	66 ± 7	66 ± 7

Sources: Kang EJ et al. Korean J Radiol 2017, Stolzmann P et al. Eur Radiol 2008, Kawel-Boehm N et al. J Cardiovasc Magn Reson 2020 [1, 6, 7]

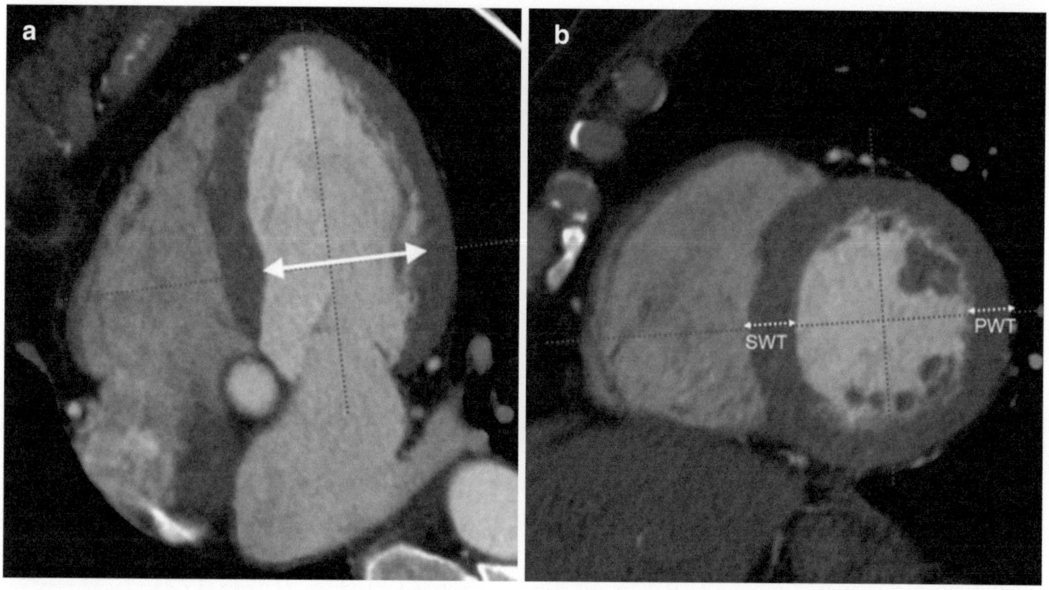

Fig. 17.4 Measurements of LV dimension and wall thickness at end-diastolic phase. (**a**) LV inner dimension was measured on 4-chamber MPR at chorda level (arrow). (**b**) LV wall thickness on septum (SWT) and posterior wall (PWT) were measured on short-axis MPR at chorda level

17.5 Left Ventricular Anatomy and Variants

Cardiac CT provides a comprehensive evaluation of the cardiac anatomy with the use of cardiac imaging planes (short-axis, 4-chamber, 2-chamber, etc.) that are easily created with MPR images [8].

17.5.1 LV Anatomy

- Anatomically, the LV consists of the inlet, apical, and outlet portions. The inlet contains the mitral valve and its apparatus and the outlet portion leads to the aortic valve (Fig. 17.5).
- The trabeculae of the LV are more densely packed than those of the right ventricle (RV); thus, the LV cavity reveals a smooth endocardial border. The LV contains two prominent papillary muscles, the anterior and posterior papillary muscles, which attach to each mitral valvular leaflet by the chordae tendinea.
- The interventricular septum typically bulges toward the right ventricle due to pressure differences between the chambers. Therefore, the LV cavity shows a round configuration on the short-axis image, and a bullet shape on 4- or 2-chamber MPR images.
- The LV lateral free wall is normally thickest at the base and granularly thinned toward the apex.
- The interventricular septum is divided into the muscular and membranous septum. The membranous portion of the septum lies beneath the right coronary and non-coronary cusp. Most ventricular septal defects (VSD) involve the membranous septum, and occasionally a membranous septal aneurysm, or latent form of remnant lesion leading to a closed VSD, may be detected incidentally.

17.5.2 Myocardial Segmentation

- For standardized assessment of LV segments with assigned coronary artery supply territories, the 17 myocardial segments model recommended by the American Heart Association is widely used in clinical practice [9].

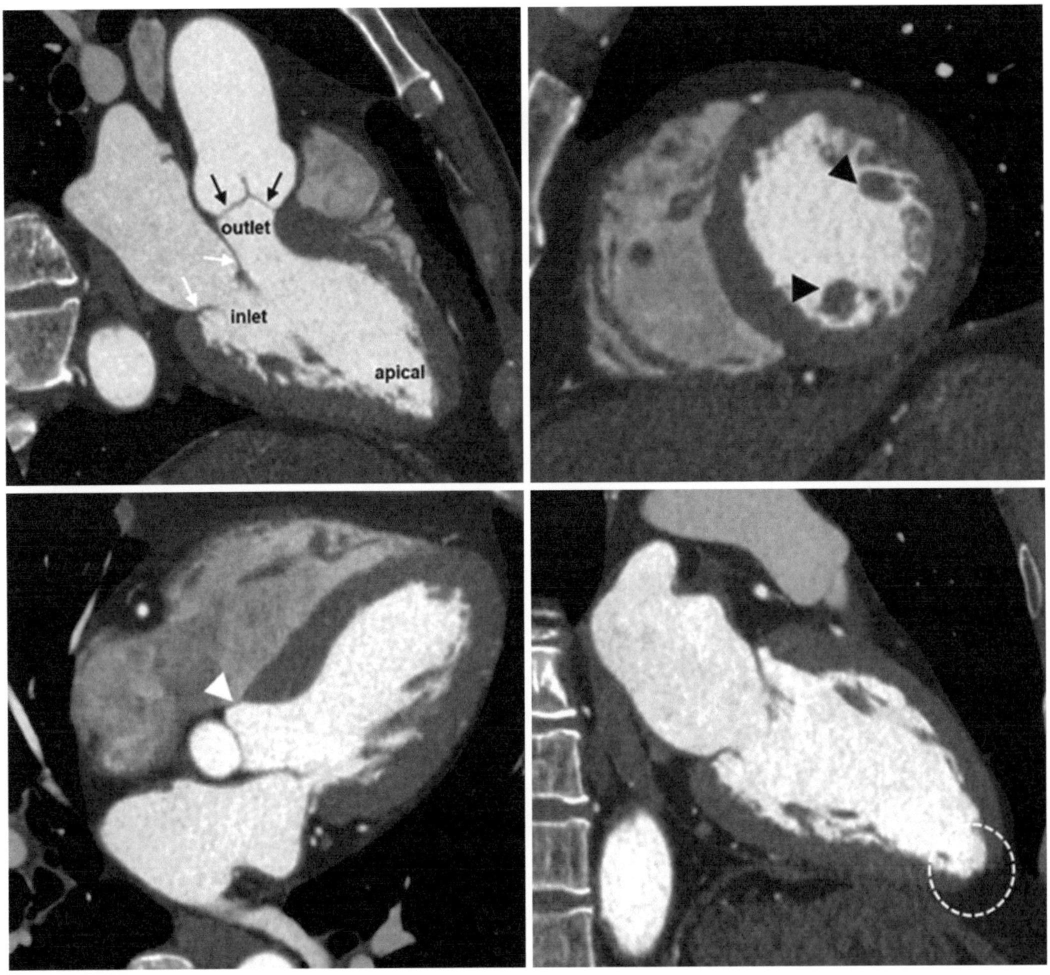

Fig. 17.5 Anatomy of left ventricle (LV). The LV consists of the inlet (contains mitral valve; white arrows), apical, and outlet portions (leads to the aortic valve; black arrows), and contains two prominent papillary muscles (arrowheads in middle); the anterior and posterior papillary muscles. The interventricular septum typically bulges toward the right ventricle (RV). Note that thin membranous septum (white arrowhead). The LV apex is normally extremely thin at the tip portion (circle)

- According to this model, the LV is divided into equal thirds, perpendicular to the long axis; basal, mid-cavity, and apical. (1) The basal third is the area from the mitral annulus to the tips of the papillary muscles; (2) the mid-cavity is the region containing the papillary muscles of the LV; and (3) the apical third refers to the area beyond the papillary muscles, to just before the end of the cavity. The LV apex or apical cap is the area of the myocardium that is beyond the end of the LV cavity.
- The circumferential locations in the basal and mid-cavity are divided into six segments, and the apical myocardium is divided into 4-segments. Figure 17.6 shows the location and names of the 17 myocardial segments on a bull's eye display.

17.5.3 Anatomic Pitfalls or Variants

- The LV apex is normally extremely thin at the tip portion and does not thicken significantly

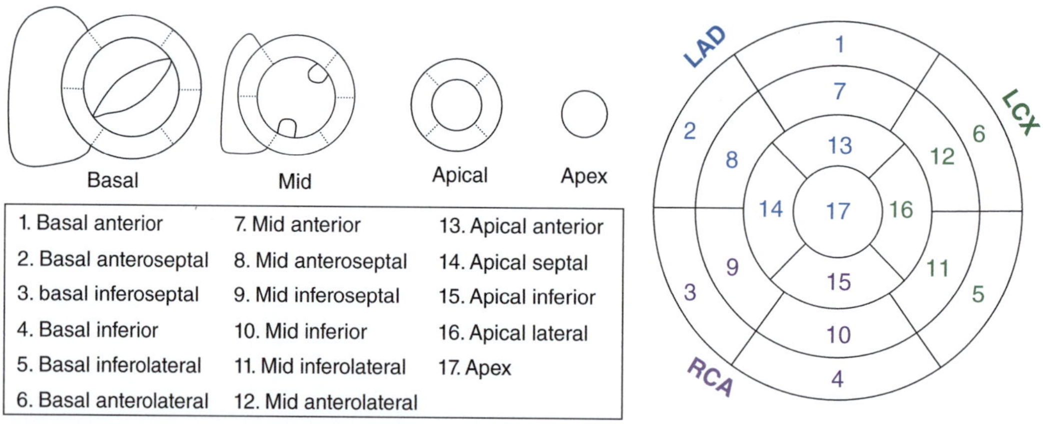

Fig. 17.6 Bull's-Eye map for 17 segments of the left ventricle according to the AHA (American Heart Association)

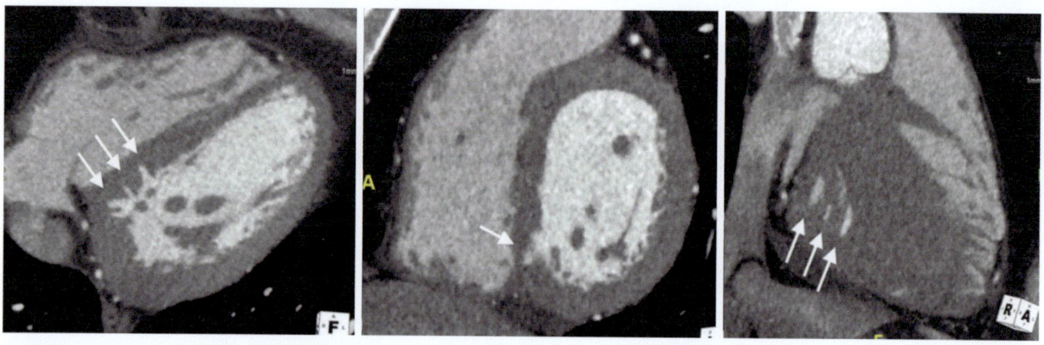

Fig. 17.7 Incidentally found multiple LV crypts (arrows) in 40-year-old, healthy man

during the cardiac cycle. This should not be confused with myocardial scarring from an old infarction.

- The thin membranous septum can be misinterpreted as a VSD on cardiac CT. To confirm a VSD, a definite visualization of shunt flow between the two ventricles is necessary.
- A LV crypt means a focal myocardial penetration (>50% of the myocardial thickness) on a normal compacted myocardium. This commonly involves the mid to basal inferior or septal segment of the LV and is completely obliterated during the systole phase. It is more frequently found in the patients with a thickened myocardium, such as hypertensive cardiomyopathy or hypertrophic cardiomyopathy (HCMP). According to a recent study [10], LV crypts are relatively frequent in the general population (9.1% incidence) and are not associated with major adverse cardiovascular events (Fig. 17.7).
- A congenital LV diverticulum is a rare cardiac malformation, and mostly found in the LV apical area. It may be confused with a LV apical aneurysm. A LV diverticulum is characterized by a well-defined finger-like outpouching sac that maintains normal contractility (synchronous with LV myocardium). Although this finding does not usually provoke any cardiac symptoms and is incidentally found, it is associated with a risk of systemic embolization, fatal ventricular arrhythmias and cardiac death [11].

17.6 Cardiac CT for the Assessment of Cardiomyopathy

- There are many classifications of cardiomyopathies proposed by various professional societies, WHO, etc.

- We focus on terminology practitioners commonly use in clinical practice.

17.6.1 Ischemic Cardiomyopathy

Ischemic cardiomyopathy is defined as LV systolic dysfunction due to coronary artery disease, e.g., in the setting of prior myocardial infarction, and/or severe coronary arterial lumen narrowing [12]. Cardiac CT allows an assessment of coronary artery disease severity, identification of associated myocardial territories, delineation of myocardial infarcts, as well as identification of myocardial perfusion abnormalities.

17.6.1.1 Myocardial Infarction

- Infarcted myocardium undergoes numerous changes which may be appreciated by cardiac CT.
- Reduced myocardial perfusion can be recognized by hypo-attenuated density, compared with a remote, normal myocardium.
- Infarcted myocardium may be detected by increased contrast uptake on delayed imaging owing to contrast accumulation in the increased extracellular space.
- Regional wall thinning, fat infiltration, calcification, and/or aneurysm may be evident in chronic, old infarcts.
- Functional imaging may reveal wall motion abnormalities,.
- A comprehensive CT analysis for the detection of an acute myocardial infarction, based on matching hypo-attenuated segments and regional wall motion abnormalities, may yield a precise diagnosis for the culprit lesion.
- The severity of myocardial thinning may be associated with poor prognosis, and LV end-diastolic wall thickness < 6 mm is defined as irreversible myocardial damage (nonviable myocardium) (Fig. 17.8).

17.6.1.2 Left Ventricular Aneurysm and Pseudoaneurysm

- Anterior or apical infarcts may lead to the development of aneurysms with nonviable thinned myocardium.
- Features of a true aneurysm include focal saccular protrusions of thin-walled myocardium, containing the full thickness of the myocardial layer, possibly linked to ballooning outward during systole. Fatty replacements or calcifications of the myocardial wall, or intraventricular thrombus may be present.
- The differentiation of a LV aneurysm from a pseudoaneurysm is clinically important, as the therapeutic management and clinical prognosis differ.
- LV pseudoaneurysms result from the partial or complete rupture of the LV free wall and are covered by adherent pericardium or scar tissue. Wall rupture may occur as result of excessive tissue damage from infarction but may also be seen as result of surgical instrumentation (iatrogenic).
- Pseudoaneurysms with narrow necks carry an increased risk of rupture. Ventricular pseudoaneurysm should prompt consultation with cardiothoracic surgery specialists.

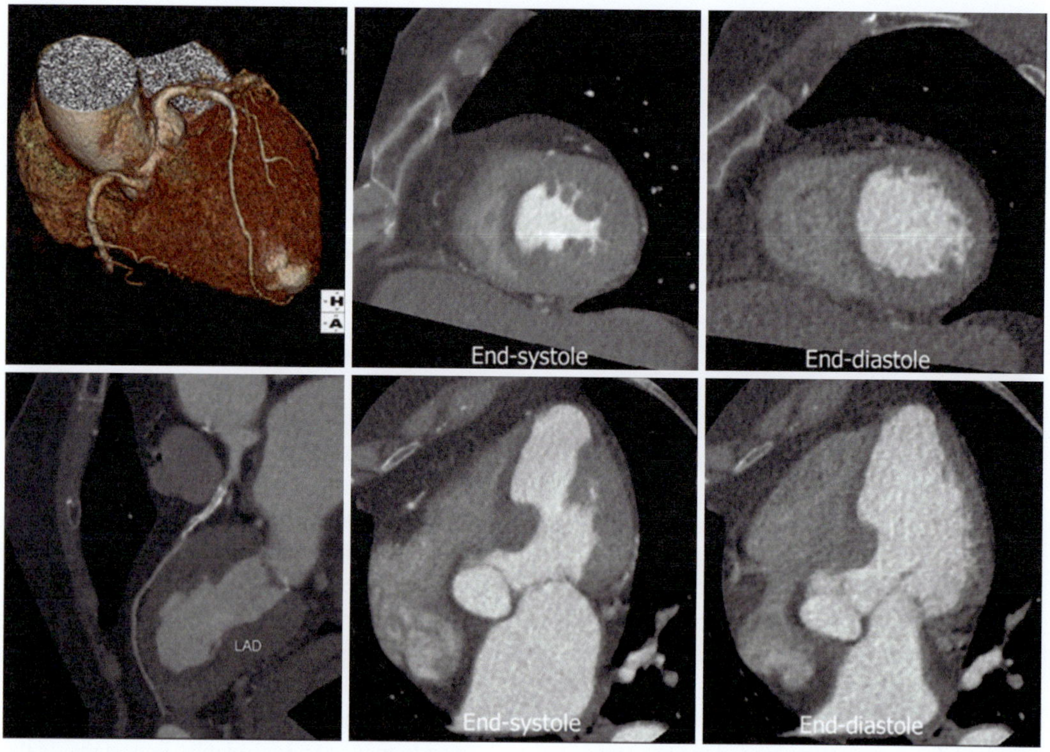

Fig. 17.8 Case example of severe luminal narrowing in the LAD with associated myocardial infarction in a 68-year-old woman. Significant myocardial thinning with aneurysm formation and subendocardial hypo-attenuation in the mid-anteroseptal and apical left ventricular segments are consistent with CT findings of myocardial infarction

17.7 Nonischemic Cardiomyopathy

- Although echocardiography and CMR remain the mainstay in the diagnosis of cardiomyopathies, cardiac CT may have a role in the morphologic assessment of disease, particularly in cases of suboptimal echocardiography or where a preceding CMR is contraindicated due to ferromagnetic devices.
- Cardiac CT can discriminate between ischemic and nonischemic causes of cardiomyopathy, and also play a potential role in the assessment of particular nonischemic cardiomyopathy, such as dilated cardiomyopathy (DCMP), hypertrophic cardiomyopathy (HCMP), LV noncompaction, and arrhythmogenic right ventricular cardiomyopathy.

17.7.1 Dilated Cardiomyopathy (DCMP)

- DCMP is characterized by LV dilation with systolic dysfunction (ejection fraction <40%), with or without RV dysfunction.
- About 50% of cases are idiopathic, the remaining are due to infectious, metabolic, toxic, mechanic, or endocrine causes with DCMP regarded as the end point of various disorders associated with myocardial injury.
- CT findings of DCMP are characterized by diffuse ventricular dilatation and impaired systolic function (EF <40%) in the absence of coronary artery disease. The thickness of the LV wall is usually normal or reduced. It is often difficult to differentiate between the various causative etiologies of DCMP (Fig. 17.9).

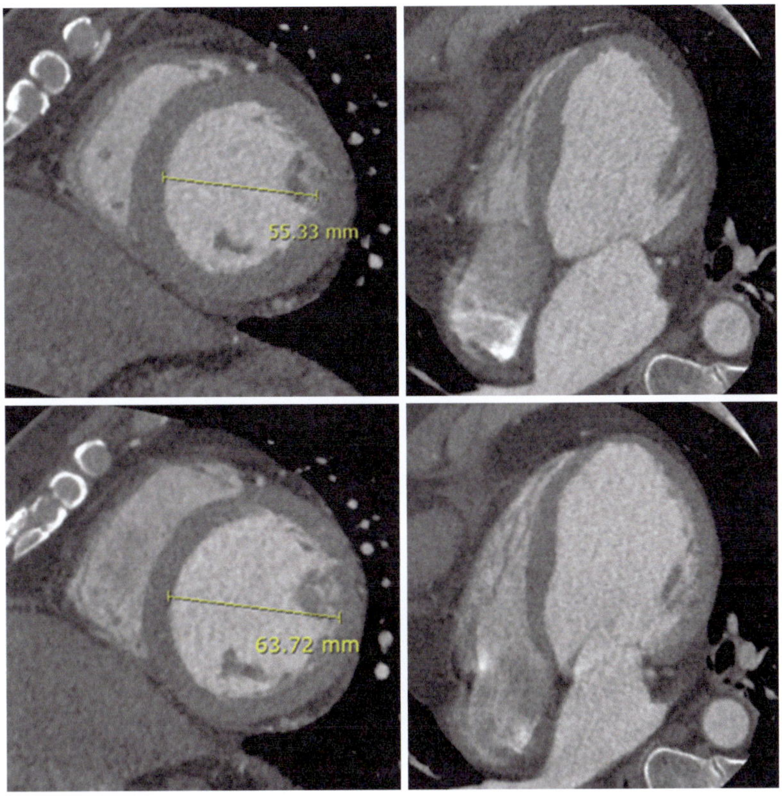

Fig. 17.9 End-systole (upper) and end-diastole (lower) images of a DCMP in a 59-year-old man with evidence of left ventricular dilatation and systolic dysfunction (LVEDV 175 mL, LVESV 128 mL, EF 27%)

17.7.2 Hypertrophic Cardiomyopathy (HCMP)

- HCMP is the most common heritable cardiovascular disorder (usually autosomal dominant inheritance) and characterized by unprovoked myocardial hypertrophy without compensatory LV dilatation, and normal or supranormal systolic function [13].
- HCMP exhibits a wide range of clinical manifestation, from asymptomatic mutation carriers to sudden cardiac death, particularly in young athletes (10–35 years).
- LV myocardial thickness > 15 mm is a common diagnostic threshold for HCMP, and > 30 mm is associated with poor prognosis (such as risk of sudden cardiac death).
- Morphological phenotypes include asymmetric septal (most common type), concentric, apical, mid-ventricular, and mass-like (or localized) types (Fig. 17.10).
- Cardiac CT offers detailed assessment of LV morphology in HCMP patients and is of particular value in patients with suboptimal echocardiography windows, contraindications to CMR, and those referred for concomitant CAD evaluation.
- Suspected HCMP on CCTA for the evaluation of CAD should prompt consideration of the acquisition phase within cardiac cycle to avoid misdiagnosis in systole or mid-diastole vs. to end-diastole .

17.7.3 LV Noncompaction

- LV noncompaction is characterized by a prominent trabecular meshwork in the lining of the LV due to the arrested development of endomyocardial compaction, without other structural heart disease.
- Clinically, LV noncompaction is revealed in a wide range of manifestations from asymptomatic to impaired LV systolic function, and other complications, such as thromboembolism and arrhythmia.

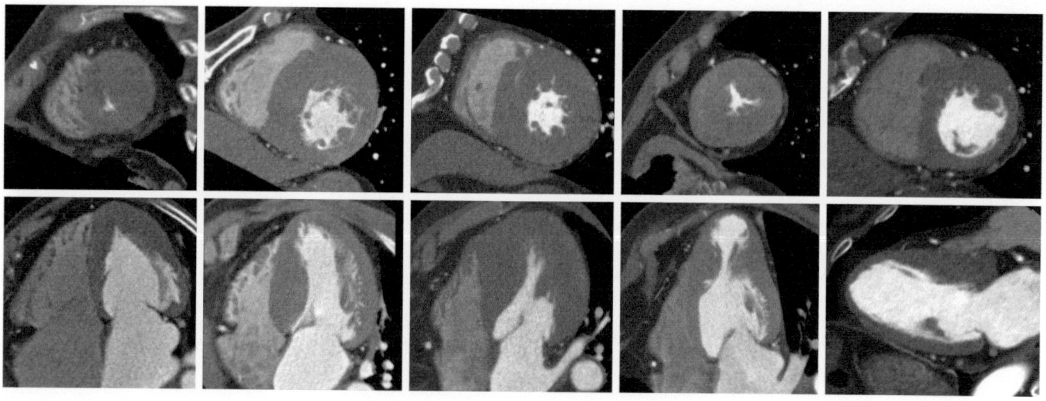

Fig. 17.10 Different morphologic types of HCMP: apical, asymmetric septal, concentric, mid-ventricular, and mass-like types (left to right)

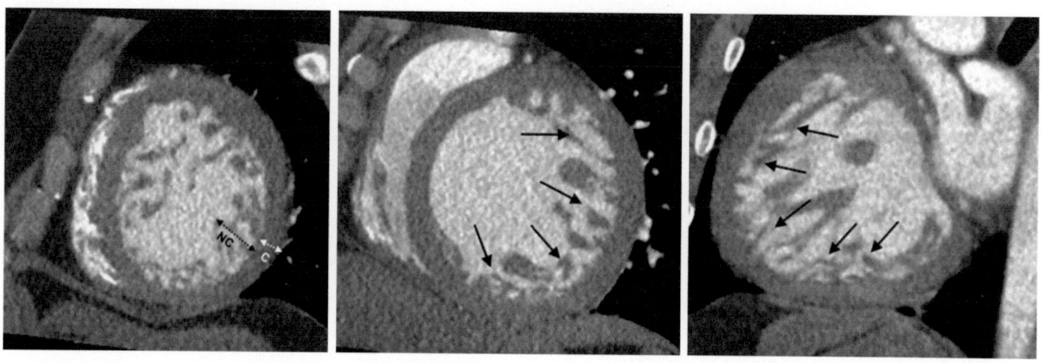

Fig. 17.11 Short axis and 2-chamber MPR CT images demonstrating LV noncompaction. Non-compacted trabeculation is evident in the apical and the mid-lateral LV segments (arrows). The ratio of non-compacted and compacted myocardial thickness (NC/C ratio) exceeds 2.3, which is diagnostic of LV concompaction

- Embryologically, the compaction process of the myocardium progresses from the epicardium to the endocardium, base to apex, and septum to LV free wall. Therefore, the LV apical segment is always involved in LV noncompaction and the mid-inferior and lateral segments are also frequently involved.
- The prominent LV trabeculation in the apical and mid-segment of the LV, with the ratio of non-compacted to compacted myocardium (NC/C ratio) > 2.3 at the end-diastole, together with global LV hypokinesia, are diagnostic hallmarks of LV noncompaction by CMR.
- Since cardiac CT can delineate the characteristic two-layered myocardium of the LV with excellent visualization of the LV trabeculation and can provide precise measurements of the myocardial thickness as well as provide systolic functional images, several papers suggest that the diagnosis of LV noncompaction by cardiac CT is accurate [14, 15] (Fig. 17.11).

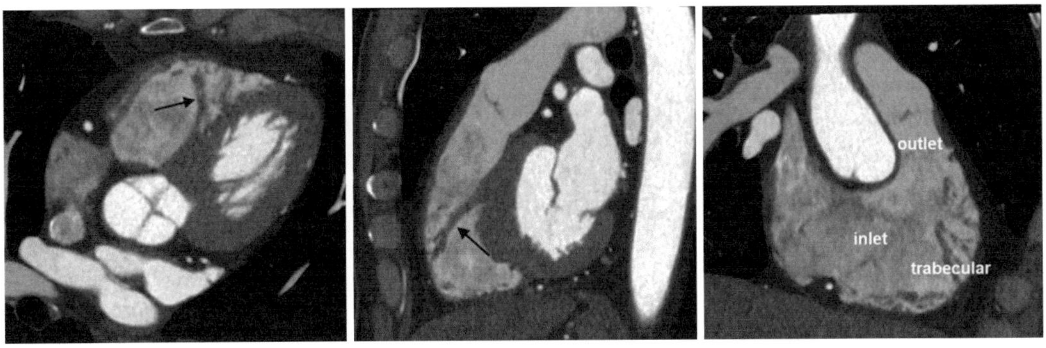

Fig. 17.12 Normal anatomy of the right ventricle (RV). The RV exhibits coarser trabeculae (including the moderator band, arrows), a lack of fibrous continuity between its inlet and outflow valves, and a relatively thinner wall compared to the left ventricle. The RV may be divided into three anatomic components: the inlet, trabeculated apical myocardium, and infundibulum (outlet). Note the RV chamber in this example is filled with saline contrast mixture, which is an appropriate for RV assessment

17.8 Right Ventricular Assessment

Since the right ventricle (RV) has a complex, irregular geometry, CT and CMR are better suited to evaluated its anatomy than conventional two-dimensional echocardiography. Providing true three-dimensional, high-resolution images, CT is a valid alternative to CMR for RV assessment and function.

17.8.1 Anatomic Considerations

- The RV exhibits coarser trabeculae (including the moderator band), a lack of fibrous continuity between its inlet and outflow valves, and a thinner wall than the LV owing to its lower loading requirements [16].
- The RV may be divided into three anatomic components: the inlet, trabeculated apical myocardium, and infundibulum (conus or outlet, Fig. 17.12). In clinical practice, the RV is often divided into the apical, mid, and basal segments, akin to LV segmentation.
- Owing to its complex morphology, the RV exhibits a triangular shape in the coronal plane and a crescent shape in the transversal plane [17].
- The normal RV wall measures 3–4 mm in thickness and is thicker at the base than at the apex. Although the RV volume is typically larger than the LV, the RV muscle mass is only one-sixth of the LV mass.
- The posterior wall of the RV (interventricular septum) is normally concave toward the LV in both the systole and diastole phases.
- RV normal anatomical reference values vary depending on age, gender, race, etc., and there are significant differences among diagnostic modalities (Echocardiography, MRI, CT), hindering adequate comparison.
- A meta-analysis on RV normal reference values by 3D ecocardiography by Wang et al. [18] revealed the following values: RV end-diastolic volume, 100.71 mL [95% confidence interval (CI), 90.92–110.51 mL); RV end-systolic volume, 44.19 mL (95% CI, 39.05–49.33 mL); RV end-diastolic volume indexed, 57.01 mL/m^2 (95% CI, 51.93–62.08 mL/m^2); RV end-systolic volume indexed, 25.41 mL/m^2 (95% CI, 22.58–28.24 mL/m^2); and RVEF, 56.20% (95% CI, 54.59–57.82%).
- A meta-analysis on RV normal reference values by CMR by Kawel-Boehm et al. reported reference ranges (normal value) for RV parameters in the adult for men (papillar included in RV volume) as follows: RV end-diastolic volume, 166 ± 39 mL (87–244 mL); RV end-systolic volume, 73 ± 22 mL (29–117 mL); RV end-diastolic volume

indexed, 88 ± 17 mL/m^2 (53–123 mL/m^2); RV end-systolic volume indexed, 38 ± 11 mL/m^2 (17–59 mL/m^2); and RVEF, 57 ± 8% (42–72%).

17.8.2 Acquisition and Reconstruction Techniques

- Standard injection techniques used for coronary CT angiography are optimized for the left heart chamber and aorta, resulting in varying levels of enhancement of the right chamber.
- Therefore, to examine the RV, the contrast injection protocol has to be modified to maintain adequate contrast on the right side of the heart during image acquisition.
- A multiphasic infusion protocol (that combines contrast media, saline contrast mixture, and saline flush) is recommended, using a rapid flow rate throughout the injection period to minimize the effect of venous return from the IVC (Fig. 17.13). If simultaneous pulmonary opacification is desired, the saline flush should be omitted [19].
- For post-processing, the horizontal 4-chamber and short-axis views are most useful for right heart analysis. The measurements of RV myocardial thickness and internal dimensions have not been standardized for CT. In general, however, a transverse RV diameter of more than 45 mm is considered abnormal.
- As with LV functional assessment, RV function can be assessed with retrospective ECG-gated cardiac CT acquisition. Multiple studies have reported reliable functional RV assessment by CT compared with other imaging techniques. Compared to CMR, cardiac CT may slightly overestimate RV volumes due to different respiratory cycles during the image acquisition (end-inspiration for CT, end-expiration for CMR), and as well as contour detection techniques.

17.8.3 RV Pathology

17.8.3.1 Arrhythmogenic RV Cardiomyopathy (ARVC)

- ARVC is a rare genetic cardiomyopathy associated with gradual demise of RV myocytes and subsequent fibro-fatty replacement. It confers an increased risk of ventricular tachyarrhythmia, RV failure and sudden cardiac death.
- The diagnosis by imaging is challenging given the subtle changes within the thin RV wall and there is no gold standard other than endomyocardial biopsy. Thus, a multi-disciplinary approach is typically required for a diagnosis, including ECG findings, cardiac rhythm/depolarization/repolarization analysis, tissue characterization, family history, and imaging data.
- The revised criteria proposed by the Task Force of the European Society of Radiology and the Scientific Council on Cardiomyopathies of the International Society and Federation of Cardiology in 2010 confirm a role of imaging by 2D-echcardiography and CMR for the diagnosis of ARVC but does not explicitly discuss CT [20].
- Cardiac CT is capable of evaluating most of the major and minor features of the Task Force criteria, and several researchers have recently demonstrated the utility of CT for ARVC assessment. However quantitative thresholds for ARVC diagnosis in consensus guidelines derived from CMR values may not be fully applicable to cardiac CT.
- By cardiac CT, diffuse dilatation of the RV (EDVI >110 mL/m^2 males and > 100 mL/m^2 females) with prominent trabeculation, focal wall thinning due to aneurysms, and RVOT dilatation are morphologic characteristics of ARVC. Occasionally, a RV intramyocardial fat deposition may be detected. On retrospective ECG-gated cardiac CT imaging, the presence of RV systolic dysfunction (RVEF <40%) or wall motion abnormality may be evaluated (Fig. 17.13).

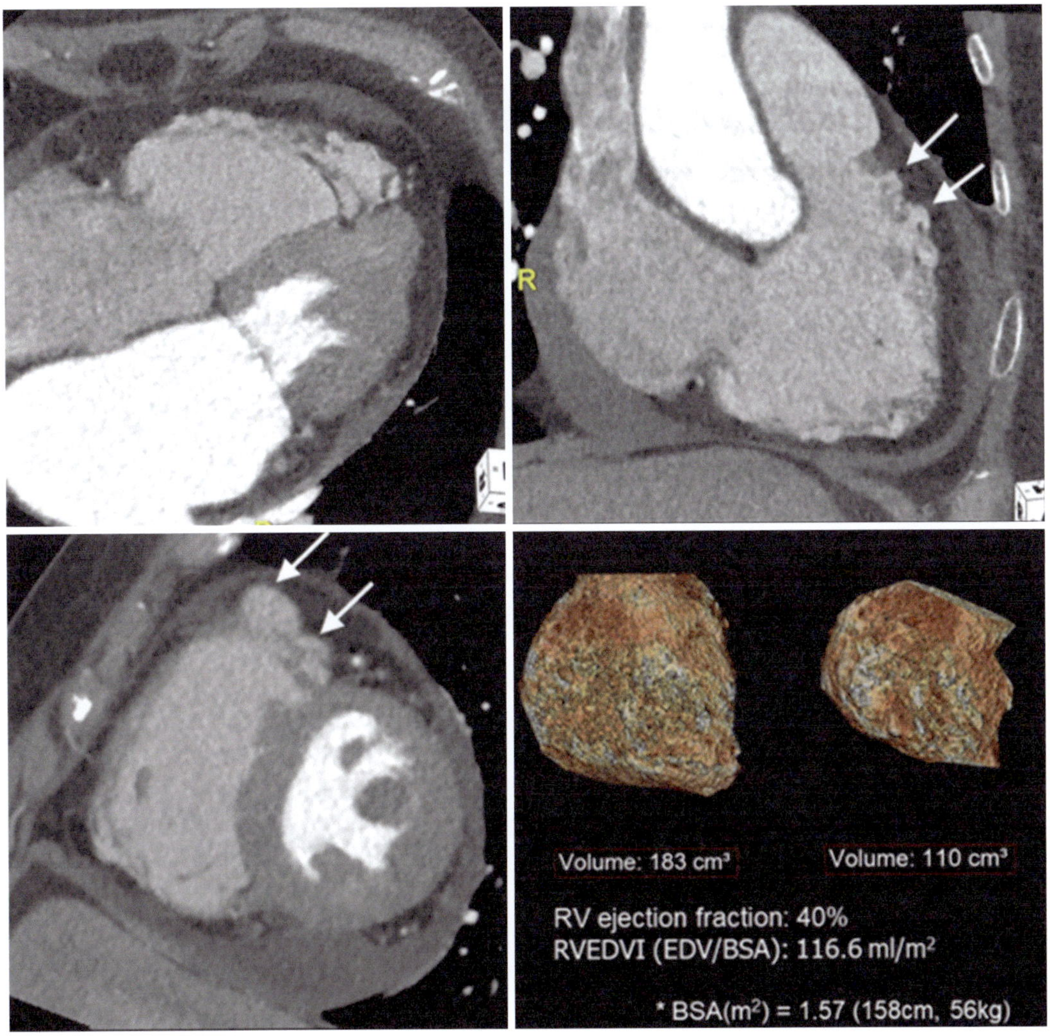

Fig. 17.13 A case example of ARVC in 77-year-old women. Diffuse dilatation of the RV chamber with a scalloped margin in the RV lateral wall, multifocal linear fat depositions in the RV trabeculation and septal wall. Note that multiple small aneurysm formations (arrows) along the RVOT, increased RV volume, and decreased ejection fraction, are compatible with ARVC

17.8.4 RV Involvement of Ischemic Heart Disease

- The RV is generally less susceptible to ischemic injury than the LV, due to a lower demand for oxygen, a greater oxygen reserve during hemodynamic stress, and a right coronary circulation that has more extensive collateral flow and perfusion during both systole and diastole [21].
- Involvement of the RV occurs in 50% of inferior, and in 33% of anterior LV myocardial infarctions.
- RV dilatation, abnormal wall motions, and paradoxical motion of the interventricular septum are imaging features on RV infarction (Fig. 17.14).

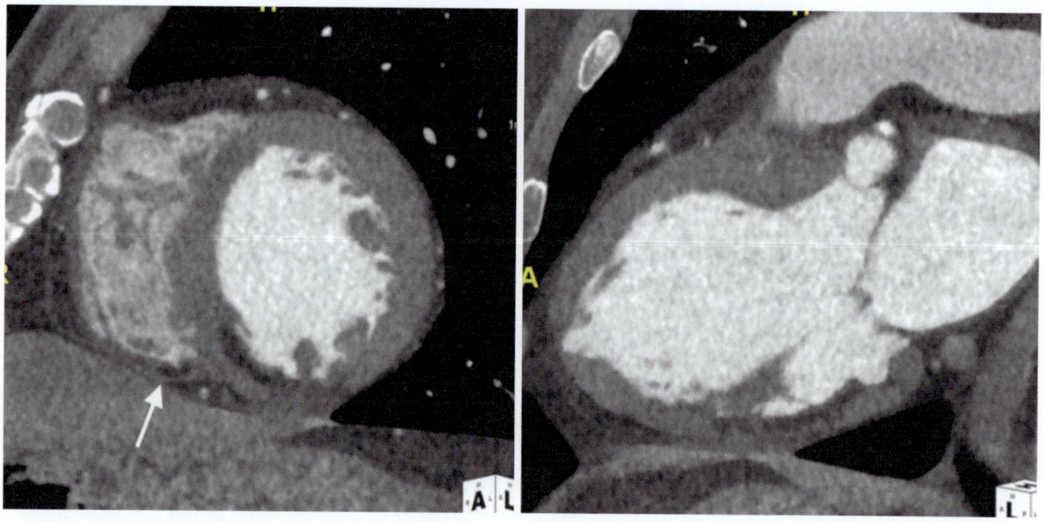

Fig. 17.14 A case example of an old myocardial infarction in the RCA territory involving both the LV and RV inferior wall in a 57-year-old man. Myocardial thinning and linear subendocardial fat infiltrations are evident in both the LV and RV inferior walls (arrow)

17.9 Evaluation of Cardiac Masses

- Echocardiography remains the preferred initial imaging modality for the evaluation of cardiac masses. Cardiac CT is an alternative option in the setting of poor echocardiographic windows or if CMR is contraindicated/not available.
- Cardiac CT may be particularly helpful to evaluate calcified or fatty masses, and to detect metastasis for cancer staging. Non-contrast CT and/or delayed contrast enhancing CT may be needed in addition to standard CTA for selected cases.
- Cardiac masses are uncommon entities and they may be categorized as non-neoplastic or neoplastic. Primary cardiac tumors are rare and about 75% of these are benign. Myxoma is the most common benign tumor (50%), followed by papillary fibroelastoma (20%), lipoma (20%), and hemangioma (5%) [22]. The most common malignant tumors of the heart are metastases from other primary origins.

17.9.1 Malignant Tumors

- Cardiac sarcoma is the most common primary malignant cardiac tumor. The most common phenotype of a cardiac sarcoma is an angiosarcoma. Although other types of sarcomas usually occur in the left atrium, angiosarcomas are commonly detected in the right atrium (80%). On cardiac CT, sarcomas reveal a broad-based low attenuation mass with enhancement, and often invasion to the myocardium or large vessels.
- Cardiac lymphoma is extremely rare. In cardiac CT, lymphomas present as hypo- or iso-attenuated, infiltrative soft-tissue masses, in comparison with the myocardium and can involve one or multiple chambers.

17.9.2 Thrombus

- Thrombus is the most common type of intracardiac mass and is usually found in the left atrial appendage.

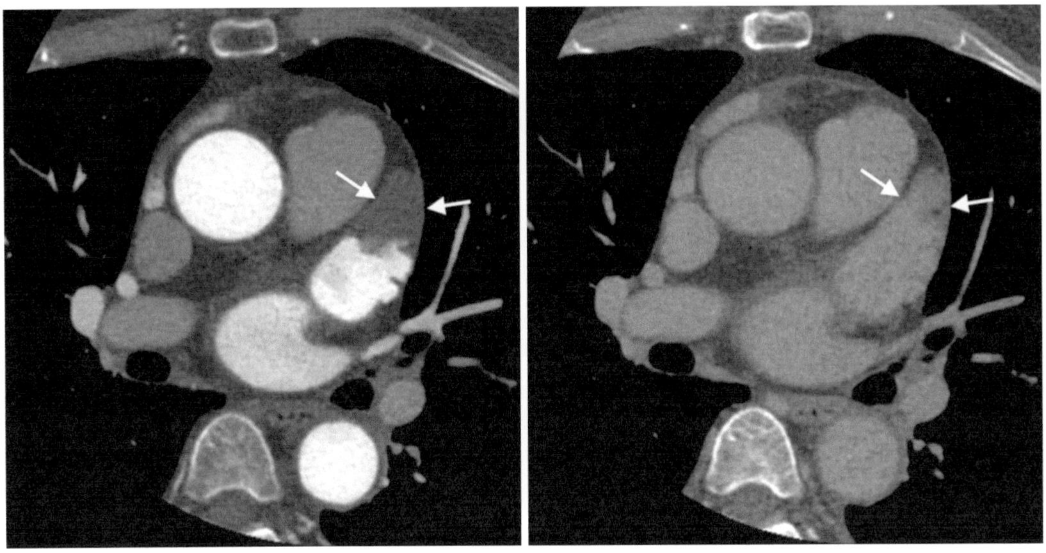

Fig. 17.15 A case example of delayed left atrial appendage contrast filling, mimicking thrombus. Note that the contrast filling defect (arrows on the left) completely resolved on delayed CT imaging (arrows on right), excluding the diagnosis of thrombus

- It may be associated with a hypercoagulable state, atrial fibrillation, mitral valve disease, severe LV dysfunction following myocardial infarction, or implantation of metallic devices.
- In atrial fibrillation, left atrial "thrombus" may be mimicked by circulatory stasis (spontaneous echo contrast on echocardiography), and delayed CT (30 s after the first scan) should be performed for differentiation (Fig. 17.15).
- For the differential diagnosis between a thrombus and a tumor, clinical knowledge of predisposing risk factors, the location and shape of the lesion, and appearance by delayed enhancement may be helpful.

17.9.3 Myxoma

- Myxoma is the most common benign cardiac tumor found in the heart.
- It is usually seen in the left atrium, attached to the fossa ovalis (60–75%) or the right atrium. However, it can also be detected in other cardiac structures (inferior vena cava, valvular leaflets).
- A myxoma commonly presents as well-defined, low attenuation intracavitary mass with lobular contours. It has smooth or lobular margins and is usually heterogeneously enhanced on delayed CT. The internal density depends on chronicity and tumor components (such as necrosis or hemorrhage).
- A mobile or huge myxoma occasionally prolapses into the ventricular chamber and the atrioventricular valves, causing obstruction (Fig. 17.16).

17.9.4 Lipoma

- A lipoma is a benign mesenchymal tumor composed of mature adipose tissue and can be located at various sites.
- Given the fatty density of lipoma, it is easily detected by CT, which is a highly specific image modality for its diagnosis.
- In cases where the fatty mass contains thickened or nodular septa, a liposarcoma should be considered in the differential diagnosis and images should be inspected for non-adipose

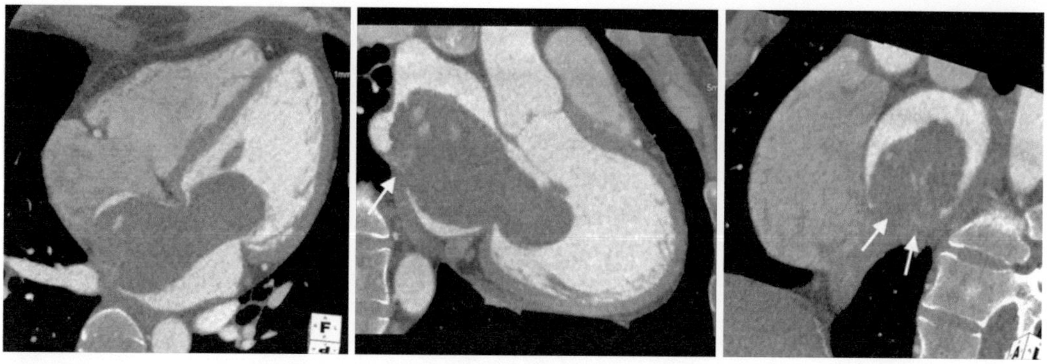

Fig. 17.16 A case example of a large myxoma in the left atrium with a small stalk attached to the LA inferior wall (arrows) with patchy central enhancement. The 4-chamber and 3-chamber images show the mass prolapsing into the left atrium across the mitral valve

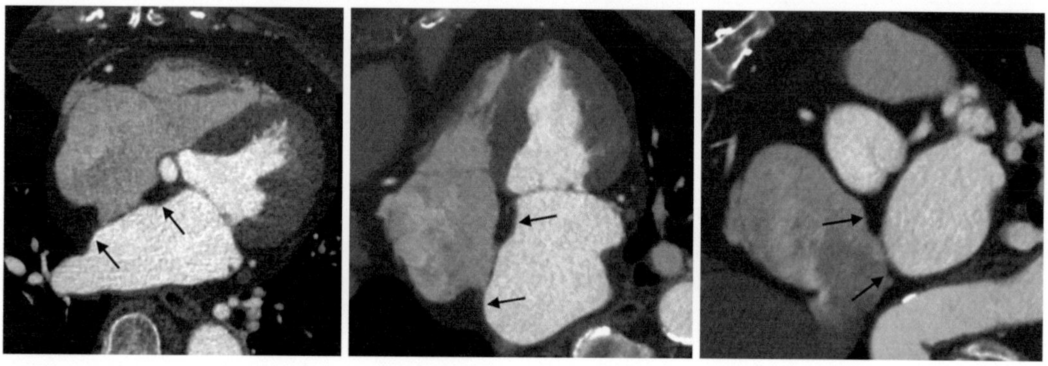

Fig. 17.17 Lipomatous hypertrophy of the interatrial septum in a 75-year-old obese woman. Transaxial images show the typical dumbbell-shaped, low attenuation mass (arrows) of the interatrial septum with sparing of the fossa ovalis. Note that the mass is confined to the interatrial septum, and that the cephalad portion is thicker than the caudal portion

density lesions which are often contrast enhanced on delayed imaging [23].

- Lipomatous hypertrophy of the interatrial septum is a non-neoplastic accumulation of fat cells in the interatrial septum, which may mimic a lipoma. This lesion is associated obesity and is easily recognized by its typical location and shape (dumbbell-shaped mass with sparing of the fossa ovalis) (Fig. 17.17).
- Nonspecific myocardial fat (cardiac physiologic fat) is often detected incidentally and increases with age as part of the aging process [24]. It occurs predominantly in the RV, particularly involving the anterolateral free wall and outflow tracts of the RV, and sometimes in the RV trabeculation and LV apex. Consideration of the patient's age, the characteristic location of the lesion, and the preservation of the normal myocardial thickness as well as ventricular size are diagnostic clues assisting with differentiating nonspecific from pathologic myocardial fat (Fig. 17.18).

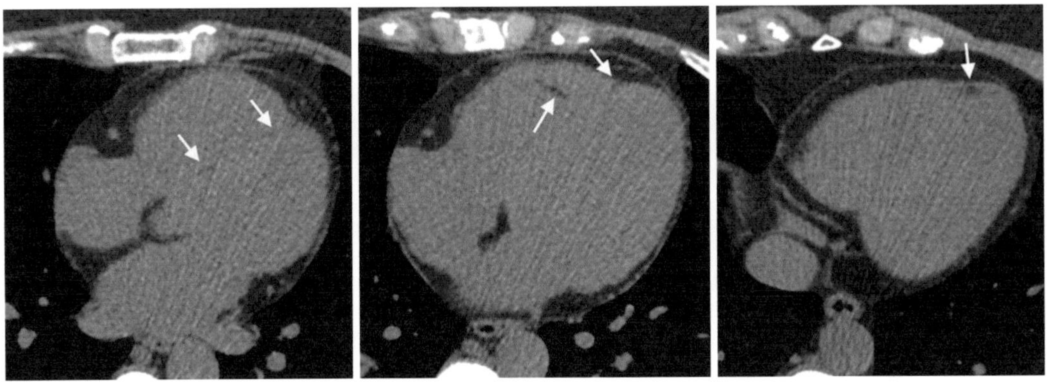

Fig. 17.18 Multifocal, nonspecific myocardial fat (arrows) detected in a 41-year-old woman without cardiac symptoms and with normal cardiac chamber size/mass

References

1. Kawel-Boehm N, Hetzel SJ, Ambale-Venkatesh B, et al. Reference ranges ("normal values") for cardiovascular magnetic resonance (CMR) in adults and children: 2020 update. J Cardiovasc Magn Reson. 2020;22(1):87. https://doi.org/10.1186/s12968-020-00683-3.
2. Clemente A, Seitun S, Mantini C, et al. Cardiac CT angiography: normal and pathological anatomical features-a narrative review. Cardiovasc Diagn Ther. 2020;10(6):1918–45. https://doi.org/10.21037/cdt-20-530.
3. Yamamuro M, Tadamura E, Kubo S, et al. Cardiac functional analysis with multi-detector row CT and segmental reconstruction algorithm: comparison with echocardiography SPECT, and MR imaging. Radiology. 2005;234(2):381–90. https://doi.org/10.1148/radiol.2342031271.
4. Belge B, Coche E, Pasquet A, et al. Accurate estimation of global and regional cardiac function by retrospectively gated multidetector row computed tomography. Eur Radiol. 2006;16(7):1424–33. https://doi.org/10.1007/s00330-006-0169-6.
5. Clayton B, Roobottom C, Morgan-Hughes G. Assessment of the myocardium with cardiac computed tomography. Eur Heart J Cardiovasc Imaging. 2014 Jun;15(6):603–9. https://doi.org/10.1093/ehjci/jeu028.
6. Kang EJ, Lee KN, Choi WJ, et al. Left ventricular functional parameters and geometric patterns in Korean adults on coronary CT angiography with a 320-detector-row CT scanner. Korean J Radiol. 2017;18(4):664–73. https://doi.org/10.3348/kjr.2017.18.4.664.
7. Stolzmann P, Scheffel H, Leschka S, et al. Reference values for quantitative left ventricular and left atrial measurements in cardiac computed tomography. Eur Radiol. 2008;18(8):1625–34. https://doi.org/10.1007/s00330-008-0939-4.
8. O'Brien JP, Srichai MB, Hecht EM, Kim DC, Jacobs JE. Anatomy of the heart at multidetector CT: what the radiologist needs to know. Radiographics. 2007;27(6):1569–82. https://doi.org/10.1148/rg.276065747.
9. Cerqueira MD, Weissman NJ, Dilsizian V, Jacobs AK, Kaul S, Laskey WK, Pennell DJ, Rumberger JA, Ryan T, Verani MS. American Heart Association writing group on myocardial segmentation and registration for cardiac imaging. Standardized myocardial segmentation and nomenclature for tomographic imaging of the heart. A statement for healthcare professionals from the cardiac imaging Committee of the Council on clinical cardiology of the American Heart Association. Circulation. 2002;105(4):539–42. https://doi.org/10.1161/hc0402.102975.
10. Sigvardsen PE, Pham MHC, Kühl JT, et al. Left ventricular myocardial crypts: morphological patterns and prognostic implications. Eur Heart J Cardiovasc Imaging. 2021;22(1):75–81. https://doi.org/10.1093/ehjci/jeaa020.
11. Ohlow MA. Congenital left ventricular aneurysms and diverticula: definition, pathophysiology, clinical relevance and treatment. Cardiology. 2006;106(2):63–72. https://doi.org/10.1159/000092634.
12. Felker GM, Shaw LK, O'Connor CM. A standardized definition of ischemic cardiomyopathy for use in clinical research. J Am Coll Cardiol. 2002;39(2):210–8. https://doi.org/10.1016/s0735-1097(01)01738-7.
13. Ko SM, Kim TH, Chun EJ, Kim JY, Hwang SH. Assessment of left ventricular myocardial diseases with cardiac computed tomography. Korean J Radiol. 2019;20(3):333–51. https://doi.org/10.3348/kjr.2018.0280.
14. Melendez-Ramirez G, Castillo-Castellon F, Espinola-Zavaleta N, Meave A, Kimura-Hayama ET. Left ventricular noncompaction: a proposal of new diagnostic criteria by multidetector computed tomography. J Cardiovasc Comput Tomogr. 2012;6(5):346–54. https://doi.org/10.1016/j.jcct.2012.07.001.

15. Fuchs TA, Erhart L, Ghadri JR, et al. Diagnostic criteria for left ventricular non-compaction in cardiac computed tomography. PLoS One. 2020;15(7):e0235751. https://doi.org/10.1371/journal.pone.0235751.
16. Wang S, Wang S, Zhu Q, et al. Reference values of right ventricular volumes and ejection fraction by three-dimensional echocardiography in adults: a systematic review and meta-analysis. Front Cardiovasc Med. 2021;8:709863. https://doi.org/10.3389/fcvm.2021.709863.
17. Sheehan F, Redington A. The right ventricle: anatomy, physiology and clinical imaging. Heart. 2008;94(11):1510–5. https://doi.org/10.1136/hrt.2007.132779.
18. Kochav J, Simprini L, Weinsaft JW. Imaging of the right heart—CT and CMR. Echocardiography. 2015;32(Suppl 1):S53–68. https://doi.org/10.1111/echo.12212.
19. Gopalan D. Right heart on multidetector CT. Br J Radiol. 2011;84:S306–23. https://doi.org/10.1259/bjr/59278996.
20. Marcus FI, McKenna WJ, Sherrill D, et al. Diagnosis of arrhythmogenic right ventricular cardiomyopathy/dysplasia: proposed modification of the task force criteria. Eur Heart J. 2010;31(7):806–14. https://doi.org/10.1093/eurheartj/ehq025.
21. Galea N, Carbone I, Cannata D, et al. Right ventricular cardiovascular magnetic resonance imaging: normal anatomy and spectrum of pathological findings. Insights Imaging. 2013;4(2):213–23. https://doi.org/10.1007/s13244-013-0222-3.
22. Kassop D, Donovan MS, Cheezum MK, Nguyen BT, Gambill NB, Blankstein R, Villines TC. Cardiac masses on cardiac CT: a review. Curr Cardiovasc Imaging Rep. 2014;7(8):9281. https://doi.org/10.1007/s12410-014-9281-1.
23. Shu S, Yuan H, Kong X, Wang J, Wang J, Zheng C. The value of multimodality imaging in diagnosis and treatment of cardiac lipoma. BMC Med Imaging. 2021;21(1):71. https://doi.org/10.1186/s12880-021-00603-6.
24. Kimura F, Matsuo Y, Nakajima T, et al. Myocardial fat at cardiac imaging: how can we differentiate pathologic from physiologic fatty infiltration? Radiographics. 2010;30(6):1587–602. https://doi.org/10.1148/rg.306105519.

18 Myocardial Perfusion and Viability CT Imaging

Omar Chehab, Henrique Doria De Vasconcellos, and Joao Lima

Abstract

This chapter summarizes the methods of computed tomography (CT) myocardial perfusion imaging for comprehensive anatomical and functional assessment of coronary heart disease. Options include static myocardial CT perfusion, either using a single or dual energy source, and dynamic myocardial CT perfusion. While static CT myocardial perfusion has been the traditional approach for detecting myocardial ischemia, dynamic CT myocardial perfusion is emerging as an attractive alternative given the potential for estimating absolute myocardial blood flow/reserve and myocardial fibrosis using extracellular volume. This chapter lists protocols and discusses advantages and disadvantages of various approaches to CT myocardial perfusion imaging.

Keywords

Stress myocardial perfusion · Computed tomography perfusion · Coronary artery disease · Coronary computed tomography angiography · Myocardial blood flow · Risk assessment · Functional assessment · Static myocardial perfusion · Dynamic myocardial perfusion

O. Chehab · H. D. De Vasconcellos · J. Lima (✉)
Department of Medicine, Division of Cardiology, The Johns Hopkins University School of Medicine, Baltimore, MD, USA
e-mail: ochehab1@jhu.edu; hvascon1@jhu.edu; jlima@jhmi.edu

Abbreviations

BMI	Body mass index
CAD	Coronary artery disease
CCTA	Coronary computed tomographic angiography
CMD	Coronary microvascular disease
CTP	Myocardial perfusion imaging
DECT	Dual energy CT
ECG	Electrocardiogram
INOCA	Ischemia and non-obstructive coronary artery disease
MBF	Myocardial blood flow
MRI	Magnetic resonance imaging
PET	Positron emission tomography
SECT	Single energy CT
TAC	Time attenuation curve
TPR	Transmural Perfusion Ratio

18.1 Introduction

- The prevalence of coronary artery disease (CAD) continues to increase [1].
- At least 60% of patients with signs and symptoms of CAD referred for invasive coronary

A. A. Zadeh, J. Hoe (eds.), *Practical Guide to Cardiac CT*,
https://doi.org/10.1007/978-981-97-6919-3_18

angiography have non-obstructive coronary artery disease [2].

- Patients with normal coronary computed tomographic angiography (CCTA) findings have an excellent prognosis and do not require further testing for CAD [3].
- However, like invasive coronary angiography, CCTA, usually in the form of stress testing [4–6].
- Stress testing is commonly done by exercise or pharmacologic "stress" with electrocardiographic monitoring and often myocardial perfusion imaging (MPI) using single-photon emission computed tomography (SPECT), and positron emission tomography (PET) or detection of abnormal contraction by echocardiography [7].
- Ideally, we attain both anatomic and functional information with one test but CCTA alone has limitations for gaging hemodynamic significant CAD in the setting of severe calcifications [8] which may lead to consideration of revascularization with no hemodynamic or functional significance [9–11].
- With the lack of functional assessment by CCTA, the ability to accurately stratify patients of intermediate lesions or patients with ischemia and non-obstructive coronary artery disease (INOCA) or "microvascular disease" is limited.
- CT myocardial perfusion or CTP has emerged a new non-invasive functional imaging modality to accurately identify hemodynamic significance in patients with CAD [12].
- CTP can be performed by either single or dual energy (SECT or DECT) modalities. Moreover, CTP can be performed as either "static" or "dynamic" (Fig. 18.1). Advantages and disadvantages of each myocardial CTP are summarized in Table 18.1.

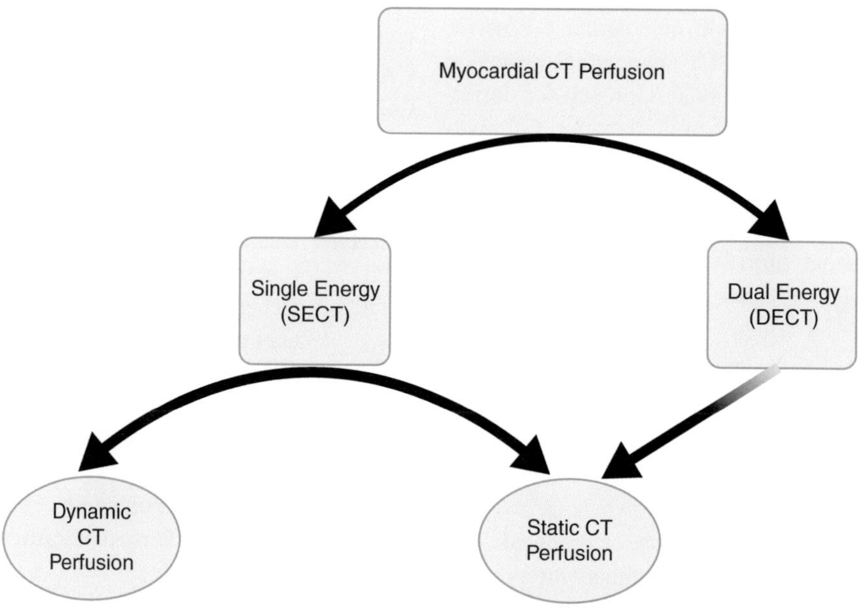

Fig. 18.1 Flow diagram describing the different forms of myocardial CT perfusion

Table 18.1 Advantages and Disadvantages of CT Myocardial Perfusion Imaging Modalities: Single Energy Static CTP—Dual Energy Static CTP—Dynamic CTP

	Single energy static CTP	Dual energy static CTP	Dynamic CTP
Timing	Rapid	Rapid	Longer secondary to breath holds increasing risk for cardiac motion artifacts
Diagnosis	(a) Qualitative (b) Semi-quantitative	(a) Qualitative (b) Semi-quantitative	(a) Qualitative (b) Semi-quantitative (c) Fully quantitative
Radiation	Lowest radiation	Similar radiation dose as single energy	Higher radiation than SECT and DECT
Simplicity	• Timing is critical for acquisition • Susceptible to motion and beam hardening artifacts	• Depends on specific vendor technology • Reduces beam hardening artifacts	• Complex and needs more time for analysis • Given this is retrospective acquisition, timing is less essential compared to static CTP and ability reduce artifacts through observation of "first pass" of myocardial perfusion • High image noise
Evidence	Highest level of evidence	Less number of studies compared to single energy static CTP	Emerging imaging modality with less number of studies compared to single energy static CTP

18.2 Static CTP

18.2.1 Single Energy Static CTP

- It has been more than a decade since the introduction of CTP in animal and preliminary human studies [13–18]. To date, the results of single energy CTP have been demonstrated in single and multicenter trials [12, 19].
- The static CTP method samples a snapshot of the iodine distribution in the blood pool and the myocardium over a short period of time, targeting either the upslope or the peak of contrast bolus. Static myocardial perfusion permits a qualitative and semi-quantitative assessment of differences in contrast densities where hypoperfusion is defined as areas of reduced densities but does not allow for direct quantification of the myocardial blood flow (MBF), unlike dynamic CTP [20, 21].
- The static CTP method samples a snapshot of the iodine distribution in the blood pool and the myocardium over a short period of time, targeting either the upslope or the peak of contrast bolus. At the upslope of the contrast, the difference in attenuation value of the ischemic and remote myocardium is at the maximum which enables qualitative and semi-quantitative assessment of myocardial perfusion defects [22].
- A disadvantage of static CTP is the acquisition of only one data sample and the possibility of mistiming the contrast bolus that may result in poor contrast-to-tissue ratios by missing the peak attenuation [23]. Output and flow rate of the contrast material may affect bolus timing. In addition, the acquisition of data from sequential heartbeats affects the attenuation gradient and may result in a heterogeneous iodine distribution, mimicking perfusion defects [24].
- Static CTP is limited in detecting balanced ischemia, where the perfusion of the entire myocardium is impaired and therefore there is no reference remote myocardium for comparison for semi-quantitative or qualitative static methods of CTP interpretation [25].
- Clinical trial data in support of CTP suggest similar accuracy for detecting myocardial perfusion defect as other non-invasive methods [26] [27].
- A systematic review and meta-analysis of 12 studies found an incremental increase in specificity with no difference in sensitivity for static CTP compared to CTA alone [19].
- When comparing static vs. dynamic CTP, dynamic CTP has higher sensitivity [while static CTP had higher specificity [12]].

18.2.2 Dual Energy CTP

- One of the main limitations of single energy static CTP is beam hardening artifacts which may mimic a perfusion defect [28–30]. The use of dual energy CTP has decreased the rates of beam hardening artifacts with vendors offering different solutions in acquisition with different tube voltages [31, 32].
- Spectral imaging refers to analyzing images from different energy levels. Initially, polychromatic images are obtained, and then either an evaluation by material decomposition through iodine contrast and assess difference in iodine density in the myocardium or through monochromatic imaging evaluation or reconstruction where we can analyze images from different energies [33].
- By analyzing images through material decomposition using iodine maps, dual energy CTP measures the amount of iodine in the myocardial wall, where patients with normal scans will have a homogeneous uptake, signaling normal perfusion. By analyzing two areas a hypodensity can be referenced to a known normal area, allowing distinction between artifacts and true perfusion defects [33, 34].
- Clinical studies found improved diagnostic accuracy of dual energy CT [35, 36].

18.3 Dynamic CTP

- One of the main limitations of static CTP is the inability to provide quantitative assessment of myocardial ischemia. Myocardial blood flow (MBF), measured by cardiac magnetic resonance perfusion and by PET myocardial perfusion (the gold standard), has been consistently found to be an independent predictor of worse cardiovascular outcomes [37, 38].
- Dynamic CTP has emerged as a new imaging modality that highly correlates with rubidium-82 PET [39].
- Dynamic CT perfusion imaging entails continuous myocardial imaging to record the kinetics of "wash in" and "wash out" of iodinated contrast in the arterial blood pool and myocardium.
- This technique allows for multiple sampling of the myocardium and the blood pool and creating time attenuation curves (TAC) by measuring the change in CT attenuation over time. Mathematical modeling of TACs permits for direct quantification of MBF. In addition, dynamic CTP provides additional quantitative measures such as time to peak, mean transit time, and blood volumes.
- Dynamic CTP is ideally acquired using wide detector CT to capture perfusion throughout the entire myocardium but a shuttle mode may be used with scanners of less coverage where the table will move back and forth to get a complete acquisition of left ventricle [40–42].
- The key limitation of dynamic CTP acquisition is high radiation dose due to extending scan time.
- Wide detector CTP acquisition allows lower scan times and radiation doses [42–44].
- Another major limitation of dynamic CTA is the lack of standardization between the different vendors [45].
- Diagnostic accuracy of dynamic CTP revealed an overall sensitivity of 0.85 (95% CI: 0.76–0.92) and a specificity of 0.81 (95% CI: 0.64–0.93) in a meta-analysis [12].
- Dynamic CTP improves diagnostic accuracy when added to CCTA alone [46, 47] (Fig. 18.2).

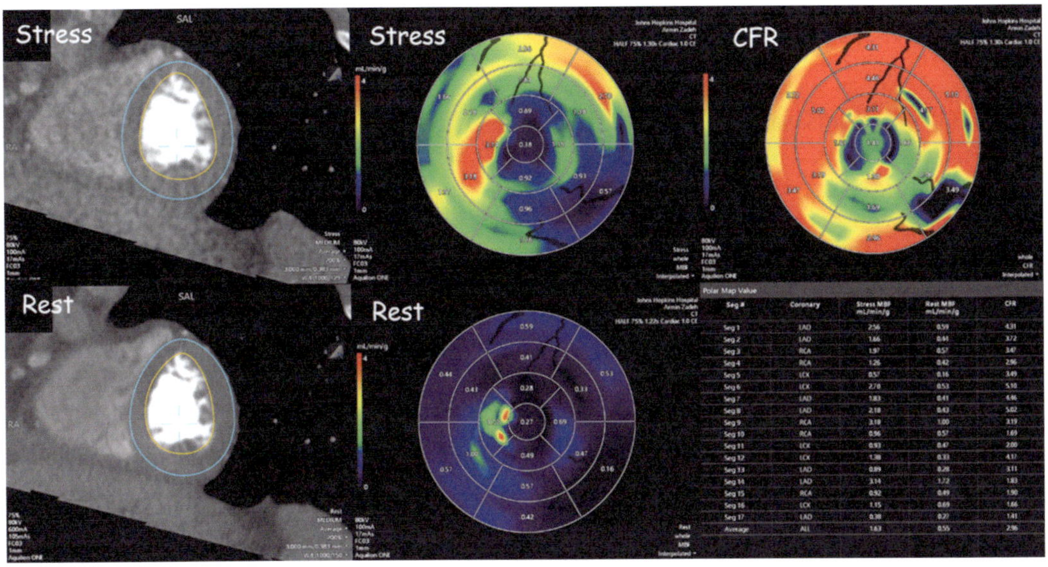

Fig. 18.2 Dynamic CTP study in a 75-year-old man with past medical history of hyperlipidemia, who presented with atypical chest pain. Rest CCTA reveals severe coronary artery calcification with a calcium score of 1349, mild left main disease (30% stenosis), moderate to severe LAD, LCx, and RCA atherosclerotic disease (up to 50–60% stenosis). Dynamic CTP showing a very mild perfusion defect in the apical region (CFR < 2)

18.4 How to Perform CTP: Protocols

18.4.1 Contraindications

- Like all stress imaging, CTP studies are contraindicated in the setting of unstable angina, acute myocardial infarction (less than 4 days), uncontrolled arrhythmias, uncontrolled hypertension (blood pressure greater than 200/100 mmHg), severe aortic stenosis, acute pulmonary embolism, acute myocarditis or pericarditis, acute aortic dissection, severe pulmonary hypertension, or high-degree of atrial-ventricular block.

18.4.2 Technical Requirements

- CTP can be acquired either with a rest/stress or a stress/rest method. If the stress images are acquired first, images are not affected by residual contrast (from the rest images) and beta-blockers can be held until the end of stress phase. However, heart rate control after the stress acquisition may be challenging. With first acquiring rest images, CCTA allows to identify patients without significant disease, thus eliminating the need of CTP and reducing radiation risks to patients [32].

18.4.3 Exam Preparation

- Patients should be fasting for at least 4 h and refrain from caffeine, aminophylline, and theophylline for 24 h prior to the scan.
- Heart rate controlling medication is ideally given the night before the exam and adjusted as needed 1 h before the exam, e.g., metoprolol 50–150 mg, with a target heart rate of 55–60 beats per minute.
- As with CCTA, intravenous (IV) access is required, ideally with a 18 gage cannula.
- Intravenous hydration with 0.5 L of normal saline may be given to avoid dehydration.
- A 12-lead electrocardiogram (ECG) is required before and at the end of the scan.
- Continuous ECG and blood pressure monitoring are recommended throughout the procedure.

18.4.4 "Stressor" Agents

- Three commonly used agents for CTP are the vasodilators dipyridamole, adenosine, and regadenason.
- Dipyridamole is inexpensive and the most commonly used agent throughout the world, particularly in regions where drug costs are a consideration. It acts as an adenosine deaminase and phosphodiesterase inhibitor, promoting its vasodilator effects via adenosine accumulation. It is used via a 4-minute intravenous (IV) infusion at a dose of 0.56 mg/Kg. Due its long half-life and risk of bronchospasm, reversion of its effect with IV aminophylline may be required.
- Adenosine is a non-specific adenosine receptor agonist with an ultra-short action time (half-life less than 10 s), used via 4–6-min intravenous infusion. Adenosine may increase heart rate by an average of 20 beats per minute. Side effects are facial flushing, bronchospasm, chest pain, and atrioventricular (AV) block, which are mostly reversible after terminating drug infusion.
- Regadenason is a more recently introduced, more costly vasodilator with a selective A_{2A} agonist effect, providing a higher safety and reliability when compared with the other agents. It is used via a 10 s injection as a single dose of 400 μg in prefilled syringe, with a biological half-life of 2–4 min. Average heart rate increase is 25 beats per minute but it is unlikely to cause bronchospasm or AV block.

18.4.5 Scan Acquisition

- Details regarding scan protocols are being provided in Tables 18.2 and 18.3.

18.4.6 Image Reconstruction and Analysis

- If the rest imaging was performed first, the initial step should be the assessment of CAD with potential hemodynamic significance (e.g., > 50% stenosis).
- Evaluating the CTA first provides the opportunity to match the coronary anatomy with perfusion territories and thus avoid false positive results.
  - The scan reconstruction intervals should be every 2–5% of the R—R interval.
  - Window Width / Window Level should be set to 300/150 or 200/100 to optimize myocardial assessment.
  - Images should be screened for motion, beam hardening, cone beam, and reconstruction artifacts.
  - The CTP phase with the least myocardial motion should be selected for analysis.

Table 18.2 Suggested static CTP protocol for rest acquisition

	Dual source	64 slice	Wide detector
Scout	Scout	Chest	Chest
Scan range	To cover the myocardium	To cover the myocardium	To cover the myocardium
Bolus gating	Automatic	Automatic	Automatic
ECG gating	Heart rate less than 70 prospective Heart rate greater than 70 retrospective	Heart rate less than 70 prospective Heart rate greater than 70 retrospective	Prospective
Exposure window for peak current	Low HR: Diastole only High HR: Systole and diastole	Low HR: Diastole only High HR: Systole and diastole	Low HR: Diastole only High HR: Systole and diastole
kVp	BMI ≤ 25, 100 BMI >25, 120	BMI ≤ 25, 100 BMI >25, 120	BMI ≤ 25, 100 BMI >25, 120
mA	Patient size specific	Patient size specific	Patient size specific
Gantry rotation speed	0.33 s	0.33–0.40 s (fast as possible)	Fast as possible

Table 18.3 Suggested static CTP protocol for stress acquisition

	Dual source	64 slice	Wide detector
Scout	Scout	Chest	Chest
Scan range	To cover the myocardium	To cover the myocardium	To cover the myocardium
Bolus gating	Automatic	Automatic	Automatic
ECG gating	Heart rate less than 70 prospective Heart rate greater than 70 retrospective	Heart rate less than 65 prospective Heart rate greater than 65 retrospective	Prospective
Exposure window for peak current	75–95% R—R interval	75–95% R—R interval	75–95% R—R interval
kVp	BMI ≤ 25, 100 BMI >25, 120	BMI ≤ 25, 100 BMI >25, 120	BMI ≤ 25, 100 BMI >25, 120
mA	Patient size specific	Patient size specific	Patient size specific
Gantry rotation speed	0.33 s	0.33–0.40 s (fast as possible)	Fast as possible

- A true perfusion deficit must occupy more than one myocardial segment and be confirmed on two or more views.
- Semi-quantitative metrics maybe be used to aid the CTP interpretation, but the final read should be confirmed by visual assessment. Quantitative attenuation values may be inaccurate in the presence of chronic myocardial infarction—results should be consistent with rest/stress phases and myocardial pathology.
- Semi-quantitative metrics include contrast maps, the transmural perfusion index, and the perfusion index.
- The contrast map or polar map is a representation of myocardial CT attenuation according to myocardial segments and is very useful for comparing rest and stress phases. It provides an evaluation of attenuation in the myocardium by color and a numerical scale.
- The transmural perfusion ratio (TPR) is a ratio between subendocardial attenuation over subepicardial attention, with an abnormal value <0.99.

18.5 Future Perspectives of CT Myocardial Perfusion

18.5.1 Microvascular Disease

- Some patients continue to have significant symptoms despite optimal medical therapy, i.e., refractory angina [48–50].
- Approximately half of patients with stable angina have non-obstructive or no evidence of significant coronary artery disease [2, 51, 52] while still be at risk of morbidity and mortality [53, 54] with high rates of multiple hospitalizations and significant resource utilization [55–61] (Fig. 18.3).
- Coronary microvascular disease (CMD) is being implicated in many of these cases and accumulating evidence suggests that attrition of the myocardial microvasculature occurs progressively in the ischemic myocardium, which compounds the loss of macrovascular supply, and that interventions that protect or restore microvascular integrity can improve perfusion and function without altering the macrovascular circulation [62, 63].
- The coronary microcirculation can be evaluated using invasive procedures (such as invasive coronary angiography with measurements of fractional flow reserve, coronary flow reserve, and index of microcirculatory resistance) and non-invasive imaging modalities (using cardiac positron emission tomography (PET) though assessment of coronary flow reserve or cardiac magnetic resonance through myocardial perfusion reserve index) [64].
- Assessment of coronary microvascular dysfunction by CTP revealed that about a quarter of patients without significant stenosis by CCTA have myocardial perfusion defects [65].

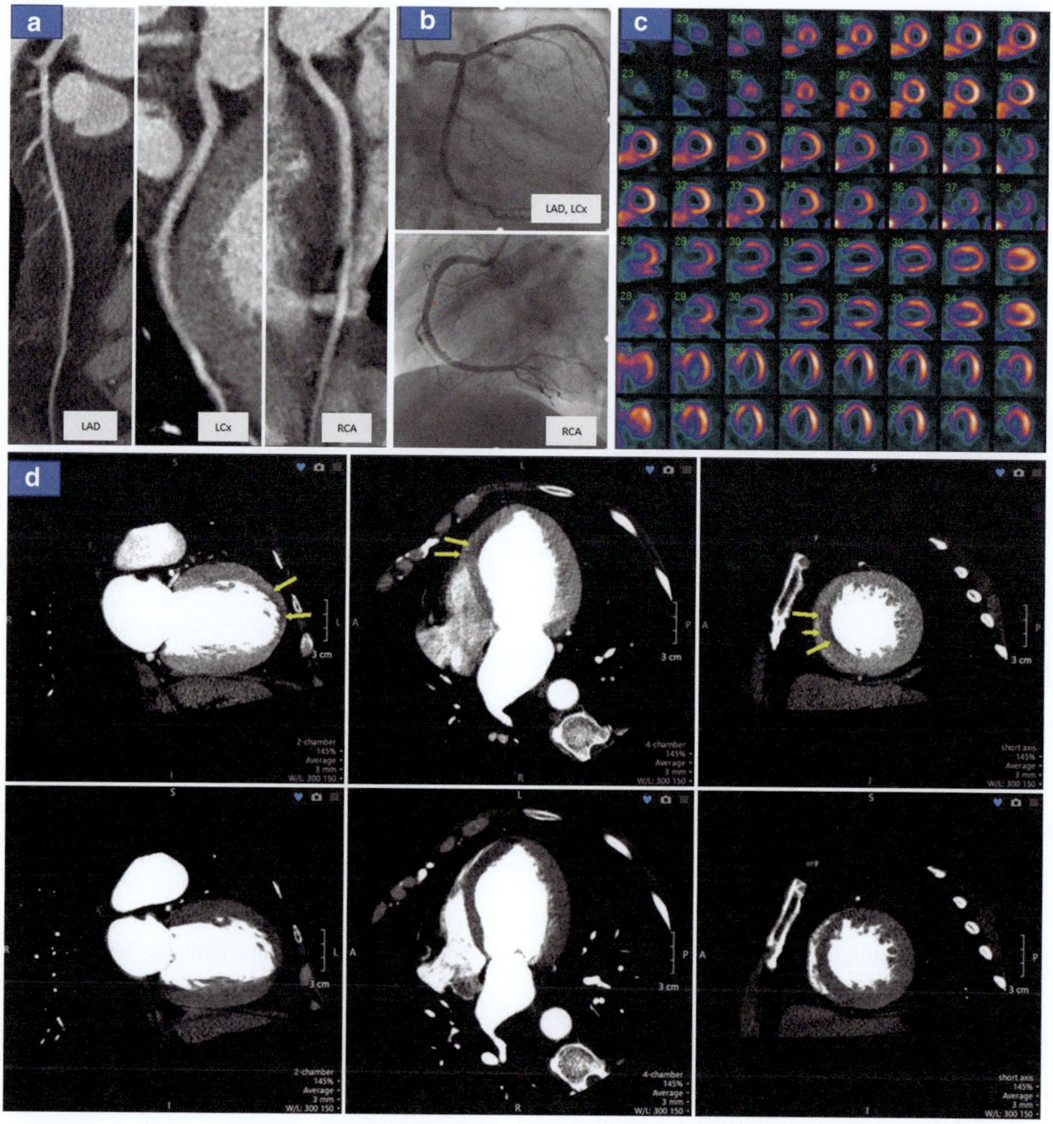

Fig. 18.3 CTA (**a**), cardiac angiography (**b**), SPECT (**c**), and static CTP (**d**) studies done in a 59-years-old female with a past medical history of hypertension and dyslipidemia who presented with typical cardiac chest pain. The anatomical cardiac exam tests (CTA and cardiac angiography) were normal. However, the functional (SPECT and static CTP) studies showed a perfusion defect in the anteroseptal mid-apical walls (arrows) on the stress phase indicated the presence of ischemia with no obstructive coronary artery disease (INOCA)

- Using animal models, dynamic CTP derived quantification of myocardial blood flow strongly correlates with the gold standard of microsphere measurements [66, 67] and PET [68].
- Some studies suggest an incremental prognostic value of myocardial blood flow data over conventional predictors for cardiovascular outcome [69].
- Future studies may utilize dynamic CTP for phenotyping coronary artery disease based on MBF and may stratify medical therapy accordingly, as suggested by the CoRMicA Trial [70].
- The role of the microcirculation may also be investigated in other pathologies such as aortic stenosis and hypertrophic cardiomyopathy [71].

18.5.2 Extracellular Volume Quantification and Myocardial Blood Flow

- Extracellular volume quantification can be obtained by MRI but CT has been found to be accurate in comparison, including for detecting myocardial fibrosis [72].
- Application of extracellular volume quantification has shown promise for characterization of cardiomyopathies [73].

References

1. Roth GA, Mensah GA, Johnson CO, Addolorato G, Ammirati E, Baddour LM, et al. Global burden of cardiovascular diseases and risk factors, 1990-2019: update from the GBD 2019 study. J Am Coll Cardiol. 2020;76(25):2982–3021.
2. Patel MR, Peterson ED, Dai D, Brennan JM, Redberg RF, Anderson HV, et al. Low diagnostic yield of elective coronary angiography. N Engl J Med. 2010;362(10):886–95.
3. Abdulla J, Asferg C, Kofoed KF. Prognostic value of absence or presence of coronary artery disease determined by 64-slice computed tomography coronary angiography a systematic review and meta-analysis. Int J Cardiovasc Imaging. 2010;27:413.
4. Gallagher MJ, Ross MA, Raff GL, Goldstein JA, O'Neill WW, O'Neil B. The diagnostic accuracy of 64-slice computed tomography coronary angiography compared with stress nuclear imaging in emergency department low-risk chest pain patients. Ann Emerg Med. 2007;49(2):125–36.
5. Goldstein JA, Gallagher MJ, O'Neill WW, Ross MA, O'Neil BJ, Raff GL. A randomized controlled trial of multi-slice coronary computed tomography for evaluation of acute chest pain. J Am Coll Cardiol. 2007;49(8):863–71.
6. Goldstein JA, Chinnaiyan KM, Abidov A, Achenbach S, Berman DS, Hayes SW, et al. The CT-STAT (coronary computed tomographic angiography for systematic triage of acute chest pain patients to treatment) trial. J Am Coll Cardiol. 2011;58(14):1414–22.
7. Miller TD, Askew JW, Anavekar NS. Noninvasive stress testing for coronary artery disease. Cardiol Clin. 2014;32(3):387–404.
8. Mushtaq S, Conte E, Pontone G, Baggiano A, Annoni A, Formenti A, et al. State-of-the-art-myocardial perfusion stress testing: static CT perfusion. J Cardiovasc Comput Tomogr. 2020;14(4):294–302.
9. Maron DJ, Hochman JS, Reynolds HR, Bangalore S, O'Brien SM, Boden WE, et al. Initial invasive or conservative strategy for stable coronary disease. N Engl J Med. 2020;382(15):1395–407.
10. Iqbal J, Zhang YJ, Holmes DR, Morice MC, Mack MJ, Kappetein AP, et al. Optimal medical therapy improves clinical outcomes in patients undergoing revascularization with percutaneous coronary intervention or coronary artery bypass grafting: insights from the synergy between percutaneous coronary intervention with TAXUS and cardiac surgery (SYNTAX) trial at the 5-year follow-up. Circulation. 2015;131(14):1269–77.
11. Pijls NH, Fearon WF, Tonino PA, Siebert U, Ikeno F, Bornschein B, et al. Fractional flow reserve versus angiography for guiding percutaneous coronary intervention in patients with multivessel coronary artery disease: 2-year follow-up of the FAME (fractional flow reserve versus angiography for multivessel evaluation) study. J Am Coll Cardiol. 2010;56(3):177–84.
12. Celeng C, Leiner T, Maurovich-Horvat P, Merkely B, de Jong P, Dankbaar JW, et al. Anatomical and functional computed tomography for diagnosing hemodynamically significant coronary artery disease: a meta-analysis. JACC Cardiovasc Imaging. 2019;12(7 Pt 2):1316–25.
13. Kurata A, Mochizuki T, Koyama Y, Haraikawa T, Suzuki J, Shigematsu Y, et al. Myocardial perfusion imaging using adenosine triphosphate stress multi-slice spiral computed tomography: alternative to stress myocardial perfusion scintigraphy. Circulation J. 2005;69(5):550–7.
14. Cury RC, Nieman K, Shapiro MD, Butler J, Nomura CH, Ferencik M, et al. Comprehensive assessment of myocardial perfusion defects, regional wall motion, and left ventricular function by using 64-section multidetector CT. Radiology. 2008;248(2):466–75.
15. Hoffmann U, Millea R, Enzweiler C, Ferencik M, Gulick S, Titus J, et al. Acute myocardial infarction: contrast-enhanced multi-detector row CT in a porcine model. Radiology. 2004;231(3):697–701.
16. Mahnken AH, Bruners P, Katoh M, Wildberger JE, Günther RW, Buecker A. Dynamic multi-section CT imaging in acute myocardial infarction: preliminary animal experience. Eur Radiol. 2006;16(3):746–52.
17. Nieman K, Shapiro MD, Ferencik M, Nomura CH, Abbara S, Hoffmann U, et al. Reperfused myocardial infarction: contrast-enhanced 64-section CT in comparison to MR imaging. Radiology. 2008;247(1):49–56.
18. Ruzsics B, Lee H, Zwerner PL, Gebregziabher M, Costello P, Schoepf UJ. Dual-energy CT of the heart for diagnosing coronary artery stenosis and myocardial ischemia-initial experience. Eur Radiol. 2008;18(11):2414–24.
19. Sorgaard MH, Kofoed KF, Linde JJ, George RT, Rochitte CE, Feuchtner G, et al. Diagnostic accuracy of static CT perfusion for the detection of myocardial ischemia. A systematic review and meta-analysis. J Cardiovasc Comput Tomogr. 2016;10(6):450–7.
20. Ostovaneh MR, Vavere AL, Mehra VC, Kofoed KF, Matheson MB, Arbab-Zadeh A, et al. Diagnostic accuracy of semi-automatic quantitative metrics as an alternative to expert reading of CT myocardial per-

fusion in the CORE320 study. J Cardiovasc Comput Tomogr. 2018;12(3):212–9.
21. George RT, Silva C, Cordeiro MA, DiPaula A, Thompson DR, McCarthy WF, et al. Multidetector computed tomography myocardial perfusion imaging during adenosine stress. J Am Coll Cardiol. 2006;48(1):153–60.
22. Assen MV, Vonder M, Pelgrim GJ, Von Knebel Doeberitz PL, Vliegenthart R. Computed tomography for myocardial characterization in ischemic heart disease: a state-of-the-art review. Eur Radiol Exp. 2020;4(1):36.
23. Bischoff B, Bamberg F, Marcus R, Schwarz F, Becker H-C, Becker A, et al. Optimal timing for first-pass stress CT myocardial perfusion imaging. Int J Cardiovasc Imaging. 2013;29(2):435–42.
24. Danad I, Szymonifka J, Schulman-Marcus J, Min JK. Static and dynamic assessment of myocardial perfusion by computed tomography. Eur Heart J-Card Img. 2016;17(8):836–44.
25. Andreini D, Mushtaq S, Pontone G, Conte E, Collet C, Sonck J, et al. CT perfusion versus coronary CT angiography in patients with suspected in-stent restenosis or CAD progression. JACC Cardiovasc Imaging. 2020;13(3):732–42.
26. Rochitte CE, George RT, Chen MY, Arbab-Zadeh A, Dewey M, Miller JM, et al. Computed tomography angiography and perfusion to assess coronary artery stenosis causing perfusion defects by single photon emission computed tomography: the CORE320 study. Eur Heart J. 2014;35(17):1120–30.
27. Pontone G, Baggiano A, Andreini D, Guaricci AI, Guglielmo M, Muscogiuri G, et al. Stress computed tomography perfusion versus fractional flow reserve CT derived in suspected coronary artery disease: the PERFECTION study. JACC Cardiovasc Imaging. 2019;12(8 Pt 1):1487–97.
28. Balabanoff C, Gaffney CE, Ghersin E, Okamoto Y, Carrillo R, Fishman JE. Radiographic and electrocardiography-gated noncontrast cardiac CT assessment of lead perforation: modality comparison and interobserver agreement. J Cardiovasc Comput Tomogr. 2014;8(5):384–90.
29. van der Wall EE, Schuijf JD, Bax JJ, Jukema JW, Schalij MJ. CT perfusion angiography; beware of artifacts! Int J Cardiovasc Imaging. 2010;26(3):355–8.
30. Rodríguez-Granillo GA, Rosales MA, Degrossi E, Rodriguez AE. Signal density of left ventricular myocardial segments and impact of beam hardening artifact: implications for myocardial perfusion assessment by multidetector CT coronary angiography. Int J Cardiovasc Imaging. 2010;26(3):345–54.
31. Matsumoto K, Jinzaki M, Tanami Y, Ueno A, Yamada M, Kuribayashi S. Virtual monochromatic spectral imaging with fast kilovoltage switching: improved image quality as compared with that obtained with conventional 120-kVp CT. Radiology. 2011;259(1):257–62.
32. Vliegenthart R, Pelgrim GJ, Ebersberger U, Rowe GW, Oudkerk M, Schoepf UJ. Dual-energy CT of the heart. AJR Am J Roentgenol. 2012;199(5 Suppl):S54–63.
33. Johnson TR, Krauss B, Sedlmair M, Grasruck M, Bruder H, Morhard D, et al. Material differentiation by dual energy CT: initial experience. Eur Radiol. 2007;17(6):1510–7.
34. McCollough CH, Leng S, Yu L, Fletcher JG. Dual- and multi-energy CT: principles, technical approaches, and clinical applications. Radiology. 2015;276(3):637–53.
35. Carrascosa P, Deviggiano A, de Zan M, Capunay C, Campisi R, Rodriguez-Granillo GA. Improved discrimination of myocardial perfusion defects at low energy levels using virtual monochromatic imaging. J Comput Assist Tomogr. 2017;41(4):661–7.
36. Carrascosa PM, Cury RC, Deviggiano A, Capunay C, Campisi R, López de Munain M, et al. Comparison of myocardial perfusion evaluation with single versus dual-energy CT and effect of beam-hardening artifacts. Acad Radiol. 2015;22(5):591–9.
37. Knott KD, Seraphim A, Augusto JB, Xue H, Chacko L, Aung N, et al. The prognostic significance of quantitative myocardial perfusion: an artificial intelligence-based approach using perfusion mapping. Circulation. 2020;141(16):1282–91.
38. Patel KK, Spertus JA, Chan PS, Sperry BW, Al Badarin F, Kennedy KF, et al. Myocardial blood flow reserve assessed by positron emission tomography myocardial perfusion imaging identifies patients with a survival benefit from early revascularization. Eur Heart J. 2020;41(6):759–68.
39. Alessio AM, Bindschadler M, Busey JM, Shuman WP, Caldwell JH, Branch KR. Accuracy of myocardial blood flow estimation from dynamic contrast-enhanced cardiac CT compared with PET. Circ Cardiovasc Imaging. 2019;12(6):e008323.
40. Danad I, Szymonifka J, Schulman-Marcus J, Min JK. Static and dynamic assessment of myocardial perfusion by computed tomography. Eur Heart J Cardiovasc Imaging. 2016;17(8):836–44.
41. Schuleri KH, George RT, Lardo AC. Applications of cardiac multidetector CT beyond coronary angiography. Nat Rev Cardiol. 2009;6(11):699–710.
42. Valdiviezo C, Ambrose M, Mehra V, Lardo AC, Lima JA, George RT. Quantitative and qualitative analysis and interpretation of CT perfusion imaging. J Nucl Cardiol. 2010;17(6):1091–100.
43. Kikuchi Y, Oyama-Manabe N, Naya M, Manabe O, Tomiyama Y, Sasaki T, et al. Quantification of myocardial blood flow using dynamic 320-row multi-detector CT as compared with 15O-H2O PET. Eur Radiol. 2014;24(7):1547–56.
44. Fujita M, Kitagawa K, Ito T, Shiraishi Y, Kurobe Y, Nagata M, et al. Dose reduction in dynamic CT stress myocardial perfusion imaging: comparison of 80-kV/370-mAs and 100-kV/300-mAs protocols. Eur Radiol. 2014;24(3):748–55.

45. Rossi A, Wragg A, Klotz E, Pirro F, Moon JC, Nieman K, et al. Dynamic computed tomography myocardial perfusion imaging: comparison of clinical analysis methods for the detection of vessel-specific ischemia. Circ Cardiovasc Imaging. 2017;10(4):e005505.
46. Nous FMA, Geisler T, Kruk MBP, Alkadhi H, Kitagawa K, Vliegenthart R, et al. Dynamic myocardial perfusion CT for the detection of hemodynamically significant coronary artery disease. JACC Cardiovasc Imaging. 2021;15:75.
47. Kitagawa K, Nakamura S, Ota H, Ogawa R, Shizuka T, Kubo T, et al. Diagnostic performance of dynamic myocardial perfusion imaging using dual-source computed tomography. J Am Coll Cardiol. 2021;78(20):1937–49.
48. Henry TD, Satran D, Jolicoeur EM. Treatment of refractory angina in patients not suitable for revascularization. Nat Rev Cardiol. 2014;11(2):78–95.
49. Mannheimer C, Camici P, Chester MR, Collins A, DeJongste M, Eliasson T, et al. The problem of chronic refractory angina; report from the ESC joint study group on the treatment of refractory angina. Eur Heart J. 2002;23(5):355–70.
50. Povsic TJ, Henry TD, Ohman EM. Therapeutic approaches for the no-option refractory angina patient. Circ Cardiovasc Interv. 2021;14(2):e009002.
51. Ong P, Athanasiadis A, Borgulya G, Mahrholdt H, Kaski JC, Sechtem U. High prevalence of a pathological response to acetylcholine testing in patients with stable angina pectoris and unobstructed coronary arteries. The ACOVA study (abnormal COronary VAsomotion in patients with stable angina and unobstructed coronary arteries). J Am Coll Cardiol. 2012;59(7):655–62.
52. Sara JD, Widmer RJ, Matsuzawa Y, Lennon RJ, Lerman LO, Lerman A. Prevalence of coronary microvascular dysfunction among patients with chest pain and nonobstructive coronary artery disease. JACC Cardiovasc Interv. 2015;8(11):1445–53.
53. Maddox TM, Stanislawski MA, Grunwald GK, Bradley SM, Ho PM, Tsai TT, et al. Nonobstructive coronary artery disease and risk of myocardial infarction. JAMA. 2014;312(17):1754–63.
54. Shaw LJ, Merz CN, Pepine CJ, Reis SE, Bittner V, Kip KE, et al. The economic burden of angina in women with suspected ischemic heart disease: results from the National Institutes of Health—National Heart, Lung, and Blood Institute—sponsored Women's Ischemia Syndrome Evaluation. Circulation. 2006;114(9):894–904.
55. Mukherjee D, Comella K, Bhatt DL, Roe MT, Patel V, Ellis SG. Clinical outcome of a cohort of patients eligible for therapeutic angiogenesis or transmyocardial revascularization. Am Heart J. 2001;142(1):72–4.
56. Povsic TJ, Broderick S, Anstrom KJ, Shaw LK, Ohman EM, Eisenstein EL, et al. Predictors of long-term clinical endpoints in patients with refractory angina. J Am Heart Assoc. 2015;4(2):e001287.
57. Reynolds MW, Frame D, Scheye R, Rose ME, George S, Watson JB, et al. A systematic review of the economic burden of chronic angina. Am J Manag Care. 2004;10(11 Suppl):S347–57.
58. Henry TD, Satran D, Hodges JS, Johnson RK, Poulose AK, Campbell AR, et al. Long-term survival in patients with refractory angina. Eur Heart J. 2013;34(34):2683–8.
59. Serruys PW, Morice MC, Kappetein AP, Colombo A, Holmes DR, Mack MJ, et al. Percutaneous coronary intervention versus coronary-artery bypass grafting for severe coronary artery disease. N Engl J Med. 2009;360(10):961–72.
60. Boden WE, O'Rourke RA, Teo KK, Hartigan PM, Maron DJ, Kostuk WJ, et al. Optimal medical therapy with or without PCI for stable coronary disease. N Engl J Med. 2007;356(15):1503–16.
61. Tonino PA, De Bruyne B, Pijls NH, Siebert U, Ikeno F, Van't Veer M, et al. Fractional flow reserve versus angiography for guiding percutaneous coronary intervention. N Engl J Med. 2009;360(3):213–24.
62. Arbab-Zadeh A, Fuster V. The myth of the "vulnerable plaque": transitioning from a focus on individual lesions to atherosclerotic disease burden for coronary artery disease risk assessment. J Am Coll Cardiol. 2015;65(8):846–55.
63. Nicholls SJ, Puri R, Anderson T, Ballantyne CM, Cho L, Kastelein JJ, et al. Effect of Evolocumab on progression of coronary disease in statin-treated patients: the GLAGOV randomized clinical trial. JAMA. 2016;316(22):2373–84.
64. Taqueti VR, Di Carli MF. Coronary microvascular disease pathogenic mechanisms and therapeutic options: JACC state-of-the-art review. J Am Coll Cardiol. 2018;72(21):2625–41.
65. Schuijf JD, Matheson MB, Ostovaneh MR, Arbab-Zadeh A, Kofoed KF, Scholte AJHA, et al. Ischemia and no obstructive stenosis (INOCA) at CT angiography, CT myocardial perfusion, invasive coronary angiography, and SPECT: the CORE320 study. Radiology. 2020;294(1):61–73.
66. Bamberg F, Hinkel R, Marcus RP, Baloch E, Hildebrandt K, Schwarz F, et al. Feasibility of dynamic CT-based adenosine stress myocardial perfusion imaging to detect and differentiate ischemic and infarcted myocardium in an large experimental porcine animal model. Int J Cardiovasc Imaging. 2014;30(4):803–12.
67. George RT, Jerosch-Herold M, Silva C, Kitagawa K, Bluemke DA, Lima JA, et al. Quantification of myocardial perfusion using dynamic 64-detector computed tomography. Investig Radiol. 2007;42(12):815–22.
68. Tomizawa N, Chou S, Fujino Y, Matsuoka S, Yamamoto K, Inoh S, et al. Impact of abnormal remote stress myocardial blood flow by dynamic CT perfusion on clinical outcomes. Sci Rep. 2020;10(1):10244.
69. Nakamura S, Kitagawa K, Goto Y, Omori T, Kurita T, Yamada A, et al. Incremental prognostic value of myocardial blood flow quantified with stress dynamic

computed tomography perfusion imaging. JACC Cardiovasc Imaging. 2019;12(7 Pt 2):1379–87.
70. Ford TJ, Stanley B, Good R, Rocchiccioli P, McEntegart M, Watkins S, et al. Stratified medical therapy using invasive coronary function testing in angina: the CorMicA trial. J Am Coll Cardiol. 2018;72(23 Pt A):2841-55:2841.
71. Zhou W, Sun YP, Divakaran S, Bajaj NS, Gupta A, Chandra A, et al. Association of Myocardial Blood Flow Reserve with Adverse Left Ventricular Remodeling in patients with aortic stenosis: the microvascular disease in aortic stenosis (MIDAS) study. JAMA Cardiol. 2021;7:93.
72. Nacif MS, Kawel N, Lee JJ, Chen X, Yao J, Zavodni A, et al. Interstitial myocardial fibrosis assessed as extracellular volume fraction with low-radiation-dose cardiac CT. Radiology. 2012;264(3):876–83.
73. Deux JF, Nouri R, Tacher V, Zaroui A, Derbel H, Sifaoui I, et al. Diagnostic value of extracellular volume quantification and myocardial perfusion analysis at CT in cardiac amyloidosis. Radiology. 2021;300(2):326–35.

19 Noncoronary Cardiac CT Assessment

Dong Hyun Yang

Abstract

Cardiac CT has evolved into a valuable modality for assessing cardiac valves and pericardium with a critical role for guiding valve replacement or repair. In certain scenarios, cardiac CT yields better image quality than echocardiography for delineating disease. This chapter will review imaging techniques for the assessment valves and pericardium, normal valvular and pericardial anatomy, valvular and pericardial pathology, and prosthetic valvular heart disease.

Keywords

CT · Heart · Valves · Pericardium · Infective Endocarditis · Prosthetic Valve

Abbreviations

AR	Aortic regurgitation
AS	Aortic stenosis
AV	Aortic valve
BAV	Bicuspid aortic valve
CCTA	Coronary computed tomography angiography
CT	Computed tomography
ECG	Electrocardiography
LA	Left atrium
MR	Mitral regurgitation
MV	Mitral valve
MVP	Mitral valve prolapse
PVL	Paravalvular leakage
RV	Right ventricle
TAVR	Transarterial aortic valve replacement
TV	Tricuspid valve
VHD	Valvular heart disease
3D	Three-dimensional

19.1 Valvular Heart Disease

19.1.1 Disease Burden

- A reported prevalence of valvular heart disease (VHD) is 2.5% in the USA [1].
- The prevalence of VHD increased considerably with age, from 0.3% of the 18–44 year old to 11.7% of those aged 75 years and older [2].
- Valvular disease is the cause of 10–20% of cardiac surgical procedures performed in the USA [3].

D. H. Yang (✉)
Asan Medical Center, University of Ulsan College of Medicine, Seoul, Republic of Korea

A. A. Zadeh, J. Hoe (eds.), *Practical Guide to Cardiac CT*,
https://doi.org/10.1007/978-981-97-6919-3_19

19.1.2 Role of Computed Tomography [2]

- Cardiac computed tomography (CT) is a valuable modality to evaluate various forms of VHD. Facility and expertise personnel of cardiac CT are essential for the structure of primary and comprehensive valve centers [4].
- Direct planimetry at the level of the aortic valve (AV) tip can be performed to estimate aortic stenosis (AS) [5].
- Using noncontrast CT for aortic valve calcium scoring, an Agatston of >2065 in men and > 1274 in women is predictive of severe AS and adverse patient outcome [6].
- In the setting of aortic regurgitation (AR), the presence of a coaptation defect can be evaluated by depicting AV closure during diastole [7].
- Mitral valve prolapse can be assessed similarly to methods by three-dimensional (3D) transesophageal echocardiography [8].
- In patients with prosthetic heart valve disease, CT can help evaluate valvular thrombi, pannus formation, and paravalvular leakage [9–11].
- With suspicion for infective endocarditis, CT can identify paravalvular lesions such as pseudoaneurysm, abscess, or fistula, as well as vegetation itself [11, 12].
- CT can contribute to the preoperative evaluation, including the thoracic aorta (e.g., dilatation, calcification, arch branches), coronary orifice (e.g., high take-off, anomalous origin), thoracic wall (e.g., kyphoscoliosis, a surgical port in endoscopic or robotic surgery), vascular access, and sternal reentry site for redo thoracotomy [13].
- Cardiac CT has become an essential tool for preprocedural guidance and postprocedural evaluation for many structural heart disease interventions, including transarterial aortic valve replacement (TAVR; see Chap. XXIII), arrhythmia ablation, and occlusion of left atrial appendage (see Chap. XXIV),

19.1.3 Scan Protocols for Cardiac Valve Assessment

- Scan coverage
  - Electrocardiography (ECG)—synchronized CT of the heart (with aortic root) and non-ECG-synchronized CT angiography of the aorto/ilio/femoral vasculature can be performed for comprehensive preoperative or preprocedural evaluation.
- ECG - synchronized CT protocol [8, 14]
  - In CT systems with limited detector coverage, spiral/helical acquisition with retrospective ECG-gated image reconstruction is often more feasible for valvular assessment than prospective scan triggering. ECG-based tube current modulation (e.g., full tube current for 20–70% R-R interval; 20% of tube current for late diastole and early systole) may be helpful to reduce radiation dose.
  - In CT systems with whole-heart coverage prospective ECG-triggered axial one-beat acquisition is preferred.
- Intravenous Contrast Administration Protocol [8, 14]
  - High intra-arterial opacification is required for optimal images, and attenuation values should be >250 Hounsfield units.
  - Dual-head injector and antecubital intravenous access are recommended with bolus tracking in the ascending aorta for accurate scan timing. In general, 4–6 mL/s flow rate and 50–100 cc iodinated contrast agent are recommended but the protocol should be tailored to patient characteristics and available scanning system.
  - For homogeneous enhancement of the right ventricle (RV), a triphasic injection protocol is helpful (first, 60–70 mL of contrast media; second, 20 mL of 70:30 saline-contrast mixture; and third, 40 mL of saline chaser) [15].

19.1.4 Image Reconstruction

- Cardiac CT may provide anatomical detail of the cardiac valves and adjacent structures for helping clinical decision-making and surgical planning.
- Cine display function, translating and rotating imaging plane in any direction, various modes of image display (e.g., volume rendering, thin- or thick-slab multiplanar reformatted image) are key advantages of cardiac CT.
- An example of various CT image reconstructions in a patient with Marfan syndrome with annulo-aortic ectasia (Fig. 19.1; supplementary movie 1–https://youtu.be/keZF-I9xWJ8) shows that CT can provide detailed anatomical information of the aorta as well as valve leaflet. In addition, CT can easily demonstrate a surgeon's view, which is more intuitive and correlated well with the surgical findings than an echocardiographic imaging plane [16]. In this chapter, all enface views of the aortic and mitral valve are surgeon's view (Fig. 19.2a, b).

19.1.5 Normal Anatomy of the Cardiac Valves

19.1.5.1 Aortic Valve (Fig. 19.2)

- The aortic root comprises the AV leaflets and their hinge lines, the sinuses, the interleaflet triangles, the ventriculo-arterial junction, and the sinutubular junction [17].
- The virtual ring joining the basal attachment of the AV leaflets corresponds to the "aortic annulus" in the sizing of the aortic root. The basal attachment of the AV leaflets to the ventricular myocardium is proximal to the ventriculo-arterial junction. The sinutubular junction forms a circle joining the peaks of the commissures.
- The interleaflet triangle between the right- and noncoronary sinuses incorporates the membranous interventricular septum. The interleaflet triangle between the left- and the noncoronary sinuses forms part of the aortic-mitral valvular curtain.
- The bulged aortic wall outlines the sinus of Valsalva forms a trilobed configuration in a

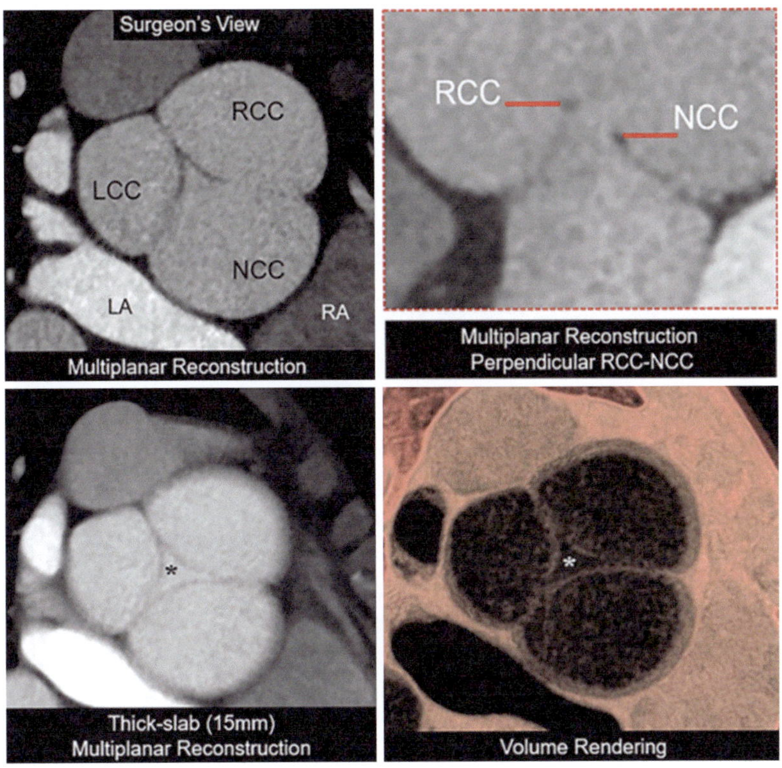

Fig. 19.1 Image Reconstruction Methods in a Patient with Marfan Syndrome with Annulo-aortic Ectasia. Case example of a 29-year-old man with Marfan syndrome. Surgeon's view of multiplanar reconstruction and volume rendering show central coaptation defect (asterisks). In the perpendicular view of the right coronary cusp (RCC) and noncoronary cusp (NCC), the different heights of the leaflet tips are revealed. This detailed anatomical information may help surgeons who are planning valve repair surgery. *LCC* left coronary cusp

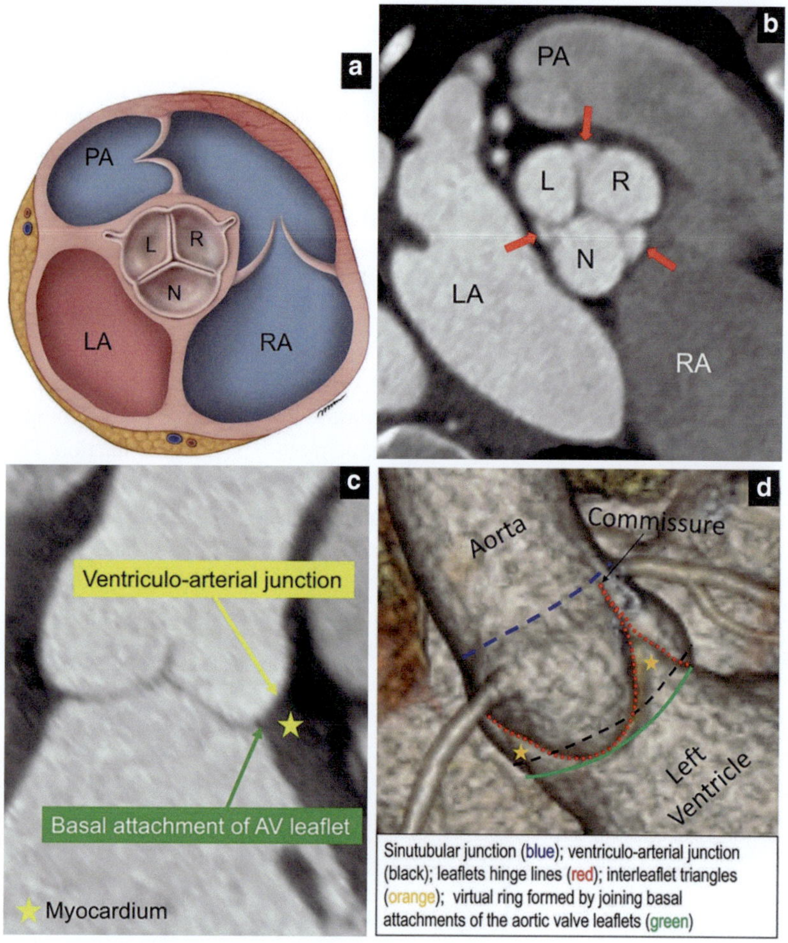

Fig. 19.2 Normal Anatomy of the Aortic Root. **Panels (a–d). Panel (a)** Surgeon's view of the aortic root. The noncoronary sinus (N) is in front of the interatrial septum. **Panel (b)** Surgeon's view of the aortic root in CT image. Arrows mean interleaflet triangles. **Panel (c)** Relationship of the ventriculo-arterial junction and basal attachment of AV leaflet. The ventriculo-arterial junction is more distal than the basal attachment of the AV leaflet. **Panel (d)** CT volume rendering image shows leaflet's hinge lines and the virtual ring formed by joining basal attachments of the AV leaflets

cross-sectional image. The left coronary sinus was slightly smaller than the other two sinuses, and the aortic root size increased with age [18].

19.1.5.2 Mitral Valve (Fig. 19.3)

- The MV apparatus comprises valvular leaflets, mitral annulus, tendinous cords (chordae tendineae), and papillary muscles [17].
- The mitral annulus consists of two horns (peaks) separated by the medial and lateral fibrous trigones and forms a saddle-shaped configuration. The anterior horn proceeds with fibrous continuity between aortic and mitral valves, also known as "aortomitral continuity" or the "intervalvular fibrosa" (Fig. 19.4). The posterior horn runs along with insertion points of mitral valve leaflets to the junction of the atrial and ventricular myocardium.
- The MV has two leaflets: the anterior (or aortic) leaflet and the posterior (or mural) leaflet. The anterior mitral leaflet occupies about one-third of the annular circumference, whereas the posterior mitral leaflet occupies the residual two-third. Each mitral leaflet can be subdivided into three scallops using the surgeon's terminology (Carpentier nomenclature). Each scallop can be denoted from lateral (A1 or P1) to medial (A3 or P3).
- The papillary muscle anchors the tendinous cords from the MV leaflet to the left ventricular wall. It comprises anterolateral papillary muscle and posteromedial papillary muscle.

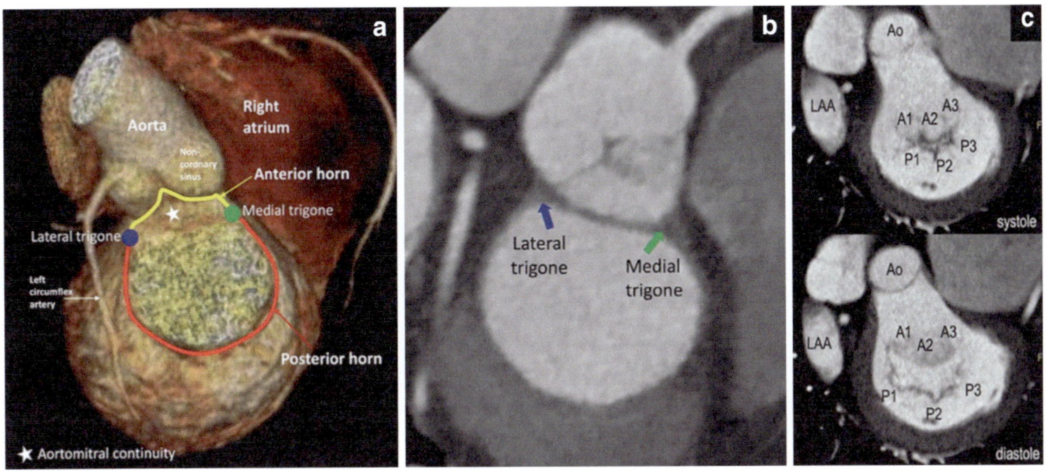

Fig. 19.3 Normal Anatomy of Mitral Valve. Normal Mitral Valve Anatomy. (**a**) Mitral annulus displayed on a volume rendering image (**b**) Lateral and medial trigones. (**c**) Scallops of mitral valve leaflets. Left atrial appendage (LAA) indicates the lateral direction of the mitral annulus on the surgeon's view of the CT image. Ao, aorta; A1/A2/A3/P1/P2/P3 mean scallops of the MV

Fig. 19.4 Aortomitral Continuity in Normal vs. Subaortic Conus in a Patient with ccTGA. (**a**) Aortomitral continuity (green arrow) in the normal heart. (**b**) Subaortic conus (red arrow) in the congenitally corrected transposition of the great artery (ccTGA)

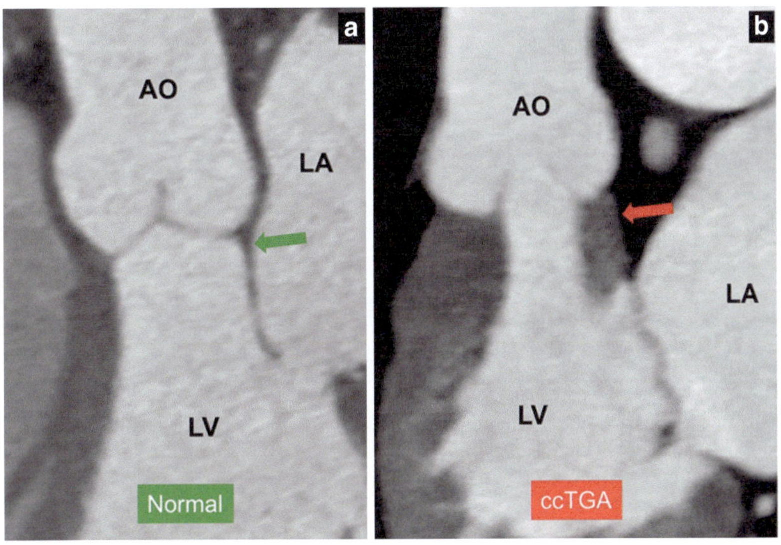

19.1.5.3 Tricuspid Valve (Fig. 19.5)

- The tricuspid valve (TV) apparatus comprises three leaflets (anterior, septal, and posterior), tricuspid annulus, tendinous cords, and papillary muscles, similar to the MV [17].
- The tricuspid annulus has straight septal and curved mural components, nearly mirrors the mitral annulus.
- The anterior leaflet is the largest, and the posterior leaflet is the smallest. The septal leaflet has some interesting anatomical features: 1) The hinge of the septal leaflet shows a more apical location than that of the mitral leaflet. This offset arrangement of two atrioventricular valves results in a muscular atrioventricular septum—also referred to as "atrioventricular fibrofatty sandwich" to address the anatomic composition of this region [19] (Fig. 19.5a, b). The septal leaflet attached to the membranous septum bisects into the atrioventricular and interventricular components.

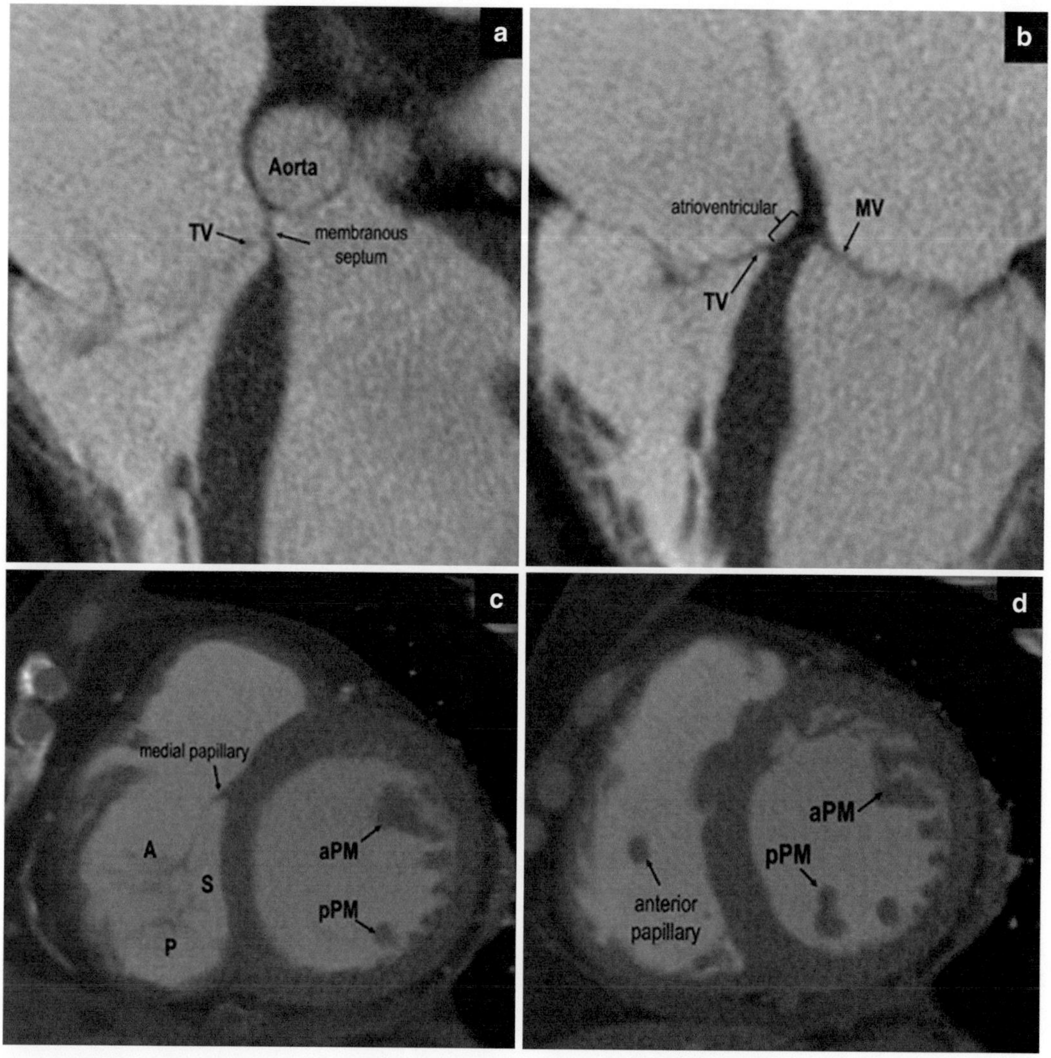

Fig. 19.5 Tricuspid Valve Anatomy. Normal Tricuspid Valve Anatomy. (**a**) Septal leaflet of TV bisects membranous septum. (**b**) Septal leaflet of TV attached more apical location than the MV leaflet. Therefore, atrioventricular septum between the right atrium and left ventricle could be formed. Note the "fibrofatty sandwich" in the atrioventricular septum. (**c**, **d**) Short-axis image in systole shows TV leaflets (*A* anterior, *S* septal, *P* posterior) and LV papillary muscles (aPM, anterolateral; pPM, posteromedial)

- Three papillary muscles support the tricuspid valve leaflets. The anterior papillary muscle, the largest one, supports the anterior leaflet and arises from the moderator band. The medial papillary muscle, usually very small, supports the anteroseptal commissure and inserts into the ventricular septum (Fig. 19.5c, d). Finally, the posterior leaflet is supported by several small papillary muscles from the diaphragmatic wall of the right ventricle.

19.1.5.4 Pulmonary Valve

- The pulmonary valve locates anterior, superior, and slightly to the left of the aortic valve [17].
- The pulmonary valve is identical in design with a semilunar shape. Two of the three sinuses of the pulmonary valve face the aortic sinuses. (Fig. 19.6).
- The pulmonary valve is separated from the tricuspid valve because of the subpulmonary infundibulum.

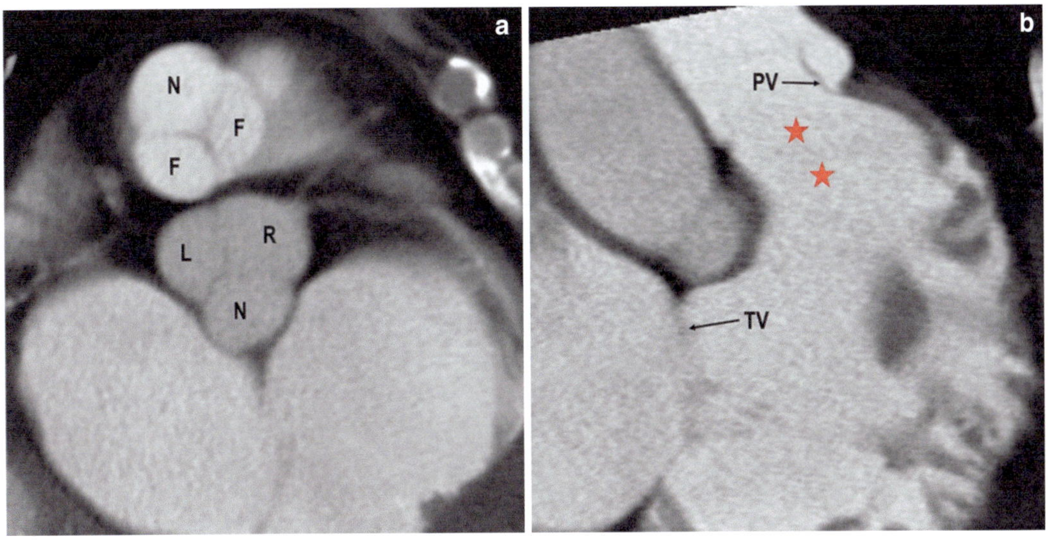

Fig. 19.6 Pulmonary Valve. Normal Pulmonary Valve Anatomy. (**a**) Normal pulmonary valve (PV) has three sinuses (*F* facing sinus, *N* non-facing sinus) with a similar design to the AV (*L* left coronary; *R* right coronary; *N* non-coronary). (**b**) Unlike aortomitral continuity, PV and TV are separated by subpulmonary infundibulum (stars)

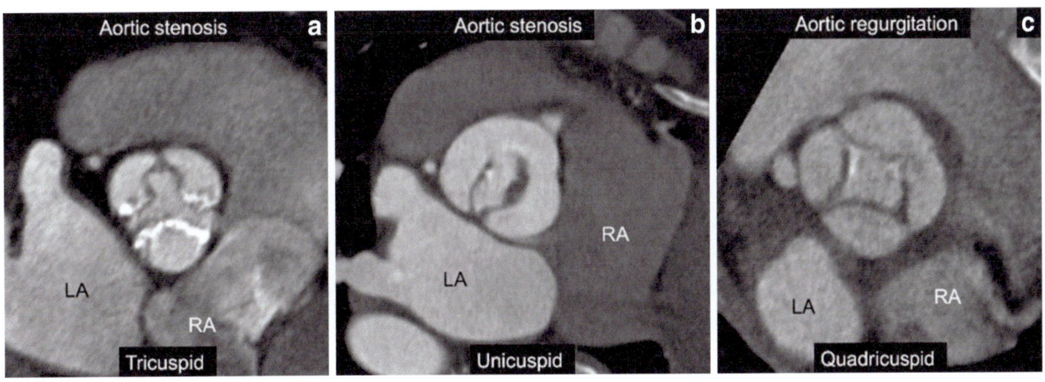

Fig. 19.7 Tricuspid, Unicuspid, and Quadricuspid Aortic Valves. Aortic Stenosis. (**a**) Calcific aortic valve stenosis with tricuspid valve in an 84-year-old man. (**b**) Unicuspid aortic valve with opening limitation in a 61-year-old man. (**c**) Quadricuspid aortic valve with severe AR in a 45-year-old man. *LA* left atrium, *RA* right atrium

19.1.6 Valvular Pathology

19.1.6.1 Aortic Stenosis

Overview [2]

- Among persons older than 75, 3.4% (95% confidence interval 1.1% to 5.7%) have severe aortic stenosis (AS).
- Valvular AS has three principal etiologies (Fig. 19.7): a congenitally bicuspid aortic valve (BAV), calcific aortic valve disease, and rheumatic disease. Rare causes of valvular AS include severe atherosclerosis, rheumatoid involvement, and ochronosis with alkaptonuria.

19.1.6.2 Calcific Aortic Valve Disease

- Calcific (formerly “senile” or “degenerative”) AV disease is the most common cause of AS and may affect both congenitally BAV and the normal trileaflet valve (Fig. 19.7a).

- Other than mechanical stress to the valve leaflet, biological factors (e.g., inflammation, lipid infiltration, and procalcific stimuli) underlying the initiation and progression of the calcific aortic valve disease have been revealed. When using noncontrast CT for aortic valve calcium scoring, an Agatston score of more than 2065 in men and more than 1274 in women is associated with severe AS and a poor patient outcome [6].
- Chronic pressure overload by the valvular obstruction leads to hypertrophic myocardial remodeling, ventricular dysfunction, and pulmonary and systemic vasculature changes.

19.1.6.3 Bicuspid Aortic Valve Disease

- Congenital bicuspid aortic valve disease (BAV) is found in approximately 1–2% of the population. In patients who underwent aortic valve replacement, bicuspid valve disease was present in more than 50% [20].
- BAV types are defined as fused BAV, two-sinus BAV, and partial-fusion BAV as per the international evidence-based nomenclature and classification consensus 2021 [20]. (Fig. 19.8).
- In order of frequency, clinical manifestations of typical valvulo-aortopathy are AS, ascending aorta dilatation, aortic regurgitation (AR), mitral valve prolapse (MVP), infective endocarditis, and aortic dissection [2].

19.1.6.4 Rheumatic Aortic Stenosis

- As a consequence of rheumatic fever, adhesion and fusions of the valve commissures and cusps may result in rheumatic AS. In addition, retraction and stiffening of the free borders of the cusps may occur (Fig. 19.9). As a result, the rheumatic valve is frequently regurgitant as well as stenotic [2].
- Patents with rheumatic AS invariably have mitral valve rheumatic involvement [2].
- With the decline in rheumatic fever in developed countries, rheumatic AS is becoming less common, though it remains a major problem on a global scale [2].

19.1.6.5 Role of CT

- CT is increasingly used for clinical decision-making, preprocedural evaluation (e.g., TAVR), and surgical planning (Table 19.1).

19.1.6.6 Stages of Valvular Aortic Stenosis (Table 19.2)

19.1.7 Aortic Regurgitation (Insufficiency)

19.1.7.1 Overview

- Aortic regurgitation (AR) results from valvular leaflet abnormality or the aortic root and ascending aorta dilatation.
- Etiologies of AV leaflet abnormality.
  - Young adults (20–40 years old) with non-calcified BAVs with incomplete closure or prolapse of a valve leaflet (Fig. 19.10).
  - Older patients with calcific AV disease may have combined aortic stenosis.
  - Other leaflet abnormalities include infective endocarditis, trauma-induced leaflet abnormality, rheumatic valve disease, the myxomatous proliferation of the AV, and congenital leaflet abnormality (e.g., unicuspid, bicuspid, and quadricuspid valves, Fig. 19.7).
  - Associated with congenital heart disease (e.g., aortic valve prolapse combined with subaortic ventricular septal defect).
- Disease of the aortic root and ascending aorta.
  - Chronic hypertension, Marfan syndrome, annulo-aortic ectasia, aortic dissection (Fig. 19.11), osteogenesis imperfecta, atherosclerotic aneurysm, syphilitic aortitis, and other systemic inflammatory disorders (e.g., giant cell aortitis, Behcet disease) (Fig. 19.12).

19.1.7.2 Mechanisms of Aortic Regurgitation by Echocardiography

- Type 1: normal cusps but insufficient coaptation due to dilatation of the aortic root with central jet.
- Type 2: aortic cusp prolapse with eccentric jet.
- Type 3: retraction with poor cusp tissue quality and large central or eccentric jet.

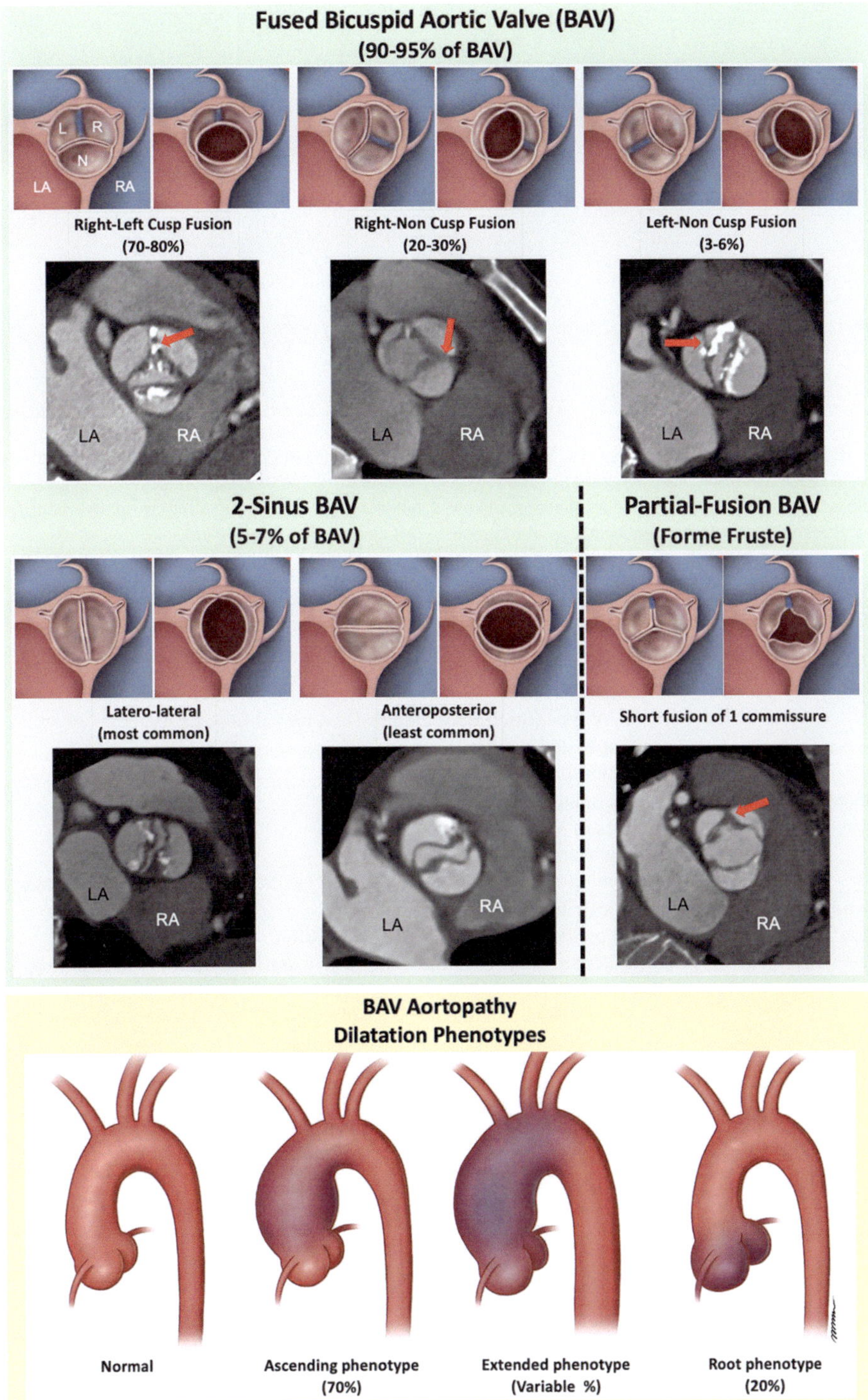

Fig. 19.8 Bicuspid Aortic Valve and Aortopathy (international evidence-based nomenclature and classification consensus 2021) [18]. Bicuspid Aortic Valve Pathology

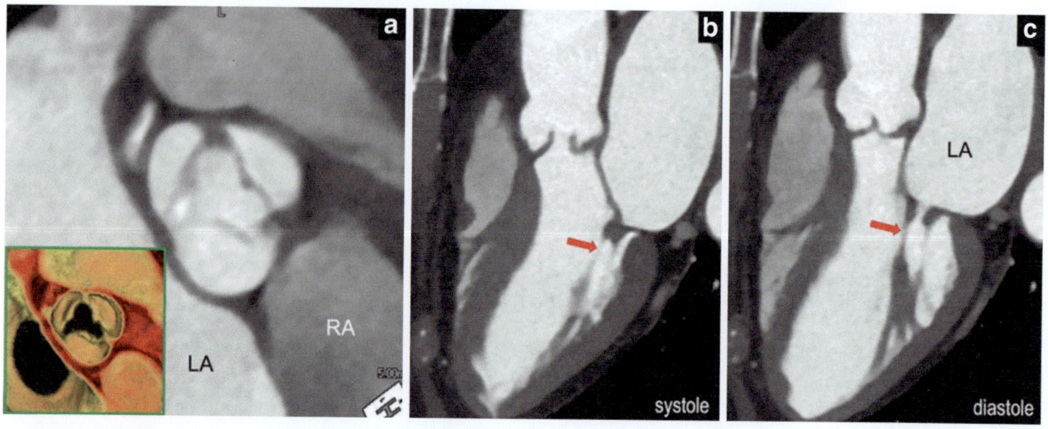

Fig. 19.9 Rheumatic Aortic Stenosis. Case Example of Rheumatic Aortic Stenosis. (**a**) Rheumatic AS in a 63-year-old woman. CT images show commissural fusion and leaflet thickening (volume rendering in the green box). (**b**, **c**) This patient has mitral valve involvement of rheumatic valve disease, hockey stick appearance of MV anterior leaflet, and subvalvular involvement (arrow). *LA* left atrium, *RA* right atrium

Table 19.1 Comprehensive Assessment of Valve and Aorta in Patients with Aortic Stenosis

Etiology of AS	Calcific/Bicuspid/Rheumatic/Others
Valve morphology	Tricuspid Bicuspid • BAV type (fused BAV, 2-sinus BAV, partial-fusion BAV) • Raphe and symmetry Quadricuspid or unicuspid
Measurement of aortic dimensions	Aortic annulus Sinuses of Valsalva Sinutubular junction Ascending aorta tubular portion (usually at the level of the right pulmonary artery)
Location and extent of valve calcification	Valve calcification • To predict the rate of disease progression • When the severity of the stenosis is in doubt, particularly in low-flow, low-gradient AS • For decision-making of surgical and interventional AV replacement
Preoperative of preprocedural evaluation	Valve sizing/access route/porcelain aorta
Evaluation of coronary artery	Coronary artery disease Coronary artery anomaly (e.g., high take-off, anomalous origin)
Potential obstruction to left ventricular outflow	Supravalvular stenosis Subvalvular stenosis Dynamic subaortic obstruction (e.g., hypertrophic cardiomyopathy)

19.1.8 Role of CT

- CT is recommended to assess the maximum diameter of the aortic root and ascending aorta for surgical decision-making.
- Ascending aorta surgery should be considered in patients with the maximal ascending aortic diameter [13]:
  - ≥55 mm in all patients
  - ≥45 mm in the presence of Marfan syndrome and additional risk factors
  - ≥50 mm in the presence of a BAV and additional risk factors
  - The additional risk factors include family history of aortic dissection, severe aortic or mitral regurgitation, desire for pregnancy, uncontrolled systemic arterial hypertension, or aortic size increase >3 mm/year.

Table 19.2 Stages of Valvular Aortic Stenosis

Stage	Definition	Valve hemodynamics
A	At risk of AS	Aortic V_{max} < 2 m/s with normal leaflet motion
B	Progressive AS	**Mild AS:** Aortic V_{max} 2.0–2.9 m/s or mean ΔP <20 mmHg **Moderate AS:** Aortic V_{max} 3.0–3.9 m/s or mean ΔP 20–39 mmHg
C	Asymptomatic severe AS	
C1	Asymptomatic severe AS	**Severe AS:** Aortic V_{max} ≥ 4 m/s or mean ΔP ≥40 mmHg AVA ≤1 cm^2 (or AVAi ≤0.6 cm^2/m^2) **Very severe AS:** Aortic V_{max} ≥ 5 m/s or mean ΔP ≥60 mmHg
C2	Asymptomatic severe AS with LV systolic dysfunction	Aortic V_{max} ≥ 4 m/s or mean ΔP ≥40 mmHg AVA typically ≤1 cm^2 (or AVAi ≤0.6 cm^2/m^2) but is not required to define severe AS LV systolic dysfunction (LVEF<50%)
D	Symptomatic severe AS	
	Symptomatic severe high-gradient AS	**Severe AS:** Aortic V_{max} ≥ 4 m/s or mean ΔP ≥40 mmHg AVA ≤1 cm^2 (or AVAi ≤0.6 cm^2/m^2), but may be larger with mixed AS/AR
	Symptomatic severe low-flow, low-gradient AS with reduced LVEF	AVA ≤1 cm^2 with resting aortic V_{max} < 4 m/sec, or mean ΔP <40 mmHg **Dobutamine stress echo:** AVA ≤1 cm^2 with aortic V_{max} ≥ 4 m/sec at any flow rate
	Symptomatic severe low-gradient AS with normal LVEF or paradoxical low-flow severe AS	AVA ≤1 cm^2 (or AVAi ≤0.6 cm^2/m^2) with an aortic V_{max} < 4 m/s, or mean ΔP <40 mmHg **AND** Stroke volume index <35 mL/m^2 Measured when patients are normotensive

Note—Stages are summarized from the 2020 AHA/ACC guideline [4]

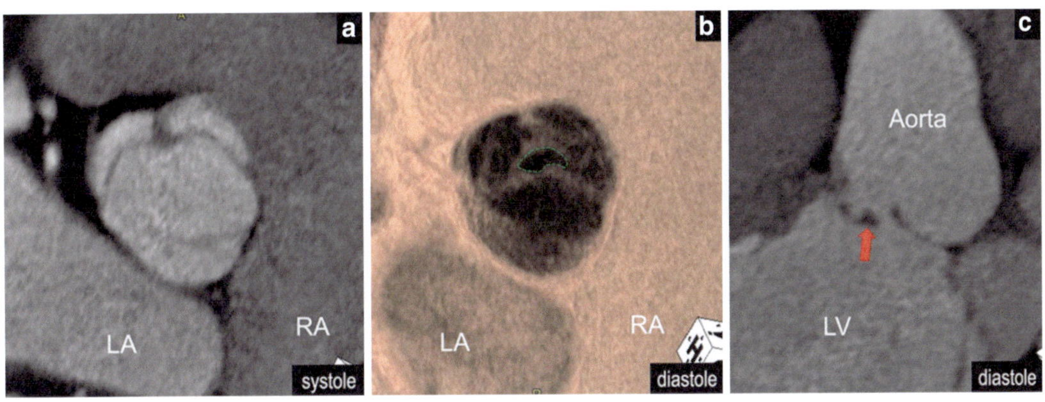

Fig. 19.10 Bicuspid Aortic Valve with Prolapse of Anterior Leaflet. Case Example of Aortic Regurgitation. (**a**) BAV with severe aortic regurgitation due to prolapse of the anterior leaflet in a 48-year-old man. (**b**) Volume rendering image shows significant coaptation defect (green dot lines). (**c**) Anterior leaflet of the BAV was prolapsed and thickened (arrow). *LA* left atrium, *LV* left ventricle, *RA* right atrium

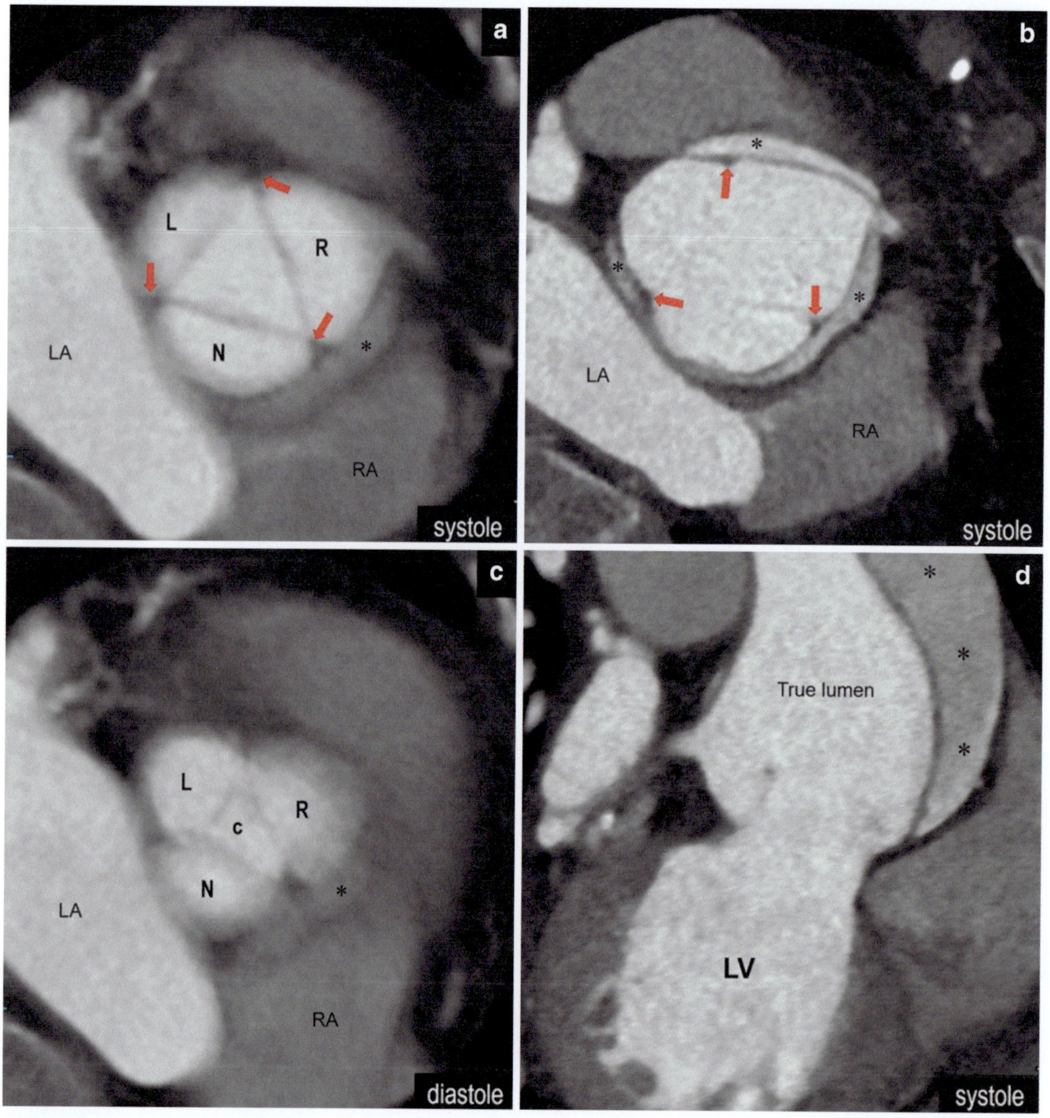

Fig. 19.11 Aortic Dissection Related Aortic Regurgitation. Aortic Regurgitation due to Aortic Dissection. (**a**, **b**) Commissural detachment (arrows) of the AV resulted from aortic dissection in a 61-year-old woman. Asterisks mean false lumen. (**c**) The diastole image noted a significant central coaptation defect (**c**). (**d**) Long axis image delineates the extent of the false lumen

  - The upper normal range (97.5th percentile) of the aortic root and ascending aorta in the Copenhagen general population study is as follows [21]:Sinus of Valsalva (cusp-to-commissure): 40 mm in men, 34 mm in women.
  - Sinutubular junction at the narrowest level: 38 mm in men, 33 mm in women.
  - Ascending aorta at the pulmonary artery trunk level: 41 mm in men, 38 mm in women.
- CT may be helpful for the evaluation of AV cusp anatomy and its suitability for valve repair (e.g., leaflet prolapse, perforation, retraction, and calcification).

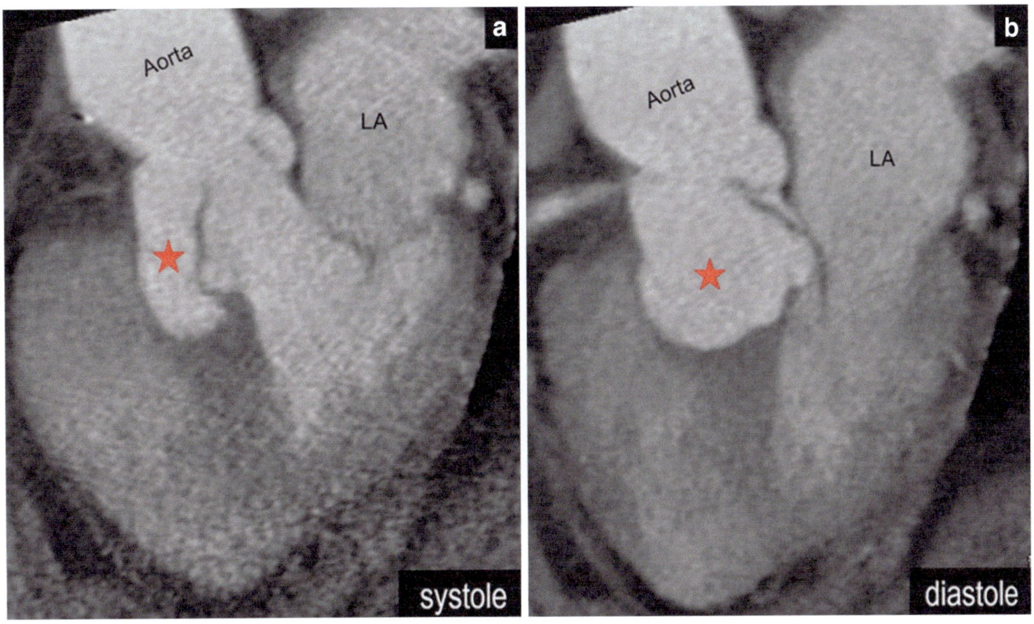

Fig. 19.12 Behcet Disease with Aortic Regurgitation and Pseudoaneurysm Extended to the Interventricular Septum. Aortic Regurgitation due to Behcet Disease. (**a, b**) A 54-year-old man confirmed Behcet disease based on clinical symptoms and pathology of the aortic root. Note the large pseudoaneurysm (stars) bulged out to the myocardium. *LA* left atrium

19.1.8.1 Stages of Chronic Aortic Regurgitation [4] (Table 19.3)

19.1.9 Mitral Stenosis

19.1.9.1 Overview

- Mitral valve disease is the most common involvement site in rheumatic heart disease. Rheumatic mitral stenosis (MS) is a significant cause of heart disease in low- and middle-income countries.
- Degenerative MS is relatively common in high-income countries and is mainly associated with mitral annular calcification (MAC).
- The MAC may be found between 9% and 15% of the general population. Almost half of the patients with severe aortic stenosis who underwent TAVR have MAC. Severe MAC may result in mitral stenosis or mitral regurgitation, or both (more frequently MS) [13].
- Although MAC was initially thought to be an age-related degenerative process, evidence is mounting that other mechanisms, such as atherosclerosis and abnormal calcium-phosphorus metabolism, also play a role in its development [22]. MAC may be linked to a higher risk of cardiovascular disease, MV disease, arrhythmias, stroke, and mortality [22].

19.1.9.2 Imaging Findings and Role of CT

- Echocardiography is the primary diagnostic modality in MS [2]. In addition, cardiac CT can provide anatomical and functional information regarding valve morphology, MAC, thrombi in the left atrium (LA), and changes of cardiac chambers.
- The CT is beneficial in determining the precise location and extent of MAC, mitral leaflet calcification, myocardial extension of calcification, and for detecting caseous calcification of the mitral annulus [23].
- Features of Rheumatic MS (Fig. 19.9).
  - Fused commissures are the hallmark of the rheumatic MS (a fish-mouth appearance).
  - Hockey stick appearance of the anterior leaflet.

Table 19.3 Stages of Chronic Aortic Regurgitation

Stage	Definition	Valve hemodynamics
A	At risk of AR	AR severity none or trace
B	Progressive AR	**Mild AR:** Jet width < 25% of LVOT Vena contracta <0.3 cm Regurgitant volume < 30 mL/beat Regurgitant fraction <30% ERO <0.10 cm^2 Angiography grade 1 **Moderate AR:** Jet width 26%–64% of LVOT Vena contracta 0.3–0.6 cm Regurgitant volume 30–59 mL/beat Regurgitant fraction 30–49% ERO 0.10–0.29 cm^2 Angiography grade 2
C	Asymptomatic severe AR	**Severe AR:** Jet width ≥ 65% of LVOT Vena contracta ≥0.6 cm Holodiastolic flow reversal in the proximal abdominal aorta Regurgitant volume ≥ 60 mL/beat Regurgitant fraction ≥50% ERO ≥0.3 cm^2 Angiography grade 3–4 In addition, diagnosis of chronic severe AR requires evidence of LV dilation.
D	Symptomatic severe AS	**Severe AR: Same as above**

Note—Stages are summarized from the 2020 AHA/ACC guideline [4]

  - Matted and retracted chordae resulted from fibrosis and fusion to the subvalvular apparatus.
- Features of degenerative MS related to MAC (Fig. 19.13).
  - No commissural fusion or subvalvular involvement, unlike rheumatic MS.
  - Severely restricted posterior leaflet due to significant calcification; but the tips of both leaflets are spared and mobile.

19.1.9.3 Stages of Mitral Stenosis (Table 19.4)

19.1.10 Mitral Regurgitation

19.1.10.1 Etiology

- The major causes of MR are myxomatous degeneration (MVP and ruptured chordae), rheumatic heart disease, infective endocarditis, hypertrophic cardiomyopathy, annular calcification, dilated cardiomyopathy, and ischemic heart disease [2].

19.1.10.2 Primary Vs. Secondary Mitral Regurgitation

- Primary MR is caused by disrupting one or more parts of the mitral valve apparatus. Degenerative etiology (fibroelastic deficiency and Barlow disease) is most frequent in Western countries [13].
- In secondary MR, the regurgitation results from an imbalance between closing and tethering forces secondary to alterations in LV and LA geometry [13]. The valve leaflets and chordae are structurally normal in the secondary MR. The two main etiologies of secondary MR are annular dilatation or iatrogenic MR and leaflet tethering from a ventricular disease (e.g., dilated or ischemic cardiomyopathy) [2].

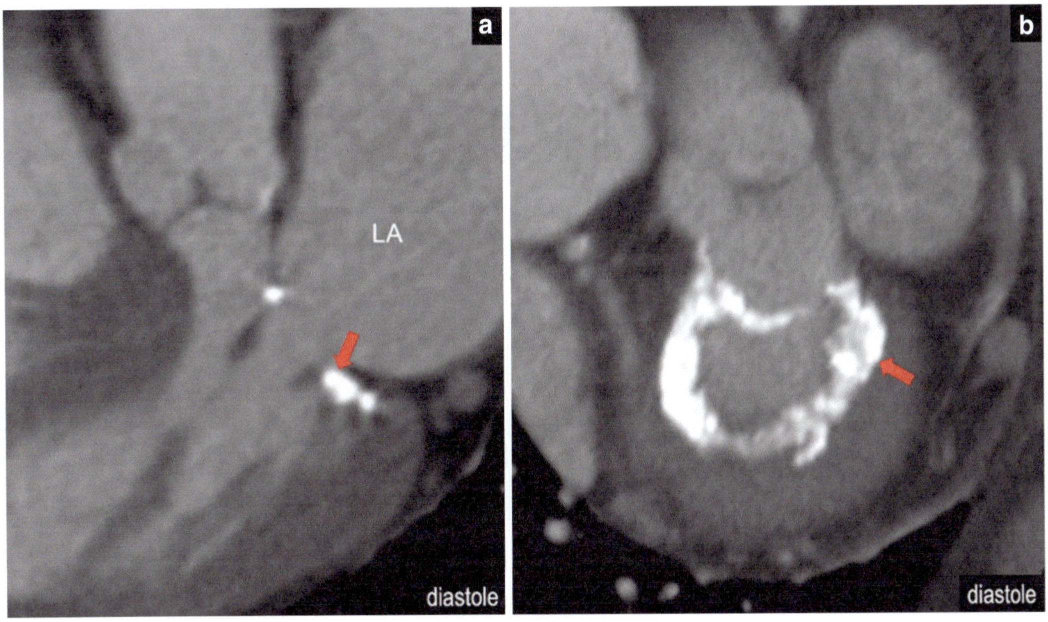

Fig. 19.13 Degenerative Mitral Stenosis with Extensive Mitral Annular Calcification. (**a**, **b**) Case Example of degenerative Mitral Stenosis. Degenerative MS in an 84-year-old woman with severe mitral annular calcification (arrows). *LA* left atrium

Table 19.4 Stages of Mitral Stenosis

Stage	Definition	Valve Hemodynamics
A	At risk of MS	Normal transmitral flow velocity
B	Progressive MS	Increased transmitral flow velocities Mitral valve area > 1.5 cm^2 Diastolic pressure half-time < 150 ms
C	Asymptomatic severe MS	Mitral valve area ≤ 1.5 cm^2 Diastolic pressure half-time ≥ 150 ms
D	Symptomatic severe MS	Same as above

Note—Stages are summarized from the 2020 AHA/ACC guideline [4]

19.1.10.3 The Morphological Classification for MR Based on Leaflet Mobility [24]

- Type I - normal leaflet motion with poor coaptation due to annular dilatation or leaflet perforation or cleft (cause: ischemic cardiomyopathy, dilated cardiomyopathy, endocarditis, congenital [e.g., MV cleft]) (Fig. 19.14).
- Type II - increased leaflet motion or leaflet prolapse or leaflet flail) (cause: degenerative disease [i.e., fibroelastic deficiency, Marfan syndrome, Barlow disease], rheumatic disease, endocarditis, trauma, ischemic cardiomyopathy, Ehlers-Danlos syndrome).
- Type III - decreased leaflet motion in diastolic and systolic [type IIIA] or just systolic [type IIIB] (cause of type IIIA: rheumatic heart disease, carcinoid, radiation-induced, and MAC-related MR; cause of type IIIB: LV enlargement and displacement of papillary muscles away from the mitral annulus [e.g., ischemic cardiomyopathy, dilated cardiomyopathy]).

19.1.10.4 Imaging Findings and Role of Cardiac CT

- Cardiac CT may be useful for providing the precise anatomical information of the regurgitant MV leaflet, annulus, and subvalvular

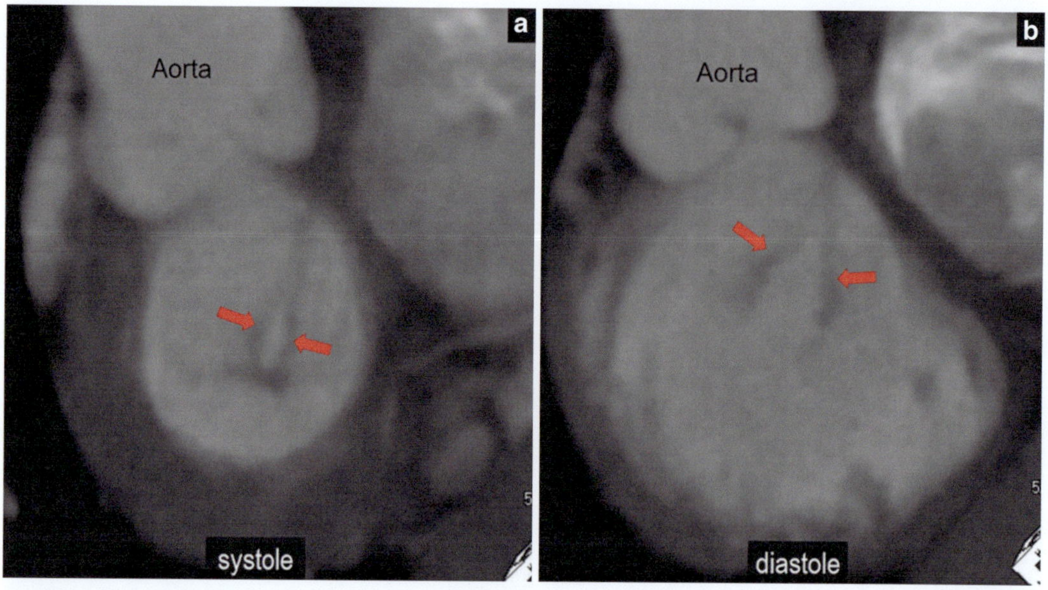

Fig. 19.14 (**a**, **b**) Mitral valve cleft (arrows) in a 7-year-old boy who underwent arterial switch operation and closure of the ventricular septal defect

apparatus [2, 8]. In addition, for percutaneous MV replacement, CT can be helpful for annulus sizing and for evaluating annular calcification [25].

- Demonstration of MVP—a step-by-step approach [8, 26]: (Fig. 19.15).
  - Selection of the best cardiac phase: The best cardiac phase for demonstrating the prolapsed MV scallop can be determined by reviewing four-dimensional multiphase CT data. Typically, the best-quality images can be obtained during the 20–40% of R-R among the multiphase CT data [8].
  - Determination of prolapsed scallop (anterior or posterior leaflet): The sagittal view of the MV coaptation plane is similar to the three-chamber view of the heart. The prolapsed leaflet (anterior versus posterior) can be localized in the sagittal images perpendicular to the MV coaptation line.
  - Determination of prolapsed scallop (medial, middle, or lateral scallop): In the coronal images along the coaptation line of MV leaflet, the localization of the MVP—lateral, middle, or medial scallop—can be possible. In this coronal image, the left atrial appendage is an anatomical landmark indicating lateral direction, while the coronary sinus is a marker of medial direction.
  - Surgeon's view of the MV: Using a thick-slab multiplanar reformatted image or volume rendering image (typically 15–20 mm of slab thickness), the prolapsed scallop can be demonstrated on the surgeon's view of the MV. In this image, the extent and location of the MVP can be determined.

19.1.10.5 Stages of Chronic Mitral Regurgitation (Table 19.5)

19.1.11 Tricuspid Valve Disease

19.1.11.1 Tricuspid Stenosis

- Tricuspid stenosis (TS) is almost always associated with rheumatic heart disease [2].
- Other rare etiologies are congenital tricuspid atresia, right atrial tumors, and iatrogenic (e.g., a fusion of device leads and valve apparatus).
- Rheumatic TS resembles the morphologic changes of rheumatic MS (i.e., diastolic doming, thickening and restricted motion of leaflet, commissural fusion).

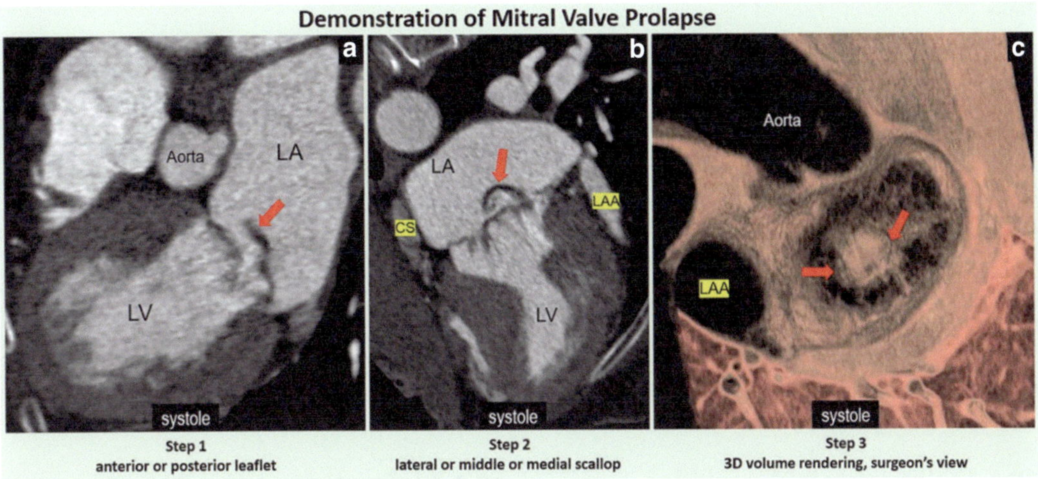

Fig. 19.15 Demonstration of Mitral Valve Prolapse. (**a**–**c**) Stepwise Approach to Diagnosing Mitral Valve Prolapse. Case example of mitral valve prolapse in a 73-yearold woman. *CS* coronary sinus, *LA* left atrium, *LAA* left atrial appendage, *LV* left ventricle

Table 19.5 Stages of Chronic Mitral Regurgitation

Stage	Definition	Valve Hemodynamics (Primary MR)	Valve Hemodynamics (Secondary MR)
A	At risk of MR	No MR jet or small central jet area < 20% LA on Doppler Small vena contracta <0.3 cm	No MR jet or small central jet area < 20% LA on Doppler Small vena contracta <0.3 cm
B	Progressive MR	Central jet MR 20–40% LA or late systolic eccentric jet MR Vena contracta <0.7 cm Regurgitant volume < 60 mL Regurgitant fraction <50% ERO <0.40 cm^2 Angiography grade 1+ to 2+	Regurgitant volume < 60 mL Regurgitant fraction <50% ERO <0.40 cm^2
C	Asymptomatic severe MR	Central jet MR >40% LA or holosystolic eccentric jet MR Vena contracta ≥0.7 cm Regurgitant volume ≥ 60 mL Regurgitant fraction ≥50% ERO ≥0.40 cm^2 Angiography grade 3+ to 4+	Regurgitant volume ≥ 60 mL Regurgitant fraction ≥50% ERO ≥0.40 cm^2
D	Symptomatic severe MR	Same as above	Same as above

Note—Stages are summarized from the 2020 AHA/ACC guideline [4]

19.1.11.2 Tricuspid Regurgitation

- The most common cause of tricuspid regurgitation (TR) is dilation of the right ventricle and the tricuspid annulus (i.e., secondary TR) [2].
- The primary TR may result from rheumatic heart disease, infective endocarditis, prolapse of TV, Epstein anomaly, distortion of the TV leaflet by device leads, trauma, carcinoid, drugs, and irradiation.
- Isolated TR is associated with atrial fibrillation and has LVEF >60%, pulmonary artery systolic pressure < 50 mmHg, and no left-sided valve disease, with normal-appearing tricuspid valve leaflets [4].
- Stages of tricuspid regurgitation (Table 19.6).

Table 19.6 Stages of Tricuspid Regurgitation

Stage	Definition	Valve hemodynamics
B	Progressive TR	Central jet <50% RA Vena contracta <0.7 cm ERO <0.40 cm^2 Regurgitant volume < 45 mL
C	Asymptomatic severe TR	Central jet ≥50% RA Vena contracta ≥0.7 cm ERO ≥0.40 cm^2 Regurgitant volume ≥ 45 mL Dense continuous wave signal with a triangular shape Hepatic vein systolic flow reversal
D	Symptomatic severe TR	Same as above

Note—Stages are summarized from the 2020 AHA/ACC guideline [4]

19.1.12 Infective Endocarditis

19.1.12.1 Overview

- Infective endocarditis (IE) is often fatal unless treated appropriately (in-hospital mortality rate is 15–20%) [4].
- The modified Duke criteria are the current standard for diagnosis of IE [2, 4]. Two major criteria in the modified Duke criteria are (1) blood culture positive for IE and (2) evidence of endocardial involvement [4].
- The evidence of endocardial involvement includes (1) echocardiogram positive for IE (i.e., oscillating intracardiac mass on valve or supporting structures, abscess, or new partial dehiscence of the prosthetic valve) and (2) new valvular regurgitation [4].

19.1.12.2 Anatomical and Echocardiographic Definitions in IE (Table 19.7)

19.1.12.3 Role of Cardiac CT

- CT may help evaluate complications of IE, particularly in patients with suspected paravalvular infection (abscess/pseudoaneurysm formation) (Fig. 19.16).
- In right-sided IE, CT is useful for detecting septic pulmonary infarcts or abscesses [4].
- In patients with prosthetic heart valves, cardiac CT is less susceptible to shadowing artifacts, possibly obscuring paravalvular lesions or infected vegetation/thrombus attached to the prosthetic valve leaflet [4, 11].

19.1.13 Prosthetic Valve Disease

19.1.13.1 Overview

- Mechanical valve stenosis may be occurred by thrombus formation, pannus ingrowth, or a combination of both [4]. Biological valve stenosis may be caused by leaflet deterioration attributed by degeneration, thickening, calcification, thrombosis, endocarditis, and pannus [4].
- Cine CT images help measure the opening and closing angle of a mechanical valve and detect pannus or thrombus formation on or adjacent to the valve [4, 9]. When prosthetic valve stenosis is suspected, cardiac CT is recommended for treatment planning [4, 13, 27].
- Paravalvular leakage (PVL) may be occurred by suture line disruption related to a technical error, annular disruption, or endocarditis [4, 10].

19.1.14 Pannus and Thrombus Formation

- Pannus and thrombus in a prosthetic heart valve have different clinical and imaging findings [27]. Compared to thrombus formation, pannus shows a gradual increase of pressure gradient (Fig. 19.17). In addition, pannus formation is occurred in the subvalvular area along the valve strut ring, while thrombus shows an irregular low attenuated mass lesion with sub- or supravalvular location. A recent prospective trial found that thrombus had a

Table 19.7 Anatomical and Echocardiographic Definitions in Infective Endocarditis

Term	Surgery/necropsy [12]	Echocardiography [12]	CT [11]
Vegetation	An infected mass attached to an endocardial structure or on implanted intracardiac material.	Oscillating or non-oscillating intracardiac mass on valve or other endocardial structures or on implanted intracardiac material	An irregular-shaped soft tissue lesion that is attached to valves or paravalvular structures and distinct from the endocardium[a]
Abscess	Perivalvular cavity with necrosis and purulent material not communicating with the cardiovascular lumen	Thickened, a non-homogeneous perivalvular area with echodense or echolucent appearance	A perivalvular fluid collection showing 0–40 HU with a layer of thickened inflammatory enhancing tissue or irregular inhomogeneous paravalvular areas surrounding the fluid.
Pseudoaneurysm	Perivalvular cavity communicating with the cardiovascular lumen	Pulsatile perivalvular echo-free space, with color-Doppler flow detected	A space filled with contrast or blood that has communication with cardiac chambers or the aortic root; located near the paravalvular or periannular region, possibly extending to the myocardium or pericardium.
Dehiscence of a prosthetic valve	Dehiscence of the prosthesis	Paravalvular regurgitation identified by echocardiography, with or without rocking motion of the prosthesis	Tearing of any part of the stitch site that has formed a hole connecting two different chambers, without or without rocking motion of the prosthesis

[a]Should be found in more than two different dimensional views

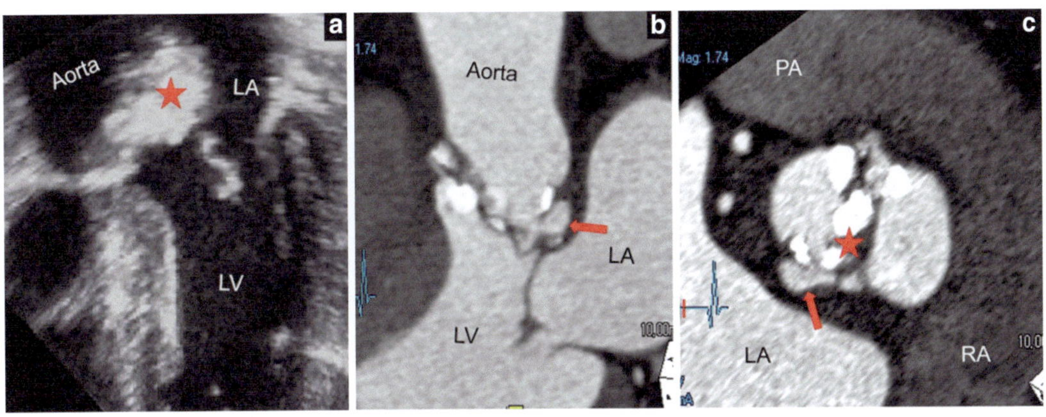

Fig. 19.16 Infective Endocarditis with Pseudoaneurysm in the Mitral-Aortic Intervalvular Fibrosa. Case Example of Infectious Endocarditis. Infective endocarditis in a 78-year-old man. (**a**) On echocardiography, extensive calcified vegetation (stars) obscured the pseudoaneurysm (arrows in Panels B and C) found on CT. (**b**, **c**) Pseudoaneurysm was extended to the mitral-aortic intervalvular fibrosa, a critical structure for surgical decision-making. *LA* left atrium, *LV* left ventricle, *RA* right atrium

mean attenuation value of 87 HU compared to 322 HU for pannus. The researchers suggested a cut-off point of >145 HU for distinguishing pannus from thrombus, with a sensitivity of 88% and specificity of 96% [28].

- The extent of pannus formation measured by CT increased over time and is correlated with transvalvular pressure gradient by echocardiography [9, 29, 30]. Furthermore, the association between pannus formation and increased

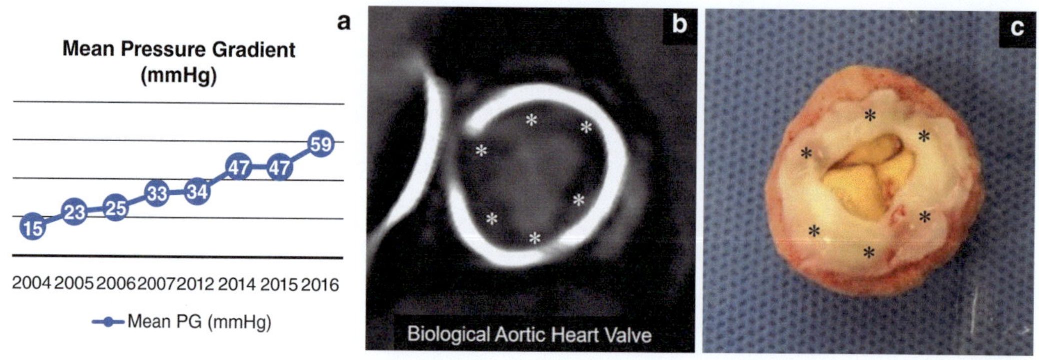

Fig. 19.17 Pannus Formation in the Biological Aortic Valve. Aortic Valve Pannus. (**a**) Gradual increase of transvalvular pressure gradient in a 41-year-old woman. The mean pressure gradient was 15 mmHg immediately after operation. X-axis means years from 2004 to 2016. (**b**) Circumferential low attenuated pannus (asterisks) was observed just below the valve strut in CT. (**c**) Surgical specimen shows the extent of pannus formation, which was well matched with the preoperative CT image

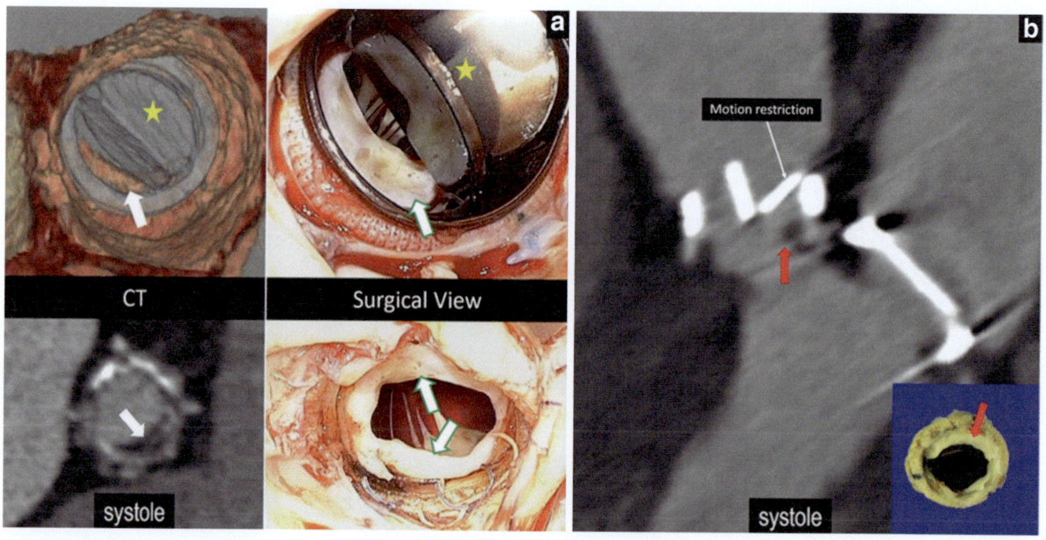

Fig. 19.18 Pannus Formation in the Mechanical Aortic Valve with Leaflet Motion Restriction. Case Examples of Pannus Formation with Mechanical Aortic Valves. (**a**): Pannus formation (arrows) in a 68-year-old patient with a mechanical valve (stars). The extent of the pannus formation is matched well with surgical photography. (**b**): Leaflet motion restriction of a mechanical valve resulted from the hemodynamic effect of the subvalvular pannus (arrow) in a 54-year-old woman. There was no motion restriction in the mechanical valve in the surgical field

transvalvular pressure gradient has been demonstrated in clinical [29–31] and experimental studies [32, 33]. Of interest, subvalvular pannus formation may result in a decreased opening angle of the mechanical valve by hemodynamic change (e.g., flow oscillation and decreased torque to leaflet) around the valve leaflet [32, 33] (Fig. 19.18). In almost all modern valves, the opening angle of the mechanical valve as measured by cardiac CT should be greater than 75 degrees [34].

19.1.14.1 Paravalvular Leakage

- Although 2D and 3D echocardiography are key imaging techniques for assessing the PVL, cardiac CT may complement clinical decision-making. Assessment of morphological factors should be included in the evalua-

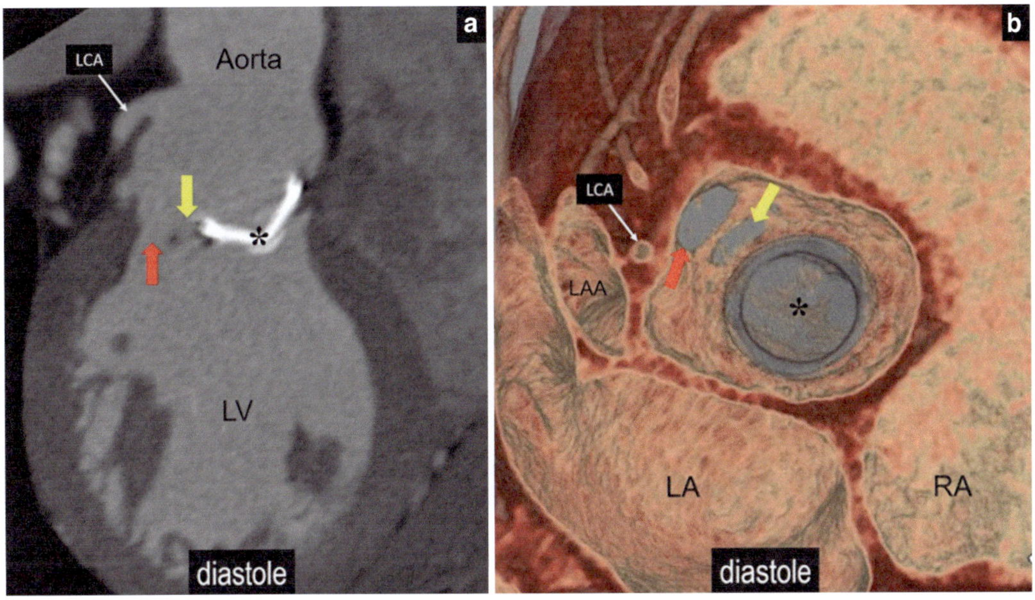

Fig. 19.19 Paravalvular Leakage around Mechanical Aortic Valve. Case Example of Paravalvular Leakage. (**a**) Paravalvular leakage (arrows) in a 47-year-old man with a prothetic aortic valve (asterisk). A band-like lesion bisects the leakage site. (**b**) Volume rendering image with surgeon's view help understand overall shape and location of the lesion. *LA* left atrium, *LCA* left coronary artery, *LV* left ventricle, *RA* right atrium

tion of PVL: (1) precise location of the defect, (2) precise dimensions, (3) orientation of the defect concerning the sewing ring and prosthetic valve occluders or leaflets, and (4) location and orientation of the subvalvular structures [4].

- In addition to the anatomic detail of PVL, cardiac CT may provide a surgeon's view or fluoroscopic view for helping surgeons or interventionists, respectively [10, 16] (Fig. 19.19).

19.1.15 Cardiac Tumors—Valves

- Papillary fibroelastoma is a typical benign cardiac tumor involving valve leaflets [2]. The AV is the most common site, followed by MV. Grossly, the fibroelastoma may show sea anemone appearance on its surface. Due to the high likelihood of an embolic event in left-sided papillary fibroelastoma, surgical resection is recommended. Differential diagnosis includes vegetation, myxoma (rare), and lipoma (rare) (Fig. 19.20). Carcinoid heart disease may manifest as diffuse thickening of the tricuspid and/or pulmonary valves, leading in right-sided heart failure [35].

19.2 Pericardium

19.2.1 Normal Pericardial Anatomy and CT Findings [36, 37]

- The heart is enclosed within a fibro-serous pericardial pouch, the pericardium [38]. The fibrous outer layer (**fibrous pericardium**) is tough and reflects onto great vessels (Fig. 19.21). The **serous pericardium** lines the inner aspect of the fibrous pericardium (**parietal layer**), which then reflects on the heart as epicardium (**visceral layer**) [38]. These two serous layers form the **pericardial cavity (sac).**
- The small amount of fluid (25–50 mL) between two layers allows for friction-free motion from the beating heart [29]. The visceral layer is a monolayer of mesothelial cells and is closely adhered to the heart and

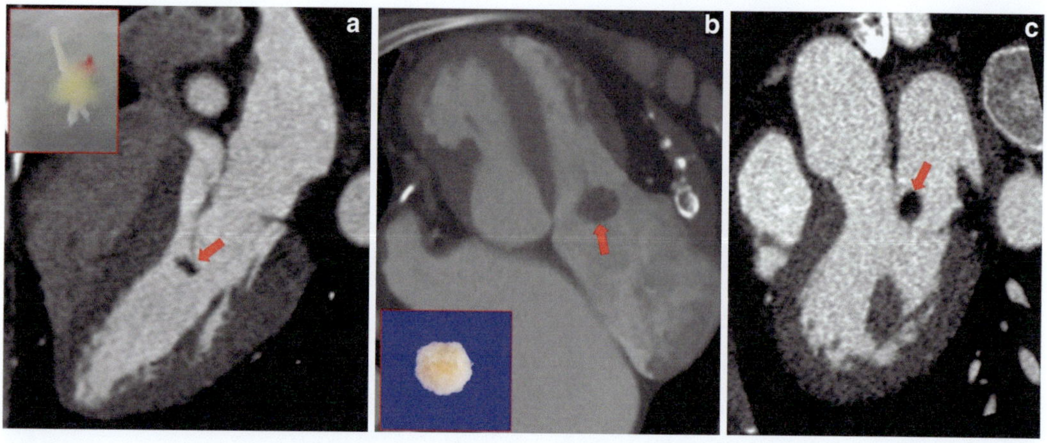

Fig. 19.20 Cardiac Tumors involving Valve Leaflets. Case Example of Tumors Associated with Cardiac Valves. (**a**): Papillary fibroelastoma in the tricuspid valve. (**b, c**) Well-differentiated liposarcoma in the mitral valve anterior leaflet

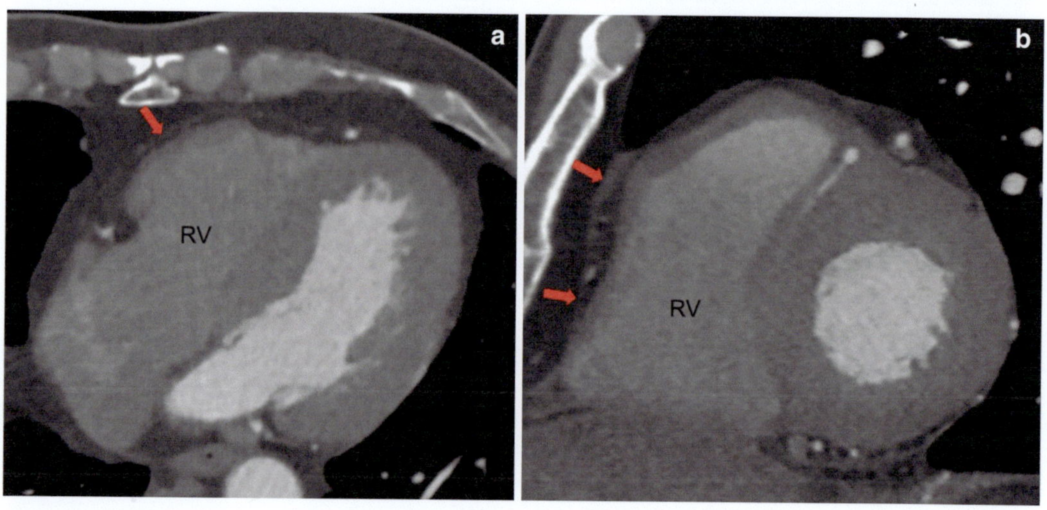

Fig. 19.21 Normal Pericardium. Normal Pericardium. Normal pericardium (arrows) can be easily observed using standard axial and coronal planes. *RV* right ventricle

the overlying epicardial fat and coronary arteries [36].

- The fibrous pericardium is attached to the mediastinum and is relatively stationary. ECG-synchronized acquisitions with intravenous contrast enhancement are preferred for pericardial evaluation, and a section thickness of greater than 3 mm is recommended. Although dynamic evaluation of ventricular septal motion to assess constrictive physiology is theoretically possible with ECG-synchronized CT, real-time functional imaging with echocardiography and MR imaging is much easier and more accurate [37].
- In CT, the thickness of the pericardium is the combination of the fibrous pericardium, serous pericardium, and normal pericardial fluid [36]. **Normal pericardial thickness** ranges from 0.7 to 2.0 mm on CT images [37] (Fig. 19.21).

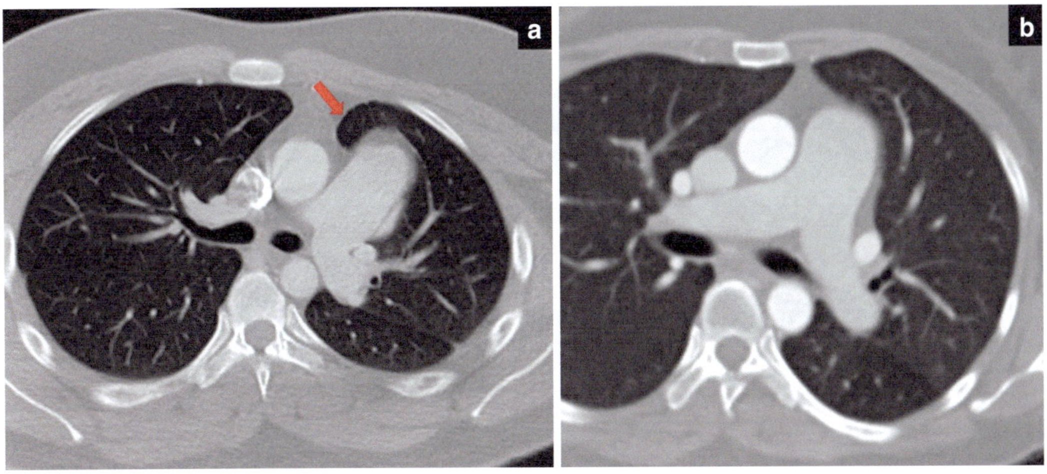

Fig. 19.22 Congenital Absence of the Pericardium. Case Example of Congenital Absence of the Pericardium. **Panel** (**a**) Congenital absence of the pericardium in a 19-year-old man. Note the interposed lung (arrow) between the aorta and the pulmonary artery. The heart and great vessels show slightly levodisplacement. **Panel** (**b**) Normal control for comparison

- **Pericardial fat** refers to the fat covering the fibrous pericardium's outside. **Epicardial fat** refers to the fat over the heart's surface, inside the visceral layer (epicardium) [36]. The epicardial fat is increased in obesity, and there is accumulating evidence that epicardial fat is associated with coronary atherogenesis [37].
- **Pericoronary adipose tissue** mapping with the coronary CT angiography (CCTA)-derived fat attenuation index is a recently developed approach to noninvasively detect coronary inflammation and atherosclerotic alterations at CCTA, with incremental prognostic value beyond established risk variables [39]. However, criteria for clinical use have not been established.
- Two major sinuses (pericardial spaces): **The transverse sinus** is the space posterior to the aorta and pulmonary trunk above the LA. **The oblique sinus** is immediately posterior to the LA and anterior to the esophagus [36, 38].
- CT may be helpful to differentiate the pericardial thickening [36]: nodularity and contrast enhancement may be suggestive of metastasis or malignancy; calcification may indicate chronic pericarditis; smoothly thickened pericardial contour may be suggestive of pericardial effusion [36].

19.2.2 Congenital Anomalies of the Pericardium

- **A pericardial cyst** is a benign congenital lesion typically found at the right or left cardiophrenic angle as an incidental finding. On CT, cysts appear as round or elliptical cystic lesions without contrast enhancement [2]. Surgery is not recommended without symptoms or complications (e.g., infection, bleeding).
- **Congenital absence (defect) of the pericardium** is a very rare anomaly. Most defects are partial and involve a defect over the left atrial appendage [36, 37]. While usually asymptomatic, herniation or torsion of the heart or great vessel might occur and significant consequences [2]. Because CT may not delineate normal pericardium on the left side, direct detection of the "defect" of the pericardium could be problematic in CT imaging. **Radiological signs of the pericardial defect** [36] are: (1) a prominent notch between the aorta and the pulmonary artery, which is filled with interposed lung; (2) lung between heart and the diaphragm; (3) continuity of the pericardial space with the pleural cavity on CT; and (4) lung between the right atrium and the right ventricular outflow tract (Fig. 19.22).

19.2.3 Pericardial Effusion

- **Etiologies**: heart failure, renal and liver insufficiency, inflammation, infection, neoplastic disease, trauma, and myocardial infarction [37].
- **Amount of effusion**: In general, a pericardial effusion thickness greater than 4 mm is regarded as abnormal [37]. The pericardium normally contains between 15 and 50 mL of fluid. Small pericardial effusions are very common on routine CCTA, usually near the right heart border or below the RV. A pericardial space greater than 5 mm anterior to the RV is considered to be moderate effusion [40]. The relationship between the measured width and the total volume of fluid is unclear because the pericardial fluid could be accumulated in the pericardial recesses or sinuses. Roughly, a pericardial space anterior to the RV exceeding 5 mm corresponds to a moderate effusion of 100–500 mL of fluid [37].
- **Characterization of fluid:** A simple pericardial effusion typically has CT numbers of 10–20 HU. When attenuation of the effusion exceeds 40 HU, complicated effusion (e.g., hemopericardium, malignancy, purulent exudates, or hypothyroid-related effusion) should be suspected [36, 37]. Conversely, low-attenuation of the effusion may be chylopericardium [37].

19.2.4 Pericarditis

- **Etiologies** [2]: idiopathic, infectious pericarditis (viral, bacterial [tuberculosis, purulent, others]), neoplastic (5–9–35% [in tertiary referral centers]), autoimmune (2–24%), other noninfectious causes.
- **Imaging Findings** [37]: Echocardiography is the diagnostic modality of choice. On CT, pericardial layers may be thickened and show contrast enhancement. In addition, signs of cardiac tamponade might be present (diastolic collapse of the RV free wall due to exceeded pericardial pressure). In chronic inflammatory pericarditis, pericardial layers show irregularly thickened, and loculation of the effusion may present. Occasionally, prominent epicardial fat may be seen as a chronic inflammatory response (Fig. 19.23) [41].

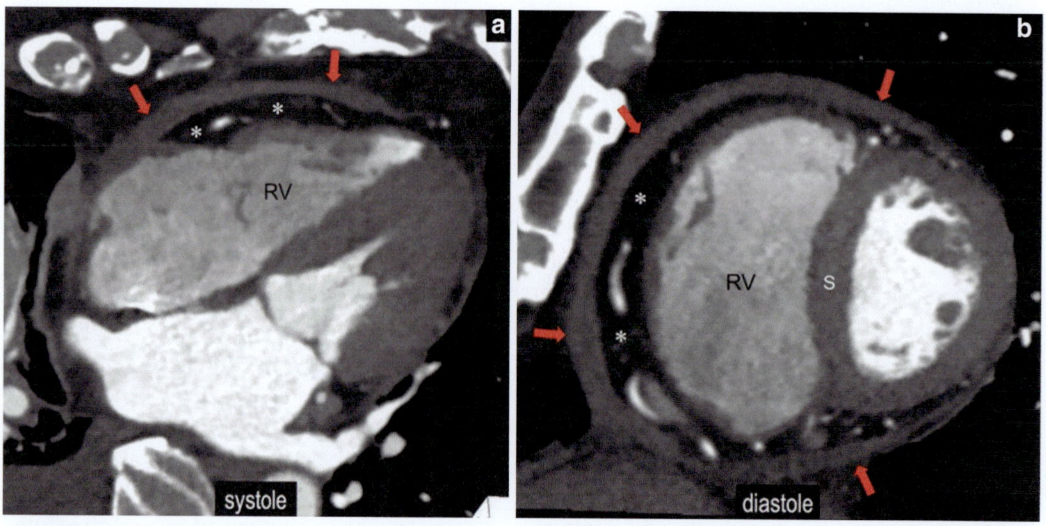

Fig. 19.23 Chronic Inflammatory Pericarditis**.** Case Example of Chronic Pericarditis. **Panel** (**a**) Chronic constrictive pericarditis in a 73-year-old man. Diffuse pericardial thickening and effusion were observed (arrows). Note the prominent epicardial fat (asterisks) reflecting chronic inflammatory process. **Panel** (**b**) In diastole, the interventricular septum (S) is flattened. *RV* right ventricle

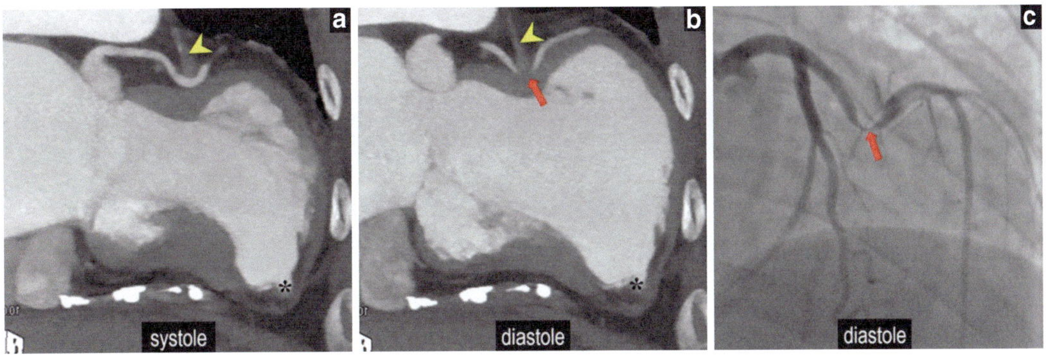

Fig. 19.24 Entrapment of the Left Anterior Descending Coronary Artery by Band-like Thickening of the Pericardium. Coronary Entrapment as Result of Pericarditis. **Panel** (**a**, **b**) Chronic constrictive pericarditis in a 55-year-old woman. The mid-portion of the left anterior descending coronary artery (arrow) was compression by thickened pericardium (arrowheads) in diastole. Note the subendocardial low attenuated lesion (asterisks) in the LV apex, suggestive of ischemic insult. The dynamic narrowing of the coronary artery was confirmed on angiography (**Panel c**)

19.2.5 Constrictive Pericarditis

- **Etiologies (2)**: Constrictive pericarditis represents the end-stage of the inflammatory process of the pericardium. Common etiologies are idiopathic, post-surgical, and radiation injury in developed countries. Tuberculosis is still an important etiology in a developing country.
- **Pathophysiology** [2]: Ventricular interdependence and dissociation of intrathoracic and intracardiac pressure are the key pathophysiological findings in patients with constrictive pericarditis. Echocardiography is the diagnostic modality of choice for evaluating constrictive physiology.
- **Role of CT** [2]: ECG-synchronized CT may have an important additive role to echocardiography in evaluating constrictive pericarditis: (1) CT is well-suited for preoperative planning because CT helps detect calcified foci of the thickened pericardium. (2) CT helps obviate the need for invasive angiography. (3) Cine CT may be useful for detecting constrictive physiology (i.e., septal 'bounce,' ventricular interaction) (Fig. 19.23). (4) Other additional findings are distorted ventricular contours, hepatic venous congestion, ascites, and pleural effusion. In addition, rarely localized calcified pericarditis may induce the entrapment of the coronary artery (Fig. 19.24) [42].

19.2.6 Pericardial Masses

- Pericardial masses include cystic lesions (e.g., bronchogenic cyst), hematomas, organized effusions, primary and secondary malignancies [37].
- Primary tumors are more frequently malignant and include mesothelioma (Fig. 19.25), angiosarcoma, liposarcoma, and lymphoma (Fig. 19.26). The malignant mesothelioma may show pericardial nodular lesions or heterogeneously enhancing mass with hemorrhagic effusions [43].
- Benign tumors include fibroma, teratoma, hemangioma, lipoma, paraganglioma, and germ-cell tumor [43].

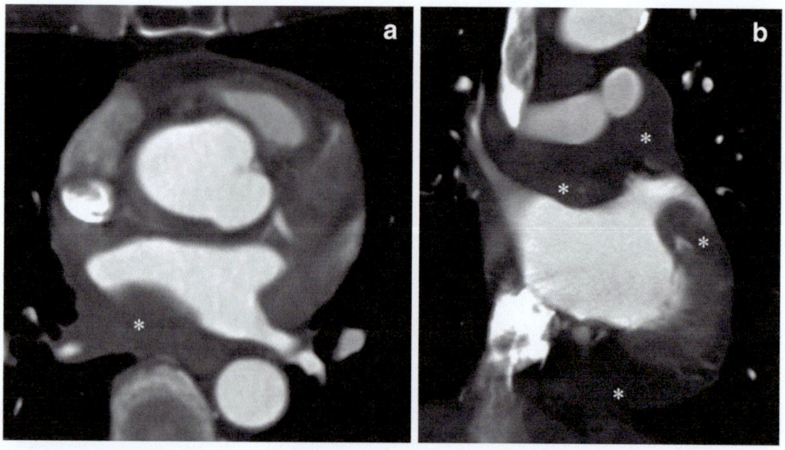

Fig. 19.25 Pericardial Mesothelioma. Pericardial Tumor. Case example of a pericardial mesothelioma in a 69-year-old man. (**a**, **b**) Multifocal masses (asterisks) in the pericardial space compress the left atrium, left atrial appendage, and pulmonary veins

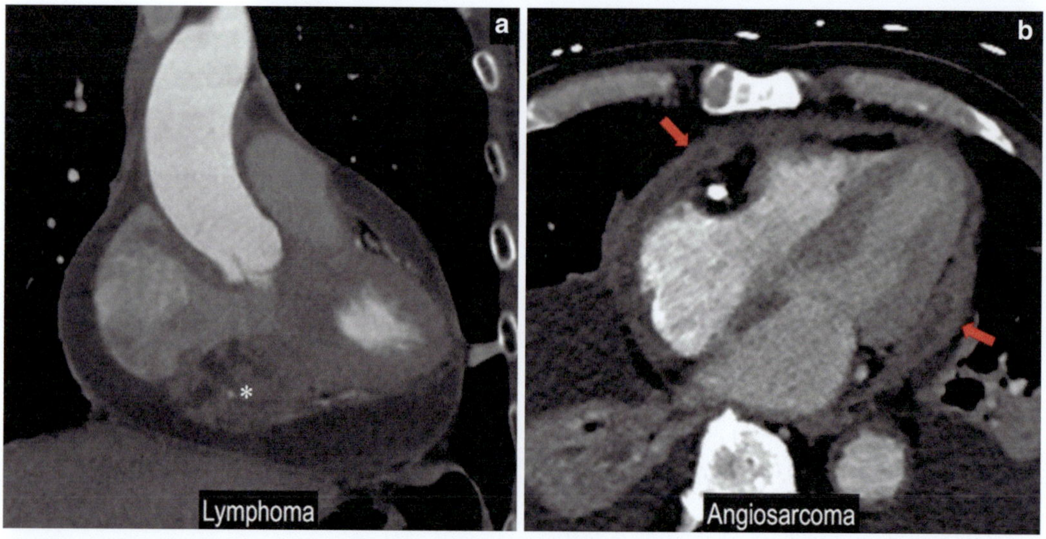

Fig. 19.26 Other Malignant Tumors of the Pericardium. Case Examples of Pericardial Tumors. **Panel** (**a**) Malignant pericardial effusion with lymphoma (asterisks) in a 78-year-old man. **Panel** (**b**) Angiosarcoma of the pericardium in a 67-year-old man. There was irregular thickening (arrows) and enhancement of the pericardium on CT

References

1. Nkomo VT, Gardin JM, Skelton TN, Gottdiener JS, Scott CG, Enriquez-Sarano M. Burden of valvular heart diseases: a population-based study. Lancet. 2006;368(9540):1005–11.
2. Libby P. Braunwald's heart disease: a textbook of cardiovascular medicine. Twelfth edition ed. Amsterdam: Elsevier; 2021. 2 volumes: illustrations (black and white, and colour).
3. Maganti K, Rigolin VH, Sarano ME, Bonow RO. Valvular heart disease: diagnosis and management. Mayo Clin Proc. 2010;85(5):483–500.
4. Writing Committee M, Otto CM, Nishimura RA, Bonow RO, Carabello BA, Erwin JP 3rd, et al. 2020 ACC/AHA guideline for the Management of Patients with Valvular Heart Disease: a report of the American College of Cardiology/American Heart Association joint Committee on clinical practice guidelines. J Am Coll Cardiol. 2021;77(4):e25–e197.
5. Ahn Y, Choi SJ, Lim S, Kim JB, Song J-M, Kang D-H, et al. Classification of severe aortic stenosis and outcomes after aortic valve replacement. Sci Rep. 2022;12(1):1–13.
6. Pawade T, Clavel MA, Tribouilloy C, Dreyfus J, Mathieu T, Tastet L, et al. Computed tomography aortic valve calcium scoring in patients with aortic stenosis. Circ Cardiovasc Imaging. 2018;11(3):e007146.

7. Koo HJ, Kang JW, Kim JA, Kim JB, Jung SH, Choo SJ, et al. Functional classification of aortic regurgitation using cardiac computed tomography: comparison with surgical inspection. Int J Cardiovasc Imaging. 2018;34(8):1295–303.
8. Koo HJ, Yang DH, Oh SY, Kang JW, Kim DH, Song JK, et al. Demonstration of mitral valve prolapse with CT for planning of mitral valve repair. Radiographics. 2014;34(6):1537–52.
9. Han K, Yang DH, Shin SY, Kim N, Kang JW, Kim DH, et al. Subprosthetic pannus after aortic valve replacement surgery: cardiac CT findings and clinical features. Radiology. 2015;276(3):724–31.
10. Koo HJ, Lee JY, Kim GH, Kang JW, Kim YH, Kim DH, et al. Paravalvular leakage in patients with prosthetic heart valves: cardiac computed tomography findings and clinical features. Eur Heart J Cardiovasc Imaging. 2018;19(12):1419–27.
11. Koo HJ, Yang DH, Kang JW, Lee JY, Kim DH, Song JM, et al. Demonstration of infective endocarditis by cardiac CT and transoesophageal echocardiography: comparison with intra-operative findings. Eur Heart J Cardiovasc Imaging. 2018;19(2):199–207.
12. Habib G, Lancellotti P, Antunes MJ, Bongiorni MG, Casalta JP, Del Zotti F, et al. 2015 ESC guidelines for the management of infective endocarditis: the task force for the Management of Infective Endocarditis of the European Society of Cardiology (ESC). Endorsed by: European Association for Cardio-Thoracic Surgery (EACTS), the European Association of Nuclear Medicine (EANM). Eur Heart J. 2015;36(44):3075–128.
13. Vahanian A, Beyersdorf F, Praz F, Milojevic M, Baldus S, Bauersachs J, et al. 2021 ESC/EACTS guidelines for the management of valvular heart disease. Eur Heart J. 2021;42:4207.
14. Blanke P, Weir-McCall JR, Achenbach S, Delgado V, Hausleiter J, Jilaihawi H, et al. Computed tomography imaging in the context of transcatheter aortic valve implantation (TAVI) /transcatheter aortic valve replacement (TAVR): an expert consensus document of the Society of Cardiovascular Computed Tomography. J Cardiovasc Comput Tomogr. 2019;13(1):1–20.
15. Ahn Y, Koo HJ, Kang JW, Yang DH. Tricuspid valve imaging and right ventricular function analysis using cardiac CT and MRI. Korean J Radiol. 2021;22(12):1946–63.
16. Koo HJ, Yang DH, Kang JW, Han K, Chung CH, Song JK, et al. Demonstration of prosthetic aortic valve dehiscence in a patient with noninfectious aortitis by multimodality imaging: findings of echocardiography and computed tomography. Circulation. 2013;128(7):759–61.
17. Faletra FF, Faletra FF, Pandian NG, Ho SY, Dawsonera C, Dawsonera. Anatomy of the heart by multislice computed tomography. Oxford; Hoboken, NJ: Wiley-Blackwell; 2008.
18. Yang DH, Kim DH, Handschumacher MD, Levine RA, Kim JB, Sun BJ, et al. In vivo assessment of aortic root geometry in normal controls using 3D analysis of computed tomography. Eur Heart J Cardiovasc Imaging. 2017;18(7):780–6.
19. Saremi F, Hassani C, Sanchez-Quintana D. Septal atrioventricular junction region: comprehensive imaging in adults. Radiographics. 2016;36(7):1966–86.
20. Michelena HI, Della Corte A, Evangelista A, Maleszewski JJ, Edwards WD, Roman MJ, et al. International consensus statement on nomenclature and classification of the congenital bicuspid aortic valve and its aortopathy, for clinical, surgical, interventional and research purposes. J Thorac Cardiovasc Surg. 2021;162(3):e383–414.
21. Pham MHC, Ballegaard C, de Knegt MC, Sigvardsen PE, Sorgaard MH, Fuchs A, et al. Normal values of aortic dimensions assessed by multidetector computed tomography in the Copenhagen general population study. Eur Heart J Cardiovasc Imaging. 2019;20(8):939–48.
22. Abramowitz Y, Jilaihawi H, Chakravarty T, Mack MJ, Makkar RR. Mitral Annulus Calcification. J Am Coll Cardiol. 2015;66(17):1934–41.
23. Eleid MF, Foley TA, Said SM, Pislaru SV, Rihal CS. Severe mitral annular calcification: multimodality imaging for therapeutic strategies and interventions. JACC Cardiovasc Imaging. 2016;9(11):1318–37.
24. Carpentier A. Cardiac valve surgery—the "French correction". J Thorac Cardiovasc Surg. 1983;86(3):323–37.
25. Weir-McCall JR, Blanke P, Naoum C, Delgado V, Bax JJ, Leipsic J. Mitral valve imaging with CT: relationship with Transcatheter mitral valve interventions. Radiology. 2018;288(3):638–55.
26. Koo HJ, Kang JW, Oh SY, Kim DH, Song JM, Kang DH, et al. Cardiac computed tomography for the localization of mitral valve prolapse: scallop-by-scallop comparisons with echocardiography and intraoperative findings. Eur Heart J Cardiovasc Imaging. 2019;20(5):550–7.
27. Tanis W, Habets J, van den Brink RB, Symersky P, Budde RP, Chamuleau SA. Differentiation of thrombus from pannus as the cause of acquired mechanical prosthetic heart valve obstruction by non-invasive imaging: a review of the literature. Eur Heart J Cardiovasc Imaging. 2014;15(2):119–29.
28. Gunduz S, Ozkan M, Kalcik M, Gursoy OM, Astarcioglu MA, Karakoyun S, et al. Sixty-four-section cardiac computed tomography in mechanical prosthetic heart valve dysfunction: thrombus or pannus. Circ Cardiovasc Imaging. 2015;8(12):e003246.
29. Koo HJ, Ha H, Kang JW, Kim JA, Song JK, Kim HJ, et al. Impact of pannus formation on hemodynamic dysfunction of prosthetic aortic valve: pannus extent and its relationship to prosthetic valve motion and degree of stenosis. Clin Res Cardiol. 2018;107(7):554–64.
30. Park MY, Koo HJ, Ha H, Kang J-W, Yang DH. Extent of subprosthetic pannus after aortic valve replacement: changes over time and relationship with

echocardiographic findings. J Korean Soc Radiol. 2020;81(5):1151–63.
31. Suh YJ, Kim YJ, Lee S, Hong YJ, Lee HJ, Hur J, et al. Utility of cardiac computed tomography for evaluation of pannus in mechanical aortic valve. Int J Cardiovasc Imaging. 2015;31(6):1271–80.
32. Kim W, Choi H, Kweon J, Yang DH, Kim YH. Effects of pannus formation on the flow around a bileaflet mechanical heart valve. PLoS One. 2020;15(6):e0234341.
33. Ha H, Koo HJ, Huh HK, Kim GB, Kweon J, Kim N, et al. Effect of pannus formation on the prosthetic heart valve: in vitro demonstration using particle image velocimetry. PLoS One. 2018;13(6):e0199792.
34. Suh YJ, Kim YJ, Hong YJ, Lee HJ, Hur J, Im DJ, et al. Measurement of opening and closing angles of aortic valve prostheses in vivo using dual-source computed tomography: comparison with those of Manufacturers' in 10 different types. Korean J Radiol. 2015;16(5):1012–23.
35. Ram P, Penalver JL, Lo KBU, Rangaswami J, Pressman GS. Carcinoid heart disease: review of current knowledge. Tex Heart Inst J. 2019;46(1):21–7.
36. Boxt LM, Abbara S. Cardiac imaging: the requisites. 4th ed. Philadelphia, Pennsylvania: Elsevier; 2016.
37. Bogaert J, Francone M. Pericardial disease: value of CT and MR imaging. Radiology. 2013;267(2):340–56.
38. John TH. Netter's clinical anatomy. Amsterdam: Elsevier; 2019.
39. Kluner LV, Oikonomou EK, Antoniades C. Assessing cardiovascular risk by using the fat attenuation index in coronary CT angiography. Radiol Cardiothorac Imaging. 2021;3(1):e200563.
40. O'Leary SM, Williams PL, Williams MP, Edwards AJ, Roobottom CA, Morgan-Hughes GJ, et al. Imaging the pericardium: appearances on ECG-gated 64-detector row cardiac computed tomography. Br J Radiol. 2010;83(987):194–205.
41. Rajiah P. Cardiac MRI: part 2, pericardial diseases. AJR Am J Roentgenol. 2011;197(4):W621–34.
42. Gaur S, Jensen JM, Terkelsen CJ, Holm NR, Norgaard BL. Entrapment of the left anterior descending coronary artery by localized calcific pericarditis: from dynamic to fixed coronary stenosis. Circulation. 2013;128(3):e30–1.
43. Restrepo CS, Vargas D, Ocazionez D, Martinez-Jimenez S, Betancourt Cuellar SL, Gutierrez FR. Primary pericardial tumors. Radiographics. 2013;33(6):1613–30.

CT for Diseases of the Great Vessels

20

Abdullah Al Khalifah, Muhammad Umair, and Stefan L. Zimmerman

Abstract

Evaluation of the aorta and its major branches by CTA requires providing consistent and accurate measurements. This chapter reviews guidelines and technical tips on how to appropriately measure vascular dimensions. Recognition of normal anatomy and anatomic variation is critical to differentiate normal findings from pathologies of similar appearance. Diseases of the aorta and its major branches may have congenital, inflammatory, infectious, traumatic, or post-operative etiologies. A correct diagnosis is essential for identifying the appropriate management.

Keywords

Aortic dissection · Aortic coarctation · Aortic aneurysm · Marfan Syndrome · Takayasu Arteritis · Intramural hematoma · Mycotic aneurysm · Penetrating atherosclerotic ulcer · Acute aortic syndrome

A. Al Khalifah · M. Umair · S. L. Zimmerman (✉)
Johns Hopkins University, Baltimore, MD, USA
e-mail: Abdullah.AlKhalifah@JHAH.COM; mumair2@jhmi.edu; stefan.zimmerman@jhmi.edu

Abbreviations

LVOT	Left ventricular outflow tract
MIP	Magnetic Resonance Imaging, Maximum intensity projection
MPR	Multiplanar reformation

20.1 Thoracic Aorta

1. **Normal Anatomy:** The thoracic aorta can be divided into four segments (Fig. 20.1):
    - Aortic root: extends from the ventricular-aortic junction (annulus) to the sino-tubular junction.
    - Ascending thoracic aorta: it extends from the sino-tubular junction to the origin of the right brachiocephalic (also known as innominate) artery.
    - Aortic arch: it extends from the origin of the right brachiocephalic artery to the attachment of the ligamentum arteriosum.
    - The descending aorta extends from the ligamentum arteriosum distally to the diaphragmatic hiatus approximately at the T12 vertebral body level.

A. A. Zadeh, J. Hoe (eds.), *Practical Guide to Cardiac CT*,
https://doi.org/10.1007/978-981-97-6919-3_20

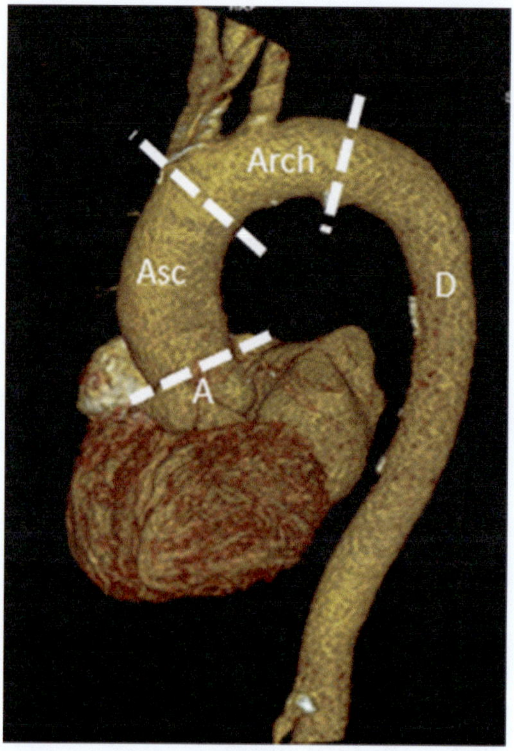

Fig. 20.1 Conventional thoracic aortic anatomy on a volume rendered 3D image. The parts of the thoracic aorta are the root (R), ascending thoracic aorta (Asc), arch (Arch), and descending thoracic aorta (D)

20.2 Measurement of the Thoracic aorta [1–3]

- Technical considerations: There are many technical variables that could introduce variation in the measurement between individuals including planes, modalities, cardiac cycle timing, and anatomical location. In addition, there are morphological factors that could affect the normal diameter measurements such age, race, and gender.
- Most ascending thoracic aorta reference measurements have used 2D echocardiographic values to establish the basis of surgical repair recommendations.
- Echocardiogram has limitations related to the operator's technical skills and availability of clear imaging windows, which can be difficult in patients with large body habitus or with electronic devices, which reduces the reproducibility of measurements.
- The three-chamber or left ventricular outflow tract (LVOT) plane on cardiac CT (Computed Tomography) or MRI (Magnetic Resonance Imaging) is the closest equivalent view to the two-dimensional parasternal long axis echocardiographic plane used for measurements of the aortic root and ascending aorta. However, CT and MRI with volumetric 3-D acquisitions and double orthogonal/oblique measurements are more accurate than standard echocardiography.
- ECG-gated CT angiography (CTA) is preferred over ungated scans to minimize cardiac motion and pulsation artifact, especially affecting the ascending aorta, improving the accuracy and reducibility.
- A double oblique multiplanar reformation (MPR) perpendicular to the longitudinal axis of the aorta is the most accurate plane to perform measurements of the ascending aorta.
- Typical anatomical locations for cross-sectional diameter measurements of the thoracic aorta includes the following (Fig. 20.2):
  - Aortic annulus.
  - Sinus of Valsalva.
  - Sino-tubular junction.
  - Mid-ascending aorta at the level of right pulmonary artery.
  - Arch and at the level of isthmus.
  - Descending aorta at the level of right pulmonary artery.

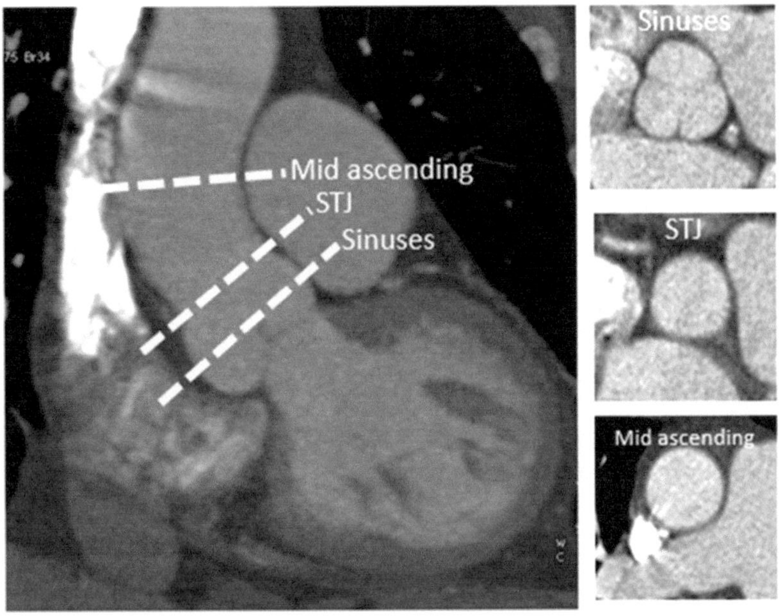

Fig. 20.2 Typical measurements of the thoracic aorta. Sagittal Oblique MIP of the aortic root shows typical levels for measurements and their corresponding double oblique MPR planes (mid sinus, sino-tubular junction (STJ), and mid-ascending aorta at the level of the right pulmonary artery)

20.3 Image Analysis and Reporting

- Additional anatomical locations that may be helpful in certain scenarios, depending upon location of aortic pathology include:
  - High ascending aorta just below the brachiocephalic origin
  - Mid-aortic arch
  - Diaphragmatic hiatus
- On follow-up studies, both new measurements and repeat measurements of the aorta on the previous study are recommended to minimize interobserver variability.
- Indexing aortic diameter by body surface area has been suggested as a standardizing method to account for differences in body size by some authors. In clinic practice, decisions management decisions often rely on a single maximal diameter threshold (see surveillance section below) rather than normalized thresholds although aortic size strongly correlates with body surface area, revealing up to 3-mm variation among patient sizes [2].

20.4 Coarctation [4, 5]

- Definition: Focal narrowing of the thoracic aorta, just distal to the origin of the left subclavian artery (Fig. 20.3).
- Sub-types:
  - Preductal: proximal to the insertion site of the ductus arteriosus.
  - Ductal: at the insertion site of the ductus arteriosus.
  - Post ductal: distal to the insertion site of the ductus arteriosus.
- Clinical features:
  - More common in males. Male to female = 2:1.
  - Rare, 226 per 10,000 births. Associated with Turner syndrome, bicuspid valve, VSD, PDA, and cerebral aneurysm.
  - Maybe asymptomatic or can present with lower extremity claudication, angina pectoralis, or severe hypertension.
  - Pregnant patients with a history of coarctation are at high risk for aortic dissection or aneurysm before treatment and for miscarriage and preeclampsia after treatment.

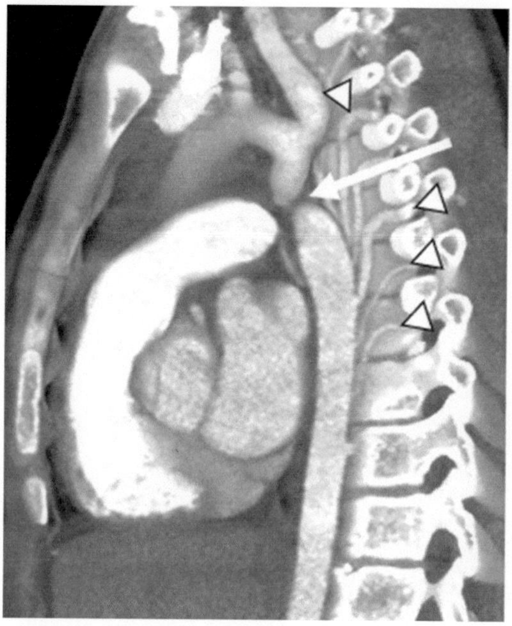

Fig. 20.3 Aortic coarctation. Sagittal oblique volume rendered image in a 15-year-old female patient showing the typical appearance of a coarctation with severe narrowing at the isthmus, just distal to the left subclavian artery (arrow), and multiple enlarged intercostal arteries due to collateral flow (arrowheads)

- CT findings: Evaluate the location and degree of coarctation, the presence of dilated intercostal artery and internal mammary collaterals, and look for bicuspid aortic valve (Fig. 20.3).
- Other imaging modalities –.
  - MRA: Suitable to evaluate the morphology and function of coarctation and other complications such as aneurysms. Flow velocities before, at and after the level of coarctation and flow measurements before and after the level of coarctation and flow measurements at the level of diaphragmatic hiatus (utilizing 4D flow or 2D phase contrast MRI) can provide insightful information into the hemodynamic significance and shunting volume across the intercostal and other collaterals.
  - Longer acquisition time.
  - Catheter Angiography: Suitable to measure the pressure gradient. A pressure gradient >20 mmHg may suggest the need for surgical intervention.

20.5 Pseudocoarctation

- Congenital or acquired secondary to underlying atherosclerosis.
- Focal kinking or apparent narrowing of the thoracic aorta without clinical signs and symptoms, pressure gradient, or dilated collaterals (Fig. 20.4).

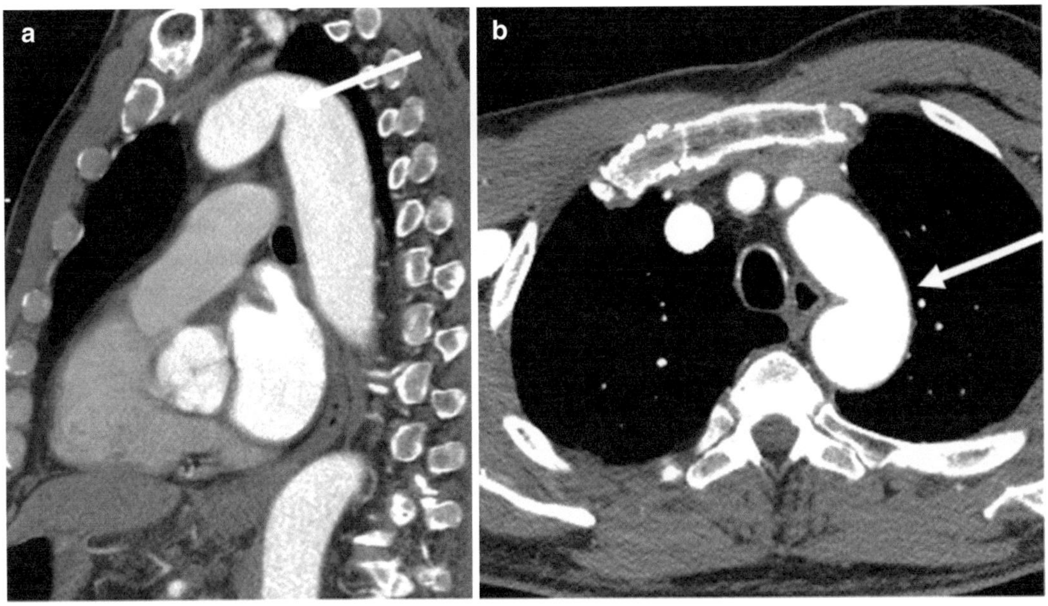

Fig. 20.4 Pseudocoarctation. Sagittal (**a**) and axial (**b**) CT angiographic images in a 73-year-old woman showing a tortuous aorta with focal kinked appearance on sagittal imaging (arrow, **a**) but no significant narrowing on axial image (arrow, **b**). There are no dilated intercostal arteries to indicate collateral flow around the kinking

20.6 Double Aortic arch [4]

- Overview:
  - Two distinct aortic arches with varying amounts of hypoplastic or atretic arch tissue.
  - Two separate ipsilateral subclavian and carotid arteries arise from each side.
  - The left arch can be fully patent and functional or hypoplastic and atretic distal to the left subclavian artery origin (complete versus incomplete double aortic arch).
- Clinical presentation:
  - Symptomatic patients usually present during early childhood with respiratory symptoms due to tracheal compression: dyspnea, wheezing, stridor, and coughing.
  - In adults, it could be an incidental finding in asymptomatic patients or associated with difficulty in swallowing.
- CT findings:
  - Useful to evaluate arch anatomy for surgical planning and define tracheal abnormalities.
  - Can define which side of arch is larger (dominant). Dominant right is most common (75–80%) (Fig. 20.5), then codominant (25%), and finally dominant left (5%).
  - The double arches join to form a single descending aorta that is usually on the left.
- Other imaging modalities: Radiographs may reveal upper mediastinal widening and bilateral paratracheal soft tissue on posteroanterior view and posterior tracheal indentation on lateral views.

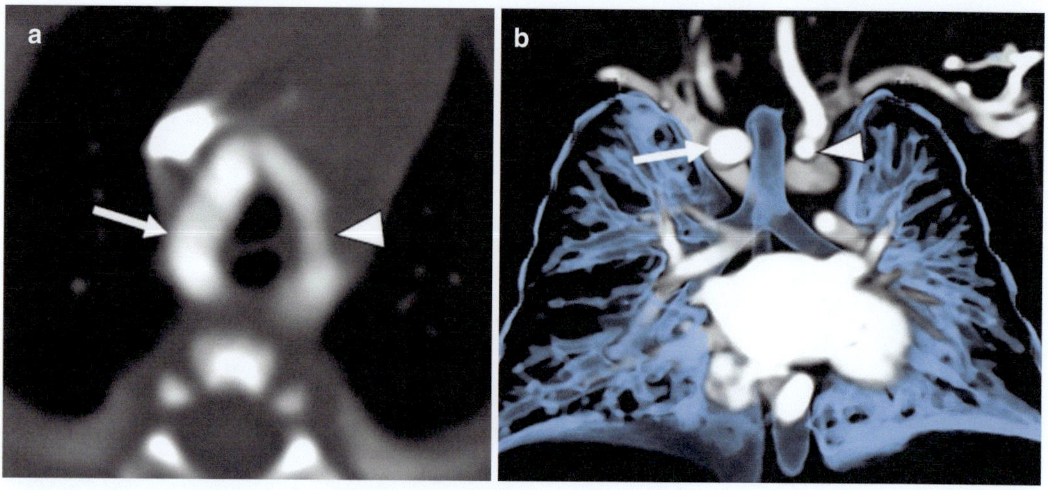

Fig. 20.5 Double aortic arch. Axial (**a**) and VR (**b**) images from a CT angiogram obtained in a 1-day-old male with a complete double aortic arch. The right arch is dominant (arrow), which is the most common pattern. The left arch is smaller (arrowhead) and both surround the trachea, shaded blue in B

20.7 Branch Vessel Variants [5]

- Common origin of the brachiocephalic and the left common carotid arteries—most common arch variant, ~10–20% of the general population.
- Variant origin of vertebral arteries directly from the arch–most often characterized by direct origin of the left vertebral artery from the arch between the left common carotid artery and the left subclavian artery.
- Common origin of both common carotid arteries.
- Aberrant right subclavian artery, which arises from the distal arch near the isthmus, beyond the left subclavian origin, and takes a retroesophageal course to the right upper extremity.
- Aberrant left subclavian artery, which is always associated with a right aortic arch, take-off distal to the right subclavian artery, and a retroesophageal course (Fig. 20.6).
- Diverticulum of Kommerell is a finding that may be present with aberrant subclavian artery origins in either right or left aortic arches. It corresponds to a fusiform dilation of the origin of the aberrant vessel at its attachment to the aorta (Fig. 20.6).
- Thyroidea ima artery—present in 7.5%—a rare vascular variant of thyroid arterial supply that usually arises from the brachiocelphalic trunk and is associated with absent inferior thyroid arteries.

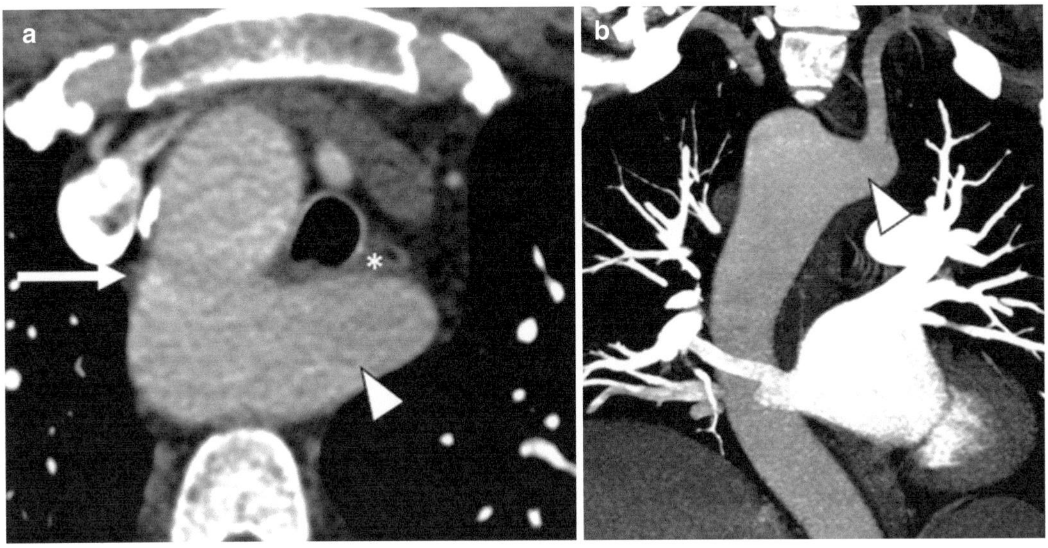

Fig. 20.6 Right aortic arch with aberrant left subclavian artery and diverticulum of Kommerell. Axial CT angiogram (**a**) and coronal MIP (**b**) show the right arch (arrow) with aberrant left subclavian artery (arrowhead) that courses behind the esophagus (asterisk) and is dilated at its origin at the diverticulum of Kommerell

20.8 Patent Ductus Arteriosus [6]

- Overview:
  - The ductus arteriosus is a fetal vascular structure developed from the sixth aortic arch, which connects the aorta with the pulmonary arterial system in utero. Upon birth and resultant increase in systemic pressure this ductal structure closes spontaneously within 48 hours.
  - A patent ductus arteriosus (PDA) beyond 48 hrs of life can be essential to ensure pulmonic blood flow in the setting of congenital heart disease, such as Tetralogy of Fallot, pulmonary atresia, or hypoplastic left heart syndrome.
  - On imaging, a blood vessel is seen connecting the inferior surface of the distal aortic arch with either the main or proximal left pulmonary artery (Fig. 20.7).
- Clinical presentation:
  - 1 in 2000 full-term neonates
  - More common in females, F:M ratio of 2:1
  - Loud continuous machine-like murmur on auscultation

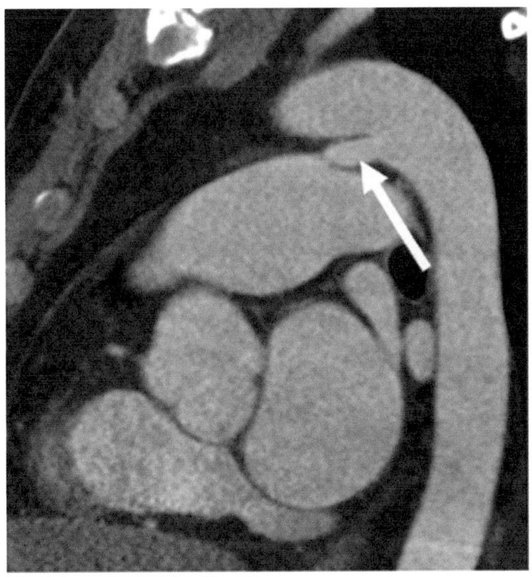

Fig. 20.7 Patent ductus arteriosus. Sagittal MPR of the thoracic aorta from an ECG-gated CT angiogram shows a small patent ductus arteriosus extending from the undersurface of the arch to the roof of the main pulmonary artery (arrow)

20.9 Aortic Aneurysm

- Definition: Enlargement of the diameter of the aorta by 1.5 times above the upper limit of the normal value. Enlargement 1.1–1.4 times greater than average size but less than the threshold of aneurysm is considered aortic dilatation [7, 8].
- Epidemiology: More common in males (M:F = 3:1); age: usually 50–60 years.
- Risk factors:
  - Atherosclerosis of aorta.
  - Connective tissue diseases (although different guidelines and treatment thresholds followed for aortic dilations and aneurysms associated):
  - Marfan syndrome.
  - Ehlers-Danlos syndrome.
  - Loeys-Dietz syndrome.
  - Inflammatory aortitis.
  - Syphilis.
  - Takayasu disease.
  - Rheumatoid arthritis.
  - Ankylosing spondylitis.
  - Bicuspid aortic valve (Fig. 20.8).
- Imaging features [9, 10]:
  - Nonenhanced CT: Helpful to evaluate for attenuation of the aortic wall, hemorrhage, and calcification (see DD intramural hematoma below). Can also be used to follow external aortic diameters for stable, low risk aortic dilation.
  - CT angiography [9]: Gold standard requires rapid contrast injection (5–7 mL/s) through a large bore IV (ideally 18 gauge) with acquisition during the arterial phase of enhancement for maximum image quality.
  - Key components of imaging assessment of thoracic aortic aneurysm:

    Size: Sac dimensions, luminal diameter, length of aneurysmal segment, and the vicinity and the size of proximal/distal vessels adjacent to the aneurysm.

    Shape: fusiform or saccular.

    Aortic wall: Wall thickness, periaortic wall stranding, mural thrombus, or calcification.

    Mural thrombus is a common finding that occurs primarily in large aneurysms of the descending thoracic aorta and in the abdominal aorta and is secondary to layering intraluminal thrombi that form an organized clot along the wall of the dilated vessel (Fig. 20.8).

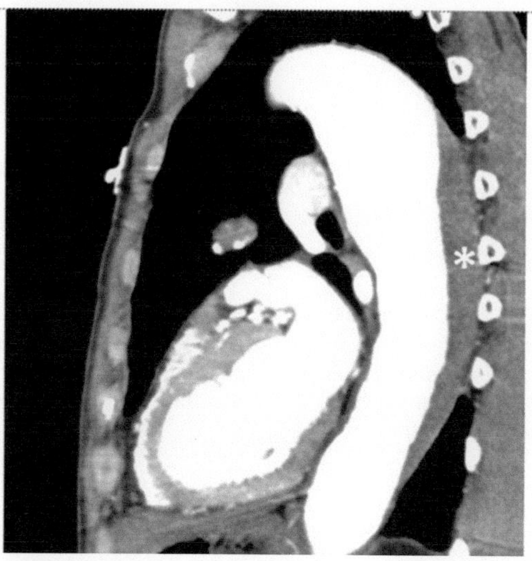

Fig. 20.8 Sagittal image from CT angiogram showing descending thoracic aortic aneurysm with mural thrombus (asterisk)

- Other imaging modalities:
  - Plain radiographs show an enlarged aorta as mediastinal widening, which must be differentiated to other mediastinal pathologies, such as hemorrhage, mediastinal masses, or lymphadenopathies.
  - Magnetic resonance angiography (MRA) [10] is a valid alternative to CT and may be preferred in younger patients or for surveillance to avoid X-ray exposure.
- Surveillance of thoracic aortic aneurysms:

For patients without history of high-risk conditions (e.g., Marfan syndrome, Loeys-Dietz syndrome, Ehlers-Danlos syndrome, Turner syndrome, Familial Thoracic aortic aneurysms):

- TTE and CTA or MRA at baseline and 6 months.
- If TAA is smaller than 5 cm in diameter and stable, then yearly.
- If TAA is equal to or greater than 5 cm or growing more than 0.5 cm/year, then every 6 months and refer to the vascular surgeon.

For patients with high-risk conditions:

- TTE and CTA or MRA at baseline and 6 months.
- If TAA is smaller than 5 cm in diameter and stable (growing less than 0.3 cm per year), then TTE yearly and CTA or MRA every 2 years.
- If TAA is equal to or greater than 5 cm or growing more than 0.5 cm/year, then every 6 months and refer to the vascular surgeon.
- Follow-up after initial diagnosis: If less than 4.5 cm in diameter and stable (growing less than 0.3 cm per year), then TTE and CTA or MRA yearly. Otherwise, every 6 months and refer to vascular surgery.

Special consideration for high-risk conditions:

- Index dimensions by body surface area are useful to monitor patients with Turner syndrome. If indexed diameter > 2 cm/m^2, then repeat MRA or CTA yearly. Otherwise, every 2 years.
- A lower diameter threshold is recommended to follow-up with Ehlers-Danlos syndrome compared to other high-risk condition using 4 cm cutoff instead of 4.5 cm.
- Surgical options include open repair, combined open and endovascular repair, endovascular repair.
- Indications for initial surgery [7]:

For ascending thoracic aortic aneurysms:

- Symptomatic.
- Evidence of rupture.
- Aortic diameter > 5.5 cm.
- Aortic diameter > 4.5 cm in patients with bicuspid aortic valves or with connective tissue disorders (syndromic and non-syndromic aortopathies).

For the descending thoracic aortic aneurysms:

- Aortic diameter > 5.5 cm.
- Aortic diameter > 5.0 cm in patients with connective tissue disorders.
- Aortic diameter > twice the diameter of the non-aneurysmal aorta in smaller patients (including women).
- Annual growth rate of aortic diameter > 0.5 cm/year.

20.10 Marfan Syndrome

- Autosomal dominant mode of inheritance with 25–30% de novo mutation.
- Known association with FBN1 gene mutation located in the 15q21 chromosome, resulting in a defect in Fibrillin 1 protein, an important extracellular structural protein.
- Diagnosis is based on a combination of criteria (known as the Ghent nosology [11]) with or without associated family history.
- Aortic root dilation is a common criterion (Z-score ≥ 2) (Fig. 20.9). Z-score calculations

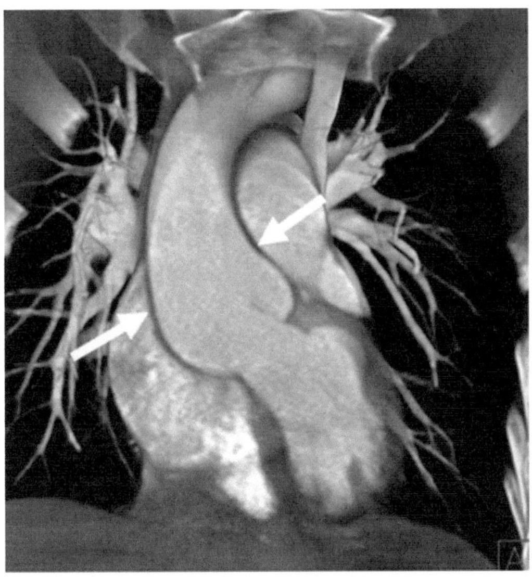

Fig. 20.9 Thoracic aortic aneurysm in a patient with Marfan syndrome. Coronal volume rendered image from a CT angiogram of the chest showing a dilated aortic root with typical effacement of the sino-tubular junction (arrows), known as a tulip bulb deformity

are based on the degree of aortic root dilation relative to normal means obtained by two-dimensional echocardiography and available through an online calculator (marfan.org/dx/z--score-adults). Please note that two-dimensional echocardiographic measures are obtained using parasternal long axis views and measured from leading-edge to leading edge [12]. CT measurements to assess for root dilation in Marfan syndrome should use similar techniques.

- Mitral valve prolapse is a common cardiovascular co-morbidity.
- Acute presentations: Spontaneous pneumothorax, aortic dissection.
- Other diagnostic criteria include:
  - Ectopia lentis (lens dislocation),
  - pectus carinatum,
  - hindfoot deformity,
  - protrusion acetabuli,
  - scoliosis,
  - facial dysmorphia (dolichocephaly, enophthalmos, downslanting palpebral fissures, malar hypoplasia, retrognathia),
  - reduced upper segment to lower body segment ratio,
  - increased arm length/height,
  - dural ectasia (dilation of the cerebrospinal fluid spaces around the neural formina).

20.11 Inflammatory/Infectious Aortic Disease

- Mycotic aneurysm.
  - Definition: Aneurysm due to infection of the aortic wall.
  - Clinical presentation: Usually seen with cases of systematic bacteremia, often caused by Salmonella or Staphylococcus aureus.
  - Risk factors include infective endocarditis, endovascular stent/graft or arterial device infection, trauma, immunosuppression, IV drug use.
  - Imaging features include periaortic inflammatory changes, including fat stranding, enhancing soft tissue, gas, high attenuating fluid.
  - Focal saccular aneurysm are typical, narrow-necked and asymmetric, with lobulated contour, usually more than 1 cm (Fig. 20.10).
  - A rim-enhancing periaortic abscess may be seen in some cases.
  - A focal calcified lesion with other inflammatory changes may suggest syphilis etiology.
- Takayasu Arteritis
  - Characterized by chronic granulomatous vasculitis of the large vessels [13].
  - It predominantly affects the aorta and its major branches (Fig. 20.11).
  - The left subclavian artery is the most common involved artery.
  - Clinical features [13]: more common in females (M: F = 1:9), Asian race, and younger patients <50-year-old.
  - Ischemic symptoms related to stenosis or occlusion.
  - Imaging features include circumferential aortic wall thickening and post-contrast enhancement.

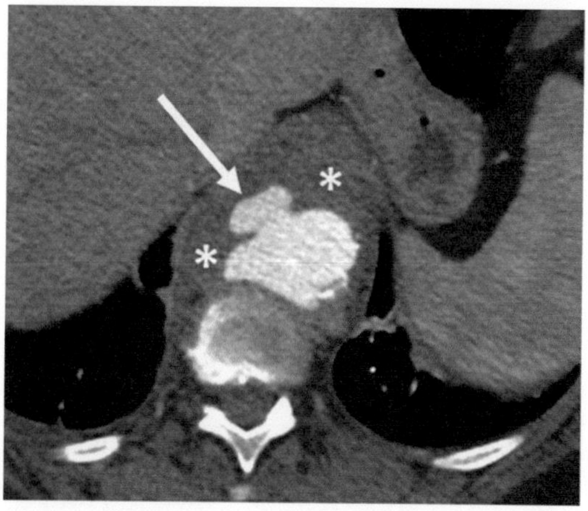

Fig. 20.10 Mycotic aneurysm. Axial CT angiogram images obtained in a 61-year-old woman with staphylococcus aureus-related mycotic aneurysm of the descending thoracic aorta revealing a dilated thoracic aorta with a focal narrow-necked aneurysm (arrow) and low attenuation soft tissue thickening surrounding the aorta (asterisks), compatible with inflammatory phlegmon

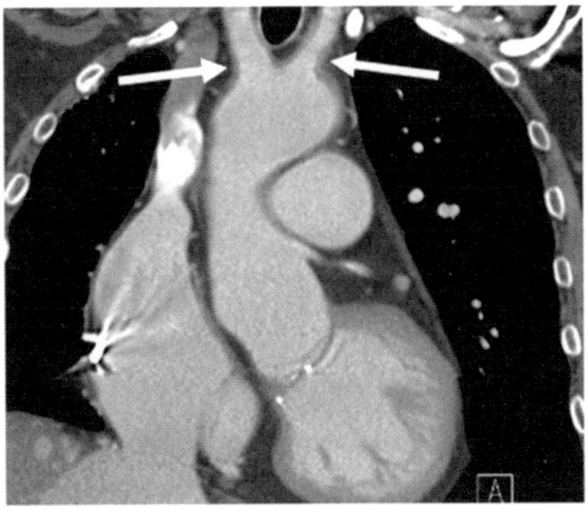

Fig. 20.11 Takayasu Arteritis. Coronal CT angiogram images in a 54-year-old male with Takayasu Arteritis and previous surgical aortic valve repair showing diffuse thickening of the wall of the ascending aorta and the aortic arch branch vessels due to extensive inflammatory changes (arrows)

- Coronary artery involvement in approximately 10%.
- Complications: Stenosis, occlusion, or aneurysm.
- Differential diagnosis [13]: Giant cell arteritis which has a similar radiological appearance but tends to affect patients older than 50 years.

20.12 Acute Aortic Syndromes

20.12.1 Overview

Spectrum of aortic pathologies that present with acute chest pain and abnormalities of the aortic wall ranging from hematoma to dissection to frank rupture [14].

- Aortic dissection.
- Intramural hematoma (IMH).
- Penetrating atherosclerotic ulcers (PAU).
- Aortic rupture.

20.12.2 Technical Considerations

- Contrast-enhanced CT is the exam of choice to evaluate acute aortic syndrome, typically performed without ECG-gating (unless concern over ascending aortic dissection or IMH.
- Pulsation and cardiac motion artifact might produce motion blurring of the ascending aortic wall, which might be mistakenly interpreted as a dissection or intramural hematoma.
- ECG-gated CTA is preferred to minimize pulsation and cardiac motion artifacts in cases with equivocal root abnormalities (Fig. 20.12). Pulsation artifacts can be identified by evaluating adjacent structures, such as the main pulmonary artery, which will show similar artifacts; whereas, in true dissection, the main pulmonary artery should appear normal.
- Non-contract CT phase before contrast injection may be helpful to evaluate any hyperattenuation of the aortic wall usually associated with intramural hematoma (IMH). Ideally, an ECG-gated non-contrast CT phase should be acquired if clinical suspicion for an ascending aortic IMH is high.
- If there is a suspicion for aortic dissection or aneurysmal rupture, a delayed phase should be considered in addition to the arterial phase to avoid the possibility of incomplete opacification of the aneurysmal sac or false lumen, which might be mistakenly interpreted as partial thrombosis, and to gain information about cardiac output.

20.12.3 Clinical Presentation

- Higher risk with older age (mean age of patients presented with dissection of the ascending thoracic aorta is 61 years and with intramural hematoma of the ascending thoracic aorta is 70).
- Atherosclerosis is a known risk factor.

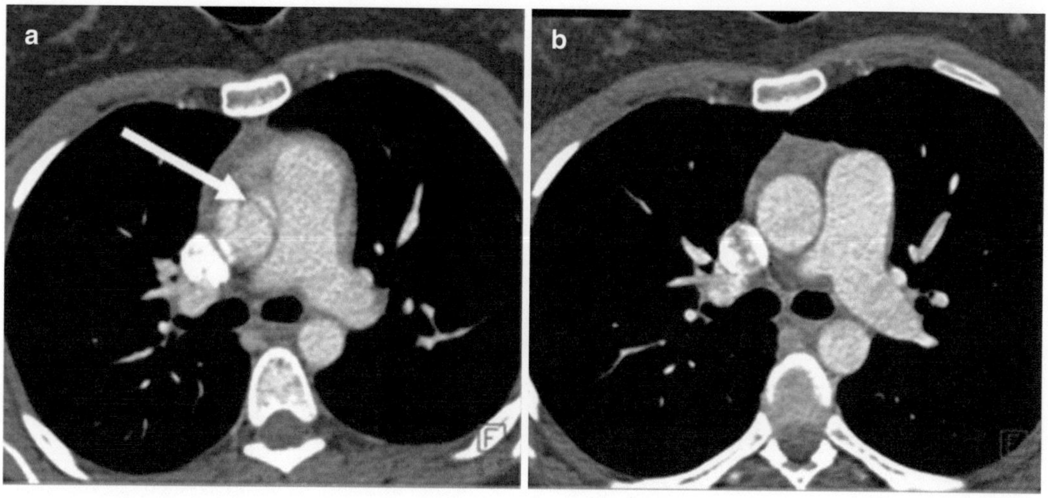

Fig. 20.12 "Pseudo-dissection" due to motion artifact in the ascending aorta on a non-gated study (arrow, **a**) which resolves on the subsequent ECG-gated scan (**b**)

- Male > female.
- Associated with hypertension which can increase intimal shear stress leading to dissection.
- Younger patients with connective tissue disorders such as Marfan or Ehlers-Danlos syndromes.
- Chest pain is presenting symptom in more than 80% of the patients.

20.12.4 Aortic Dissection

- The aorta is made up of three layers, the inner intima with thin layer of endothelium, middle media made of muscular layers, and the outer adventitia made of loose connective tissue. A dissection occurs when blood penetrates the intima and splits the media longitudinally, creating a false and a true lumen with an interposed intimal flap.
- Aortic dissections are commonly described using the Stanford Classification, Type A (involvement of the ascending aorta, Fig. 20.13) vs. Type B (other).
- Type A dissections are typically treated with surgery due to the high mortality risk of consequent coronary artery occlusion, aortic valve incompetence, or cardiac tamponade.
- Type B (Fig. 20.14) dissection may involve the aortic arch and/or descending aorta distal to the origin of the left subclavian artery [15].
- Type B dissections are commonly treated medically (blood pressure control), particularly in an asymptomatic patient.
- CT features of aortic dissection:
  - Displacement of intimal calcification into the lumen.
  - Contrast within true and false lumen (unless false lumen thrombosed).
  - Proximal and distal entry tears (Fig. 20.13).
- Ancillary findings of hemopericardium, pneumomediastinum, or hemothorax.
- Differentiation of true and false lumen:
  - False lumen: usually has a larger size, slower flow, lesser contrast enhancement.
  - Beak sign: Defines the false lumen; where the intima meets the adventitia at an acute angle.
  - Cobweb sign: Linear low attenuation filling defects representing aortic wall media remnants.
  - Mercedes-Benz sign: Triple channel dissection due to additional secondary dissection within one channel of false lumen (Fig. 20.15).

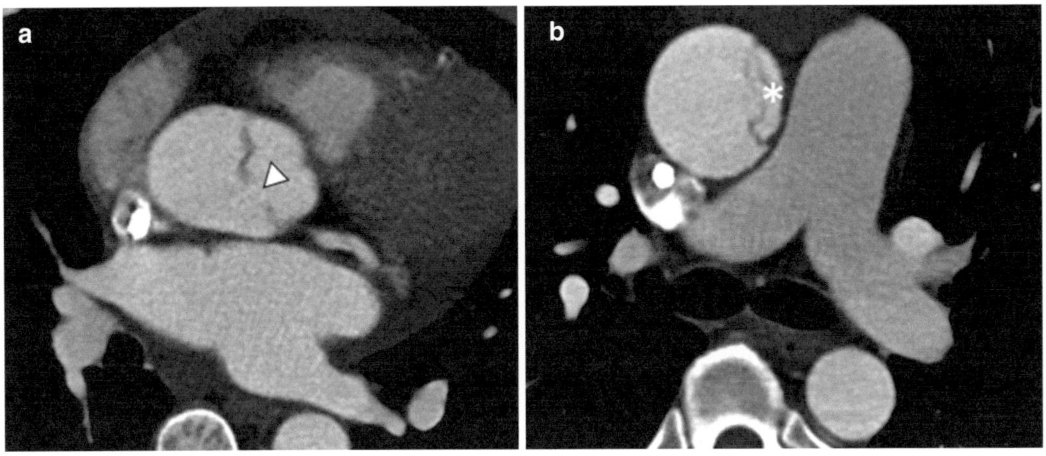

Fig. 20.13 Type A dissection. Axial CT angiographic images in a 36-year-old male who presented with acute chest pain reveal a Type A dissection in the ascending aorta with an entry site (arrowhead in **a**) in the proximal ascending aorta and a small true lumen (asterisk in **b**). Note the descending thoracic aorta is not involved in this patient

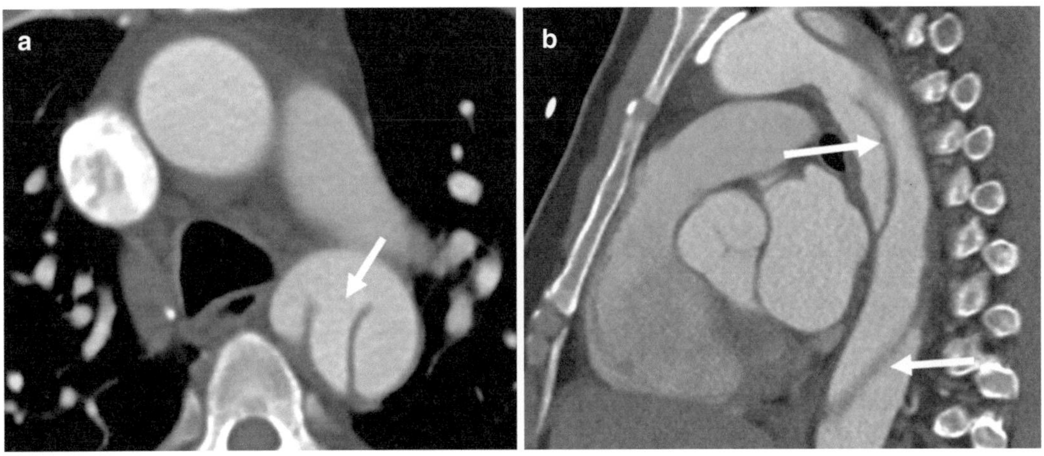

Fig. 20.14 Type B dissection. An axial image from a CT angiogram shows a false lumen and large entry tear in the proximal descending thoracic aorta (**a**, arrow). The sagittal CTA image shows the false lumen spiraling through the descending thoracic aorta (**b**, arrows)

  - True lumen: typically smaller, often with higher attenuation contrast enhancement, however, contrast enhancement differential also depends on the hemodynamic alterations associated with the dissection and the timing of the scan.
- Complications:
  - Rupture: may present as hemopericardium, hemomediastinum, or hemothorax (Fig. 20.16).
  - Pericardial tamponade.
  - Organ and extremity hypoperfusion due to major arch branch vessel involvement.
  - Acute aortic regurgitation (in the event of ascending aortic dissection extending to the sinuses/valve plane).
- Treatment:
  - Type A—urgent surgical repair.
  - Type B—conservative management for uncomplicated cases. Thoracic endovascular aortic repair to eliminate flow through the entry tear is recommended for compli-

cated cases with continued clinical symptoms, inability for medical blood pressure control, impending rupture or organ malperfusion [16].

- Indications for open repair:
  - Type A most often repaired due to higher risk of complications including tamponade and coronary occlusion.

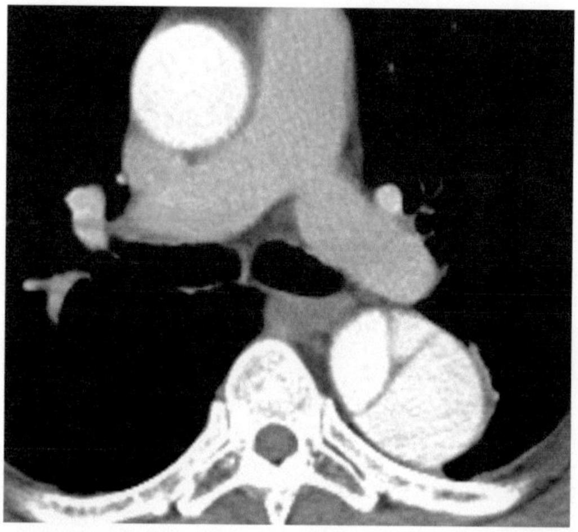

Fig. 20.15 Axial CT angiogram image from a patient with Marfan syndrome and chronic dissection showing the Mercedes-Benz sign due to an additional dissection flap within the false lumen

  - Risk of ischemia: Mesenteric, renal, arch branch vessels or extremities.
  - Hemodynamic instability.
  - Radiological progression of the disease: rupture, interval enlargement of the false lumen, descending aorta >6 cm.
  - Open surgical repair can also be considered in patients with connective tissue disorders with progression of aneurysmal disease despite optimal medical therapy.
- Percutaneous therapy (endovascular repair) may be considered in complicated cased, not suitable for open repair.

20.12.5 Intramural Hematoma

- Spontaneous hemorrhage into the aortic media due to rupture of vaso vasorum.
- May be grouped into type A and type B based on involvement of the ascending aorta, as with aortic dissection.
- Aortic wall hematoma [17] manifests as crescentic high attenuation (Fig. 20.17), wall expansion, and focal, circular contrast accumulation between the sheared arterial branches and the aortic lumen, called "intramural blood

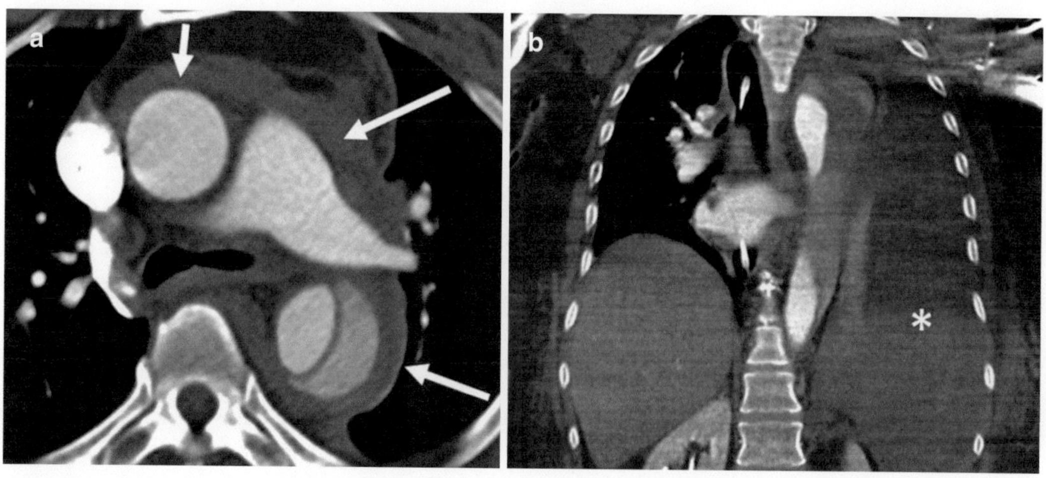

Fig. 20.16 Complications of aortic dissection. Acute type B aortic dissection in a patient presenting with chest pain revealing periaortic and mediastinal hemorrhage (arrows, **a**). Also note the beak sign in the false lumen within descending aorta (**a**). On repeat CT 2 days later, the patient developed a massive left hemothorax (asterisk, **b**). The patient underwent endovascular repair and recovered well

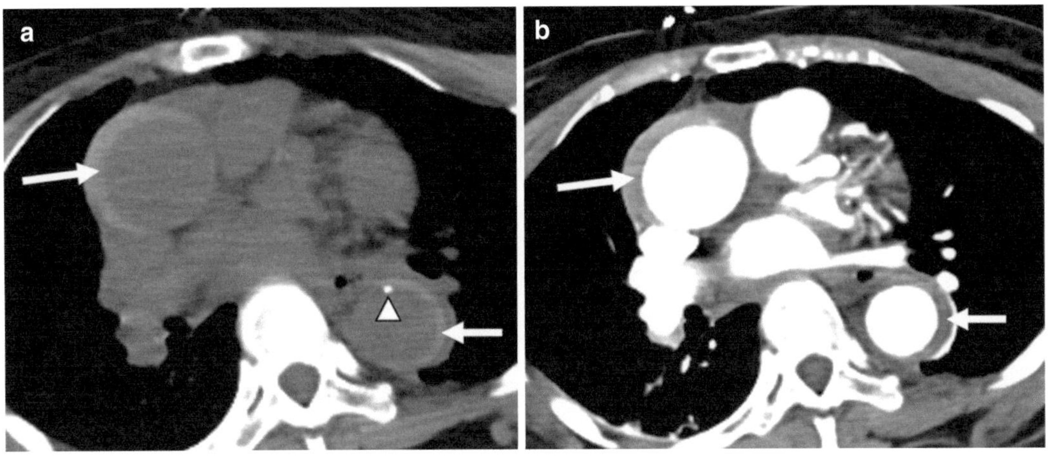

Fig. 20.17 Intramural hematoma. Axial non-contrast (**a**) and post-contrast (**b**) CT images show a crescentic type A intramural hematoma (arrows) involving both the ascending and descending thoracic aorta which is highly attenuated on the non-contrast images and lowly attenuated relative to blood pool on post-contrast images. A displaced intimal calcification is seen in the aorta on non-contrast images (arrow head)

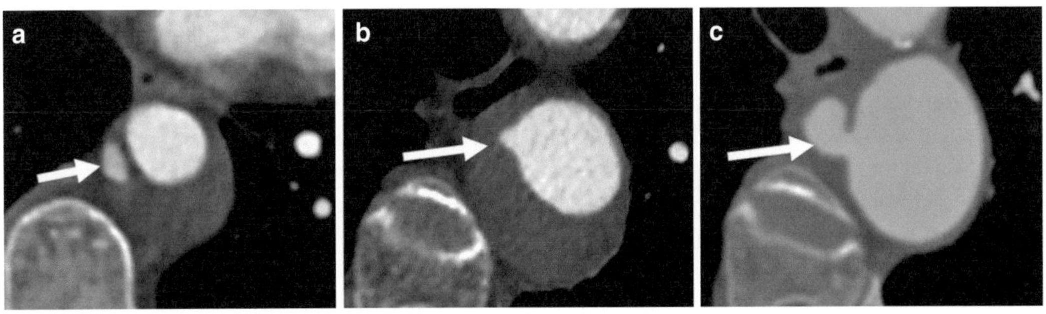

Fig. 20.18 Intramural blood pool and ulcer-like protrusion with a case of intramural hematoma. (**a**) Axial image from CTA chest in a patient with acute intramural hematoma and a small intramural blood pool within the wall (arrow), identified by intramural location and lack of communication with the lumen. (**b**) Axial image from CTA chest in a different patient with acute intramural hematoma and a small ulcer like protrusion (arrow), appearing as shallow defects in the luminal contour that extend into the wall (should be followed because of increased risk of progression to dissection or pseudoaneurysm). (**c**) Subsequent CT image in the same patient (B) 2 months later with the ulcer having evolved into a pseudoaneurysm

pools" (Fig. 20.18), also known as Chinese ring sword sign.

- Caution is advised when evaluating pooled contrast as it might mimic the appearance of contrast extravasation, which might lead to unnecessary surgical interventions.
- Ulcer-like outpouchings of contrast may indicate direct communication to the aortic lumen (unlike intramural blood pools that have no communication to the lumen) which are associated with higher risk of subsequent aneurysm and dissection formation (Fig. 20.18).

20.12.6 Penetrating Atherosclerotic Ulcer

- Defined by erosion of pre-existing atherosclerotic plaque through the intima into the media of the aortic wall with extension beyond the internal elastic lamina [14].
- Imaging findings:
  - Narrow-necked focal outpouching of contrast from the aortic lumen which bulges beyond the outer aortic contour (wide neck morphology is also possible).

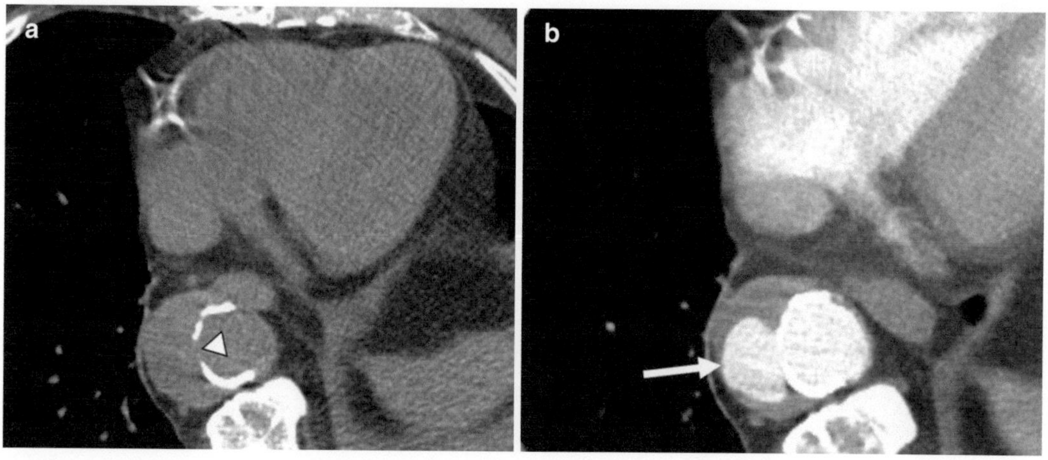

Fig. 20.19 Penetrating atherosclerotic ulcer. Axial non-contrast (**a**) and post-contrast (**b**) CT images show disrupted intimal calcification (arrowhead) and an outpouching of contrast from the aortic lumen (arrow) secondary to penetrating atherosclerotic ulcer

  - Focal disruption of atherosclerotic plaque continuity, sometimes seen as a break in calcification (Fig. 20.19).
  - Often seen intimal flap with displacement into the lumen.
- Caution should be taken to evaluate the full extent of the intima when viewing in a plane perpendicular to its long axis as the displaced intima might mimic aortic dissection (resulting in pseudo-dissection appearance).

20.13 Post-Operative Aorta

20.13.1 Thoracic Endovascular Aortic repair (TEVAR)

- Endovascular repair is the technique of choice for many patients with thoracic aortic aneurysm, particularly when disease is confined to the arch and descending thoracic aorta.
- CT is the primary modality for surveillance of aneurysm size after TEVAR.
- Post-TEVAR, aortic size should remain stable or even decrease.
- CT may also be used to evaluate for suspected post-operative complications, such as infection, stent fracture, endoleaks, stent migration.
- The imaging protocol should include a nonenhanced CT phase prior to IV contrast injection to evaluate for areas of calcification or surgical material in the aneurysm sac. Both arterial phase and delayed phase images are recommended to evaluate for aneurysm size and assess for endoleaks (some endoleaks enhance slowly and can only be identified on the delayed images, e.g., 60 seconds after the arterial phase).
- The initial arterial phase should include the entire anatomy of interest (i.e., whole chest), whereas non-contrast and delayed images may have a limited scan range of only the stented region.
- Imaging findings typically reveal shrinking aneurysm size over time (Fig. 20.20).
- Increasing aneurysm size may indicate that the aneurysm is still in communication with the stented lumen and therefore risk for aneurysm complications, e.g., aortic rupture.
- Five types of endoleaks should be differentiated:
- Type 1: Incomplete sealing of the proximal or distal stent edge, which is a particular concern with involvement of the arch stenting (due to its curvature) (Fig. 20.21).
  - Type 2: Blood flow into the aneurysm sac from retrograde flow through branch ves-

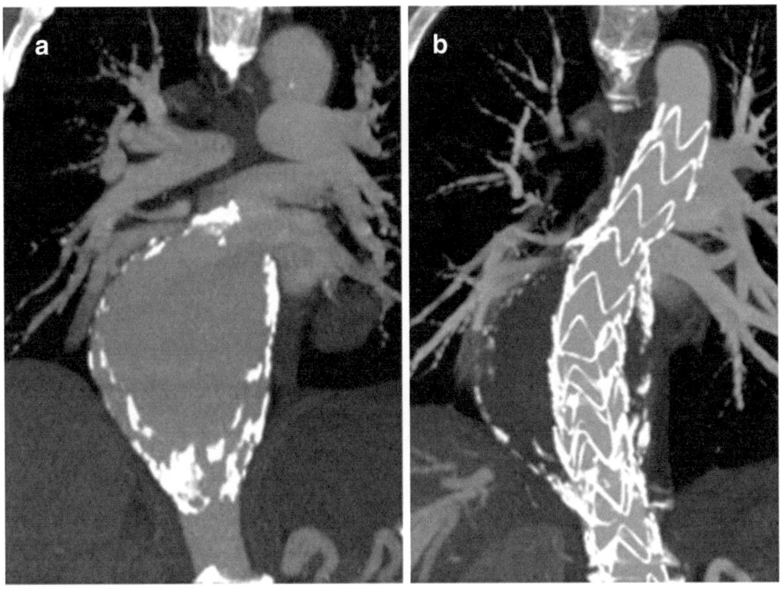

Fig. 20.20 Descending thoracic aortic aneurysm before (**a**) and after (**b**) placement of a stent graft. Note that the stent graft extends above and below the level of the aneurysm to allow for good apposition low risk of leakage

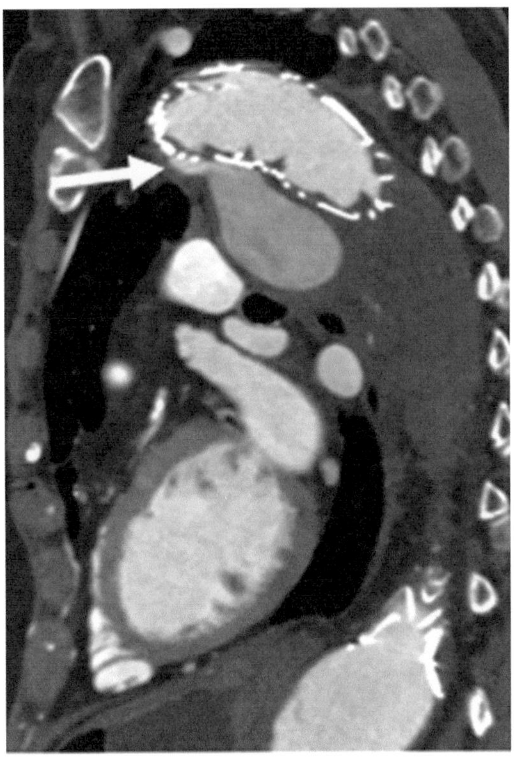

Fig. 20.21 Type I endoleak caused by incomplete seal of the proximal aspect of the thoracic aortic graft with contrast extending into the aneurysm sac from the proximal graft (arrow)

sels, most often the intercostal arteries in the thoracic aorta.

May only be seen on delayed phase

In some cases, may be selectively treated by embolization

- Type 3: Leak of blood into the aneurysm sac through a site of stent disruption, such as a stent fracture, separation of stent components (if there is more than one component), or an iatrogenically created hole in the stent fabric.
- Type 4: Slow leakage of blood/contrast from the lumen through the stent fabric into the aneurysm sac due to graft porosity. This only occurs at the time of stent placement on the immediate post-operative angiogram and is self-limited. Modern stent grafts are designed to avoid this type of endoleak.
- Type 5: Known as an endo-tension. No identifiable leak on imaging, but the aneurysm sac continues to grow.

- Other important graft findings include (Fig. 20.22):
  - Graft migration (rare).
  - Graft infection—most often identified by air within the aneurysm sac on the follow-up scans.

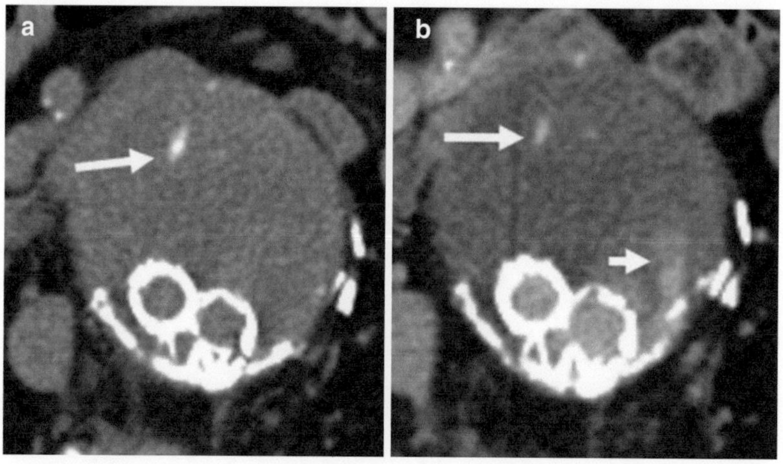

Fig. 20.22 Pre-contrast (**a**) and post-contrast delayed phase (**b**) axial CT images showing Type II endoleak in the abdominal aorta caused by retrograde flow of blood through aortic branches, likely lumbar arteries. In the thoracic aorta, retrograde flow is usually from the intercostal arteries. The leak is seen on the delayed phase (**b**, short arrow) and is important to distinguish from calcifications in the aneurysm sac (long arrow) which are seen on both pre-and post-contrast images

  - Graft fracture (rare).
  - Subclavian artery occlusion from coverage and iatrogenic embolization—in arch repair, the stent graft often covers the origin of the left subclavian artery. If this is the case, then the vessel may be purposefully occluded to prevent it acting as a source of type II endoleak. Then, a carotid to left subclavian artery bypass might be considered to ensure adequate left upper extremity blood supply (Fig. 20.23).

20.13.2 Open Surgical Repair

- CT is the modality of choice to evaluate for postsurgical complications of the aorta. Advantages include rapid acquisition time, wide availability, and the ability to perform three-dimensional reconstructions.
- The CT protocol should include a nonenhanced CT phase prior to IV contrast injection to evaluate for hyperdense surgical material that could mimic arterial bleed or pseudoaneurysm, hyperdense intramural hematoma, or blood products.

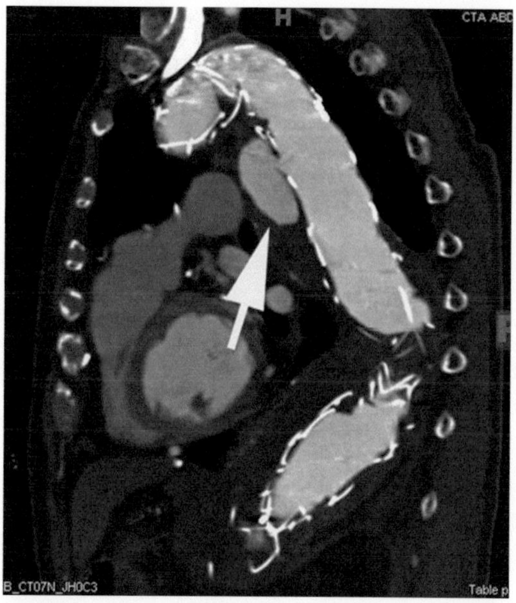

Fig. 20.23 Type III endoleak on a sagittal CTA image caused by a defect in the anterior aspect of the thoracic aortic stent graft (arrow)

- The arterial phase is the key step in evaluation for aortic complications, including active bleed, pseudoaneurysms, and dissections.
- The delayed phase could be helpful in some cases for further evaluation of suspicious find-

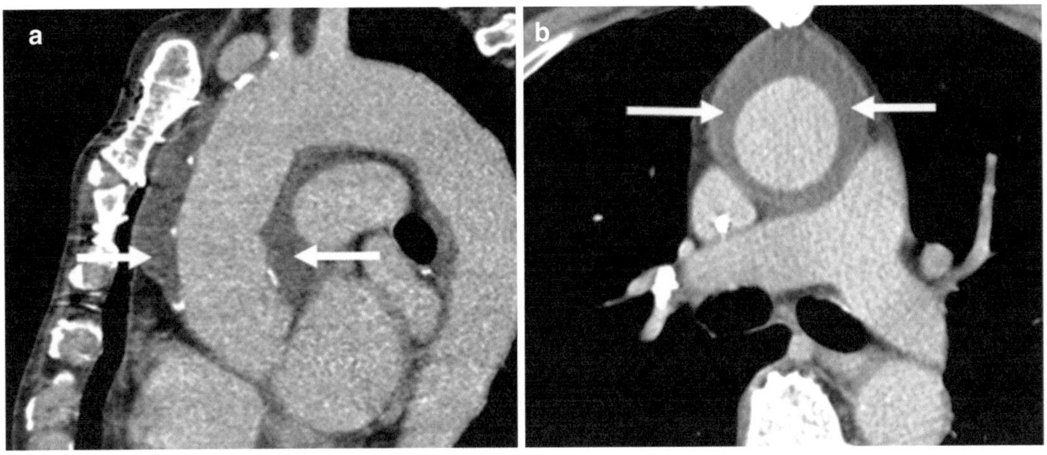

Fig. 20.24 Perigraft fluid. Axial (**a**) and coronal (**b**) CT images show low attenuation perigraft fluid in a patient with prior graft repair of the ascending aorta (arrows). This is an expected finding (as long as the fluid is confined within the excluded sac)

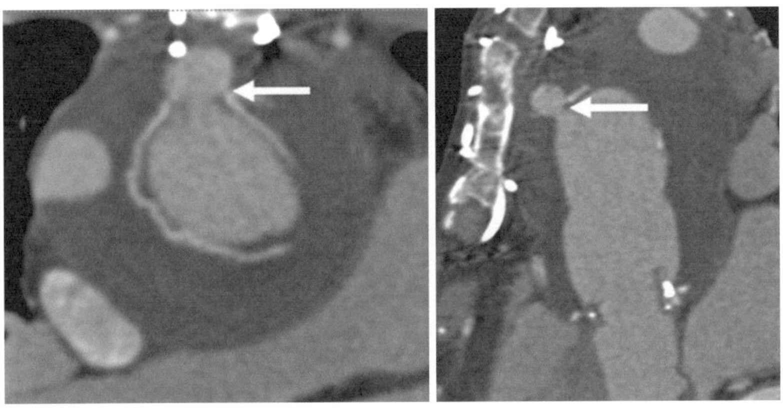

Fig. 20.25 Pseudoaneurysm. A small pseudoaneurysm developed post-operatively at the distal graft anastomosis in a patient that underwent composite graft repair of the ascending aorta and aortic valve. The pseudoaneurysm is at the anastomosis (both images below - attention at the arrow) and is secondary to a breakdown of the anastomotic site, identified by discontinuity in the surgical material (arrow)

ings such as slow leaks and false intimal flaps.

- Postsurgical complications include:
  - Substantial periaortic fluid. While some fluid surrounding the graft is a normal finding, especially in early post-operative setting, there is an increased risk of pseudoaneurysm with size >1.5 cm (Fig. 20.24).
  - Graft infection. Enlarging air-fluid collection surrounding the aortic graft, inflammatory changes in the surrounding tissues, and fistulas to adjacent structures, are concerning for infection.
  - Pseudoaneurysm, characterized by narrow-necked outpouching of contrast, most often from a leak of contrast/dehiscence in the post-operative aorta which usually develops at the graft anastomosis or at sites of intraoperative cannula placement. The finding is associated with risk of subsequent rupture and should be reported immediately. (Fig. 20.25).
- With surgical repair, the diseased aorta is replaced with a synthetic graft.
- Several different graft approaches are used and vary depending on whether there is also

replacement of the aortic valve (composite), root, or there is sparing of the native valve [18, 19].

- Two common techniques for thoracic aortic aneurysm surgeries include:
  - Interposition technique which entails replacement of the completely excised affected native aorta with a synthetic or biologic graft and yield better surgical outcomes and decreased rate of complications.
  - Inclusion technique with placement of a synthetic or biologic graft within the diseased aortic lumen, wrapping the native aorta around the graft, and creation of new space between the native aorta and graft, which may be a nidus for complications, e.g., aneurysm.
- Common surgical approaches include:
  - Supracoronary Grafts: used for ascending thoracic aortic aneurysms due to atherosclerosis with normal sinus of Valsalva. The ascending aorta is replaced distal to the coronary ostia.
  - Composite (artificial and biologic) grafts.
  - Bentall technique, i.e., implantation of a prosthetic aortic valve incorporated into a synthetic aortic graft as a single unit (Fig. 20.26), which requires implantation of excised coronary arteries from the native aorta, including a rim of aortic tissue (sometimes called a coronary button) onto the graft.
  - Cabrol procedure, involving the coronaries to be anastomosed to a prosthetic conduit, which is then sutured to the graft in a side-to-side fashion. This approach is generally less favored due to potential complications but may be indicated in patients not suitable for a modified Bentall procedure, e.g., patients with extensive atherosclerosis near the coronary ostia, excessive proximity of the coronary ostia to the aortic annulus, or redo procedures. (Fig. 20.27).
  - Valve-Sparing procedures entail the resection of the native aorta down to the level of valve insertions within the sinuses of Valsalva, with the preservation of the native aortic valve. The sinuses are reconstructed with a scalloped polyethylene (Dacron) graft, which is then attached to the remaining aortic tissue above the valve insertion. The coronary arteries are reimplanted onto the aortic graft.

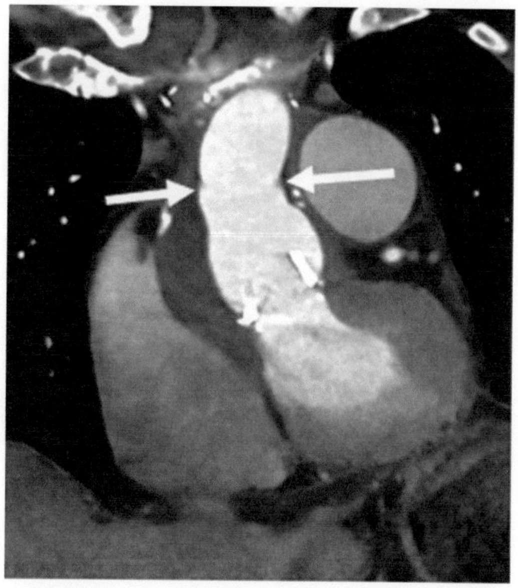

Fig. 20.26 Composite ascending aortic graft. Coronal CT angiogram image shows a composite graft with high attenuation struts of the bioprosthetic aortic valve and short synthetic graft that is anastomosed to the native distal ascending aorta (arrows)

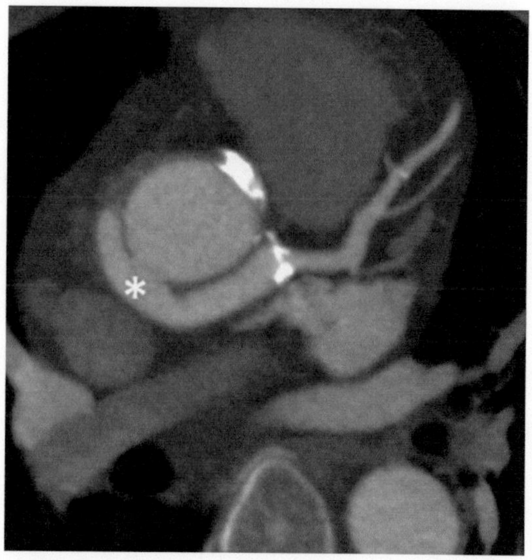

Fig. 20.27 Cabrol procedure. Axial MIP images showing changes of a Cabrol procedure, recognizable by the presence of a tubular graft supplying the left main coronary artery from the aortic graft (asterisk)

20.14 Pulmonary Artery

- The normal anatomy of the main pulmonary artery (mPA) typically reveals its origin as a continuation of the superior portion of the right ventricular outflow tract (RVOT), just distal to the pulmonary valve.
- The pulmonary artery courses posteriorly and along the left aspect of the ascending thoracic aorta and bifurcates into right and left pulmonary arteries.
- Additional smaller branches can commonly arise directly from the mPA such as the right interlobar artery.
- Normal dimensions derived from the Framingham Heart Study cohort revealed a mean mPA diameter of 25.1 ± 2.8 mm, derived from axial images just proximal to the bifurcation on a non-contrast chest CT [20].
- Dilatation of the main pulmonary artery is usually associated with pulmonary arterial hypertension (PAH).
- The 90th percentile cutoff for the mPA among men was 28.9 mm and 26.9 mm for women [20].
- For simplicity, cutoffs of 29 mm for men and 27 mm for women is a common practice in the clinical setting.
- Dilatation of the mPA is commonly reported with a diameter exceeding 33 mm or a mPA to aortic ratio (ratio of mPA to the mid-ascending aorta) of more than 1.1. However, these values vary with patient age, sex, and body surface area.
- Causes of mPA dilatation include pulmonary hypertension, left to right shunting, pulmonary arteriovenous malformation.
- Pulmonary valve stenosis may be seen with the following conditions:
  - Infection, e.g., tuberculosis, syphilis.
  - Vasculitis, e.g., Takayasu arteritis, Behcet disease.
  - Connective tissue disease, e.g., Marfan syndrome, Loeys-Dietz syndrome, Ehlers-Danlos syndrome
  - Traumatic/iatrogenic.

References

1. Hager A, Kaemmerer H, Rapp-Bernhardt U, Blücher S, Rapp K, Bernhardt TM, Galanski M, Hess J. Diameters of the thoracic aorta throughout life as measured with helical computed tomography. J Thorac Cardiovasc Surg. 2002;123(6):1060–6. ISSN 0022-5223.
2. Rogers IS, Massaro JM, Truong QA, Mahabadi AA, Kriegel MF, Fox CS, Thanassoulis G, Isselbacher EM, Hoffmann U, O'Donnell CJ. Distribution, determinants, and normal reference values of thoracic and abdominal aortic diameters by computed tomography (from the Framingham heart study). Am J Cardiol. 2013;111(10):1510–6. https://doi.org/10.1016/j.amjcard.2013.01.306. Epub 2013 Mar 13. PMID: 23497775; PMCID: PMC3644324.
3. Freeman LA, Young PM, Foley TA, Williamson EE, Bruce C, Greason KL. CT and MRI assessment of the aortic root and ascending aorta. AJR Am J Roentgenol. 2013;200(6):W581–92.
4. Ramos-Duran L, Nance JW, Schoepf UJ, et al. Developmental aortic arch anomalies in infants and children assessed with CT angiography. AJR Am J Roentgenol. 2012;198(5):W466–74. https://doi.org/10.2214/AJR.11.6982.
5. Karacan A, Türkvatan A, Karacan K. Anatomical variations of aortic arch branching: evaluation with computed tomographic angiography. Cardiol Young. 2014;24(03):485–93. https://doi.org/10.1017/S1047951113000656.
6. Morgan-Hughes GJ, Marshall AJ, Roobottom C. Morphologic assessment of patent ductus arteriosus in adults using retrospectively ECG-gated multidetector CT. AJR Am J Roentgenol. 2003;181(3):749–54. https://doi.org/10.2214/ajr.181.3.1810749.
7. Wang TKM, Desai MY. Thoracic aortic aneurysm: optimal surveillance and treatment. Cleve Clin J Med. 2020;87(9):557–68. https://doi.org/10.3949/ccjm.87a.19140-1. PMID: 32868306
8. Munden R, Carter B, Chiles C, et al. Managing incidental findings on thoracic CT: mediastinal and cardiovascular findings. A white paper of the ACR incidental findings committee. J Am Coll Radiol. 2018;15(8):1087–96. https://doi.org/10.1016/j.jacr.2018.04.029.
9. Litmanovich D, Bankier AA, Cantin L, et al. CT and MRI in diseases of the aorta. AJR Am J Roentgenol. 2009;193(4):928–40. https://doi.org/10.2214/AJR.08.2166.
10. Atar E, Belenky A, Hadad M, et-al. MR angiography for abdominal and thoracic aortic aneurysms: assessment before endovascular repair in patients with impaired renal function. AJR Am J Roentgenol. 2006;186(2):386–93. https://doi.org/10.2214/AJR.04.0449.
11. Loeys BL, et al. Revised Ghent criteria for the diagnosis of Marfan syndrome (MFS) and related con-

ditions. J Med Genet. 2010;47:476–85. https://doi.org/10.1136/jmg.2009.072785.

12. Devereux RB, de Simone G, Arnett DK, Best LG, Boerwinkle E, Howard BV, Kitzman D, Lee ET, Mosley TH Jr, Weder A, Roman MJ. Normal limits in relation to age, body size and gender of two-dimensional echocardiographic aortic root dimensions in persons ≥15 years of age. Am J Cardiol. 2012;110(8):1189–94. https://doi.org/10.1016/j.amjcard.2012.05.063. Epub 2012 Jul 6. PMID: 22770936; PMCID: PMC3462295.
13. Gulati A, Bagga A. Large vessel vasculitis. Pediatr Nephrol. 2010;25(6):1037–48.
14. Maddu KK, Shuaib W, Telleria J, Johnson JO, Khosa F. Nontraumatic acute aortic emergencies: part 1, acute aortic syndrome. AJR Am J Roentgenol. 2014;202(3):656–65. https://doi.org/10.2214/AJR.13.11437. PMID: 24555605.
15. Lombardi JV, Hughes GC, Appoo JJ, Bavaria JE, Beck AW, Cambria RP, Charlton-Ouw K, Eslami MH, Kim KM, Leshnower BG, Maldonado T, Reece TB, Wang GJ. Society for Vascular Surgery (SVS) and Society of Thoracic Surgeons (STS) reporting standards for type B aortic dissections. Ann Thorac Surg. 2020;109(3):959–81. https://doi.org/10.1016/j.athoracsur.2019.10.005. Epub 2020 Jan 27. PMID: 32000979.
16. MacGillivray TE, Gleason TG, Patel HJ, Aldea GS, Bavaria JE, Beaver TM, Chen EP, Czerny M, Estrera AL, Firestone S, Fischbein MP, Hughes GC, Hui DS, Kissoon K, Lawton JS, Pacini D, Reece TB, Roselli EE, Stulak J. The Society of Thoracic Surgeons/American Association for Thoracic Surgery clinical practice guidelines on the Management of Type B Aortic Dissection. Ann Thorac Surg. 2022;113(4):1073–92. https://doi.org/10.1016/j.athoracsur.2021.11.002. Epub 2022 Jan 25. PMID: 35090687.
17. Gutschow SE, Walker CM, Martínez-Jiménez S, Rosado-de-Christenson ML, Stowell J, Kunin JR. Emerging concepts in intramural hematoma imaging. Radiographics. 2016;36(3):660–74. https://doi.org/10.1148/rg.2016150094. PMID: 27163587.
18. Marquis KM, Naeem M, Rajput MZ, Raptis DA, Steinbrecher KL, Ohman JW, Bhalla S, Raptis CA. CT of postoperative repair of the ascending aorta and aortic arch. Radiographics. 2021;41(5):1300–20. https://doi.org/10.1148/rg.2021210026. Epub 2021 Aug 20. PMID: 34415808.
19. Prescott-Focht JA, Martinez-Jimenez S, Hurwitz LM, Hoang JK, Christensen JD, Ghoshhajra BB, Abbara S. Ascending thoracic aorta: postoperative imaging evaluation. Radiographics. 2013;33(1):73–85. https://doi.org/10.1148/rg.331125090. PMID: 23322828.
20. Truong QA, Massaro JM, Rogers IS, Mahabadi AA, Kriegel MF, Fox CS, O'Donnell CJ, Hoffmann U. Reference values for normal pulmonary artery dimensions by noncontrast cardiac computed tomography: the Framingham Heart Study. Circ Cardiovasc Imaging. 2012;5(1):147–54. https://doi.org/10.1161/CIRCIMAGING.111.968610. Epub 2011 Dec 16. PMID: 22178898; PMCID: PMC3275437.

21 CT for Congenital Heart Disease

Cristina Fuss

Abstract

Congenital heart disease (CHD) accounts for most birth defects in the USA. Many affected patients will survive to adulthood in variable stages of repair. The evaluation of CHD is challenging given the complexity of defects and small organ size, particularly in infancy. CT's excellent spatial image resolution is helpful in CHD but children require special attention to radiation exposure and contrast dose. Imaging of repaired heart disease requires knowledge of the altered physiology. This chapter provides an overview of cardiac CT's role in the evaluation and management of CHD.

Keywords

Congenital heart disease (CHD) · Critical congenital heart disease (cCHD) · Computed tomography angiography (CTA) · Tetralogy of Fallot (ToF) · Ventricle septum defect (VSD) · Atrial septum defect (ASD) · Transposition of the great arteries (TGA) · Total anomalous pulmonary venous return (TAPVR) · Anomalous left coronary artery of the pulmonary artery (ALCAPA) · Truncus arteriosus (TA)

C. Fuss (✉)
Yale University, New Haven, CT, USA
e-mail: cristina.fuss@yale.edu

Abbreviations

Ao	Aorta
aAo	Ascending aorta
ALCAPA	Anomalous left coronary artery of the pulmonary artery
ARCAPA	Anomalous right coronary artery of the pulmonary artery
AV canal	Atrioventricular canal
ASD	Atrial septal defect
CHD	Congenital heart disease
cHCD	Critical congenital heart disease
CS	Coronary sinus
CTA	Computed tomography angiography
CCTA	Cardiac computed tomography angiography
dAo	Descending aorta
DILV	Double inlet left ventricle
DORV	Double outlet right ventricle
ECG	Electrocardiography
HLHS	Hypoplastic left heart syndrome
HU	Hounsfield units
IVC	Inferior vena cava
LA	Left atrium
LPA	Left pulmonary artery
LPV	Left pulmonary veins
LSVC	Left superior vena cava
LV	Left ventricle
LVOT	Left ventricular outflow tract
MAPCA	Major aortopulmonary collateral arteries

A. A. Zadeh, J. Hoe (eds.), *Practical Guide to Cardiac CT*,
https://doi.org/10.1007/978-981-97-6919-3_21

MDCT	Multi-detector computed topography
MPA	Main pulmonary artery
MRA	Magnetic resonance angiography
PA	Pulmonary artery
PAPVR	Partial anomalous pulmonary venous return
PDA	Patent ductus arteriosus
PFO	Patent foramen oval
PV	Pulmonary veins
RA	Right atrium
RPA	Right pulmonary artery
RPV	Right pulmonary veins
RV	Right ventricle
RVOT	Right ventricular outflow tract
SVC	Superior vena cava
TA	Truncus arteriosus
TAPVR	Total anomalous pulmonary venous return
ToF	Tetralogy of Fallot
TGA	Transposition of the great arteries
VSD	Ventricle septum defect

21.1 Introduction

- More than 40,000 children are born with congenital heart disease (CHD) in the USA each year [1, 2]. This represents approximately 1% of all live births and attributes to the largest group of birth defects related mortality [3].
- Despite an overall decrease in infant mortality, the number of children born with CHD has increased over the past years from an estimated worldwide prevalence of 0.6 per 1000 live births around 1930 to 9.1 per 1000 live births after 1995 [4, 5].
- More than 97% of children born with noncritical CHD and 69% of children born with critical CHD are expected to reach adulthood.

21.2 Role of Imaging

- Initial imaging of critical CHD usually occurs during early infancy, requiring special considerations [6].
- Adequate patient preparation and close communication with the care teams are critical for successful and safe CT acquisition [7].
- Radiation doses have decreased significantly with the advent of the newer generation volume and high pitch scanners, resulting in average radiation doses of less than 1 (0.5–2) mSv in infants [8, 9].
- Diagnostic accuracy of modern CT systems can add invaluable information about existing comorbidities and therefore provide a more detailed clinical picture [10].

21.3 Scan Preparation for Infants and Children

Before the scan:

- Clear communication about the clinical question.
- Adequate intravenous access.
  - Upper extremity peripheral iv access versus central line.
  - Peripherally inserted catheters not ideal due to small caliber and resultant slow flow rates.
- Adequate sedation.
  - Can be “feed and swaddle” on a newborn but may require short sedation for older newborn.
- Positioning on the table.
  - No additional padding/blankets as they increase the radiation dose.
  - Centered within the iso-center and aligned along the z-axis.
  - ONE warm blanket may help with calming fussy patient.
- Communication with the technologist.
  - Adequate protocol tailored to clinical question. Unnecessary z-axis extension increases radiation dose.
  - Contrast dose:

    1–1.5 mL/kg body weight non-ionic iodine-based contrast, containing 300 mg iodine per mL (higher concentrated contrast media is possible; overall dose needs to be adjusted)

- Contrast injection technique:
  Manual in smaller IVs and/or suboptimal locations; for example, dorsum of hand.
  Power injector with lower flow rates (2–3 mL/s).
- ECG gating.
  - If very tachycardic, external heart beat ("chicken heart") may be applied.
- Variable set-up depending on scanner type and clinical question.

During scan:

- Close monitoring for unexpected heart rate variations.
- Sedation and vital signs.
- Depending on the size of infant, bolus triggering/time to peak may not be necessary (i.e., inject then scan). In older children, region of interest placed over ascending aorta with threshold of 150 Hounsfield Units (HU).

Scan:

- Include only necessary anatomy (Fig. 21.1).
- Know anatomic landmarks.
- Hyperdynamic infants may require immediate scan following contrast administration without further delay.

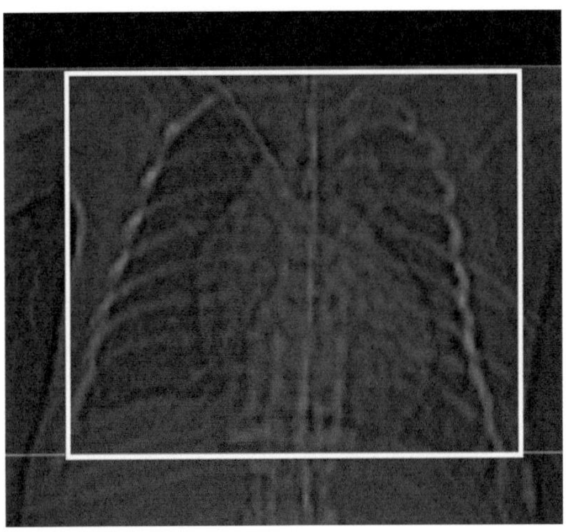

Fig. 21.1. "Scanogram" of 1-day-old infant with concern for aortic arch disease, thus including the upper thorax portion in the field-of-view. Note the scan stopped at the base of the cardiac border

- Low kV setting (80 kV) allows for optimal contrast opacification along the iodine k-edge.

Postscan processing:

- Multiple phase reconstruction determined by scan length.
  - If HR is 120 bpm, R-R interval is 500 ms. Scan time acquisition of, for example, 250 ms (volume scanner) will invariably acquire ¼ of cardiac cycle.
- Thin slice reconstruction: 1 mm or less.
- Knowledge of post-processing software, allowing for cross-sectional oblique assessment of all cardiac structures.

21.4 Evaluating Structural Cardiac Anatomy for CHD

- Evaluating CHD can be challenging and requires a structural approach to its anatomy addressing the position of the atria, ventricles, atrioventricular/ventriculoarterial connections, great vessels and associated malformations each and every time.

21.4.1 Atria

- The shape of the atrial appendages and venous connection define the right and left atrium. The right atrium is broad-based, whereas the left atrium has a narrow neck. The inferior vena cava invariably connects with the right atrium (Fig. 21.2).

21.4.2 Ventricles

- The right ventricle is defined by the presence of the moderator band; the left ventricle by the presence of the myocardium (Fig. 21.3).
- The position of the right and left ventricles defines the cardiac axis. The left ventricle has smooth walls; the right ventricular walls are trabeculated.

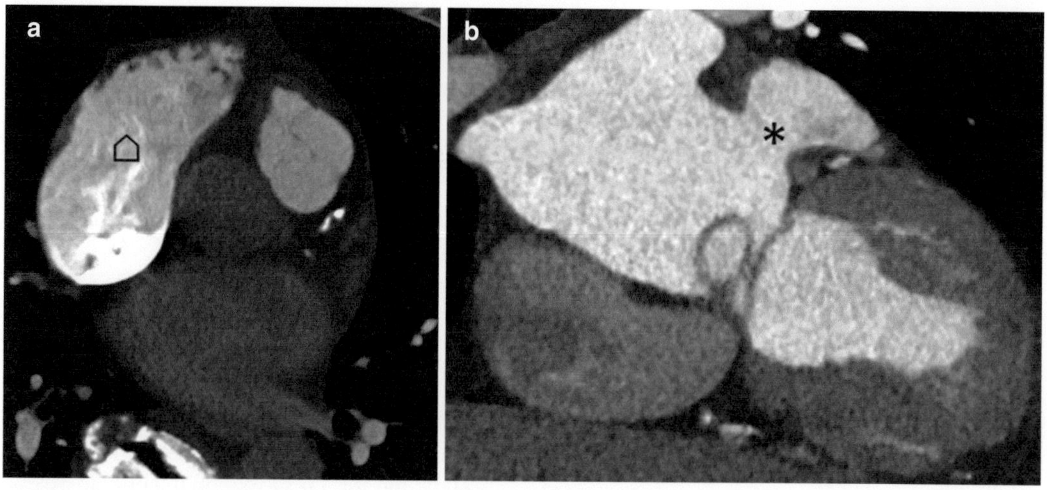

Fig. 21.2 Anatomic features of the atria. **Panel** (**a**) Axial contrast-enhanced CTA depicting broad-based right atrial appendage (⌂). **Panel** (**b**) Coronal contrast-enhanced CTA depicting narrow neck of the left atrial appendage (*)

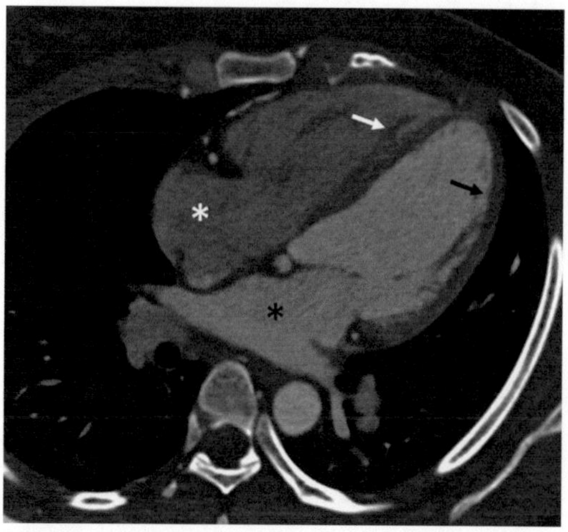

Fig. 21.3 Anatomical features of the ventricles. Axial contrast-enhanced images depicting a normal situs (Situs solitus). Right (white asterisk) and left (black asterisk) atria. Moderator band (white arrow) defining the right ventricle. Thick myocardium (black arrow) defining the left ventricle

- The right ventricle connects to a tricuspid atrioventricular valve (tricuspid valve). The left ventricle to a bicuspid atrioventricular valve (mitral valve).
- The aorto-mitral continuity is smooth without intervening myocardium (Fig. 21.4).

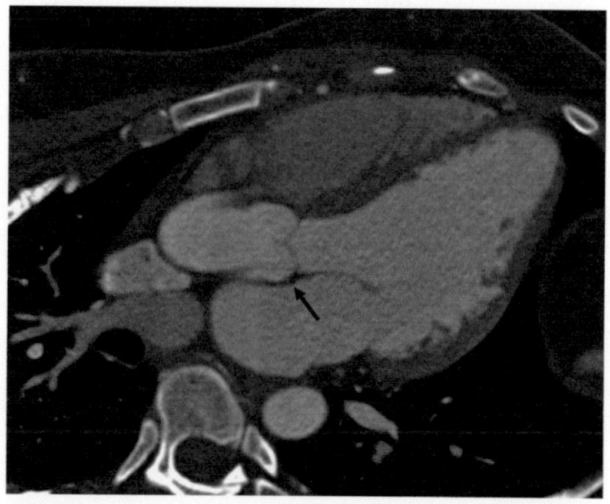

Fig. 21.4 Anatomic features of the left ventricle. Contrast-enhanced CT images of the left ventricular outflow tract demonstrating the aorto-mitral continuity (black arrow) without intervening myocardium

21.4.3 Connections

- Assess for concordance (normal) versus discordant (abnormal) atrioventricular and ventriculoarterial connections.

21.4.4 Aorta

- Describe location of ascending/descending aorta and aortic arch position.

21.4.5 Associated Abnormalities

- Atrial or ventricular septal defects, hypoplasia/aplasia of atrioventricular and pulmonic/systemic valves.

21.5 Noncritical CHD

CHD occurs as noncritical and critical (also known as cyanotic) CHD. Critical CHD presents with neonatal cyanosis and requires repair in the first year of life. Noncyanotic CHD is considered noncritical and often manifests later in life.

Common examples of noncritical CHD include:

- Ventricular septal defect (VSD) (Fig. 21.5).
- Atrial septal defect (ASD) (Fig. 21.6).
- Coronary anomalies (discussed in Chap. 10) (Fig. 21.7).
- Aortic (valve) disease (discussed in Chap. 19) (Fig. 21.8).
- Partial anomalous pulmonary venous return (Fig. 21.9, 21.10 and 21.11).
- L-transposition of the great arteries (Fig. 21.12).

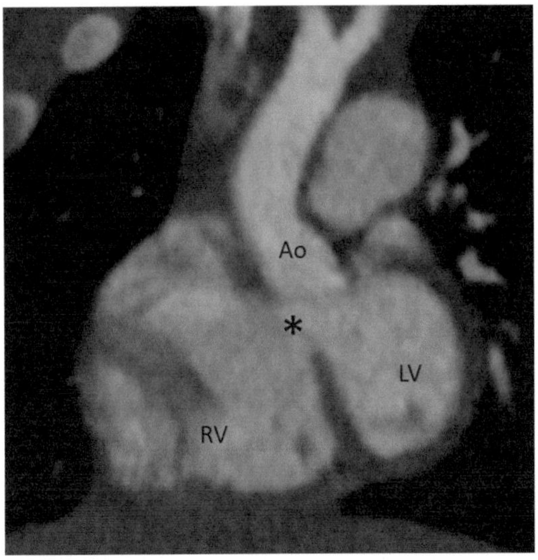

Fig. 21.5 Coronal reconstruction of contrast-enhanced CT depicting a conoventricular ventricle septum defect (VSD) (*) with right and left ventricles (RV/LV) and aorta (Ao)

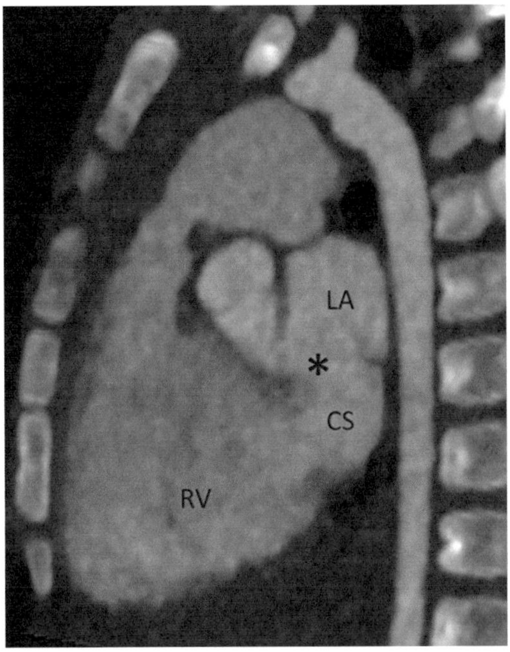

Fig. 21.6 Atrial septal defect. Case example of an unroofed coronary sinus atrial septal defect (ASD) with sagittal reconstructed image of contrast-enhanced CT depicting unroofed coronary sinus (CS) creating an ASD (*) by communicating with the left atrium (LA)

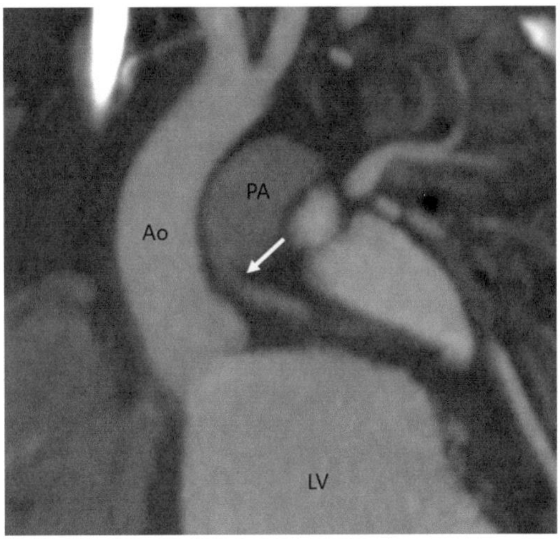

Fig. 21.7 Case example of anomalous origin of the left coronary artery from the pulmonary artery (ALCAPA). Coronal maximum-intensity-projection (MIP) image depicting anomalous origin of the left main coronary artery (white arrow) off the pulmonary artery (PA). Note that no vessel arises from the aorta (Ao)

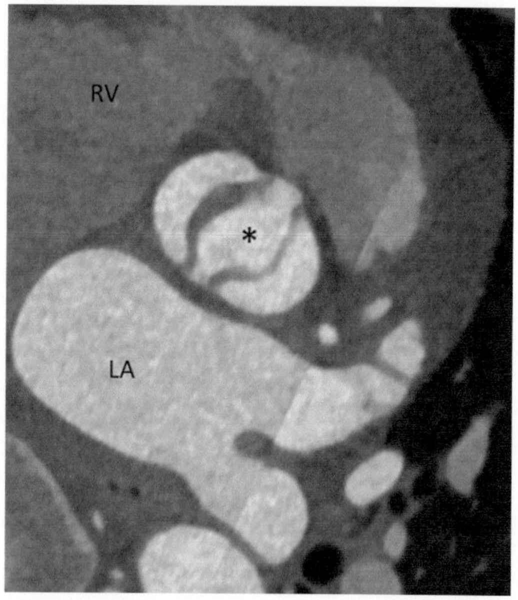

Fig. 21.8 Case example of a bicuspid aortic valve. *En face* view of the aortic valve depicting two equal sized cusps with two commissures, consistent with bicuspid aortic valve Sievers type 0 [11]

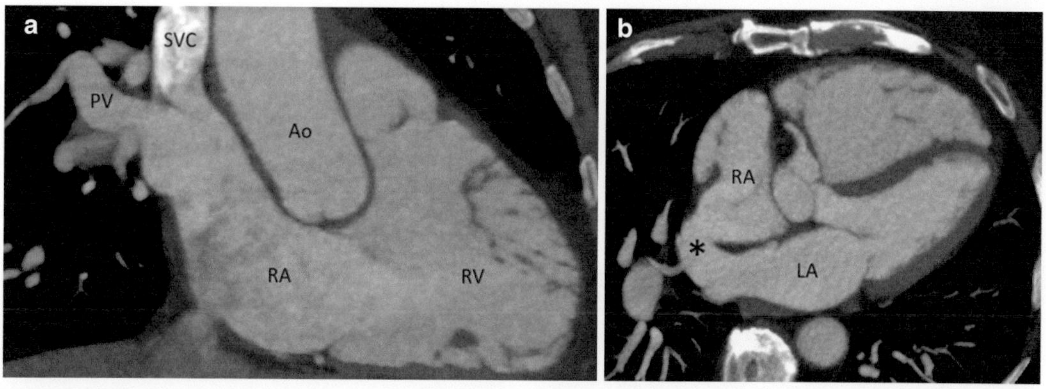

Fig. 21.9 Case example of **the** right upper lobe partial anomalous pulmonary venous return (PAPVR) associated with sinus venous ASD. Panel (**a**) shows a coronal reformatted image of contrast-enhanced CT depicting anomalous drainage of the right upper lobe pulmonary veins (PV) into the superior vena cava (SVC). Panel (**b**) shows an axial image of contrast-enhanced CT demonstrating an ASD at the level of the coronary sinus (black asterisk)

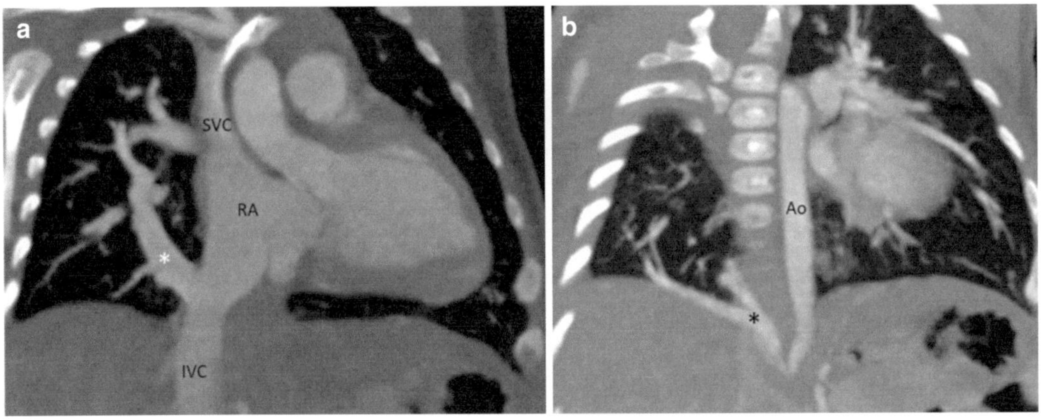

Fig. 21.10 Scimitar syndrome (veno-lobar pulmonary syndrome) [12]. Panel (**a**) shows a coronal reformatted image of contrast-enhanced CT depicting anomalous pulmonary venous drainage of the right lung (white asterisk) into the inferior vena cava (IVC). Panel (**b**) displays an oblique coronal reformatted image of contrast-enhanced CT depicting associated partial systemic arterial supply of the right lung (pulmonary sequestration) (black asterisk) and hypoplastic right lung

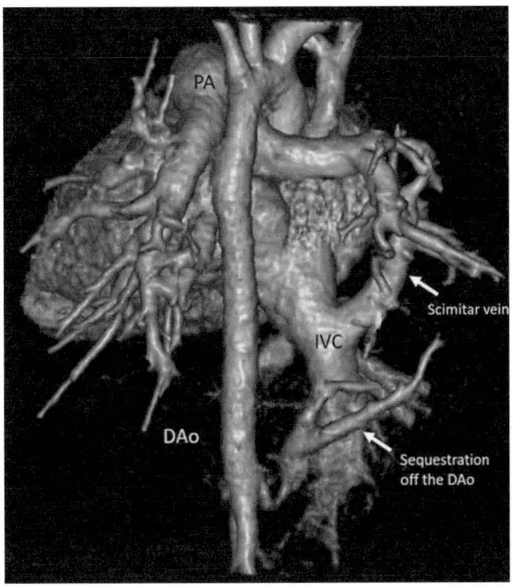

Fig. 21.11 Posterior view of 3-D reformatted contrast-enhanced CTA depicting anomalous pulmonary venous drainage of the right lung (scimitar vein) into the inferior vena cava (IVC) and associated partial systemic arterial supply of the right lung (pulmonary sequestration arising off the descending aorta)

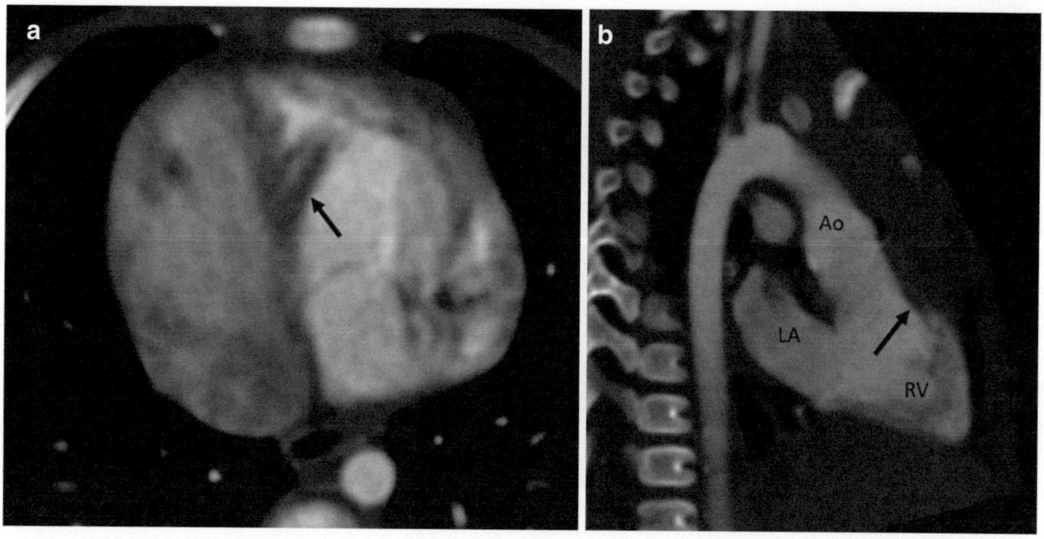

Fig. 21.12 Case example of L-transposition of the great arteries (also known as "congenitally corrected transposition"). Panel (**a**) shows an axial contrast-enhanced coronary CT image depicting the moderator band in the leftward, morphologic right ventricle serving as "systemic" ventricle. Panel (**b**) displays a three-chamber view depicting atrioventricular discordance of morphologic left atrium (LA) connecting to morphologic right ventricle (RV) and ventriculoarterial discordance of morphologic right ventricle (RV) connecting to the aorta (Ao)

21.6 Evaluation for Noncritical CHD

- While the adult heart rate usually ranges between 50 and 80 bpm, infants may have heart rates of 150 bpm or more, posing challenges to image acquisition.
- Modern CT scanners enable image acquisition with sub-millimeter special resolution and very low temporal resolution [13].
- The speed of image acquisition eliminates the need for respiratory suspension and anesthesia, while acquiring images of the entire thorax including pulmonary anatomy if desired.
- Iodinated intravenous contrast is applied in almost all scans, using 1–2 mL/kg as dose reference.
- Adverse contrast reactions are extremely rare, ranging from 0.1% to 1% in the adult and 0.18% to 0.46% in the pediatric patient population [14, 15].
- Contrast is administered preferably via the antecubital vein with bolus tracking or timing bolus to optimize scan timing [16].

21.6.1 Ventricular Septal Defect (Fig. 21.5)

- Echocardiography is the modality of choice for assessment of VSDs and ASDs. However, CTA is increasingly utilized prior to catheter guided interventions/closures of these septal defects [17].
- Most common CHD; 2.6 per 1100 live births worldwide [4, 5]·
- Often diagnosed after birth, if symptomatic; can close spontaneously [2]·
- Four VSD types [18]:
  - Conoventricular: Between the conal and ventricular septum; usually due to hypoplasia and/or malalignment of the conal septum.
  - Conal septal: Defect within the conal septum.
  - Atrioventricular canal: Complete (AV canal) or partial absence of the canal part of the septum.
  - Muscular: Myocardial defects; often close spontaneously.

21.6.2 Atrial Septal Defect (Fig. 21.6)

- Atrial septal defects represent the second most common CHD (after VSD, disregarding PFO) with 1.6 per 1100 live births worldwide [4].
- Five ASD types:

  - Patent foramen ovale (PFO, most common but not considered CHD).
  - Ostium secundum defect (most common ASD).
  - Ostium primum defect.
  - Sinus venosus defect (superior; inferior).
  - Coronary sinus ASD.

21.6.3 Coronary Anomalies (See Chap. 10)

- Acquisition and reporting parameters for coronary CTA have been published by the Society of Cardiovascular Computed Tomography (SCCT) [19, 20].
- These guidelines apply to both pediatric and adult patients for the evaluation of coronary anomalies.
- Abnormal origin, course, and terminus (Fig. 21.7).
- CT as initial diagnostic tool allows for complete assessment while observing the ALARA principle [21].

21.6.4 Aortic Valve Disease (See Chap. 19)

- Bicuspid aortic valve is the most common congenital valvular disorder, affecting 1–2% of the population.
- Bicuspid aortic valves affect more males than females and are associated with morbidity in adulthood.

21.6.5 Partial Anomalous Pulmonary Venous Return (Figs. 21.9, 21.10, 21.11)

21.6.6 L-Transposition of the Great Arteries (Fig. 21.12)

21.7 Critical (Cyanotic) CHD

- Assessment of both systemic arterial and pulmonary venous congenital anomalies has been a hallmark of CT given its high spatial and low temporal resolution [22–24].
- CTA is particularly suitable to assess the aorta before and after catheter-based therapy, such as stents and endografts [25, 26].
- Patients with both repaired and unrepaired aortic coarctation should undergo evaluation of the entire aorta and have regular follow-up by CTA or MRA [27].
- Image acquisition is tailored based on the interrogated vessel with ROI placed accordingly to optimized contrast opacification [16].

Types of Critical CHD:

- Severe aortic coarctation (Fig. 21.13).
- Double outlet right ventricle.
- D-transposition of the great arteries (Fig. 21.14).
- Epstein anomaly (Fig. 21.15).
- Hypoplastic left heart syndrome (Fig. 21.16).
- Interrupted aortic arch (Fig. 21.17).
- Pulmonary atresia.
- Single ventricle.
- Tertalogy of Fallot (Figs. 21.18 and 21.19).
- Total anomalous pulmonary venous return (Figs. 21.20 and 21.21).
- Tricuspid atresia (Fig. 21.22).
- Truncus arteriosus.

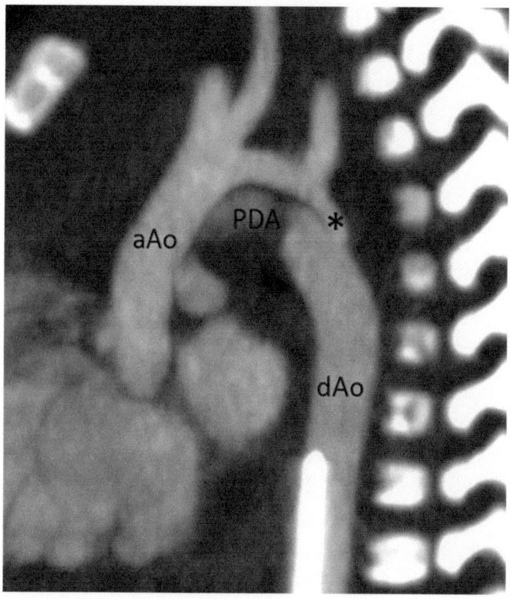

Fig. 21.13 A case example of aortic coarctation. Sagittal MIP-image depicting discrete severe aortic coarctation (asterisk) with patent ductus arteriosus (PDA) supplying blood flow to the descending aorta (dAo). Note the tip of an umbilical arterial catheter in the dAo

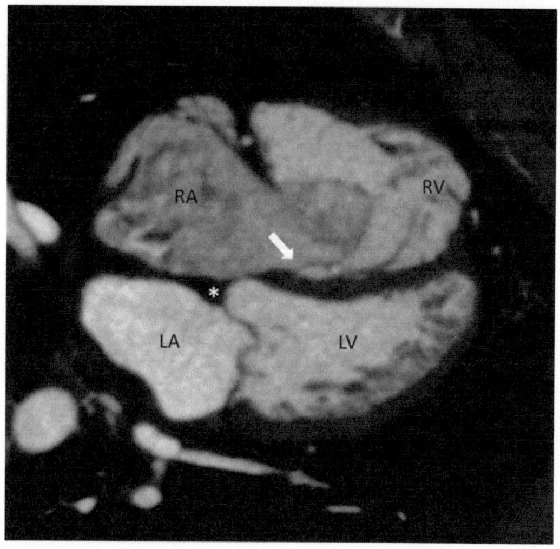

Fig. 21.15 Ebstein's anomaly. Four-chamber view of contrast-enhanced CTA depicting downward displacement of the septal tricuspid leaflet (white arrow) with respect to the septal mitral leaflet insertion (white asterisk), resulting in "atrialization" of the right ventricle (RV). Note the markedly enlarged right heart and interventricular septal straightening due to elevated right heart pressures

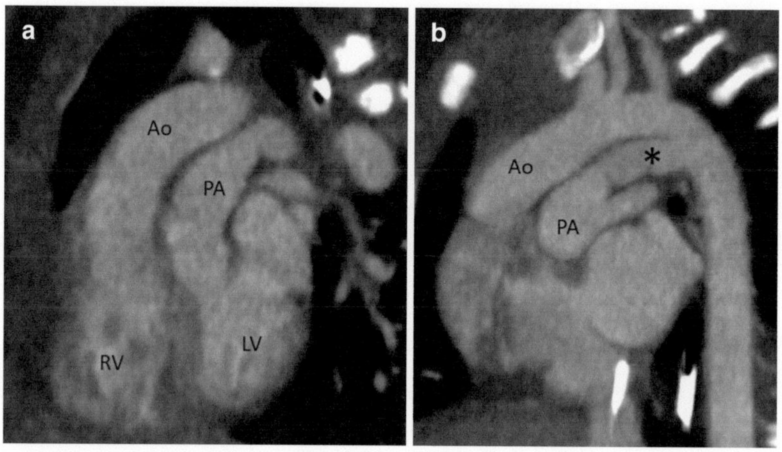

Fig. 21.14 D-Transposition of the great arteries with patent ductus arteriosus. Sagittal reformatted images of contrast-enhanced CTA depicting **a**) anterior, morphologic right ventricle (RV) giving rise to the aorta (Ao) and posterior, morphologic left ventricle (LV) giving rise to the pulmonary artery (PA) with typical "double-barrel" appearance of the great arties. **b**) Due to two separate circulations only survivable with large shunt, as in this case a patent ductus arteriosus (black asterisk)

21.7.1 Aortic Coarctation (Fig. 21.13)

- Typical location: Aortic isthmus.
- Common associated anomalies:

  - Bicuspid aortic valve.
  - PDA.
  - VSD.
  - Turner syndrome.

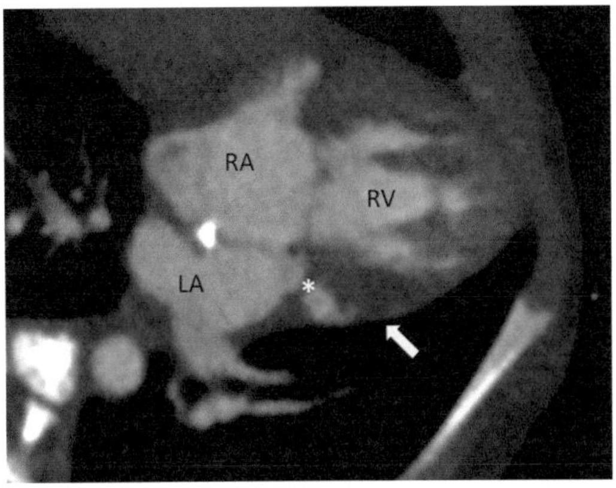

Fig. 21.16 Hypoplastic left heart syndrome (HLHS). Four-chamber view of contrast-enhanced congenital CTA depicting severely hypoplastic mitral valve (white asterisk) and left ventricle (white arrow)

21.7.2 Double Outlet Right Ventricle (DORV)

- Rare; less than 1% of all CHD [28].
- Both aorta and pulmonary arteries arise of the morphologic RV by min. 50% circumference.
- CTA for presurgical planning and assessment of comorbidities [29].
- Usually associated with large VSD; restriction of VSD determines severity.
- Four types [30, 31].
  - VSD type (24%): VSD without pulmonic stenosis.
  - TOF type (36%): VSD with pulmonic stenosis.
  - TGA/Taussig-Bing type (18%): Subpulmonic VSD with LVOT flow directed toward the PA.
  - DORV non-committed VSD type (22%).

21.7.3 D-Transposition of the Great Arteries (Fig. 21.14)

- Atrioventricular concordance with ventriculo-arterial discordance.
- Only survivable with shunt (PDA, ASD, and VSD).

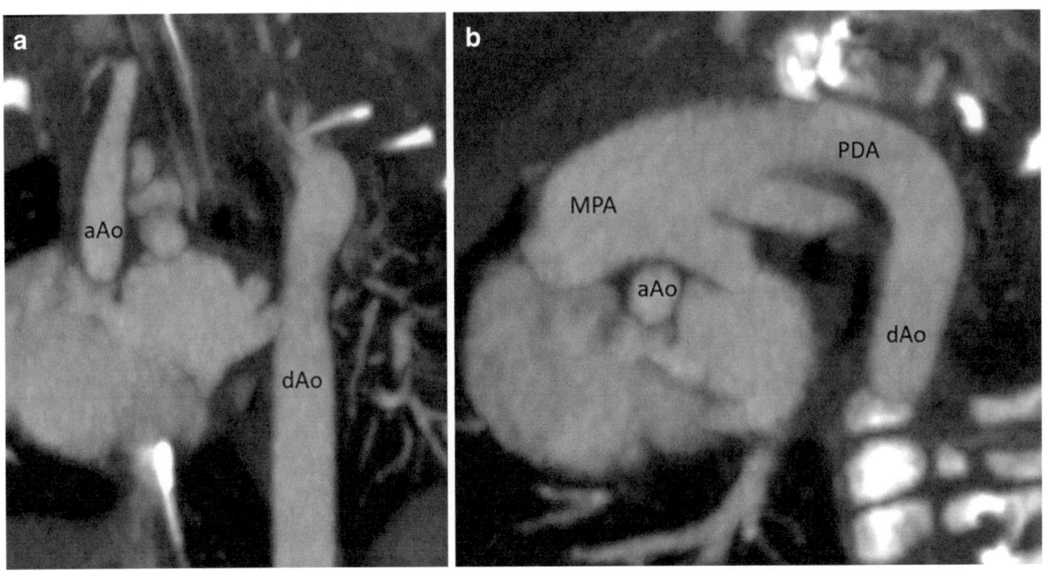

Fig. 21.17 Interrupted aortic arch (IAA) Type B. Panel (**a**) Oblique sagittal MIP images of contrast-enhanced CTA depict lack of communication between the aAo and the dAo. Panel (**b**) Oblique sagittal MIP images of contrast-enhanced CTA depicting widely patent PDA and normal caliber dAo with hypoplastic aAo

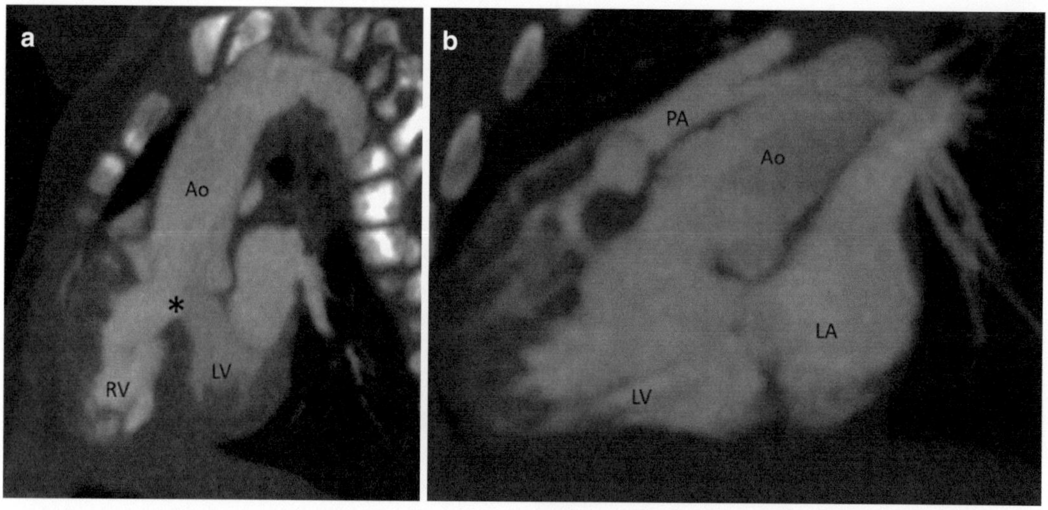

Fig. 21.18 Tetralogy of fallot with pulmonary hypoplasia. Panel (**a**) Coronal oblique reformatted contrast-enhanced CTA depicting three components of the tetralogy ("four-fold"): Malalignment VSD (black asterisk), overriding aorta (Ao), and right ventricular hypertrophy. Panel (**b**) Sagittal oblique reformatted image completes the forth component with pulmonary stenosis. Note the hypoplastic pulmonary artery (PA) adjacent to the large aortic root (Ao)

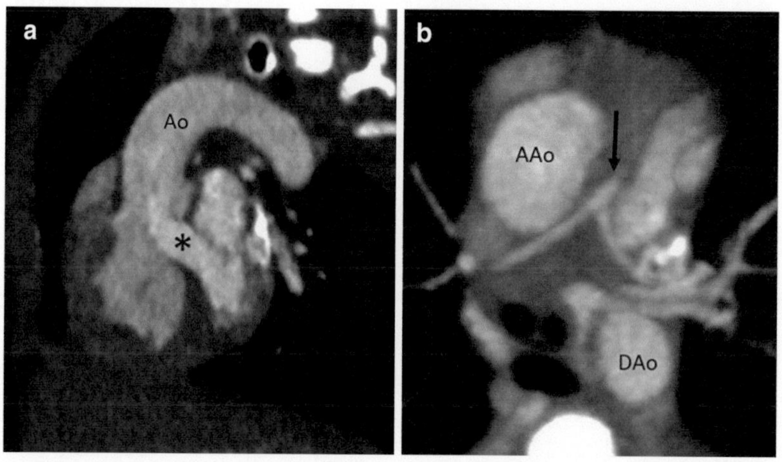

Fig. 21.19 Tetralogy of Fallot with pulmonary atresia. Panel (**a**) Coronal oblique reformatted contrast-enhanced CTA depicting three components of the tetralogy ("four-fold"): Malalignment VSD (black asterisk), overriding aorta (Ao), and right ventricular hypertrophy. Panel (**b**) Axial image depicting severely hypoplastic branch pulmonary arteries with lack of RV-PA communication (black arrow)

21.7.4 Ebstein's Anomaly (Fig. 21.15)

- Dysplasia of the posterior and septal leaflet of the tricuspid valve by greater than 8 mm/m^2 body surface area [32, 33].
- "Atrialization" of the right ventricle.
- 40% of congenital malformations of the tricuspid valve [34].

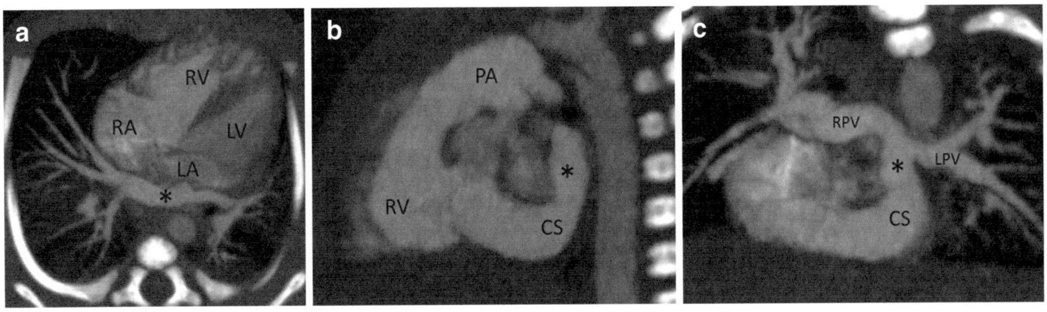

Fig. 21.20 Total anomalous pulmonary venous return (TAPVR)—cardiac type. Panel (**a**) Axial contrast-enhanced coronary CT depicting bilateral pulmonary veins forming a common channel (black asterisk) behind the left atrium (LA) without connection. Panel (**b**): Sagittal and (**c**) coronal reformatted views depicting common channel (black asterisk) of bilateral pulmonary veins (RPV-LPV) draining into the coronary sinus (CS)

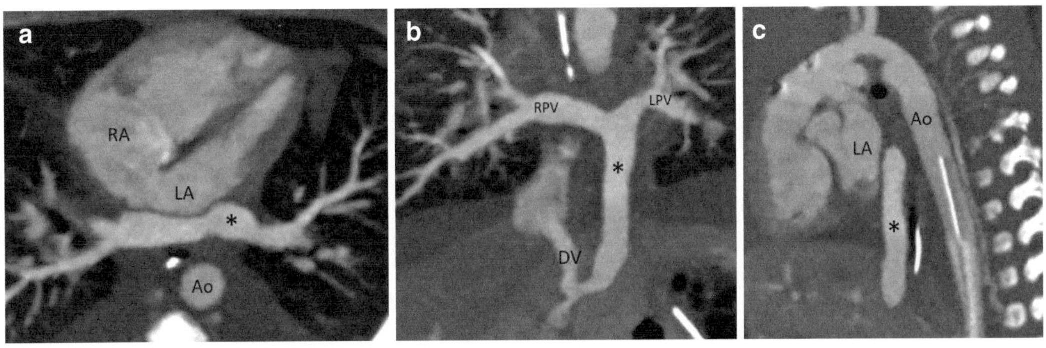

Fig. 21.21 Total anomalous pulmonary venous return (TAPVR)—infracardiac type. Panel (**a**) Axial contrast-enhanced coronary CT depicting bilateral pulmonary veins forming a common channel (black asterisk) behind the left atrium (LA) without connection. Panel (**b**) Coronal and (**c**) sagittal reformatted images depict common channel (black asterisk) of bilateral pulmonary veins (RPV-LPV) coursing below the diaphragm, draining into the portal vein/ductus venosus (DV)

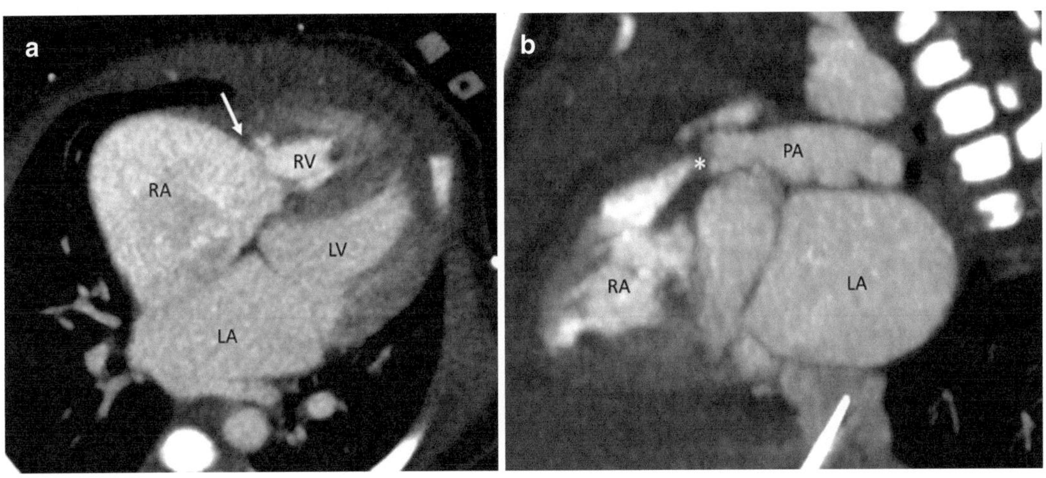

Fig. 21.22 Tricuspid atresia, RV, and pulmonic valve hypoplasia. Panel (**a**) four-chamber view of contrast-enhanced congenital CT depicting near-atretic tricuspid valve (white arrow) with hypoplastic RV. Panel (**b**) RVOT view contrast-enhanced congenital CTA depicting hypoplastic RV and pulmonic valve (white asterisk)

21.7.5 Hypoplastic Left Heart Syndrome (HLHS) (Fig. 21.16)

- Diminutive left-sided structures (mitral and aortic valves, LV, and aAo).
- Rare, but representing 1.2–1.5% of all CHD [35].
- Male predominance with increased familial risk (sibling is at 0.5% increased risk) [36].
- 25% of HLHS have genetic anomaly/syndrome (such as Turner, Holt-Oram, Noonan) [36].

21.7.6 Interrupted Aortic Arch (IAA) (Fig. 21.17)

- Loss of continuity within the aortic arch.
- Three types.
  A: Distal to the left subclavian artery.
  B: Between the left common carotid and left subclavian arteries.
  C: Between the brachiocephalic and left common carotid arteries
- Associated with Di George syndrome [37].

21.7.7 Pulmonary Atresia with Intact Ventricular Septum

- Rare CHD accounting for 1–3% of all CHD [28].
- Absence of the pulmonic valve.
- Commonly associated with PFO (shunt), coronary arteriovenous fistulae (10–50%), and tricuspid regurgitation (TR; 20%) [38, 39].

21.7.8 Double-Inlet Left Ventricle (DILV)

- Both aorta and pulmonary arteries arise of the morphologic LV by min. 50% circumference.
- Most common single ventricle CHD (70–80%).
- Often with transposed great arteries (70%) [38].

21.7.9 Tetralogy of Fallot (ToF) (Figs. 21.18 and 21.19)

- Most common critical CHD, accounting for 7 to 10% of all CHD [40–42].
- Often associated with other CHD such as right aortic arch (25%), ASD (15%), or coronary anomalies [39, 41, 42].
- Due to conal septal malposition toward the ventricular endocardial cushion with resultant abnormal septal alignment.
  - malalignment VSD,
  - pulmonary stenosis,
  - overriding aorta,
  - RV hypertrophy.
- Variant expressions of severity.
  - ToF with pulmonary atresia: Complete discontinuity between the RVOT and PA's.
  - ToF with MAPCAs (major aortopulmonary collaterals): Absent or diminutive central pulmonary arteries with large systemic collaterals.
  - ToF with absent pulmonary valve: Absence of the pulmonic valve (PV) with free PV regurgitation.

21.7.10 Total Anomalous Pulmonary Venous Return (Figs. 21.20 and 21.21)

- Rare CHD (2–3%).
- Only survivable with existing shunt (PDA, VSD, ASD).
- Four types.
  - Supracardiac
    Drainage into SVC, brachiocephalic or subclavian veins.
  - Intracardiac.
    Drainage into coronary sinus or right atrium.
  - Infracardiac.
    Drainage into the IVC, hepatic veins, ductus venous or portal vein.
  - Mixed type.
- Imaging depends on suspected type [43, 44].

21.7.11 Tricuspid Atresia (Fig. 21.22)

- 1.4% of CHD
- Agenesis or hypoplasia of the tricuspid valve and hypoplastic RV [45].
- Types dependent on associated abnormalities.
  - Normal great arteries (→increased pulmonary blood flow).
  - TGA (→decreased pulmonary blood flow).
- > VSD restriction →> cyanotic and PDA dependent [46].

21.7.12 Truncus Arteriosus (TA)

- Rare CHD (1–2% of neonates with CHD). 50% associated with genetic disorder, most commonly DiGeorge (chromosome 22q11.2 deletion syndrome) (approx. 20%) [47].
- Failure of embryonic division of the TA with resultant single trunk giving rise to the aorta and PA.
- Four types based on the location of pulmonary artery take-off [48] versus pulmonary artery take-off, aortic arch configuration, and presences of PDA including modifier "A" (plus VSD) or "B" (intact septum) [49].

References

1. Hoffman JI, Kaplan S. The incidence of congenital heart disease. J Am Coll Cardiol. 2002;39(12):1890–900. https://doi.org/10.1016/s0735-1097(02)01886-7.
2. Reller MD, Strickland MJ, Riehle-Colarusso T, Mahle WT, Correa A. Prevalence of congenital heart defects in metropolitan Atlanta, 1998-2005. J Pediatr. 2008;153(6):807–13. https://doi.org/10.1016/j.jpeds.2008.05.059.
3. Centers for Disease C, Prevention. Trends in infant mortality attributable to birth defects—United States, 1980–1995. MMWR Morb Mortal Wkly Rep. 1998;47(37):773–8. https://www.ncbi.nlm.nih.gov/pubmed/9769135.
4. van der Linde D, Konings EE, Slager MA, et al. Birth prevalence of congenital heart disease worldwide: a systematic review and meta-analysis. J Am Coll Cardiol. 2011;58(21):2241–7. https://doi.org/10.1016/j.jacc.2011.08.025.
5. Botto LD, Correa A, Erickson JD. Racial and temporal variations in the prevalence of heart defects. Pediatrics. 2001;107(3):E32. https://doi.org/10.1542/peds.107.3.e32.
6. Goo HW, Park IS, Ko JK, et al. CT of congenital heart disease: normal anatomy and typical pathologic conditions. Radiographics. 2003;23:S147–65. https://doi.org/10.1148/rg.23si035501.
7. De Oliveira NM, Witt DR, Casey SA, et al. Multi-institution assessment of the use and risk of cardiovascular computed tomography in pediatric patients with congenital heart disease. J Cardiovasc Comput Tomogr. 2021;15(5):441–8. https://doi.org/10.1016/j.jcct.2021.01.003.
8. Westwood M, Al M, Burgers L, et al. A systematic review and economic evaluation of new-generation computed tomography scanners for imaging in coronary artery disease and congenital heart disease: Somatom definition flash, Aquilion ONE, brilliance iCT and discovery CT750 HD. Health Technol Assess. 2013;17(9):1–243. https://doi.org/10.3310/hta17090.
9. Long CM, Long SS, Johnson PT, Mahesh M, Fishman EK, Zimmerman SL. Utility of low-dose high-pitch scanning for pediatric cardiac computed tomographic imaging. J Thorac Imaging. 2015;30(4):W36–40. https://doi.org/10.1097/RTI.0000000000000131.
10. Chandrashekhar G, Sodhi KS, Saxena AK, Rohit MK, Khandelwal N. Correlation of 64 row MDCT, echocardiography and cardiac catheterization angiography in assessment of pulmonary arterial anatomy in children with cyanotic congenital heart disease. Eur J Radiol. 2012;81(12):4211–7. https://doi.org/10.1016/j.ejrad.2012.08.010.
11. Sievers HH, Schmidtke C. A classification system for the bicuspid aortic valve from 304 surgical specimens. J Thorac Cardiovasc Surg. 2007;133(5):1226–33. https://doi.org/10.1016/j.jtcvs.2007.01.039.
12. Ho ML, Bhalla S, Bierhals A, Gutierrez F. MDCT of partial anomalous pulmonary venous return (PAPVR) in adults. J Thorac Imaging. 2009;24(2):89–95. https://doi.org/10.1097/RTI.0b013e318194c942.
13. Han BK, Rigsby CK, Hlavacek A, et al. Computed tomography imaging in patients with congenital heart Disease part I: rationale and utility. An expert consensus document of the Society of Cardiovascular Computed Tomography (SCCT): endorsed by the Society of Pediatric Radiology (SPR) and the north American Society of Cardiac Imaging (NASCI). J Cardiovasc Comput Tomogr. 2015;9(6):475–92. https://doi.org/10.1016/j.jcct.2015.07.004.
14. Hunt CH, Hartman RP, Hesley GK. Frequency and severity of adverse effects of iodinated and gadolinium contrast materials: retrospective review of 456,930 doses. AJR Am J Roentgenol. 2009;193(4):1124–7. https://doi.org/10.2214/AJR.09.2520.
15. Callahan MJ, Poznauskis L, Zurakowski D, Taylor GA. Nonionic iodinated intravenous contrast material-related reactions: incidence in large urban children's hospital—retrospective analysis of data in 12,494 patients. Radiology. 2009;250(3):674–81. https://doi.org/10.1148/radiol.2503071577.

16. Scholtz JE, Ghoshhajra B. Advances in cardiac CT contrast injection and acquisition protocols. Cardiovasc Diagn Ther. 2017;7(5):439–51. https://doi.org/10.21037/cdt.2017.06.07.
17. Ko SF, Liang CD, Yip HK, et al. Amplatzer septal occluder closure of atrial septal defect: evaluation of transthoracic echocardiography, cardiac CT, and transesophageal echocardiography. AJR Am J Roentgenol. 2009;193(6):1522–9. https://doi.org/10.2214/AJR.09.2854.
18. Praagh RV, Geva T, Kreutzer J. Ventricular septal defects: how shall we describe, name and classify them? J Am Coll Cardiol. 1989;14(5):1298–9. https://doi.org/10.1016/0735-1097(89)90431-2.
19. Leipsic J, Abbara S, Achenbach S, et al. SCCT guidelines for the interpretation and reporting of coronary CT angiography: a report of the Society of Cardiovascular Computed Tomography Guidelines Committee. J Cardiovasc Comput Tomogr. 2014;8(5):342–58. https://doi.org/10.1016/j.jcct.2014.07.003.
20. Abbara S, Blanke P, Maroules CD, et al. SCCT guidelines for the performance and acquisition of coronary computed tomographic angiography: a report of the society of cardiovascular computed tomography guidelines committee: endorsed by the north American Society for Cardiovascular Imaging (NASCI). J Cardiovasc Comput Tomogr. 2016;10(6):435–49. https://doi.org/10.1016/j.jcct.2016.10.002.
21. Malone LJ, Morin CE, Browne LP. Coronary computed tomography angiography in children. Pediatr Radiol. 2021;52:2498. https://doi.org/10.1007/s00247-021-05209-2.
22. Oh KH, Choo KS, Lim SJ, et al. Multidetector CT evaluation of total anomalous pulmonary venous connections: comparison with echocardiography. Pediatr Radiol. 2009;39(9):950–4. https://doi.org/10.1007/s00247-009-1309-3.
23. Burney K, Young H, Barnard SA, McCoubrie P, Darby M. CT appearances of congential and acquired abnormalities of the superior vena cava. Clin Radiol. 2007;62(9):837–42. https://doi.org/10.1016/j.crad.2007.04.001.
24. Zhao Q, Wang J, Yang ZG, et al. Assessment of intracardiac and extracardiac anomalies associated with coarctation of aorta and interrupted aortic arch using dual-source computed tomography. Sci Rep. 2019;9(1):11656. https://doi.org/10.1038/s41598-019-47136-1.
25. Budoff MJ, Shittu A, Roy S. Use of cardiovascular computed tomography in the diagnosis and management of coarctation of the aorta. J Thorac Cardiovasc Surg. 2013;146(1):229–32. https://doi.org/10.1016/j.jtcvs.2013.01.024.
26. Thanopoulos BD, Giannakoulas G, Giannopoulos A, Galdo F, Tsaoussis GS. Initial and six-year results of stent implantation for aortic coarctation in children. Am J Cardiol. 2012;109(10):1499–503. https://doi.org/10.1016/j.amjcard.2012.01.365.
27. Warnes CA, Williams RG, Bashore TM, et al. ACC/AHA 2008 guidelines for the Management of Adults with congenital heart Disease: executive summary: a report of the American College of Cardiology/American Heart Association task force on practice guidelines (writing committee to develop guidelines for the management of adults with congenital heart disease). Circulation. 2008;118(23):2395–451. https://doi.org/10.1161/CIRCULATIONAHA.108.190811.
28. Samanek M, Slavik Z, Zborilova B, Hrobonova V, Voriskova M, Skovranek J. Prevalence, treatment, and outcome of heart disease in live-born children: a prospective analysis of 91,823 live-born children. Pediatr Cardiol. 1989;10(4):205–11. https://doi.org/10.1007/BF02083294.
29. Chen SJ, Lin MT, Liu KL, et al. Usefulness of 3D reconstructed computed tomography imaging for double outlet right ventricle. J Formos Med Assoc. 2008;107(5):371–80. https://doi.org/10.1016/S0929-6646(08)60102-3.
30. Walters HL 3rd, Mavroudis C, Tchervenkov CI, Jacobs JP, Lacour-Gayet F, Jacobs ML. Congenital heart surgery nomenclature and database project: double outlet right ventricle. Ann Thorac Surg. 2000;69(4 Suppl):S249–63. https://doi.org/10.1016/s0003-4975(99)01247-3.
31. Lev M, Bharati S, Meng CC, Liberthson RR, Paul MH, Idriss F. A concept of double-outlet right ventricle. J Thorac Cardiovasc Surg. 1972;64(2):271–81. https://www.ncbi.nlm.nih.gov/pubmed/5048382.
32. Shiina A, Seward JB, Tajik AJ, Hagler DJ, Danielson GK. Two-dimensional echocardiographic—surgical correlation in Ebstein's anomaly: preoperative determination of patients requiring tricuspid valve plication vs replacement. Circulation. 1983;68(3):534–44. https://doi.org/10.1161/01.cir.68.3.534.
33. Malik SB, Kwan D, Shah AB, Hsu JY. The right atrium: gateway to the heart—anatomic and pathologic imaging findings. Radiographics. 2015;35(1):14–31. https://doi.org/10.1148/rg.351130010.
34. Negoi RI, Ispas AT, Ghiorghiu I, et al. Complex Ebstein's malformation: defining preoperative cardiac anatomy and function. J Card Surg. 2013;28(1):70–81. https://doi.org/10.1111/jocs.12032.
35. Bardo DM, Frankel DG, Applegate KE, Murphy DJ, Saneto RP. Hypoplastic left heart syndrome. Radiographics. 2001;21(3):705–17. https://doi.org/10.1148/radiographics.21.3.g01ma09705.
36. Boughman JA, Berg KA, Astemborski JA, et al. Familial risks of congenital heart defect assessed in a population-based epidemiologic study. Am J Med Genet. 1987;26(4):839–49. https://doi.org/10.1002/ajmg.1320260411.
37. Corsten-Janssen N, Kerstjens-Frederikse WS, du Marchie Sarvaas GJ, et al. The cardiac phenotype in patients with a CHD7 mutation. Circ Cardiovasc Genet. 2013;6(3):248–54. https://doi.org/10.1161/CIRCGENETICS.113.000054.
38. Rao PS. Diagnosis and management of cyanotic congenital heart disease: part II. Indian J Pediatr. 2009;76(3):297–308. https://doi.org/10.1007/s12098-009-0056-7.

39. Rao PS. Diagnosis and management of cyanotic congenital heart disease: part I. Indian J Pediatr. 2009;76(1):57–70. https://doi.org/10.1007/s12098-009-0030-4.
40. Zucker EJ. Computed tomography in tetralogy of Fallot: pre-and postoperative imaging evaluation. Pediatr Radiol. 2021;52:2485. https://doi.org/10.1007/s00247-021-05179-5.
41. Pandey NN, Bhambri K, Verma M, Jagia P, Kothari SS, Saxena A. Anomalies of coronary arteries in tetralogy of Fallot: evaluation on multidetector CT angiography using dual-source scanner. J Card Surg. 2021;36(7):2373–80. https://doi.org/10.1111/jocs.15572.
42. Prabhu S, Kasturi S, Mehra S, et al. The aortic arch in tetralogy of Fallot: types of branching and clinical implications. Cardiol Young. 2020;30(8):1144–50. https://doi.org/10.1017/S1047951120001705.
43. Files MD, Morray B. Total anomalous pulmonary venous connection: preoperative anatomy, physiology, imaging, and interventional Management of Postoperative Pulmonary Venous Obstruction. Semin Cardiothorac Vasc Anesth. 2017;21(2):123–31. https://doi.org/10.1177/1089253216672442.
44. Kim TH, Kim YM, Suh CH, et al. Helical CT angiography and three-dimensional reconstruction of total anomalous pulmonary venous connections in neonates and infants. AJR Am J Roentgenol. 2000;175(5):1381–6. https://doi.org/10.2214/ajr.175.5.1751381.
45. Burns SKS-F, H. Tricuspid atresia. In: White CSH, L. B.; Chen, J. J.-S.; Levsky, J. M, Rotations in radiology: cardiac imaging. New York: Oxford University Press; 2014:179–182.
46. Schweigmann G, Gassner I, Maurer K. Imaging the neonatal heart—essentials for the radiologist. Eur J Radiol. 2006;60(2):159–70. https://doi.org/10.1016/j.ejrad.2006.07.017.
47. Goldmuntz E, Clark BJ, Mitchell LE, et al. Frequency of 22q11 deletions in patients with conotruncal defects. J Am Coll Cardiol. 1998;32(2):492–8. https://doi.org/10.1016/s0735-1097(98)00259-9.
48. Collett RW, Edwards JE. Persistent truncus arteriosus; a classification according to anatomic types. Surg Clin North Am. 1949;29(4):1245–70. https://doi.org/10.1016/s0039-6109(16)32803-1.
49. Van Praagh R, Van Praagh S. The anatomy of common aorticopulmonary trunk (truncus arteriosus communis) and its embryologic implications. A study of 57 necropsy cases. Am J Cardiol. 1965;16(3):406–25. https://doi.org/10.1016/0002-9149(65)90732-0.

22 Important Non-cardiac CT Findings

Yuen Li Ng

Abstract

Incidental non-cardiac pathology is commonly noted when reporting cardiac CT results. The most frequently detected non-cardiac findings are lung nodules. While most non-cardiac findings are benign, an important proportion requires further investigation and/or treatment. These findings also may suggest alternative diagnoses for the patient's symptoms or represent important but clinically silent conditions, such as lung cancer. Cardiac CT readers should be familiar with common and significant non-cardiac findings. A systematic approach to the evaluation of non-cardiac structures is recommended, using the maximum field of view (FOV) and appropriate window level/width settings. Review of prior reference images is often critical to assess the significance of non-cardiac findings.

Keywords

Non-cardiac lesions · Extra-cardiac findings · Incidental · Field of view · Cardiac CT · Lung nodules

Y. L. Ng (✉)
Department of Radiology, Mount Elizabeth Hospital, Singapore, Republic of Singapore

Abbreviations

DICOM	Digital imaging and communication in medicine
FOV	Field of view
HU	Hounsfield unit
MRI	Magnetic resonance imaging
NCF	Non-cardiac findings

22.1 Introduction

- Concomitant evaluation of non-cardiac structures is an advantage of CT over other non-invasive cardiac imaging tests.
- The reported rates of non-cardiac findings (NCF) detected on cardiac CT imaging are highly variable, between 17.7% and 76.8%, depending on the patient population, scan protocols, and definition of reportable NCFs [1–7].
- The following are pooled estimates of NCFs from systematic reviews [8–10]:
  Total NCFs : 41–45%
  Major or clinical significant NCFs : 16–17%
  Malignant NCFs : 0.7% (70% were lung cancers)
- Some risk factors for coronary artery disease (e.g., age, male gender and smoking) are also risk factors for diseases, such as aortic disease and lung carcinoma.
- NCFs may offer alternative diagnoses for presenting symptoms (Table 22.1).

A. A. Zadeh, J. Hoe (eds.), *Practical Guide to Cardiac CT*,
https://doi.org/10.1007/978-981-97-6919-3_22

Table 22.1 Examples of non-cardiac causes of chest pain evident on cardiac CT imaging

Lung	Pneumonia, acute pulmonary embolism, pneumothorax, pleural effusion, malignancy
Mediastinum	Acute aortic syndrome, pneumomediastinum, hiatal hernia
Bone	Rib fractures, metastases

Table 22.2 Typical values of window widths and levels in Hounsfield units (HU)

Window settings	Window level (HU)	Window width (HU)
Lung	−600 to −700	1000 to 1500
Soft tissue	+ 20 to +40	450 to 500
Bone	+ 300 to +500	2000

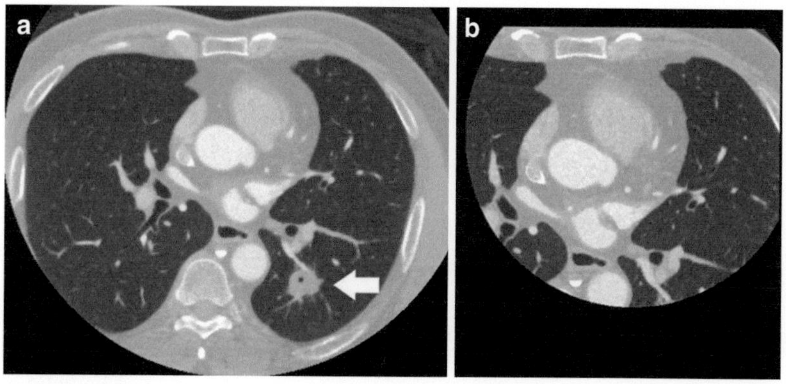

Fig. 22.1 Cardiac CT with full vs. restricted field of view. (**a**) The reconstructed image with a wider FOV shows a cavitary lung nodule in the left lower lobe *(arrow)* which was confirmed to be a primary carcinoma on histology. (**b**) The nodule is not visible on the limited FOV image

- NCFs may also represent previously undiagnosed conditions that are clinically significant and potentially treatable, including malignancy [10].

22.2 Image Reconstructions and Window Settings

22.2.1 Limited Versus Wide Field of View Image Reconstructions

- The assessment of the coronary arteries requires a limited field of view (FOV) to achieve optimal image resolution. This typically only includes about a third of the chest volume and excludes a large portion of the lung parenchyma [2].
- For the evaluation of non-cardiac structures, additional image reconstruction with a wider FOV containing the entire scan range is recommended. The same CT raw data are used and thus, the patient is not subjected to additional ionizing radiation for this assessment [2].
- The wider FOV images encompass about twice the chest volume of the cardiac FOV images and may reveal findings that are not visible on the limited FOV images focused on the heart (Fig. 22.1).
- Estimated 80% of lung nodules and lung cancers would be missed on the limited, cardiac FOV images [11, 12].

22.2.2 Window Level/Width Settings

- Review of the lungs, mediastinum, upper abdomen, and bones is performed using appropriate window width/level settings (Table 22.2) [13].
- Workstations or DICOM viewers have preset window settings which can be adjusted during scan interpretation to optimize visibility of certain structures or abnormalities of interest.

22.3 Systematic Approach to the Evaluation of Non-Cardiac Structures

22.3.1 Lung

- The lung parenchyma and airways are evaluated on the wide FOV images using lung window settings (Fig. 22.2), and ideally, reconstructed using a sharper lung reconstruction algorithm [13].

22.3.1.1 Lung Nodules

- The most commonly detected NCFs are lung nodules.
- Most of these nodules are small and require no further investigation or treatment (Fig. 22.3) [4, 15].

  Nodules <1 cm : 9.3–19.0%

  Nodules >1 cm : 0.6–2.4%
- Although many are benign, it is vital to identify nodules with risk of malignancy and manage them appropriately [14].
- The reported prevalence of lung cancer is 0.3–0.5% on cardiac CT imaging [4, 10, 11].
- Evidence-based guidelines for the management of lung nodules are available, e.g., the 2017 Fleischner Society guidelines (Table 22.3) [17], the 2015 British Thoracic Society guidelines [18], and the 2013 American College of Chest Physicians guidelines [19].
- The revised 2017 Fleischner guidelines increased the threshold for follow-up imaging to 6 mm, which has resulted in a significant decrease of follow-up CT of incidental pulmonary nodules detected on cardiac CT [20].
- Comparison with previous imaging is important.
  - For *solid* lung nodules (Fig. 22.4a), an interval stability of 2 years or more favors benign etiology.
  - *Subsolid* (part-solid and ground glass) nodules require follow-up for longer duration due to the risk of adenocarcinoma which tend to be slow-growing (Fig. 22.4b, c) [17].

22.3.1.2 Other Lung Parenchymal Findings

- Linear and dependent atelectasis are frequently encountered and are usually related to suboptimal inspiration during CT acquisition [13].
  - Dependent atelectasis is confined to the dependent areas of the lung (Fig. 22.5a) and can usually be distinguished from interstitial fibrosis.

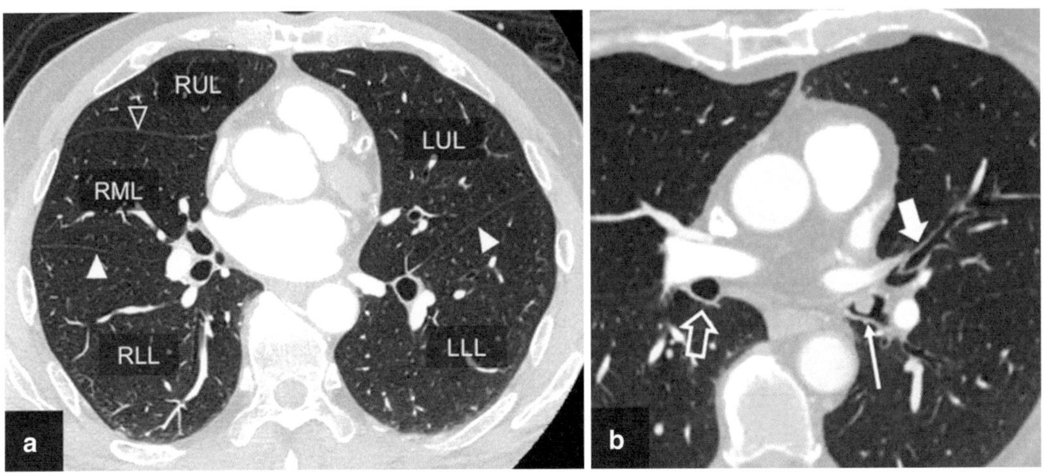

Fig. 22.2 Normal and abnormal lung findings. (**a**) Normal anatomy: Horizontal fissure (*open arrowhead*), right and left oblique fissures (*closed arrowheads*), right upper lobe (RUL), right middle lobe (RML), right lower lobe (RLL), lingular segments of the left upper lobe (LUL), left lower lobe (LLL). (**b**) Incidental endobronchial nodule in the left lower lobe bronchus (*line arrow*), bronchus intermedius (*open arrow*), lingular bronchus (*closed arrow*)

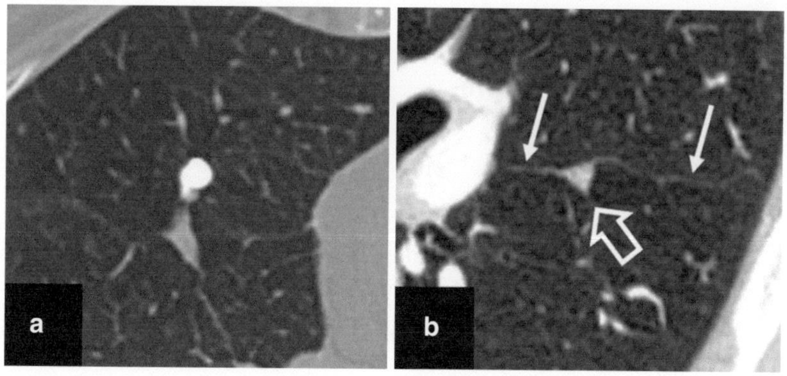

Fig. 22.3 Examples of lung nodules. (**a**) completely calcified nodule usually represents a granuloma. (**b**) triangular nodule (*open arrow*) ranging from 3 to 9 mm in size adjacent to a fissure (*arrows*) usually represents an intrapulmonary lymph node [14]

  - If there is clinical suspicion or abnormalities in the non-dependent areas of the lungs on CT, further evaluation with high resolution CT (HRCT) in supine and prone positions is helpful (Fig. 22.5b).
- Infection may manifest as consolidation and/or ground glass opacities on CT imaging (Fig. 22.5c, d) [21, 22].
  The former is more common in bacterial infection, while the latter often suggests atypical organisms, e.g., viral or fungal pneumonia.

22.3.1.3 Pleural Disease

- Pneumothorax is easily visualized using lung window settings (Fig. 22.6a) but is likely missed when viewing using soft tissue window settings.
- Pleural effusions (Fig. 22.6b) are common abnormalities detected on cardiac CT.
  Pleural effusions, pleural thickening, and masses (Fig. 22.6c) are better assessed on soft tissue window settings [13].

22.3.2 Mediastinum

- Mediastinal structures are assessed on the wider FOV images using soft tissue window settings and standard smooth reconstruction algorithm [13].

22.3.2.1 Vascular Disease

- Abnormalities of the aorta and pulmonary arteries are discussed in Chap. 20.

22.3.2.2 Mediastinal Masses

- The normal thymus gland appears in a variety of shapes and sizes, and gradually involutes with age (Fig. 22.7, Fig. 22.9a, b) [23].
- Mediastinal masses may be:
  - Benign, e.g., thymic (Fig. 22.8a), pericardial (Fig. 22.8b), bronchogenic or esophageal duplication cysts; or
  - Malignant, e.g., germ cell tumors (Fig. 22.8c), thymoma, thyroid malignancy, and lymphoma [13].
- Hiatus hernia is a common NCF and may represent an alternate cause of chest pain (Fig. 22.8d).
  The esophagus is not optimally assessed on CT and thus, further evaluation with endoscopy may be worthwhile to confirm the hernia or reflux disease, and to exclude malignant pathology.

22.3.2.3 Lymph Nodes

- Normal lymph nodes are ovoid in shape with smooth outline (Fig. 22.9a).
- Generally, lymph nodes measuring greater than 10 mm in short axis diameter are considered abnormal.
  They can be seen in conditions such as infection, congestive heart failure, collagen vascular disease, sarcoidosis (Fig. 22.9b), and malignancy [14].
- Calcified nodes are commonly related to prior granulomatous diseases, e.g., tuberculosis and histoplasmosis (Fig. 22.9c).
  Other causes include sarcoidosis, silicosis, amyloidosis, and treated lymphomas [13].

Table 22.3 Summary of clinical guidelines for evaluation and management of indeterminate solitary pulmonary nodules (modified with permission from Paez R, Kammer MN and Massion P. Risk Stratification of Indeterminate Pulmonary Nodules. Curr Opin Pulm Med 2021; 27:240–248 https://doi.org/10.1097/MCP.0000000000000780 [16]

	Subsolid	Small solid	Large solid
Fleischner Society [17]	<6 mm : No follow-up >6 mm pure ground glass : CT 6–12 months, then every 2 years until 5 years >6 mm part solid : CT 3–6 months, if unchanged and solid component <6mm, annual CT for 5 years	<6 mm : No follow-up for low risk; optional CT in 12 months for high risk 6–8 mm : CT at 6–12 months, then 18–24 months	>8 mm : CT at 3 months or PET/CT or biopsy depending on size and morphology
British Thoracic Society [18]	<5 mm : No follow-up ≥5 mm : CT at 3 months and if stable use Brock model. If risk <10%, then CT surveillance at 1, 2, and 4 years If risk >10%, consider biopsy, resection, or CT surveillance If growth at 3 months, consider resection, nonsurgical treatment, or CT surveillance	<5 mm : No follow-up 5–6 mm : CT surveillance at 1 year. Further evaluation will depend on stability 6–8 mm : CT surveillance at 3 months. If VDT ≤ 400 or clear growth, requires further investigation. If stable, repeat CT in 1 year	≥8 mm : Brock model for risk assessment. If risk <10%, CT surveillance. If risk >10%, PET/CT and apply Herder model. If <10% after Herder, CT surveillance If 10–70% after Herder, CT surveillance, or biopsy based on risk and individual preference If >70% after Herder, surgery, nonsurgical biopsy, or nonsurgical treatment
American College of Chest Physicians [19]	Pure GGN ≤5 mm : No follow-up >5 mm : Annual CT chest for 3 years >10 mm : Repeat CT in 3 months followed by biopsy if persistent Part solid ≤8 mm : CT surveillance in 3, 12, and 24 months followed by annual CT for an additional 1–3 years >8 mm : CT chest in 3 months followed by PET/CT (if solid component >8 mm) or biopsy if persistent or growing >15 mm : PET/CT or biopsy PET does not reliably identify malignant nodules in this group, particularly pure ground glass nodules TTNB has suboptimal sensitivity High likelihood of malignancy and need for longer surveillance	<8 mm : Interval follow-up CT based on size and individual risk factors for cancer (generally 6–12 months) Size divided into ≤4, 4–6, 6–8 mm Does not recommend functional imaging or biopsy given most nodules in this group are benign and unreliability of diagnostic modalities	≥8 mm : CT surveillance, PET/CT, nonsurgical biopsy, or surgical biopsy are appropriate depending on probability of cancer, surgical risk, and patient preference Low risk (<5%) : CT surveillance Intermediate risk (5–65%) : Favors PET/CT for further risk stratification High risk (>65%) : Biopsy or resection. No PET, unless staging TTNB or bronchoscopy modalities depending on nodule location and center expertise

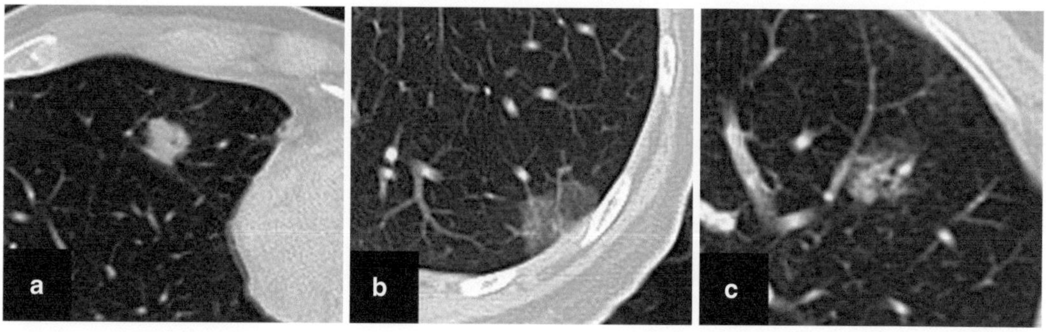

Fig. 22.4 Solid vs. subsolid lung nodules. (**a**) solid nodule completely obscures underlying vasculature. (**b**) pure ground glass nodule shows increased parenchymal attenuation but does not obscure the vasculature. (**c**) part-solid nodule contains both solid and ground glass components

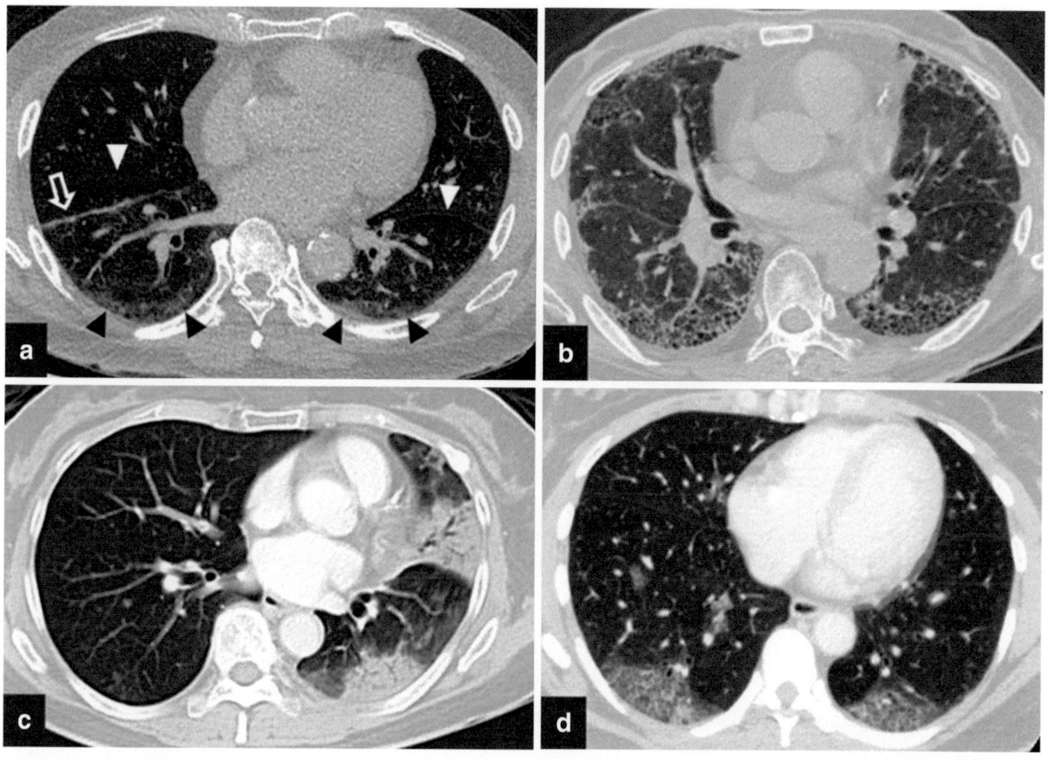

Fig. 22.5 Examples of lung parenchymal findings. (**a**) Dependent atelectasis (*black arrowheads*) in the lower lobes bilaterally, linear atelectasis (*white open arrow*) in the right lower lobe, bilateral oblique fissures (*white arrowheads*). (**b**) Interstitial fibrosis involving non-dependent areas and demonstrating honeycombing. (**c**) Consolidation in the lingula and left lower lobe with air bronchograms due to bacterial pneumonia. (**d**) Bilateral ground glass opacities in the lower lobes with septal thickening (crazy paving sign) due to viral pneumonia

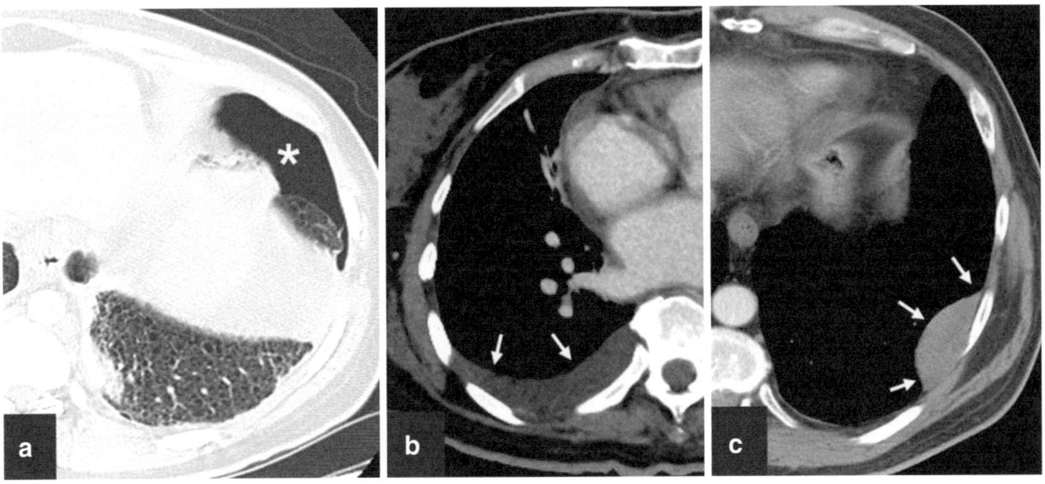

Fig. 22.6 Examples of pleural disease. (**a**) Left pneumothorax (*asterisk*). (**b**) Right basal pleural effusion (*arrows*). (**c**) Left solitary fibrous tumor (*arrows*)

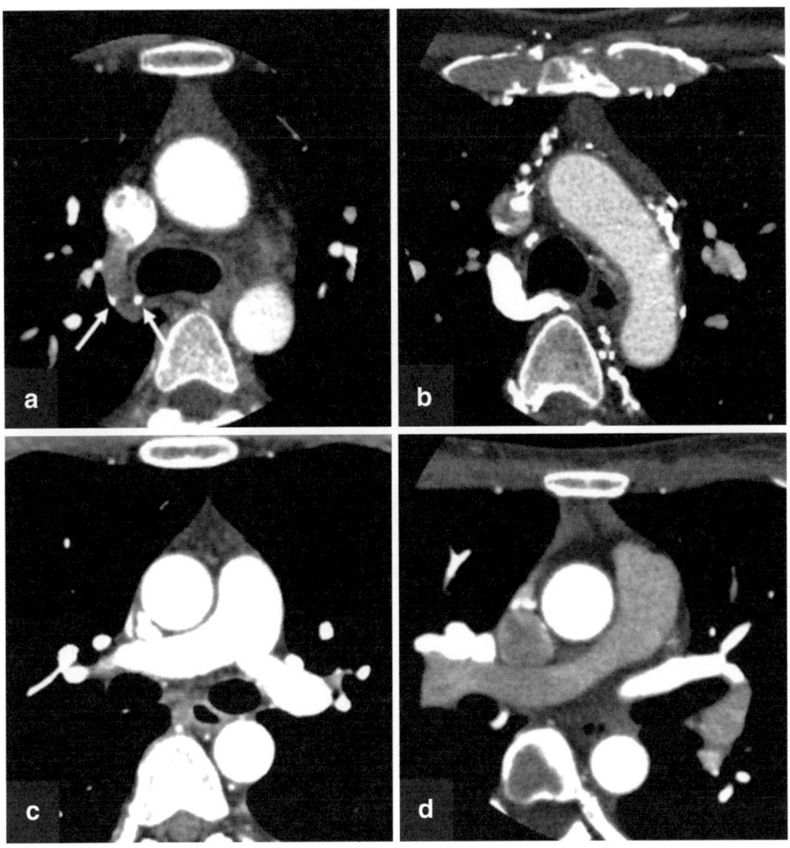

Fig. 22.7 Normal appearances of the thymus gland in the anterior mediastinum. Side note: the two small high attenuation foci in the right paratracheal region (*arrows* in **a**) represent reflux of intravenous contrast pooling in the cusps of the azygous arch valves, more frequently seen with high contrast injection rates

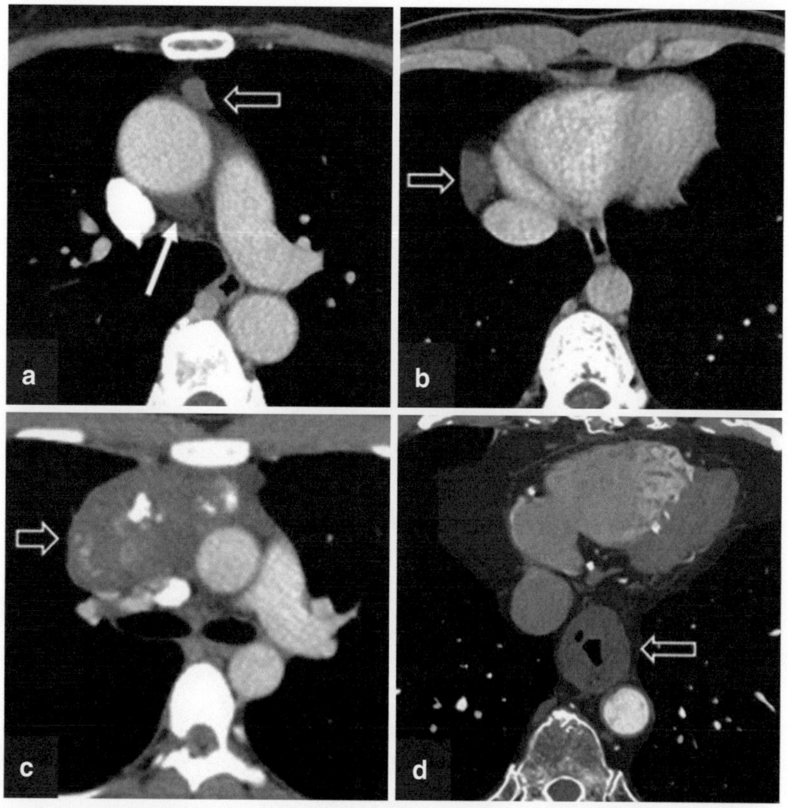

Fig. 22.8 Examples of mediastinal masses. (**a**) Small thymic cyst in the anterior mediastinum (*open arrow*), and fluid in the superior pericardial recess (*arrow*) posterior to the ascending aorta, mimicking lymphadenopathy. (**b**) Pericardial cyst (*open arrow*). (**c**) Anterior mediastinal teratoma (*open arrow*) containing calcification. (**d**) Enlarged distal esophagus (*open arrow*); the patient underwent endoscopy confirming a hiatal hernia without histological evidence of malignancy

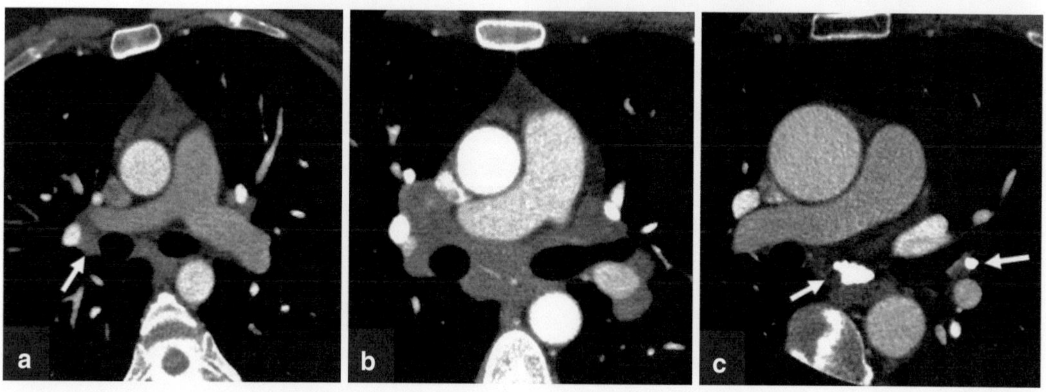

Fig. 22.9 Normal and abnormal lymph node findings. (**a**) Normal right hilar lymph node (*arrow*), measuring less than 10 mm in short axis diameter. (**b**) Subcarinal and bilateral hilar lymphadenopathy in a patient with known sarcoidosis. (**c**) Calcified subcarinal and left hilar nodes (*arrows*) due to previous tuberculosis infection

- Small amount of fluid may pool in the pericardial recesses (Fig. 22.8a) mimicking lymph nodes.
  The fluid attenuation and lack of mass effect on CT are helpful to distinguish them from lymph nodes [24].

22.3.3 Thyroid Gland

- Thyroid enlargement and thyroid nodules may be seen, especially with the larger scan range in CT imaging of coronary artery bypass grafts.

- The American Society of Thyroid Disease provides evidence-based recommendations to inform clinical decision-making in the management of thyroid nodules [25].

22.3.4 Upper Abdomen

- Findings in the upper abdomen make up a significant portion of NCFs, but many require no further follow-up or treatment [26].
- Review of previous imaging may help to demonstrate interval stability and identify benign lesions.
- Hepatic cysts are the most common intra-abdominal NCFs, accounting for approximately 5% of NCFs [7].
  - Simple cysts have fluid attenuation, without discernible wall or contrast enhancement (Fig. 22.10a). These are benign and require no further imaging.
  - Other common liver abnormalities include benign pathology, e.g., hemangioma and fatty infiltration (Fig. 22.10b).
  - For lesions that are not clearly benign, further assessment with dedicated ultrasound, multiphasic CT or magnetic resonance imaging (MRI) should be considered.
- Renal cysts are also frequently benign, requiring no further follow-up.
  - The Bosniak criteria are helpful in predicting the risk of malignancy and in guiding management of renal cysts.

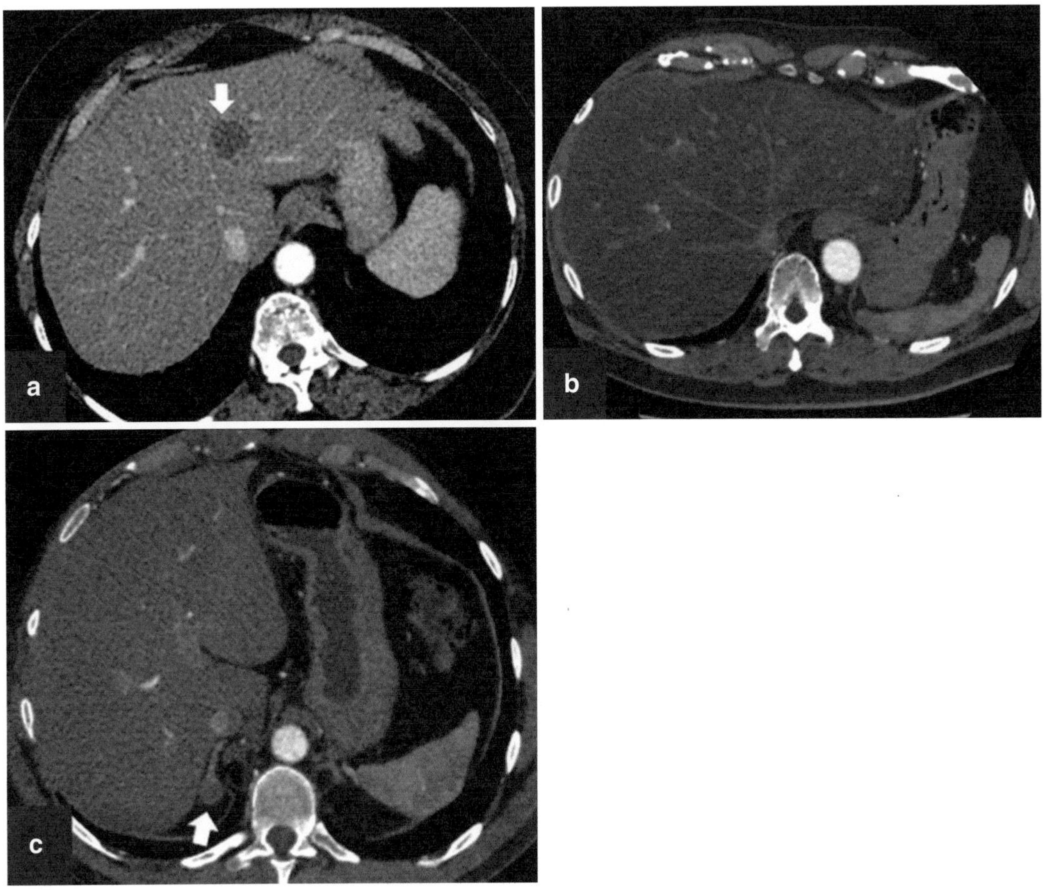

Fig. 22.10 Examples of upper abdomen incidental findings. (**a**) Simple hepatic cyst (*arrow*). (**b**) Fatty infiltration of the liver as evidenced by generalized reduced attenuation to less than 40HU. (**c**) Incidental right adrenal nodule (*arrow*), most commonly a benign adenoma

- Internal septations, contrast enhancement, calcification or soft tissue components are associated with increased the risk of malignancy [27].
- Adrenal nodules detected incidentally are mostly benign adenomas (Fig. 22.10c).
  - An attenuation of less than 10 HU on an unenhanced CT has good diagnostic accuracy for benign adenoma.
  - Evidence-based recommendations based on clinical and imaging features are helpful to guide the management of patients with adrenal incidentalomas [28, 29].
- Ascites, abnormal lymph nodes (retrocrural and gastrohepatic regions), lesions in the stomach, spleen, and pancreas are other NCFs reported in the literature [26].

22.3.5 Breast and Chest Wall

- Review of the breast tissue as well as the skin, subcutaneous fat and muscles of the chest wall included in the wider FOV images is also important.
- Breast cancer is one of the most common cancers in women.
  Nearly 30% of incidental breast lesions detected on body CT in a large series proved to be unsuspected breast cancers (Fig. 22.11a), particularly the irregular, spiculated masses [30].
- The predictive value of CT to identify breast malignancy is low.
  Further clinical review with dedicated mammography and/or breast ultrasound is often required.
- Examples of benign breast lesions include benign calcification (Fig. 22.11b), fibroadenomas, and lipomas.

22.3.6 Bones

- The bones are reviewed using bone window settings on the wider FOV images, reconstructed using sharper (lung) reconstruction algorithm.
- Certain bone lesions have classic imaging characteristics [13]:
  - Bone islands are uniformly dense with well-defined margins (Fig. 22.12a).
  - Vertebral hemangiomas have "polka dot" appearance on axial images.
- Irregular lesion margins, wide transitional zones, and bony destruction are features suggesting an aggressive lesion which requires further assessment.
  Metastases represent the most common malignant bone lesions (Fig. 22.12b).

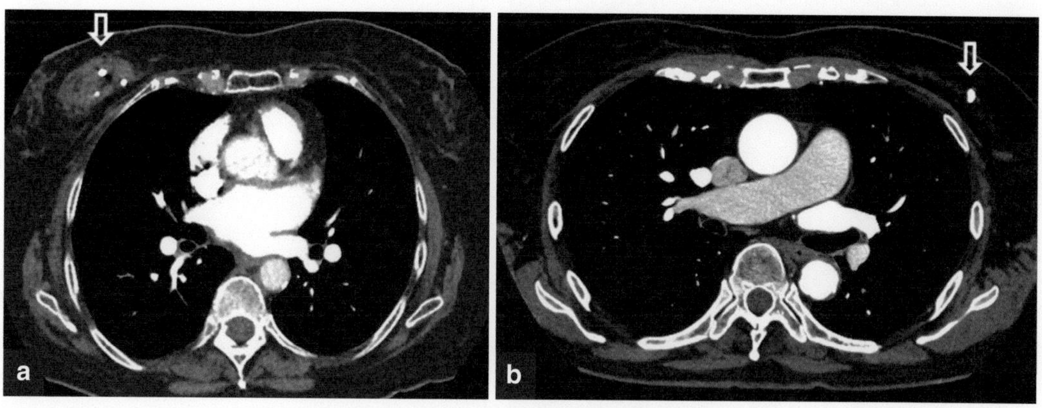

Fig. 22.11 Examples of breast tissue findings. (**a**) Right breast lobulated mass with coarse calcification, histologically confirmed as mucinous carcinoma. (**b**) Benign calcification in the left breast

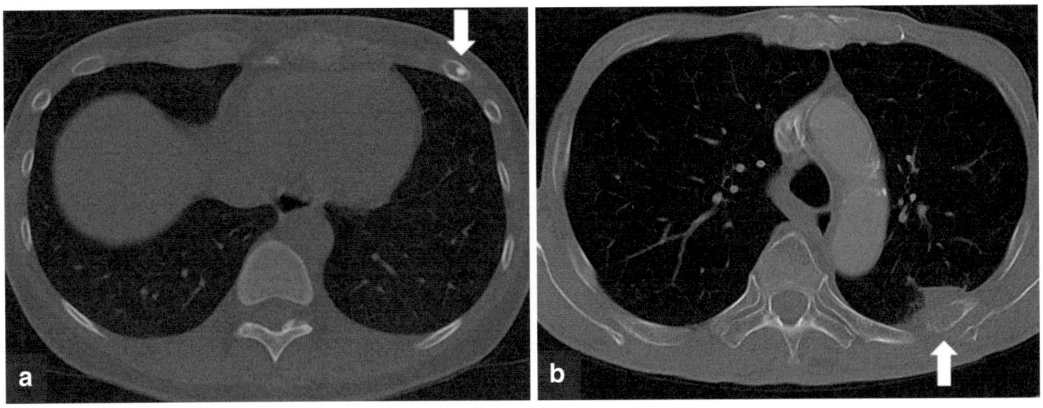

Fig. 22.12 Examples of bone pathology. (**a**) Left rib bone island (*arrow*). (**b**) Left rib metastasis demonstrating bony expansion and destruction (*arrow*)

22.4 Conclusions

The necessity of evaluating and reporting NCFs in cardiac imaging has been debated in the literature.

- Many of the NCFs are not clinically significant or may be indeterminate requiring additional investigations, leading to additional workload and increase in health-care cost.
  In addition, patients may experience unnecessary additional radiation, morbidity from complications during (invasive) workup, and added anxiety.
- On the other hand, patient may benefit from non-cardiac diagnoses or early detection of unsuspected disease that are potentially treatable, including malignancy.
  Reverse calculations estimating cost savings related to future morbidity and mortality had these findings gone undiscovered is difficult to be quantified and remain unclear [31].
- Keeping in mind our ethical duty to patients, there is wisdom in acquiring as much information from cardiac CT as possible and analyzing the full patient anatomy that has been irradiated.
  Comparison with prior imaging and using evidence-based recommendations for management where available are also prudent resource utilization.

References

1. Cho JH, Park JS, Shin DG, et al. Prevalence of extracardiac findings in the evaluation of ischemic heart disease by multidetector computed tomography. J Geriatr Cardiol. 2013;10(3):242–6.
2. Haller S, Kaiser C, Buser P, et al. Coronary artery imaging with contrast-enhanced MDCT: extracardiac findings. Am J Roentgenol. 2006;187:105–10.
3. Lee CI, Tsai EB, Sigal BM, et al. Incidental extracardiac findings at coronary CT: clinical and economic impact. Am J Roentgenol. 2010;194(6):1531–8. https://doi.org/10.2214/AJR.09.3587.
4. Onuma Y, Tanabe K, Nakazawa G, et al. Noncardiac findings in cardiac imaging with multidetector computed tomography. J Am Coll Cardiol. 2006;48:402–6.
5. Kirsch J, Araoz PA, Steinberg FB, et al. Prevalence and significance of incidental extracardiac findings at 64-multidetector coronary CTA. J Thorac Imaging. 2007;22:330–4.
6. Greenberg-Wolff I, Uliel L, Goitein O, et al. Extracardiac findings on coronary computed tomography scanning. Isr Med Assoc J. 2008;10:806–8.
7. Williams MC, Hunter A, Shah ASV, et al. Impact of noncardiac findings in patients undergoing CT coronary angiography: a substudy of the Scottish computed tomography of the heart (SCOT-HEART) trial. Eur Radiol. 2018;70(6):ii1–8.
8. Kay FU, Canan A, Abbara S. Common incidental findings on cardiac CT: a systematic review. Curr Cardiovasc Imaging Rep. 2019;12(6):21.
9. Karius P, Schuetz GM, Schlattmann P, et al. Extracardiac findings on coronary CT angiography: a systematic review. J Cardiovasc Comput Tomography. 2014;8:174–82.
10. Flor N, Di Leo G, Squarza SAC, et al. Malignant incidental extracardiac findings on cardiac CT: systematic review and meta-analysis. Am J Roentgenol. 2013;201(3):555–64.

11. Kim TJ, Han DH, Jin KN, et al. Lung cancer detected at cardiac CT: prevalence, clinicoradiologic features, and importance of full-field-of—view images. Radiology. 2010;255:369–76.
12. Northam M, Koonce J. Ravenel JG pulmonary nodules detected at cardiac CT: comparison of images in limited and full fields of view. Am J Roentgenol. 2008;191(3):878–81.
13. Webb WR, Brant WE, Major NM. Fundamentals of body CT. 4th ed. Saunders; 2014.
14. Sosnouski D, Bonsall RP, Mayer FB, et al. Extracardiac findings at cardiac CT. J Thorac Imaging. 2007;22(1):77–85.
15. Koonce J, Schoepf JU, Nguyen SA, et al. Extracardiac findings at cardiac CT: experience with 1,764 patients. Eur Radiol. 2009;19:570–6.
16. Paez R, Kammer MN, Massion P. Risk stratification of indeterminate pulmonary nodules. Curr Opin Pulm Med. 2021;27:240–8. https://doi.org/10.1097/MCP.0000000000000780.
17. MacMahon H, Naidich DP, Goo JM, Lee KS, Leung ANC, Mayo JR, et al. Guidelines for management of incidental pulmonary nodules detected on CT images: from the Fleischner society. Radiology. 2017;2017:228–43.
18. Callister MEJ, Baldwin DR, Akram AR, et al. British Thoracic Society guidelines for the investigation and management of pulmonary nodules. Thorax. 2015;70:ii1–ii54.
19. Gould MK, Donington J, Lynch WR, et al. Evaluation of individuals with pulmonary nodules: when is it lung cancer? Diagnosis and management of lung cancer, 3rd ed: American College of Chest Physicians evidence-based clinical practice guidelines. Chest. 2013;143:e93S–e120S.
20. Scoltz JW, Lu MT, Hedgire S, et al. Incidental pulmonary nodules in emergent coronary CT angiography for acute coronary syndrome: impact of revised 2017 Fleischner society guidelines. J Cardiovasc Comput Tomogr. 2018;12(1):28–33.
21. Walker CM, Abbott GF, Greene RE, et al. Imaging pulmonary infection: classic signs and patterns. Am J Roent. 2014;202(3):479–92.
22. Dueck NP, Epstein S, Franquet T, et al. Atypical pneumonia: definition, causes and imaging features. Radiographics. 2021;41(3):720–41.
23. Nasseri F, Eftekhari F. Clinical and radiologic review of the Normal and abnormal thymus: pearls and pitfalls. Radiographics. 2010;30(2):413–28.
24. Broderick LS, Brooks GN, Kuhlman JE. Anatomic pitfalls of the heart and pericardium. Radiographics. 2005;25(2):441–53.
25. Haugen BR, Alexander EK, Bible KC, Doherty GM, Mandel SJ, Nikiforov YE, et al. American Thyroid Association management guidelines for adult patients with thyroid nodules and differentiated thyroid cancer: the American Thyroid Association guidelines task force on thyroid nodules and differentiated thyroid cancer. Thyroid. 2015;2016:1–133.
26. Macmillan MT, Williams MC. Incidental Non-cardiac Findings in Cardiovascular Imaging. Curr Treat Options Cardiovasc Med. 2018;20(12):93.
27. Israel GM, Bosniak MA. An update of the Bosniak renal cyst classification system. Urology. 2005;66(3):484–8.
28. Fassnacht M, Arlt W, Bancos I, et al. Management of adrenal incidentalomas: European Society of Endocrinology Clinical Practice Guideline in collaboration with the European network for the study of adrenal tumors. Eur J Endocrinol. 2016;175(2):G1–G34.
29. Mayo-Smith WW, Song JH, Boland GL, et al. Management of Incidental Adrenal Masses: a white paper of the ACR incidental findings committee. J Am Coll Radiol. 2017;14(8):1038–44.
30. Moyle P, Sonoda L, Britton P, Sinnatamby R. Incidental breast lesions detected on CT: what is their significance? Br J Radiol. 2010;83(987):233–40.
31. Bhambhvani P. The good, bad and ugly of incidental findings on cardiovascular-computed tomography. J Nucl Cardiol. 2016;23:1275–9.

CT for TAVR Guidance

23

Muhammad Umair, Julianna Czum, and Stefan L. Zimmerman

Abstract

Cardiac CT is an important tool for pre-procedural planning and assessment of post-procedural complications in the setting of surgical and catheter-based cardiac valve repair and replacement. Dedicated software is commonly used to derive quantitative metrics for selecting the optimal device type and size for catheter-based techniques. High image quality is critical for accurate measurement. Use of cardiac CT will likely continue to expand as the field of transcatheter-based structural heart disease therapies grows.

Keywords

Transcatheter aortic valve implantation (TAVI) · Transcatheter mitral valve replacement (TMVR) · Computed tomography angiogram (CTA) · Post-processing

Abbreviations

CMPR	Curved multiplanar reformation
ECG	Electrocardiogram
LVOT	Left ventricular outflow tract
MAC	Mitral annular calcification
MPR	Multiplanar reformation
ROI	Region of interest
SAVR	Surgical aortic valve placement
TAVR	Transcatheter aortic valve replacement
TAVI	Transcatheter aortic valve implantation
TMVR	Transcatheter mitral valve replacement
ViV	Valve-in-valve
VTC	Virtual valve to coronary (distance)

M. Umair · J. Czum · S. L. Zimmerman (✉)
Johns Hopkins University, Baltimore, MD, USA
e-mail: mumair2@jhmi.edu; jczum1@jhmi.edu; stefan.zimmerman@jhmi.edu

23.1 Transcatheter Aortic Valve Replacement (TAVR)

- Transcatheter aortic valve replacement (TAVR), also called transcatheter aortic valve implantation (TAVI), is a minimally invasive interventional technique for placement of a prosthetic valve into aortic position using catheter-based vascular access under fluoroscopic guidance [1–3].

23.1.1 Preparation, Technique, and Acquisition [1, 2, 4–6]

- Patient selection is usually based on recommendations from society guidelines [1, 3–5]. Initially, only highly selected individuals with high-risk characteristics for conventional, surgical aortic valve replacement were considered. With improving experience and technology, indications for TAVR continue to expand.

A. A. Zadeh, J. Hoe (eds.), *Practical Guide to Cardiac CT*,
https://doi.org/10.1007/978-981-97-6919-3_23

- Considerations of contrast dose in the setting of renal compromise, contrast allergy/premedication, and radiation dose considerations [6] mainly follow other cardiac CT procedures and protocols (see CHAPTER V).
- Case-by-case discussions with the clinical team is encouraged for patients with complex risk–benefit considerations.
- A non-contrast CT scan prior to the injection of contrast is optional. The aortic valve calcium (Agatston) score can help differentiate moderate and severe aortic stenosis when the diagnosis is uncertain (see CHAPTER XIX). Calcium burden may add more insights into the interventional planning especially in cases with heavy annular, leaflet, and left ventricular outflow calcifications and preferred at some institutions.
- Cardiac CT with retrospective ECG-gating technique to image the whole cardiac cycle is performed during the maximal contrast opacification in the ascending aorta (most commonly using bolus tracking method; region of interest (ROI) in the ascending aorta, bolus injection rate of 4–6 mL/s), however, consistent angiographic opacification is also expected throughout the aorta and iliofemoral arteries on the subsequent non-ECG gated CT to map vasculature to select and plan vascular access route [1].
- Alternatively, a retrospective CT only limited to the coverage of the aortic valve can be obtained in cases where low dose contrast injection is recommended (e.g., advanced renal failure).
- Subsequent non-ECG synchronized CT of the whole aorta and iliofemoral vessels is performed. If available, a high-pitch dual-source technique can be useful to reduce cardiac, respiratory, and patient motion artifacts and for consistent distal arterial opacification in iliofemoral arteries.

23.1.2 Post-Processing, Measurements, and Interpretations

23.1.2.1 Valve Assessment [1, 4, 7, 8]

- Assessment of image quality is a critical first step for the interpretation of any valve planning CT case, including careful inspection for motion and artifacts.
- Post-processing performed with a dedicated software with capabilities of 3D reconstructions, multiplanar reformatting (MPR), and curved multiplanar reformatting (CMPR).
- Aortic annular measurements are obtained in end-systole per convention as they result in the largest annular dimensions. Using MPR techniques, the true orthogonal plane of the aortic annulus is selected [4, 7, 8] (Fig. 23.1).
- A drawing of the outline of the annulus is performed (different methods available depending on the post-processing software) a measurement of the perimeter, area, and maximum and minimum diameter of the annulus for that cardiac phase are determined.
- In the past, measurements of the sinuses of Valsalva and coronary heights were performed in the diastolic phase, however, in current practice, systolic phase is often used for all annulus and root measurements and the diastolic phase is considered optional (Fig. 23.2).
- Optional measurements of the sub-valvular LVOT can also be provided. Sub-valvular LVOT is a part of the landing zone of the implanted valve. Calcifications that protrude in the LVOT can make intervention challenging with increased risk of paravalvular leaks and qualitative degree of calcifications (no, mild, moderate, severe) is worthy of mention in the imaging report (Fig. 23.3).
- Heights of the left and right coronary arteries from the aortic annulus are also measured due to concern for coverage of the coronary artery ostia by the valve prosthesis. Coronary heights >10 mm above the annulus is desired [8]. However, there are no definitive thresholds to rule-out intervention (Fig. 23.4).
- The morphology of the valve (tricuspid versus bicuspid) is best determined on MPR reconstructions orthogonal with respect to the level of leaflets on dynamic cine images throughout the cardiac cycle.
- Optimal C-arm fluoroscopic projections in systole and diastole [1, 4, 8].

  By aligning the nadirs of the sinuses of Valsalva such that they are equidistant, the optimal C-arm coplanar projections without parallax can be predicted by dedicated 3D reconstruction of CT-TAVR dataset into post-

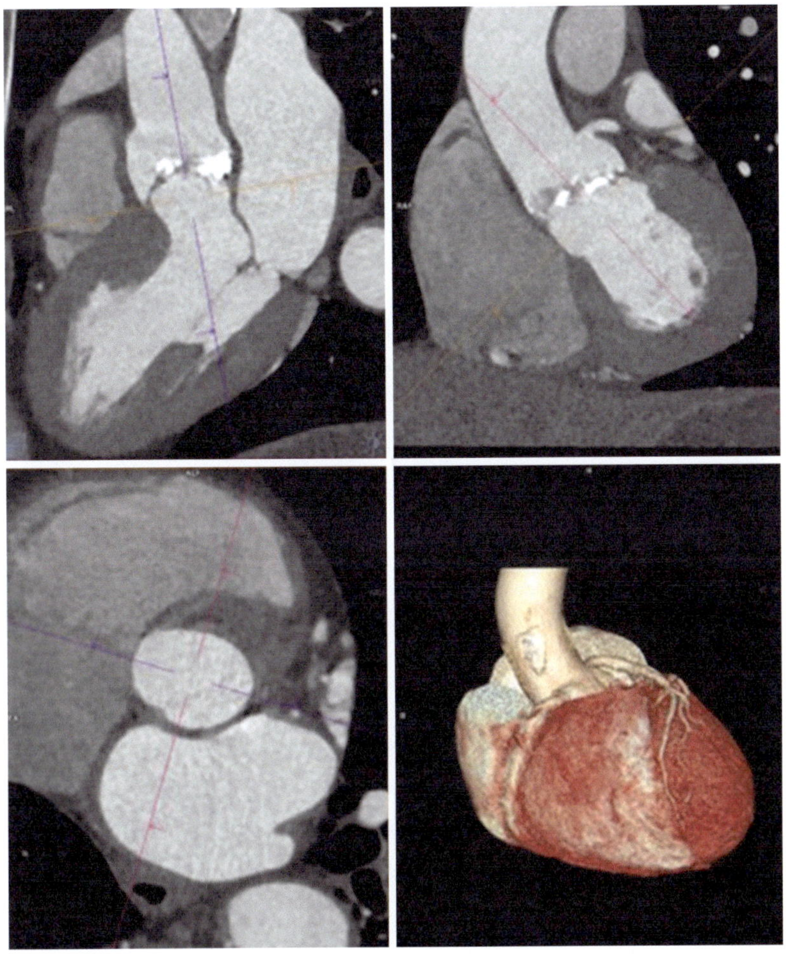

Fig. 23.1 A case demonstration of determining aortic valve annular dimensions. Multiplanar reformatted images (MPR) in orthogonal planes obtained through the aortic annulus for valve sizing in a 66-year-old male with severe aortic stenosis. The annular plane (bottom left image of panel) is the plane formed by the nadir of the three valve cusps at their attachment sites in the LVOT. Note the annular plane, prescribed by the orange line on the upper images of the panel, intersects with the nadir of the valve leaflets

processing software. The predicted projections are reported with respect to the lateral (right-left) obliquity as well as craniocaudal obliquity. This reduces the time, cost, and radiation in the angiography suite to identify these projections (Fig. 23.5).

- In select cases with high quality imaging and low atherosclerotic disease burden, an evaluation of the proximal coronary arteries is also possible. However, at present, this is not universally performed given that scans are usually performed without heart rate controlling medications or nitroglycerin in the setting of severe aortic stenosis, which limit image quality. In addition, given the advanced age of many patients, the extent and calcification of coronary artery disease is often severe, posing challenges to current CT technology.

23.1.2.2 Vascular Mapping for Guidance

Aortic Anatomy and Measurements

- The critical aortic measurements are: three diameters at the sinuses of Valsalva, two orthogonal measurements each of the sinotubular junction, mid-ascending aorta, proximal and distal aortic arch, and mid-descending aorta. An aortic aneurysm may change the procedural approach.
- The aortic arch branch pattern and disease should be described in case transfemoral access is not feasible.

23.1.2.3 Lower Extremity Access [1, 8]

- The vascular access for TAVR is primarily transfemoral unless both arteries reveal severe atherosclerotic disease or other pathologies, in

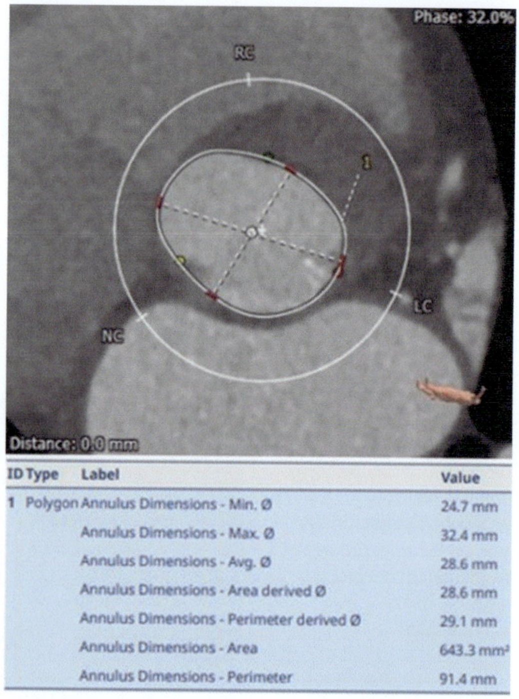

Fig. 23.2 Typical TAVR annular measurements provided by dedicated software

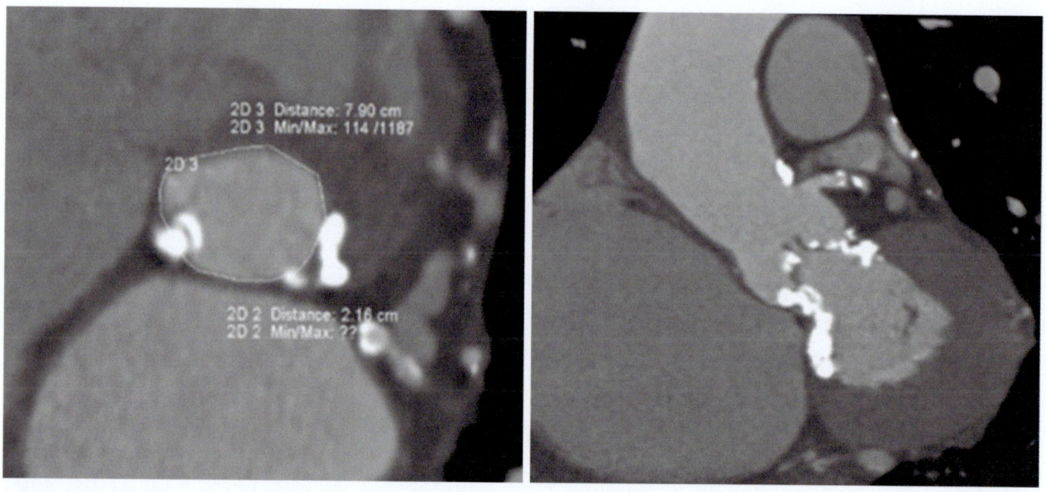

Fig. 23.3 Severe sub-valvar calcification in the left ventricular outflow tract can negatively impact stent apposition to the LVOT wall and result in paravalvular regurgitation

which event access via the carotid or subclavian arteries may be considered.

- The smallest arterial lumen diameter between the aortic valve and both common femoral arteries should be provided. Optional is the routine report of additional diameters of the bilateral common and external iliac arteries.
- The measurements may be obtained semi-automatically with the help of available post-processing software (Fig. 23.6).
- Presence and extent of aortic and ileo-femoral atherosclerosis, calcification, and lumen stenosis should be reported for assessing feasibility of access and risk of vascular dissection

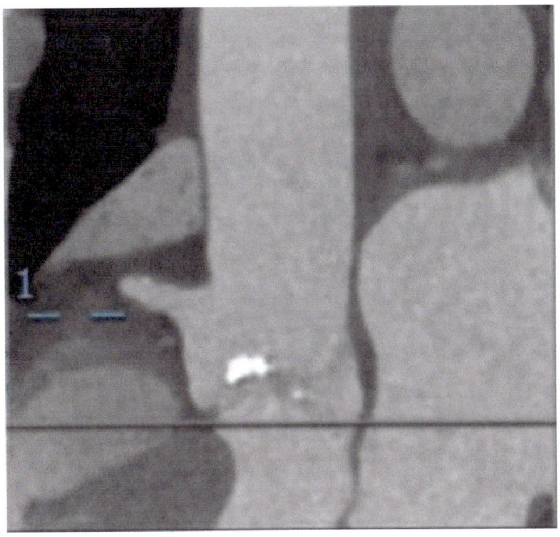

Fig. 23.4 Measurement of coronary ostial heights from the annular plane. By convention, measurements are made by drawing a line perpendicular to the annular plane to the bottom of the coronary artery at its origin, which measured 1.4 cm in this patient

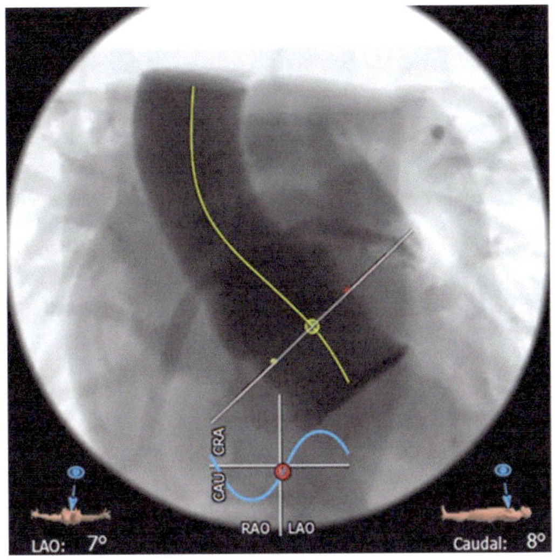

Fig. 23.5 Simulated fluoroscopic view of the aortic root for estimation of the optimal C-arm angles. These images can be obtained using post-processing software to help save fluoroscopic procedure time during valve implantation by suggesting the optimal angles of the C-arm for visualizing the root

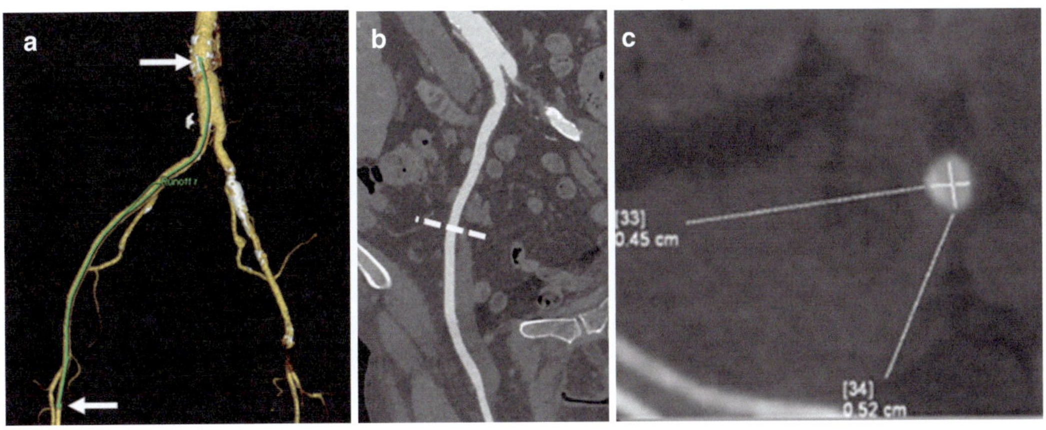

Fig. 23.6 Vascular access analysis for TAVR. Panel (**a**) shows a volume rendered 3D image of the iliac arteries with the placement of seed points proximally and distally in the right aortoiliac region. Post-processing software then traces the centerline of the vessel between these two points. Panel (**b**) shows a curved multiplanar reconstruction (CMPR) using projections in multiple angles through the centerline. Panel C shows short-axis images perpendicular to the centerline (dashed line in Panel **b**) to evaluate for minimal vessel diameters in each vascular segment

or athero-embolus during transfemoral retrograde cardiac catheterization.

- In cases where lower extremity access is expected to be suboptimal or impractical, the assessment of the stenosis, atherosclerotic plaques, occlusions, and tortuosity of the subclavian and common carotid arteries should be included in the report.
- Any significant extravascular incidental findings should also be reported, particularly, if these may affect the TAVR procedure or the patient's prognosis.

23.2 Transcatheter Mitral Valve Replacement (TMVR) [9, 10]

- Transcatheter mitral valve replacement (TMVR) is a minimally invasive approach of replacing the mitral valve using a transcatheter intravascular access under fluoroscopy.
- Open surgical valve replacement remains the procedure of choice among patients who are good surgical candidates, but TMVR has become a safe and effective option in high-risk patients, when repair may not be sufficient to address severe mitral regurgitation.
- It is likely that the clinical indication of TMVR will continue to expand, alike TAVR.

23.2.1 Technique and Acquisition [11]

- A cardiac CT examination is tailored to assess the mitral valve. A multiphasic contrast bolus administration (100% contrast first, followed by 50% saline) may be needed for optimal opacification of both right and left chambers (trans-septal access is commonly chosen).
- A bolus tracking software is used with ROI in the ascending aorta or left ventricle.
- ECG-gated retrospective CT cardiac examination is performed throughout the cardiac cycle with attention to the dynamic assessment of the mitral valve and the LVOT.
- An additional CT acquisition ranging from the carina to the pelvis (including the groin vasculature) may be obtained in the venous phase of opacification for venous access planning depending upon local expertise/preference.

23.2.2 Post-Processing, Measurements, and Interpretations [11, 12]

- Mitral valve morphology should be described, including the presence and extent of calcification of leaflets and/or annulus (mitral annular calcification [MAC]), particularly caseous MAC, leaflet thickening, prolapse or disjunction, flail leaflet, dilation of the annulus and coaptation of the leaflets.
- Similar to the CTA-TAVR cases, the optimal tube projection angles for deployment under fluoroscopy can be provided to reduce time, cost and radiation.
- Valvular measurements are being provided by dedicated software given the complex structure of the saddle shaped annulus. A simplified set of measurements may be performed for cases of D-shaped annulus with common, conventional software capable of MPR reconstructions.
- The D-shaped annulus represents the in-plane portions of the annulus with the exclusion of the part of the annulus that projects out of plane toward the aortic valve [12, 13]. This portion is truncated from the annular plane by drawing a connecting line from fibrous trigone to fibrous trigone (Fig. 23.7).
- There is no consensus on the optimal phase of the cardiac cycle for mitral annular measurements and annulus measurements are often provided in the end-diastole and end-systole given the dynamism of the annular shape and size.
- The area and perimeter of the annulus can be obtained by ROI method.
- Device over-sizing and under-sizing can cause serious complications, for example, there is a risk of annular rupture with device over-sizing or risk of compression of the circumflex artery that can lead to a circumflex territory infarct. Similarly, if undersized, there is a risk of device mal-positioning, dislodgement, or embolization.

23.2.3 LVOT Obstruction Risk Assessment [11–15]

- A possible complication of TMVR is obstruction (fixed or dynamic) of the LVOT due to the prosthesis protruding into the LVOT [11, 12, 14, 15].
- The aortomitral angulation is a key indicator for LVOT obstruction post intervention.

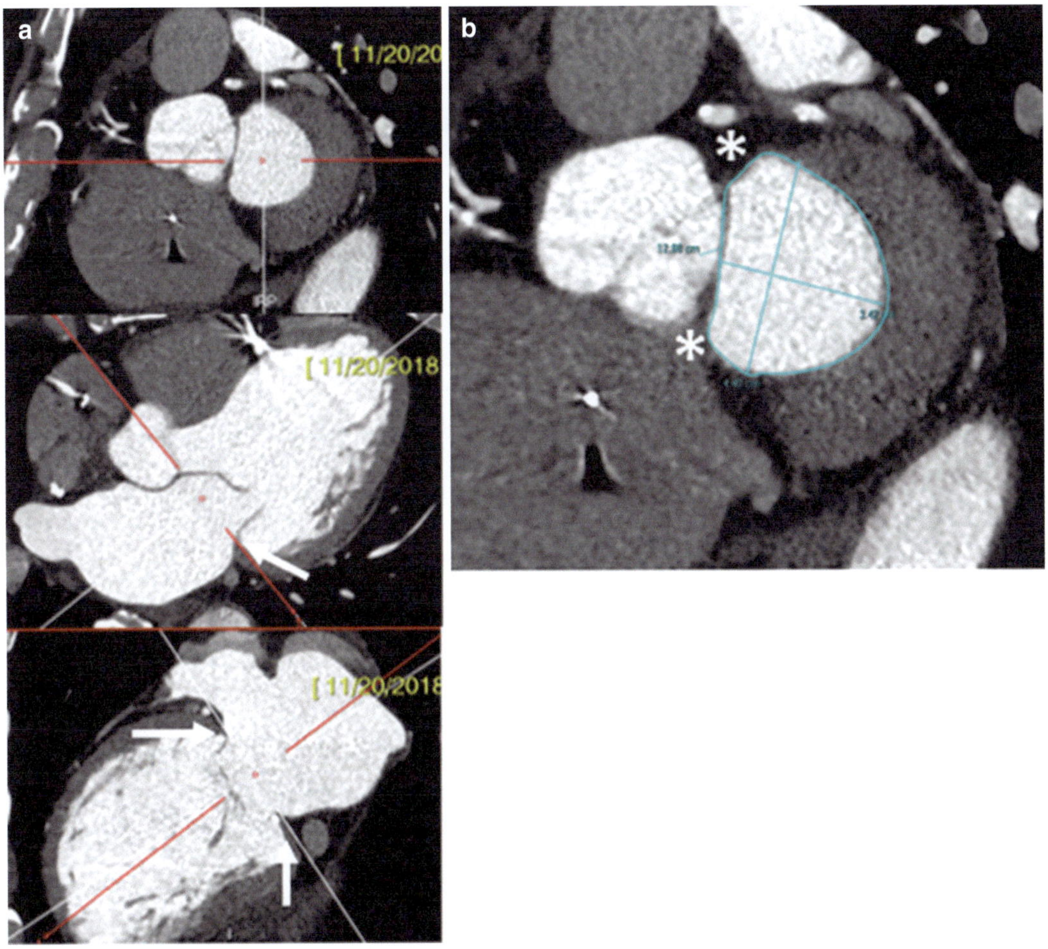

Fig. 23.7 Mitral annulus assessment for TMVR planning. Panel (**a**) Multiplanar reformatting with three orthogonal views through the junction of the mitral leaflets and the LV on the long axis views (arrows). Panel (**b**) Focused short-axis image of the D-shaped mitral annulus with perimeter measurement including the planar component of the annulus and the straight side of the "D" composed by a line connecting fibrous trigone to fibrous trigone (asterisks)

- The aortomitral angulation is measured by drawing an angle between the lines orthogonal to the mitral and aortic valve planes. Alternatively, this can be achieved by measuring the angle between lines formed parallel to the aortic and mitral annular planes on the left ventricular outflow tract reconstruction (Fig. 23.8). This can be drawn in an MPR capable software by making a true 3-chamber/LVOT view. The angle can be measured both in systole and diastole in the interest of consistency.
- Additional factors determining the risks of LVOT obstruction include the basal septal

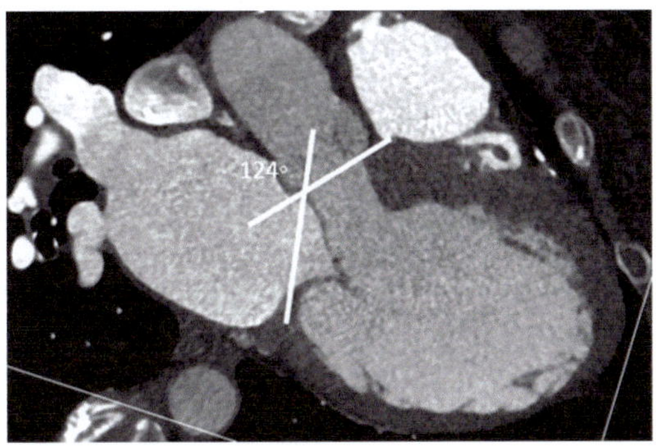

Fig. 23.8 Aortomitral angle measurement is achieved by measuring the angle between lines formed parallel to the aortic and mitral annular planes on the left ventricular outflow tract reconstruction

thickening, the dimensions of the left ventricle (minimal LV diameter) and the landing zone toward LVOT (dimensions of the LVOT in systole and diastole—perimeter, area, long and short axes) [13–15].

- The ideal valve position will be a near parallel orientation of the two axes; however, this is not often achievable. The risk of obstruction increases as the angle between these two axes becomes larger and approaches 90 degrees. No threshold for success/abort has been established and the final determination is made by the interventionalist's judgment.

23.3 Post-Valve Replacement Imaging

23.3.1 Post-Aortic Valve Replacement CT Imaging (Surgical or TAVR) [1, 8]

- Echocardiography but not CT imaging is indicated for routine follow-up for assessment of prosthetic valve function, durability, or cardiac function after TAVR.
- CT imaging, however, is well suited for evaluating suspected post-surgical complications.
- Common indications for post-TAVR cardiac CT imaging include suspected prosthetic valve thrombosis, hypoattenuating leaflet thickening (HALT), infective endocarditis, and evaluation of the structural integrity of the landing zone (pseudoaneurysm, rupture and extravasation, paravalvular leak, etc.) (Fig. 23.9).
- Assessment of the coronary artery ostia for potential obstruction by the graft is a critical finding. Adequate opacification of the coronary arteries should be noted.
- Post-operative assessment of the access vessels may be performed with a CTA of the abdomen and pelvis. If attention to both the valve and the access site is required, a combined examination similar to pre-TAVR may be performed.

23.3.1.1 Valve-in-Valve (ViV) Planning and Imaging considerations [1]

- Valve-in-valve (ViV) transcatheter replacement approach involves the implantation of a prosthetic valve inside an already implanted valve (surgical or post-TAVR).
- Among these cases, the surgical valve ring represents the narrowest fixed obstruction that

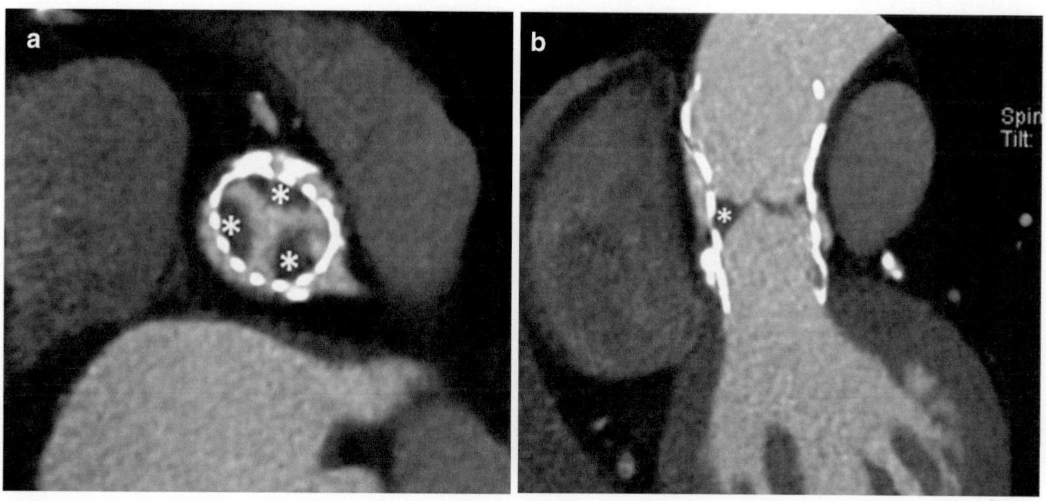

Fig. 23.9 Hypoattenuating leaflet thickening (HALT, asterisks) on short (**a**) and long axis (**b**) views of the aortic valve in a patient 3 months after TAVR, who complained of new onset dyspnea. HALT may affect leaflet mobility as well as the structural valve integrity, and is an important indicator for risk of valve failure

becomes the basis for implantation of the TAVR device.

- Measurements of the internal dimensions of the surgical valve ring are obtained to confirm the absence of significant post-operative distortion and to size the TAVR device.
- The risk of coronary ostia obstruction is an important consideration since ViV placement is more likely to affect the ostia than with primary TAVR.
- In ViV cases, the distance from the expected location of the outer edge of the planned TAVR device (which has been termed the virtual valve) to the coronary ostia in the short-axis plane should be provided (= virtual valve to coronary distance) to assess the risk of coronary obstruction.
- The virtual valve can be simulated on the short-axis CT images by creating an ROI with a diameter matching the intended transcatheter device. A virtual valve to coronary distance (VTC) of <3 mm increases the risk of coronary obstruction (Fig. 23.10).

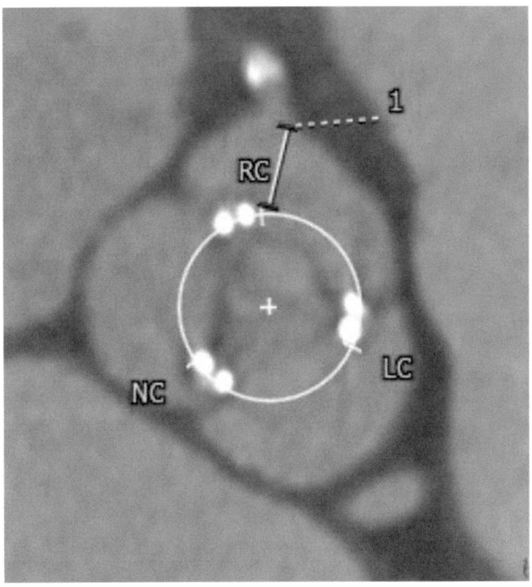

Fig. 23.10 Measurement of the virtual heart valve to coronary ostia (VTC) distance. Short-axis reconstruction through the root at the level of coronary ostia. A round region of interest with the diameter matching the diameter of the planned valve has been placed on the plane and centered on the prosthetic valve. The distance from this region of interest to the right coronary ostium has been measured [1]

- Vascular mapping of the lower extremity arterial vasculature for access assessment may be obtained if no recent prior CTA-TAVR imaging is available or if there were issues with prior access or prior vascular complications.

23.3.1.2 Post-Surgical Aortic Valve Replacement or Repair

- CT imaging post-surgical aortic valve placement (SAVR) is performed akin to post-TAVR protocols, post-processing techniques, and imaging interpretations as discussed above.
- Common indications include suspected valvular leak, pseudoaneurysm, rupture, coronary artery occlusion, valve thrombosis, leaflet degeneration, leaflet vegetations/endocarditis, assessment of structural integrity of the valve, paravalvular leaks, and mediastinal post-surgical complications.

23.3.2 Post-TMVR CT Imaging

23.3.2.1 CT for Planning Valve-in-Valve or Valve-in-Ring TMVR [12, 16]

- Prosthetic valve failure with severe mitral regurgitation is usually a long-term complication after TMVR while it is an immediate concern with valve-in-valve or valve-in-ring implantation.
- The image acquisition for CT cardiac morphology follows similar principles for the primary CT-TMVR imaging protocol.
- Structural integrity of the existing mitral annular ring as well of the prosthesis and its leaflets should be reported.
- Encroachment of the existing prosthesis into the LVOT is a pertinent finding to report (Fig. 23.11).
- Aortomitral angulation is determined by the axis of the prosthetic valve and the axis of the LVOT.
- Optimal fluoroscopic tube angle projections are not routinely needed as the existing valve is radiopaque and serves as a marker.
- Proximity of the prosthetic valve to the circumflex artery should be reported if there is

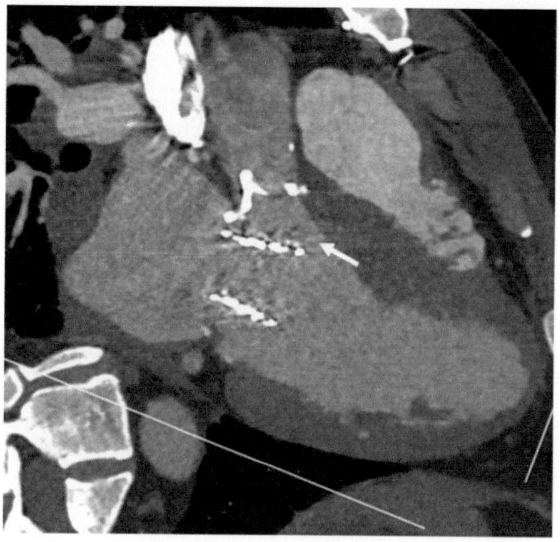

Fig. 23.11 Left ventricular outflow tract imaging in a patient post-transcatheter mitral valve replacement (TMVR) showing an aortic valve placed in the mitral position after failed prosthetic mitral valve replacement. The TMVR device projects into and narrows the LVOT (arrow)

concern for external compression (a concern with valve-in-valve mitral implantations).

23.3.3 CT Imaging of TMVR Complications [12]

- Assessment of the cardiac structure and morphology may be performed with similar techniques as for primary CT-TMVR planning, including evaluation for suspected LVOT obstruction, pseudoaneurysm, annular rupture, paravalvular leak, mal-positioning/dislodgement, or valve vegetations and/or abscess, etc.

23.4 CT Imaging for Other Valve Repair/Replacement Planning

- CT imaging for planning of tricuspid or pulmonary valve repair or replacements whether surgical or catheter based, follows similar protocols as described above (retrospective ECG-gated acquisition) with notable difference for optimizing contrast in the region of interest.
- Most such imaging protocols acquire full cardiac cycle acquisition (retrospective gating) with the coverage of the whole heart and the contrast opacification based on bolus tracking to maximize visualization of the valve in question.
- Numerous clinical trials investigating catheter-based replacement of the mitral, tricuspid, and pulmonic valve are ongoing, with CT imaging protocols and post-processing techniques usually prescribed by the device manufacturer.

References

1. Blanke P, Weir-McCall JR, Achenbach S, Delgado V, Hausleiter J, Jilaihawi H, Marwan M, Nørgaard BL, Piazza N, Schoenhagen P, Leipsic JA. Computed tomography imaging in the context of transcatheter aortic valve implantation (TAVI)/transcatheter aortic valve replacement (TAVR) an expert consensus document of the Society of Cardiovascular Computed Tomography. JACC Cardiovasc Imaging. 2019;12(1):1–24.
2. Otto C, Kumbhani D, Alexander K, et al. 2017 ACC expert consensus decision pathway for Transcatheter aortic valve replacement in the Management of Adults with Aortic Stenosis. J Am Coll Cardiol. 2017;69(10):1313–46.
3. Sundt TM, Jneid H. Guideline update on indications for transcatheter aortic valve implantation based on the 2020 American College of Cardiology/American Heart Association guidelines for management of valvular heart disease. JAMA Cardiol. 2021;6(9):1088–9.
4. Achenbach S, Delgado V, Hausleiter J, Schoenhagen P, Min JK, Leipsic JA. SCCT expert consensus document on computed tomography imaging before transcatheter aortic valve implantation (TAVI)/ transcatheter aortic valve replacement (TAVR). J Cardiovasc Comput Tomogr. 2012;6(6):366–80.
5. Leipsic JA, Blanke P, Hanley M, Batlle JC, Bolen MA, Brown RK, Desjardins B, Eberhardt RT, Gornik HL, Hurwitz LM, Maniar H. ACR appropriateness criteria® imaging for transcatheter aortic valve replacement. J Am Coll Radiol. 2017;14(11):S449–55.
6. Cohan R, Dillman JR, Hartman RP, Jafri SZ, Wang CK, Newhouse JH. American College of Radiology Manual on contrast media. American College of Radiology. Version, Reston; 2013. p. 9.
7. Pontone G, Andreini D, Bartorelli AL, Annoni A, Mushtaq S, Bertella E, Formenti A, Cortinovis S, Alamanni F, Fusari M, Bona V. Feasibility and accuracy of a comprehensive multidetector computed tomography acquisition for patients referred for balloon-expandable transcatheter aortic valve implantation. Am Heart J. 2011;161(6):1106–13.

8. Bloomfield GS, Gillam LD, Hahn RT, Kapadia S, Leipsic J, Lerakis S, Tuzcu M, Douglas PS. A practical guide to multimodality imaging of transcatheter aortic valve replacement. JACC Cardiovasc Imaging. 2012;5(4):441–55.
9. Members WC, Otto CM, Nishimura RA, Bonow RO, Carabello BA, Erwin JP III, Gentile F, Jneid H, Krieger EV, Mack M, McLeod C. 2020 ACC/AHA guideline for the management of patients with valvular heart disease: a report of the American College of Cardiology/American Heart Association joint committee on clinical practice guidelines. J Am Coll Cardiol. 2021;77(4):e25–197.
10. Gündüz S, Özkan M, Kalçik M, Gürsoy OM, Astarcioğlu MA, Karakoyun S, Aykan AÇ, Biteker M, Gökdeniz T, Kaya H, Yesin M. Sixty-four–section cardiac computed tomography in mechanical prosthetic heart valve dysfunction: thrombus or pannus. Circ Cardiovascular Imaging. 2015;8(12):e003246.
11. Blanke P, Naoum C, Webb J, Dvir D, Hahn RT, Grayburn P, Moss RR, Reisman M, Piazza N, Leipsic J. Multimodality imaging in the context of transcatheter mitral valve replacement: establishing consensus among modalities and disciplines. Cardiovasc Imaging. 2015;8(10):1191–208.
12. Ranganath P, Moore A, Guerrero M, Collins J, Foley T, Williamson E, Rajiah P. CT for pre-and postprocedural evaluation of transcatheter mitral valve replacement. Radiographics. 2020;40(6):1528–53.
13. Heiser L, Gohmann RF, Noack T, Renatus K, Lurz P, Thiele H, Seitz P, Gutberlet M. CT Planning prior to Transcatheter Mitral Valve Replacement (TMVR). RöFo. 2022;194(4):373–83.
14. Reid A, Ben Zekry S, Turaga M, Tarazi S, Bax JJ, Wang DD, Piazza N, Bapat VN, Ihdayhid AR, Cavalcante JL, Blanke P. Neo-LVOT and transcatheter mitral valve replacement: expert recommendations. Cardiovasc Imaging. 2021;14(4):854–66.
15. Blanke P, Naoum C, Dvir D, Bapat V, Ong K, Muller D, Cheung A, Ye J, Min JK, Piazza N, Theriault-Lauzier P. Predicting LVOT obstruction in transcatheter mitral valve implantation: concept of the neo-LVOT. JACC Cardiovasc Imaging. 2017;10(4):482–5.
16. Urena M, Vahanian A, Brochet E, Ducrocq G, Iung B, Himbert D. Current indications for transcatheter mitral valve replacement using transcatheter aortic valves: valve-in-valve, valve-in-ring, and valve-in-mitral annulus calcification. Circulation. 2021;143(2):178–96.

CT for Electrophysiology Applications

24

Thomas Boyle, David I. Feldman,
Roger S. Blumenthal, and Seamus P. Whelton

Abstract

The modern diagnosis and treatment of cardiac rhythm disorders relies on a broad array of multimodal cardiovascular imaging with a strong emphasis on cardiac CT, which may identify individuals at risk for arrhythmias and sudden cardiac death. CT images are the basis of the electro-anatomical voltage maps that serve as the anatomical roadmap for diagnostic and therapeutic procedures, including catheter ablation. In addition, CT is a valuable tool for procedural planning, diagnosing procedural complications, and predicting patient response to therapies. CT also has a high diagnostic accuracy for ruling out left atrial appendage thrombus prior to cardioversion of atrial fibrillation or flutter.

Keywords

Cardiac computed tomography · Electrophysiology · Cardiac structure · Left atrial appendage · Sudden cardiac death

Abbreviations

AF	Atrial fibrillation
ALCAPA	Anomalous left coronary artery from the pulmonary artery
ARVC	Arrhythmogenic right ventricular cardiomyopathy
cMRI	Cardiac magnetic resonance imaging
LAA	Left atrial appendage
MPR	Multiplanar formation
PET	Positron emission tomography
TEE	Trans-esophageal echocardiography

T. Boyle
Department of Medicine, Johns Hopkins School of Medicine, Johns Hopkins Ciccarone Center for the Prevention of Cardiovascular Disease, Baltimore, MD, USA
e-mail: tboyle5@jhmi.edu

D. I. Feldman
Division of Cardiology, Harvard University, Boston, MA, USA

Department of Medicine, Johns Hopkins School of Medicine, Johns Hopkins Ciccarone Center for the Prevention of Cardiovascular Disease, Baltimore, MD, USA

R. S. Blumenthal
Department of Medicine, Johns Hopkins School of Medicine, Johns Hopkins Ciccarone Center for the Prevention of Cardiovascular Disease, Baltimore, MD, USA
e-mail: rblument@jhmi.edu

S. P. Whelton (✉)
Department of Medicine, Johns Hopkins School of Medicine, Baltimore, MD, USA

Johns Hopkins Ciccarone Center for the Prevention of Cardiovascular Disease, Baltimore, MD, USA
e-mail: seamus.whelton@jhmi.edu

A. A. Zadeh, J. Hoe (eds.), *Practical Guide to Cardiac CT*,
https://doi.org/10.1007/978-981-97-6919-3_24

24.1 Guidance of Ablation for Atrial Fibrillation

- Atrial fibrillation (AF) is the most common arrhythmia in adults [1]. Ablation of atrial fibrillation is focused on the pulmonary veins, which are crucial to the initiation and propagation of atrial fibrillation [2–4]. The primary goal of AF ablation is to create electrical isolation of the pulmonary veins, though additional lesions may be placed to ablate ectopic foci or create preferential conduction pathways elsewhere in the atria [5–7].
- Operators must know the location of pulmonary veins so that they can accurately isolate them with ablation lines. In radiofrequency ablation, this requires a carefully placed series of focal ablation lesions just outside the pulmonary vein ostia.
- Knowledge of the anatomy is important for creating complete electrical isolation and avoiding errant ablation lesions that could lead to complications.
- There is a small risk of pulmonary vein stenosis with catheter ablation, which may result in pulmonary hypertension in severe cases [8]. This is a rare complication, occurring in <1% of cases, which can be diagnosed by CT [9, 10, 11].
- Having a pre-operative CT is helpful for establishing baseline pulmonary vein stenosis that could otherwise be attributed to the procedure or could be present in a patient with prior catheter ablation [12]. Severe stenosis is defined as >70% reduction in the ostial lumen [13].
- CT is the ideal method for determining the number and shape of pulmonary veins and ostia as well as their relationship to other structures [14–16].
- About 30% of patients with atrial fibrillation have anatomy other than the typical arrangement of two left and two right pulmonary veins (Fig. 24.1) [13, 17–19].

24.1.1 CT Protocol for Assessment of Pulmonary Veins and Left Atrium

- Imaging typically occurs at end systole (40% of the R-R cycle) with prospective scan triggering to minimize radiation dose (typically in the range of 2–4 mSv).
- X-ray tube settings may be lowered compared to coronary assessment as less detail is needed, e.g., 80–100 kV, with larger slice thickness of 1 mm to reduce noise.
- Heart rate control is not required nor is the need for nitroglycerine for vasodilation.
- Scans are being triggered with similar timing to coronary angiography.
- Common postprocessing tools help displaying the left atrial pulmonary veins with color coding (Fig. 24.1).

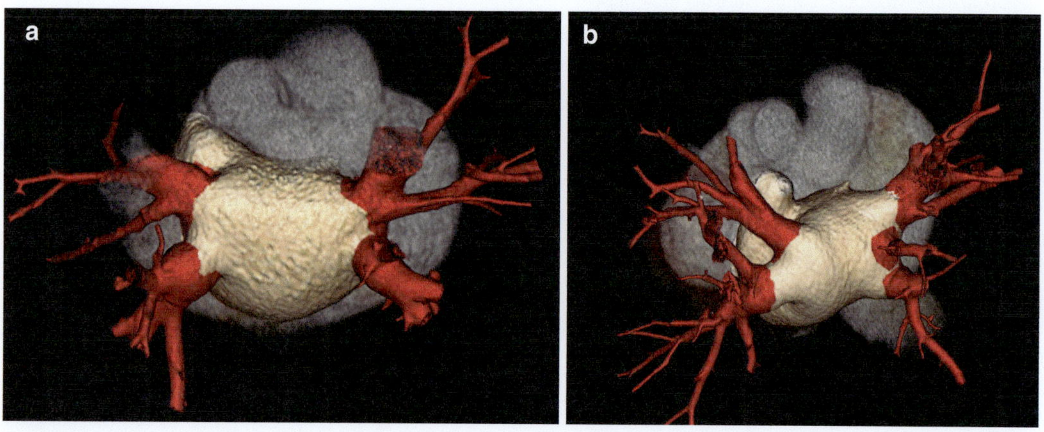

Fig. 24.1 A volume-rendered CT image of the left atrium (tan) and pulmonary vein anatomy (red). Note the normal pulmonary vein anatomy in Panel (**a**) and the normal variant anatomy in Panel (**b**), with 3 right and 2 left pulmonary veins

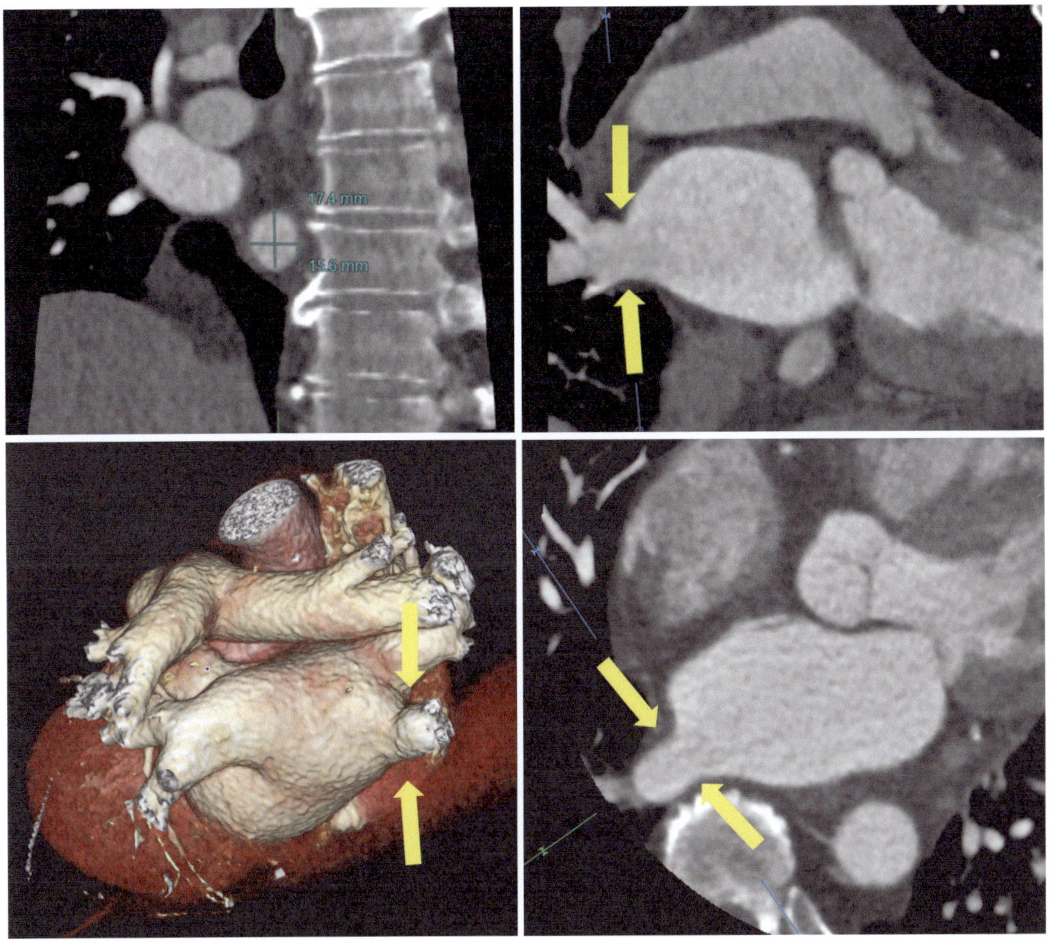

Fig. 24.2 Measurement of right inferior pulmonary vein diameter

- Each pulmonary vein should be measured cross-sectionally using double oblique MPR images at its ostium where it merges with the left atrium (Fig. 24.2).
- The two most common normal variants are the presence of three right pulmonary veins or one common left pulmonary vein.
- If there is suspicion of pulmonary vein stenosis following ablation, CT can easily confirm the diagnosis prior to treatment by angioplasty (Fig. 24.3).
- CT assessment of left atrial area and volume is a validated predictor of AF recurrence after ablation (Fig. 24.4) [21, 22].
- Measurement of left atrial area is most commonly performed in the 4-chamber view by tracing the outline of the left atrium. Care should be taken not to include the pulmonary veins in the measurement of left atrial size. Size is commonly categorized as normal <20 mm^2, mild 20–29 mm^2, moderate 30–35 mm^2, and severe ≥35mm^2.
- Left atrial volume can be measured using automated software, such as that for functional analyses. There is some variation in definitions for size by volume, but it is often categorized as normal <100 mL, mild 100–129 mL, moderate 130–149 mL, and severe ≥150 mL.

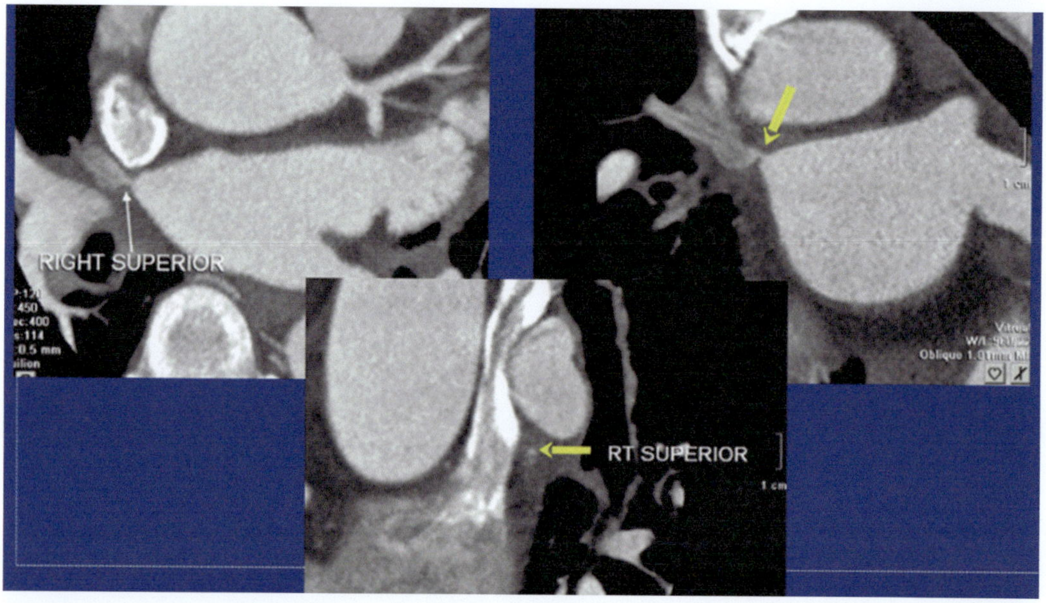

Fig. 24.3 Example of pulmonary vein stenosis (arrows)

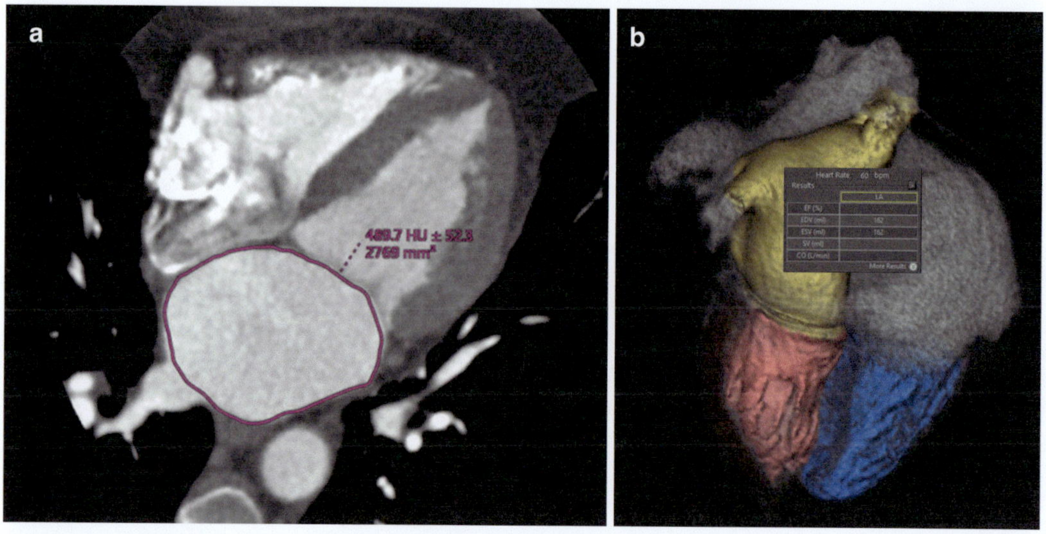

Fig. 24.4 Measurement of left atrial area (Panel **a**) and volume (Panel **b**)

24.2 Detection of Left Atrial Thrombus

- Prior to cardioversion or catheter ablation, patients need to be evaluated for intracardiac thrombus, which may be present even in a person who is continuously anticoagulated.
- Trans-esophageal echocardiography (TEE) is considered the gold standard for evaluation of left atrial appendage (LAA) thrombus, but requires sedation, can be relatively time-consuming, and while minimally invasive does have some rare, but potentially serious risks [23–25].
- CT has gained increasing recognition as an alternative to TEE for the detection of LAA thrombus and has become the procedure of choice at some institutions [26, 27].

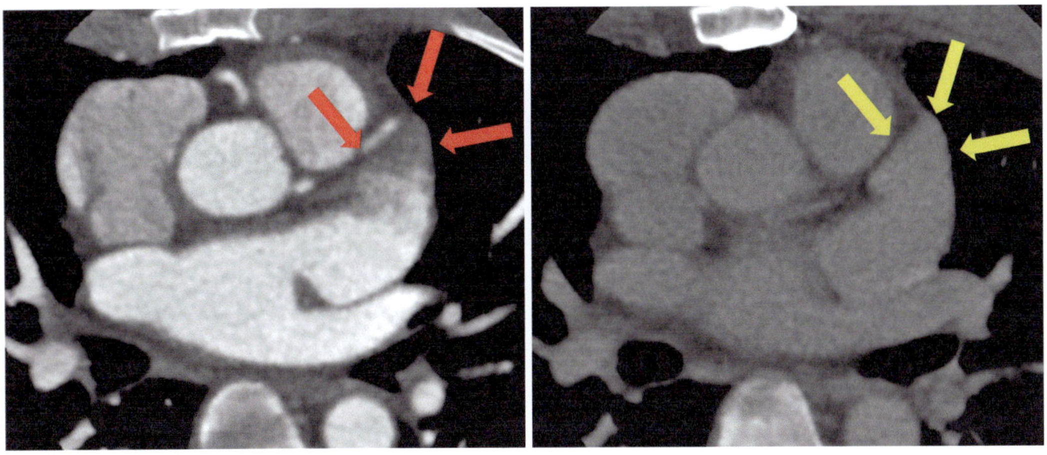

Fig. 24.5 Initial and second pass imaging for LAA thrombus evaluation by CT. Arrows denote incomplete opacification of LAA on first pass imaging (red) with subsequent complete opacification on second pass imaging (yellow)

- CT is particularly well suited as a rule out test for the presence of LAA thrombus because of its high spatial resolution and sensitivity.
- To improve specificity, CT assessment of LAA thrombus should include a second, delayed acquisition (30–60 s after the initial scan), to account for slow filling times, particularly in the setting of low cardiac output and large chamber size (Fig. 24.5).
- In a meta-analysis of 19 studies comparing CT with TEE in about 3000 patients, CT was a highly reliable alternative to TEE (sensitivity 100%; specificity 99%; positive predictive value 92%; negative predictive value 100%) [28].
- The Society for Cardiovascular Computed Tomography recommends CT with a second delayed image acquisition to ensure complete LAA opacification as an alternative to TEE for excluding LA/LAA thrombus where the risks of TEE outweigh the benefits as part of a shared decision-making discussion [29].

24.3 Reporting Pulmonary Vein and Left Atrial Scan Results

- A standardized reporting format is essential and should include:
  - Presence/absence of LAA thrombus.
  - Pulmonary vein anatomy.
  - Size of left atrium.
  - Presence of cardiac and vascular calcification (e.g. coronary artery calcium, aortic valve calcium, ascending/descending aorta calcium, etc.)
  - Noncardiac findings.

24.4 Guidance of Transcutaneous Left Atrial Appendage Occlusion

- Transcatheter occlusion of the LAA is a rapidly expanding option to reduce stroke risk in patients with atrial fibrillation who wish to avoid or cannot tolerate long-term oral anticoagulation.
- The most common transcutaneous occlusion procedure uses the WATCHMAN device (Boston Scientific, Malborough, MA) [30].
- The WATCHMAN device is shaped like an inverted umbrella and has a mesh cover that endothelializes over time. It is inserted into the LAA, where ten fixation barbs allow it to form a barrier across the ostium of the LAA. It must be carefully sized to achieve a tight seal and to prevent device migration/embolization.
- CT is well suited for ensuring proper WATCHMAN sizing by providing accurate the measurement of the LAA ostium size, landing zone size, and LAA length (Fig. 24.6).

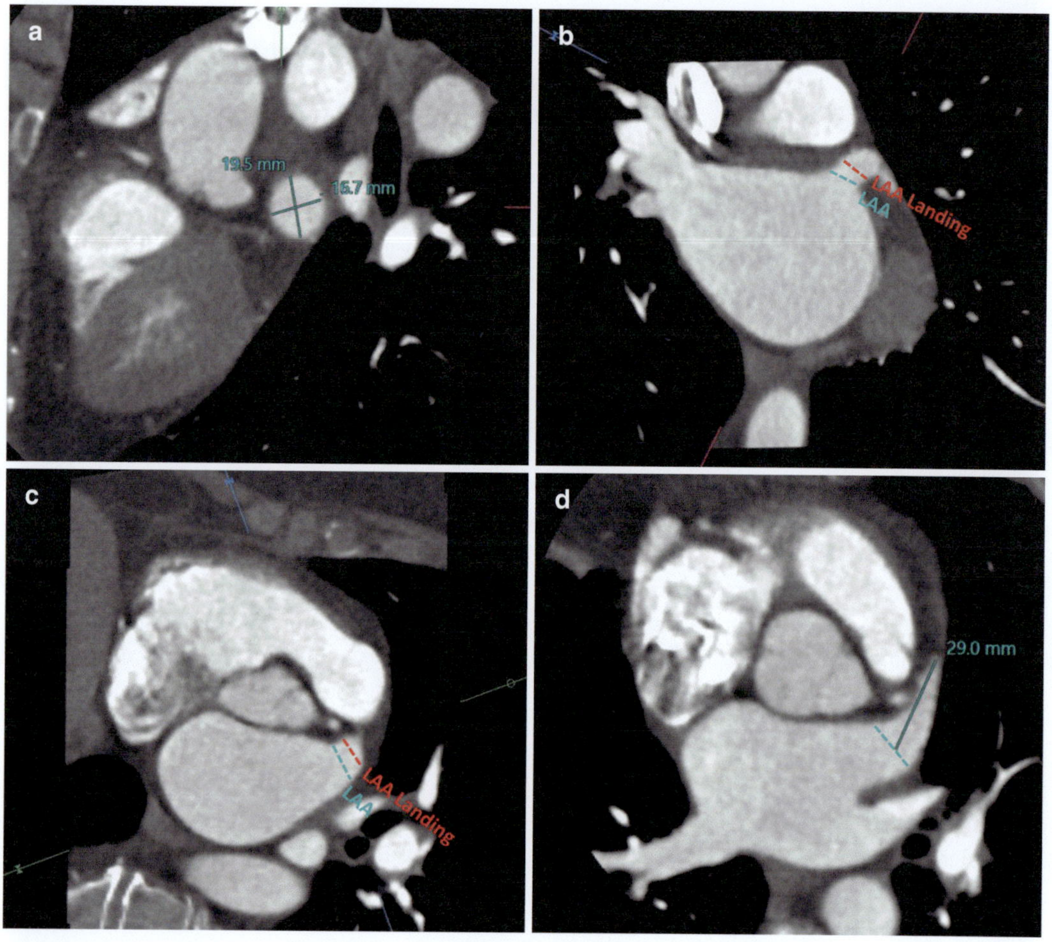

Fig. 24.6 Common measurements of left atrial appendage ostium (Panels **a–c**) and length (Panel **d**) in preparation of LAA closure

- Specific criteria for device sizing vary by operator and by device size availability but the ratio of LAA depth (measured from base to tip) (Fig. 24.6) to maximum base diameter is often used to inform feasibility of LAA closure (ratio of >1 is viewed favorably).
- In addition, CT allows for excellent visualization of the entire LAA along with its 3-dimensional structure, which can be extremely variable (Fig. 24.7).
- At least one trial has demonstrated superior WATCHMAN device selection and reduced procedure times with CT compared to TEE guidance [31].
- CT can also be used to evaluate for post procedural WATCHMAN peridevice leak.

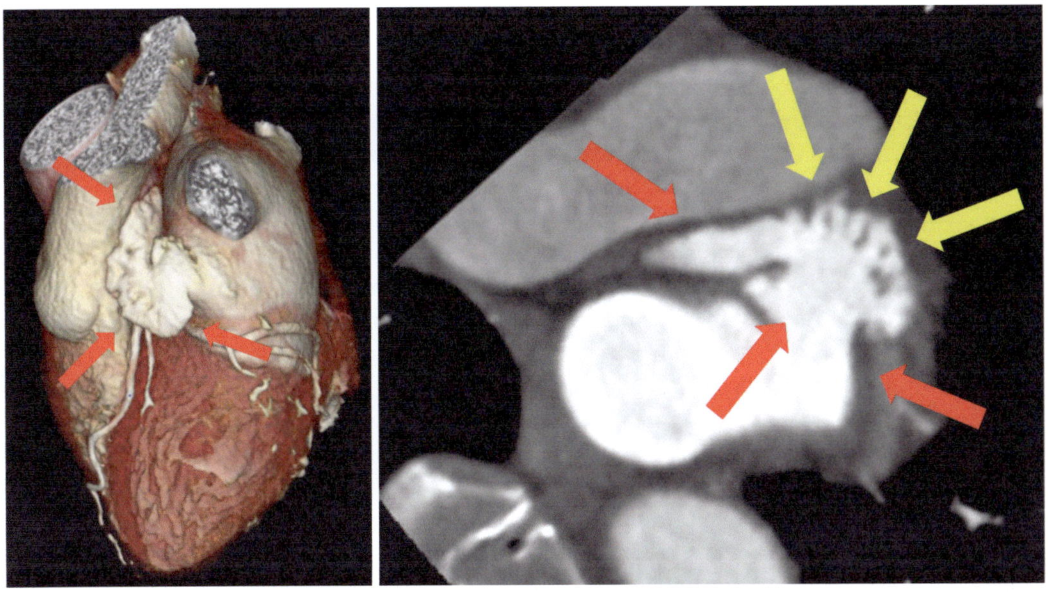

Fig. 24.7 Case example of a chicken wing shaped LAA (red arrows) with prominent pectinate muscles (yellow arrows)

24.5 Guidance of Ablation for Ventricular Arrhythmias

- Ventricular arrhythmias stem from diverse ischemic and non-ischemic etiologies. Because of the heterogeneity of substrates, pre-operative cardiac imaging is an important step in catheter ablation.
- Cardiac magnetic resonance imaging (cMRI) is the study of choice in most cases because of its sensitivity and specificity to detect myocardial scar with late-gadolinium enhancement, but it has limitations related to spatial resolution and artifact from implantable devices [32].
- CT with second pass delayed acquisition, while not as sensitive and specific as cMRI, can also be used to detect myocardial scarring, especially when cMRI cannot be performed [33].
- In a high-risk group of patients with clinical indication for catheter ablation of ventricular tachycardia and contraindication to cMRI, myocardial fibrosis was identified with excellent diagnostic accuracy (94%, 95% Confidence Interval 90.7–96.4) with cardiac CT when compared to electro-anatomical maps [34].

24.5.1 Protocol for Assessment of Left Ventricular Perfusion Defect and Scar

- Scans are typically triggered in end diastole (75%) of the R-R cycle, at which time the left ventricular cavity is at its their largest expansion.
- Second pass imaging for detecting late enhancement should be performed between 5 and 8 min after the initial acquisition, typically using 120 kV, although 100 kV can be used to reduce radiation dosing [35].
- Images are commonly reconstructed using thick slab MPRs (~4 mm) with average reconstruction projection along with window/level presets of approximately 500/200.
- When using CT to perform delayed enhancement imaging in patients with non-ischemic cardiomyopathy, delayed second pass imaging can be used to detect perfusion defects [20].

24.6 Electro-Anatomic Mapping

- Many diagnostic and therapeutic electrophysiology procedures rely on electro-anatomical mapping, which allows for the navigation of catheters and the display of real-time voltage data within a 3-D model of the heart [36–38].
- These systems integrate anatomical information obtained prior to the procedure from CT with voltage data measured by intracardiac catheters.
- There are several commercially available mapping systems that are routinely used in clinical practice: CARTO (BioSense Webster, Irvine, CA) and EnSite (Abbott, Abbott Park, IL).
- The first step in creating electro-anatomic maps is the acquisition of contrasted CT or cMRI images of the chambers of interest.
- Segmentation is the process of using software to isolate the chosen chambers from adjacent structures.
- Registration is the merging of those segmented images with electrical data obtained from catheters.
- The output of these systems is a color-coded, 3-D anatomical map that can display voltages, wavefront propagation, and real-time catheter location.
- These systems have been shown in some studies to improve outcomes during catheter ablation [39–41].
- For the purpose of creating electro-anatomical maps, CT image quality is generally equivalent to cMRI, but carries the advantages of being easier to obtain and more cost effective [36].
- One weakness of these mapping techniques is that there are invariably small differences in the cardiac and respiratory conditions between when the scan was obtained and when electro-anatomic data is incorporated [42]. Therefore, it is recommended that CT scans for this purpose be obtained within 24 h of the EP procedure, although some centers obtain these up to a week in advance. Over the course of a long procedure, alignment between the CT images and the chamber of interest may deteriorate further [43].

24.7 Identifying Patients at Risk for Arrhythmia and Sudden Cardiac Death

- CT can identify many of the structural heart diseases that place individuals at increased risk for arrhythmia and sudden cardiac death including dilated left ventricular cardiomyopathy, hypertrophic cardiomyopathy, left ventricular non-compaction, and arrhythmogenic right ventricular cardiomyopathy (ARVC).
- Out of hospital cardiac arrest leading to sudden cardiac death is most commonly due to acute coronary syndrome, with arrhythmia from cardiomyopathy, congenital arrhythmias, and ventricular failure being other common cardiovascular causes [44].
- CT can be used to evaluate for anomalous coronary artery anatomy that may cause ischemic arrhythmias leading to an cardiac death including inter-arterial course of the left main and anomalous left coronary artery from the pulmonary artery (ALCAPA) [45, 46].
- CT has emerged as a useful imaging modality for identifying VT substrate in ARVC, which is characterized by fibrofatty replacement of myocardium, scalloping of the right ventricular free wall, low attenuation trabeculation, and right ventricular dilation (Fig. 24.8) [47, 48]. Nevertheless, current ARVC diagnostic criteria do not include CT assessment.

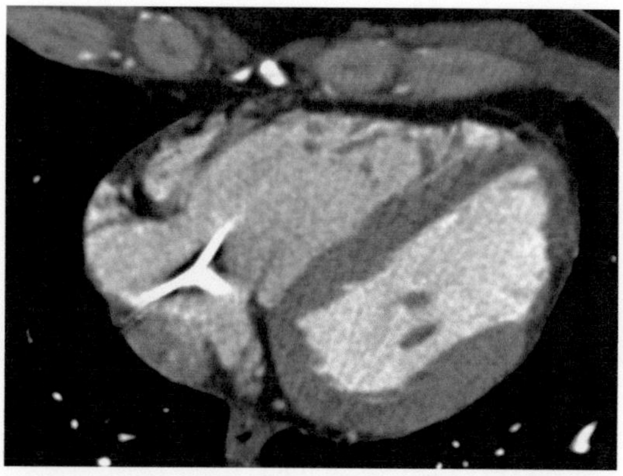

Fig. 24.8 Case example of ARVC with CT showing fibrofatty infiltration of right ventricular free wall

24.8 Pacemakers, Defibrillators, and Resynchronization Devices

- Placement of a transvenous pacemaker or implantable cardiac defibrillator in the standard positions in the right atrium or right ventricle does not require routine CT in the pre- or post-operative period [49].
- However, if a lead is believed to have been inadvertently placed in the arterial circulation, crossed through a septal defect, or created a small myocardial perforation, CT can assist in the diagnosis of these complications.
- Cardiac resynchronization therapy relies on coordinated pacing of the right and left ventricle to improve synchrony in patients with heart failure and ventricular conduction delay [50]. Left ventricular pacing is achieved by placing a lead in the coronary sinus to stimulate the left ventricular epicardium.
- Placement of the coronary sinus lead can be technically challenging and preprocedural CT can provide an invaluable anatomical roadmap to facilitate lead placement [51–53].

24.8.1 Device Infection and Lead Extraction

- One of the most common complications of cardiac implantable electronic devices is infection [54]. Infections are associated with significant morbidity and mortality and require prompt treatment, almost always involving device extraction.
- In addition to history, physical and laboratory data, positron emission tomography (PET) CT can play an important role in diagnosis. Whereas echocardiography can identify intracardiac or lead-associated vegetations, PET-CT can identify metabolically active areas associated with hardware that indicate infection [55]. In a meta-analysis, 18F-FDG PET-CT was 87% sensitive and 94% specific for the diagnosis of cardiac implanted electronic device infection [56].
- Cardiac implantable electronic device leads that malfunction, become infected, or develop thrombus may necessitate removal. The Heart Rhythm Society recommends CT prior to lead extraction to identify instances of myocardial perforation [57].
- CT has also been proposed for identifying areas of vascular adhesions. Multiple series have now found that pre-operative CT can identify adhesions in the central veins and that these are associated with significantly higher procedural complexity [58, 59].

References

1. Go AS, Hylek EM, Phillips KA, et al. Prevalence of diagnosed atrial fibrillation in adults: national implications for rhythm management and stroke prevention: the AnTicoagulation and risk factors in atrial fibrillation (ATRIA) study. JAMA. 2001;285(18):2370–5. https://doi.org/10.1001/jama.285.18.2370.
2. Fynn SP, Kalman JM. Pulmonary veins: anatomy, electrophysiology, tachycardia, and fibrillation. Pacing Clin Electrophysiol. 2004;27(11):1547–59. https://doi.org/10.1111/j.1540-8159.2004.00675.x.
3. Michaud GF, Stevenson WG. Atrial Fibrillation. N Engl J Med. 2021;384(4):353–61. https://doi.org/10.1056/NEJMcp2023658.
4. Haïssaguerre M, Jaïs P, Shah DC, et al. Spontaneous initiation of atrial fibrillation by ectopic beats originating in the pulmonary veins. N Engl J Med. 1998;339(10):659–66. https://doi.org/10.1056/NEJM199809033391003.
5. Santangeli P, Marchlinski FE. Techniques for the provocation, localization, and ablation of non-pulmonary vein triggers for atrial fibrillation. Heart Rhythm. 2017;14(7):1087–96. https://doi.org/10.1016/j.hrthm.2017.02.030.
6. Marine JE, Dong J, Calkins H. Catheter ablation therapy for atrial fibrillation. Prog Cardiovasc Dis. 2005;48(3):178–92. https://doi.org/10.1016/j.pcad.2005.06.011.
7. Voskoboinik A, Moskovitch JT, Harel N, Sanders P, Kistler PM, Kalman JM. Revisiting pulmonary vein isolation alone for persistent atrial fibrillation: a systematic review and meta-analysis. Heart Rhythm. 2017;14(5):661–7. https://doi.org/10.1016/j.hrthm.2017.01.003.
8. Robbins IM, Colvin EV, Doyle TP, et al. Pulmonary vein stenosis after catheter ablation of atrial fibrillation. Circulation. 1998;98(17):1769–75. https://doi.org/10.1161/01.cir.98.17.1769.
9. Teunissen C, Velthuis BK, Hassink RJ, et al. Incidence of pulmonary vein stenosis after radiofrequency catheter ablation of atrial fibrillation. JACC

Clin Electrophysiol. 2017;3(6):589–98. https://doi.org/10.1016/j.jacep.2017.02.003.

10. Samuel M, Khairy P, Mongeon FP, et al. Pulmonary vein stenosis after atrial fibrillation ablation: insights from the ADVICE trial. Can J Cardiol. 2020;36(12):1965–74. https://doi.org/10.1016/j.cjca.2020.10.013.
11. Packer DL, Keelan P, Munger TM, et al. Clinical presentation, investigation, and management of pulmonary vein stenosis complicating ablation for atrial fibrillation. Circulation. 2005;111(5):546–54. https://doi.org/10.1161/01.CIR.0000154541.58478.36.
12. Wongcharoen W, Tsao HM, Wu MH, et al. Preexisting pulmonary vein stenosis in patients undergoing atrial fibrillation ablation: a report of five cases. J Cardiovasc Electrophysiol. 2006;17(4):423–5. https://doi.org/10.1111/j.1540-8167.2006.00301.x.
13. Ohana M, Bakouboula B, Labani A, et al. Imaging before and after catheter ablation of atrial fibrillation. Diagn Interv Imaging. 2015;96(11):1113–23. https://doi.org/10.1016/j.diii.2014.12.011.
14. Scharf C, Sneider M, Case I, et al. Anatomy of the pulmonary veins in patients with atrial fibrillation and effects of segmental ostial ablation analyzed by computed tomography. J Cardiovasc Electrophysiol. 2003;14(2):150–5. https://doi.org/10.1046/j.1540-8167.2003.02444.x.
15. Wood MA, Wittkamp M, Henry D, et al. A comparison of pulmonary vein ostial anatomy by computerized tomography, echocardiography, and venography in patients with atrial fibrillation having radiofrequency catheter ablation. Am J Cardiol. 2004;93(1):49–53. https://doi.org/10.1016/j.amjcard.2003.09.011.
16. Jongbloed MRM, Bax JJ, Lamb HJ, et al. Multislice computed tomography versus intracardiac echocardiography to evaluate the pulmonary veins before radiofrequency catheter ablation of atrial fibrillation: a head-to-head comparison. J Am Coll Cardiol. 2005;45(3):343–50. https://doi.org/10.1016/j.jacc.2004.10.040.
17. Mansour M, Holmvang G, Sosnovik D, et al. Assessment of pulmonary vein anatomic variability by magnetic resonance imaging: implications for catheter ablation techniques for atrial fibrillation. J Cardiovasc Electrophysiol. 2004;15(4):387–93. https://doi.org/10.1046/j.1540-8167.2004.03515.x.
18. Kato R, Lickfett L, Meininger G, et al. Pulmonary vein anatomy in patients undergoing catheter ablation of atrial fibrillation: lessons learned by use of magnetic resonance imaging. Circulation. 2003;107(15):2004–10. https://doi.org/10.1161/01.CIR.0000061951.81767.4E.
19. Kaseno K, Tada H, Koyama K, et al. Prevalence and characterization of pulmonary vein variants in patients with atrial fibrillation determined using 3-dimensional computed tomography. Am J Cardiol. 2008;101(11):1638–42. https://doi.org/10.1016/j.amjcard.2008.01.053.
20. Lee HJ, Im DJ, Youn JC, et al. Assessment of myocardial delayed enhancement with cardiac computed tomography in cardiomyopathies: a prospective comparison with delayed enhancement cardiac magnetic resonance imaging. Int J Cardiovasc Imaging. 2017;33(4):577–84. https://doi.org/10.1007/s10554-016-1024-8.
21. Helms AS, West JJ, Patel A, et al. Relation of left atrial volume from three-dimensional computed tomography to atrial fibrillation recurrence following ablation. Am J Cardiol. 2009;103(7):989–93. https://doi.org/10.1016/j.amjcard.2008.12.021.
22. Hof I, Arbab-Zadeh A, Scherr D, et al. Correlation of left atrial diameter by echocardiography and left atrial volume by computed tomography. J Cardiovasc Electrophysiol. 2009;20(2):159–63. https://doi.org/10.1111/j.1540-8167.2008.01310.x.
23. Calkins H, Hindricks G, Cappato R, et al. 2017 HRS/EHRA/ECAS/APHRS/SOLAECE expert consensus statement on catheter and surgical ablation of atrial fibrillation. Heart Rhythm. 2018;20(1):e1–e160. https://doi.org/10.1093/europace/eux274.
24. Obeng-Gyimah E, Nazarian S. Advancements in imaging for atrial fibrillation ablation: is there a potential to improve procedural outcomes? J Innov Card Rhythm Manag. 2020;11(7):4172–8. https://doi.org/10.19102/icrm.2020.110701.
25. Hwang JJ, Chen JJ, Lin SC, et al. Diagnostic accuracy of transesophageal echocardiography for detecting left atrial thrombi in patients with rheumatic heart disease having undergone mitral valve operations. Am J Cardiol. 1993;72(9):677–81. https://doi.org/10.1016/0002-9149(93)90884-f.
26. Spagnolo P, Giglio M, Di Marco D, et al. Diagnosis of left atrial appendage thrombus in patients with atrial fibrillation: delayed contrast-enhanced cardiac CT. Eur Radiol. 2021;31(3):1236–44. https://doi.org/10.1007/s00330-020-07172-2.
27. Kottmaier M, Jilek C, Berglar S, et al. Exclusion of left atrial thrombus by dual-source cardiac computed tomography prior to catheter ablation for atrial fibrillation. Clin Res Cardiol. 2019;108(2):150–6. https://doi.org/10.1007/s00392-018-1333-0.
28. Romero J, Husain SA, Kelesidis I, Sanz J, Medina HM, Garcia MJ. Detection of left atrial appendage thrombus by cardiac computed tomography in patients with atrial fibrillation: a meta-analysis. Circ Cardiovasc Imaging. 2013;6(2):185–94. https://doi.org/10.1161/CIRCIMAGING.112.000153.
29. Narula J, Chandrashekhar Y, Ahmadi A, et al. SCCT 2021 expert consensus document on coronary computed tomographic angiography: a report of the Society of Cardiovascular Computed Tomography. J Cardiovasc Comput Tomogr. 2021;15(3):192–217. https://doi.org/10.1016/j.jcct.2020.11.001.
30. Kirchhof P, Benussi S, Kotecha D, et al. 2016 ESC guidelines for the management of atrial fibrillation developed in collaboration with EACTS. Eur Heart J. 2016;37(38):2893–962. https://doi.org/10.1093/eurheartj/ehw210.
31. Eng MH, Wang DD, Greenbaum AB, et al. Prospective, randomized comparison of 3-dimensional computed

tomography guidance versus TEE data for left atrial appendage occlusion (PRO3DLAAO). Catheter Cardiovasc Interv. 2018;92(2):401–7. https://doi.org/10.1002/ccd.27514.

32. Kuo L, Liang JJ, Nazarian S, Marchlinski FE. Multimodality imaging to guide ventricular tachycardia ablation in patients with non-ischaemic cardiomyopathy. Arrhythmia Electrophysiol Rev. 2020;8(4):255–64. https://doi.org/10.15420/aer.2019.37.3.
33. Esposito A, Palmisano A, Antunes S, et al. Cardiac CT with delayed enhancement in the characterization of ventricular tachycardia structural substrate: relationship between CT-segmented scar and electro-anatomic mapping. JACC Cardiovasc Imaging. 2016;9(7):822–32. https://doi.org/10.1016/j.jcmg.2015.10.024.
34. Conte E, Carbucicchio C, Catto V, et al. Live integration of comprehensive cardiac CT with electroanatomical mapping in patients with refractory ventricular tachycardia. J Cardiovasc Comput Tomogr. 2021;S1934–5925(21):00478. https://doi.org/10.1016/j.jcct.2021.12.003.
35. Ko SM, Hwang SH, Lee HJ. Role of cardiac computed tomography in the diagnosis of left ventricular myocardial diseases. J Cardiovasc Imaging. 2019;27(2):73–92. https://doi.org/10.4250/jcvi.2019.27.e17.
36. Kistler PM, Schilling RJ, Rajappan K, Sporton SC. Image integration for atrial fibrillation ablation—pearls and pitfalls. Heart Rhythm. 2007;4(9):1216–21. https://doi.org/10.1016/j.hrthm.2007.04.008.
37. LaPage MJ, Saul JP. Update on rhythm mapping and catheter navigation. Curr Opin Cardiol. 2011;26(2):79–85. https://doi.org/10.1097/HCO.0b013e3283437d48.
38. den Uijl DW, Tops LF, Tolosana JM, et al. Real-time integration of intracardiac echocardiography and multislice computed tomography to guide radiofrequency catheter ablation for atrial fibrillation. Heart Rhythm. 2008;5(10):1403–10. https://doi.org/10.1016/j.hrthm.2008.07.020.
39. Kistler PM, Rajappan K, Jahngir M, et al. The impact of CT image integration into an electroanatomic mapping system on clinical outcomes of catheter ablation of atrial fibrillation. J Cardiovasc Electrophysiol. 2006;17(10):1093–101. https://doi.org/10.1111/j.1540-8167.2006.00594.x.
40. Kistler PM, Earley MJ, Harris S, et al. Validation of three-dimensional cardiac image integration: use of integrated CT image into electroanatomic mapping system to perform catheter ablation of atrial fibrillation. J Cardiovasc Electrophysiol. 2006;17(4):341–8. https://doi.org/10.1111/j.1540-8167.2006.00371.x.
41. Martinek M, Nesser HJ, Aichinger J, Boehm G, Purerfellner H. Impact of integration of multislice computed tomography imaging into three-dimensional electroanatomic mapping on clinical outcomes, safety, and efficacy using radiofrequency ablation for atrial fibrillation. Pacing Clin Electrophysiol. 2007;30(10):1215–23. https://doi.org/10.1111/j.1540-8159.2007.00843.x.
42. Heist EK, Chevalier J, Holmvang G, et al. Factors affecting error in integration of electroanatomic mapping with CT and MR imaging during catheter ablation of atrial fibrillation. J Interv Card Electrophysiol. 2006;17(1):21–7. https://doi.org/10.1007/s10840-006-9060-2.
43. Bonso A, Fantinel M, Scalchi G, et al. Left atrial model reconstruction in atrial fibrillation ablation: reliability of new mapping and complex impedance systems. Europace. 2017;19(11):1804–9. https://doi.org/10.1093/europace/euw250.
44. Chen N, Callaway CW, Guyette FX, et al. Arrest etiology among patients resuscitated from cardiac arrest. Resuscitation. 2018;130:33–40. https://doi.org/10.1016/j.resuscitation.2018.06.024.
45. Shi H, Aschoff AJ, Brambs HJ, Hoffmann MHK. Multislice CT imaging of anomalous coronary arteries. Eur Radiol. 2004;14(12):2172–81. https://doi.org/10.1007/s00330-004-2490-2.
46. Greet B, Quinones A, Srichai M, Bangalore S, Roswell RO. Anomalous right coronary artery and sudden cardiac death. Circ Arrhythm Electrophysiol. 2012;5(6):e111–2. https://doi.org/10.1161/CIRCEP.112.978635.
47. Thiene G, Nava A, Corrado D, Rossi L, Pennelli N. Right ventricular cardiomyopathy and sudden death in young people. N Engl J Med. 1988;318(3):129–33. https://doi.org/10.1056/NEJM198801213180301.
48. Venlet J, Tao Q, de Graaf MA, et al. RV tissue heterogeneity on CT: a novel tool to identify the VT substrate in ARVC. JACC Clin Electrophysiol. 2020;6(9):1073–85. https://doi.org/10.1016/j.jacep.2020.04.029.
49. Mulpuru SK, Madhavan M, McLeod CJ, Cha YM, Friedman PA. Cardiac pacemakers: function, troubleshooting, and management: part 1 of a 2-part series. J Am Coll Cardiol. 2017;69(2):189–210. https://doi.org/10.1016/j.jacc.2016.10.061.
50. Normand C, Linde C, Singh J, Dickstein K. Indications for cardiac resynchronization therapy: a comparison of the major international guidelines. JACC Heart Fail. 2018;6(4):308–16. https://doi.org/10.1016/j.jchf.2018.01.022.
51. Mao S, Shinbane JS, Girsky MJ, et al. Coronary venous imaging with electron beam computed tomographic angiography: three-dimensional mapping and relationship with coronary arteries. Am Heart J. 2005;150(2):315–22. https://doi.org/10.1016/j.ahj.2004.09.050.
52. Jongbloed MRM, Lamb HJ, Bax JJ, et al. Noninvasive visualization of the cardiac venous system using multislice computed tomography. J Am Coll Cardiol. 2005;45(5):749–53. https://doi.org/10.1016/j.jacc.2004.11.035.
53. Van de Veire NR, Schuijf JD, De Sutter J, et al. Non-invasive visualization of the cardiac venous system in coronary artery disease patients using

64-slice computed tomography. J Am Coll Cardiol. 2006;48(9):1832–8. https://doi.org/10.1016/j.jacc.2006.07.042.
54. Voigt A, Shalaby A, Saba S. Continued rise in rates of cardiovascular implantable electronic device infections in the United States: temporal trends and causative insights. Pacing Clin Electrophysiol PACE. 2010;33(4):414–9. https://doi.org/10.1111/j.1540-8159.2009.02569.x.
55. Sarrazin JF, Philippon F, Tessier M, et al. Usefulness of fluorine-18 positron emission tomography/computed tomography for identification of cardiovascular implantable electronic device infections. J Am Coll Cardiol. 2012;59(18):1616–25. https://doi.org/10.1016/j.jacc.2011.11.059.
56. Juneau D, Golfam M, Hazra S, et al. Positron emission tomography and single-photon emission computed tomography imaging in the diagnosis of cardiac implantable electronic device infection: a systematic review and meta-analysis. Circ Cardiovasc Imaging. 2017;10(4):e005772. https://doi.org/10.1161/CIRCIMAGING.116.005772.
57. Kusumoto FM, Schoenfeld MH, Wilkoff BL, et al. 2017 HRS expert consensus statement on cardiovascular implantable electronic device lead management and extraction. Heart Rhythm. 2017;14(12):e503–51. https://doi.org/10.1016/j.hrthm.2017.09.001.
58. Lewis RK, Pokorney SD, Greenfield RA, et al. Preprocedural ECG-gated computed tomography for prevention of complications during lead extraction. Pacing Clin Electrophysiol PACE. 2014;37(10):1297–305. https://doi.org/10.1111/pace.12485.
59. Svennberg E, Jacobs K, McVeigh E, Pretorius V, Birgersdotter-Green U. Computed tomography-guided risk assessment in percutaneous Lead extraction. JACC Clin Electrophysiol. 2019;5(12):1439–46. https://doi.org/10.1016/j.jacep.2019.09.007.

25 Generating the Cardiac CT Report

Armin Arbab Zadeh

Abstract

A cardiac CT scan contains much information. The cardiac CT report must succinctly convey data for guiding effective patient management, supporting patient safety, and allowing case administration. This chapter discusses the essential components of a cardiac CT report, optional information, and suggestions for structured reporting.

Keywords

Coronary CT · Coronary CT angiography · Cardiac CT · Cardiac CT reporting

Abbreviations

BMI	Body mass index
BP	Blood pressure
CABG	Coronary artery bypass grafting
CAC	Coronary artery calcium
CAC-DRS	Coronary Artery Calcium Data and Reporting System
CAD	Coronary artery disease
CAD-RADS	Coronary artery disease data and reporting system
CCS	Coronary calcium scanning
CCTA	Cardiac computed tomography angiography
DLP	Dose-length product
FFR	Fractional flow reserve
ICD	Implantable cardioverter defibrillator
LAD	Left anterior descending artery
LCx	Left circum flex (coronary artery)
LM	Left main (coronary artery)
LVEF	Left ventricular ejection fraction
MESA	Multi-ethnic study of atherosclerosis
OM	Obtuse marginal
PCAT	Pericoronary adipose tissue attenuation
PCI	Percutaneous coronary intervention
RCA	Right coronary artery
SCCT	Society of Cardiovascular Computed Tomography

25.1 Introduction

- The cardiac CT report entails demographic, technical, and clinical information akin to most other medical tests.
- The extent and content of information should be tailored to local requirements, including institutional policies, state laws, and clinical context.
- Electronic health record platforms may provide templates for structured cardiac CT reporting.

A. A. Zadeh (✉)
Department of Medicine, Johns Hopkins University, Baltimore, MD, USA
e-mail: azadeh1@jhmi.edu

A. A. Zadeh, J. Hoe (eds.), *Practical Guide to Cardiac CT*,
https://doi.org/10.1007/978-981-97-6919-3_25

Table 25.1 Patient Demographics and Characteristics

Typically Required	Optional
Age/date of birth	Case number
Medical record number	Procedure time/duration
Accession number	Inpatient/outpatient status
Case number	
Sex	
Height/weight/BMI	
Procedure date	

Abbreviations: *BMI* body mass index

Table 25.2 Patient History and Referral Information

Typically Required	Optional
Study indication/question	Risk factors
Symptom history	Allergies
Referring provider	Primary care provider
Relevant co-morbidity	Date test ordered
Prior related studies	Relevant laboratory data

- This chapter provides general guidance for commonly required components within a cardiac CT report.
- Recommended terminology is provided from dedicated consensus statements by professional societies [1].

25.2 Patient Demographics and Characteristics

- Table 25.1 lists the demographic and other patient information typically expected in a cardiac CT report.

25.3 History and Study Indication

- Table 25.2 lists the patient history and referral information typically expected in a cardiac CT report.

25.4 Procedural Data

- Table 25.3 lists the technical information typically expected in a cardiac CT report.
- Test specification should entail which test was ordered and performed, e.g., CT coronary angiography, cardiac CT for structure and morphology, coronary calcium scanning, CT in congenital heart disease.
- Procedure description should detail the sequence of imaging, e.g., noncontrast scanning followed by contrast imaging, as well as structures imaged, key acquisition features, e.g., prospective triggering vs. retrospective gating, special features, e.g., delayed imaging or dose modulation, key limitations, and implications for availability of study results.
- Acquisition details should include the scanner specifications, e.g., 320-detector scanner, vendor identification, detector width, collimation, gantry rotation speed, gating.
- Estimated radiation dose should be reported using the dose-length-product (DLP) provided by the scanner. Given the controversy regarding the appropriate conversion factor (see Chap. 6), estimated effective dose should only be given in conjunction with the DLP to allow its derivation.
- Reconstruction details should include slice thickness and may include slice increment and kernels. Tube settings may also be provided but are not essential for the report.
- Image quality should include a graded assessment, e.g., poor, fair, good, excellent, and reasons for diminished image quality, e.g., obesity, motion, calcium, metal, etc.

Table 25.3 Procedural Information

Typically Required	Optional
Test specification	Peak tube voltage
Procedure description	Tube current
Acquisition details	Exposure window
Medications and doses given	Reconstruction kernel
Contrast type and dose	Reconstruction increment
Radiation dose (DLP)	Estimated effective radiation dose
Reconstruction details	Patient heart rates at arrival and scan time
Image quality	Patient BP at arrival & scan time
Complications	Patient heart rhythm

Abbreviations: *BP* blood pressure; *DLP* dose-length-product

Table 25.4 Noncoronary Cardiac Findings Reporting

Typically Required	Optional
Pericardium: Effusion, thickening, calcification	Epicardial fat volume, pericoronary fat attenuation
Myocardium: LV thickness, scar, LVEF (if available)	LV mass (quantitative)
Cardiac chambers: Sizes (qualitative), masses, thrombus, defects, shunts, fistulas	Chamber dimensions and volumes, including end diastole and end systole
Valves: Calcification, anomalies	Valve morphology, function (if available)
Devices: Presence and location	Identification of ICD vs. pacemaker
Aorta: Dilation, atherosclerosis, thrombus, masses, trauma, infection, deformation	Routine aortic dimensions at root, ascending aorta, arch, descending aorta

Abbreviations: *ICD* implantable cardioverter defibrillator, *LV* left ventricular, *LVEF* LV ejection fraction

- All complications should be documented, including contrast reactions, image failure, excessive radiation dose, etc.

25.5 Scan Results

25.5.1 Noncoronary Cardiovascular Findings

- Specific study questions will dictate the focus of reporting, which is covered in the respective Chapters.
- Table 25.4 lists commonly expected reporting for a cardiac CT with contrast or CT coronary angiography.

25.5.2 Noncardiac Findings

IMPORTANT: All cardiac CT scans require dedicated reporting of noncardiac findings, e.g., lung pathology, mediastinum, thorax, etc. (see Chap. 22). This report may be incorporated into the cardiac report or be provided separately. Critical findings and follow-up recommendations must be promptly communicated to providers along with documentation of date/time of communication.

25.5.3 Coronary Artery Assessment

- Cardiac CT studies for assessment of structure and morphology should include comments about the origin of the coronary arteries and qualitative assessment of the presence and extent of coronary calcification (e.g., none, mild, moderate, severe).
- For visual grading of coronary calcium, use of the Coronary Artery Calcium Data and Reporting System (CAC-DRS) is recommended (see Chap. 9) [2].
- Cardiac CT studies for the assessment of coronary artery disease should include a detailed evaluation of the coronary anatomy, presence, extent, and characteristics of coronary atherosclerotic disease, coronary lumen stenoses, and any other coronary pathology.
- The coronary CT angiography report should include a summary/impression which conveys key findings that easily translate into clinical management.

25.5.3.1 Coronary Artery Calcium Scoring

- For scans including dedicated coronary artery calcium (CAC) scoring, the Agatston score should be reported for the left main coronary artery and the three coronary arteries as well as a total score. Reporting of the volume or mass score is optional.
- We recommend to also report the Coronary Artery Calcium Data and Reporting System (CAC-DRS) score (see Chap. 9) [2].
- The calcium score percentile compared to an age and gender matched reference population should be reported.
- We recommend to include information on ethnicity to compute the percentile from MESA given its validation for more specific populations [3].
- The summary statement should include the total CAC score by Agatston along with the percentile, and grading of the score according to MESA data:

Calcium score	Severity of coronary calcium
0	None
1–99	Mild
100–299	Moderate
300–999	Severe
≥1000 or	Very severe

25.5.3.2 Coronary Arterial Anatomy by CT Angiography

- Nomenclature and coronary artery segment definitions by the SCCT are recommended for reporting the coronary arterial anatomy [4].
- Origin of the left main and right coronary arteries as well as coronary dominance should be noted.
- The caliber of the left main coronary artery (LM), left anterior descending artery (LAD), left circumflex artery (LCx), and right coronary artery (RCA) should be qualitatively reported (e.g., small, medium, large) along with the sizes of their respective branches (diagonal branches, obtuse marginal (OM) branches, posterolateral branches, and posterior descending artery).
- Graft anatomy and location of stents should be described.
- Reporting of myocardial bridging is optional as most represent normal variants without clinical implications while reporting may trigger anxiety among providers and patients. Reporting is recommended in the setting of deep bridging (e.g., > 5 mm) or significant associated lumen narrowing (>50%).
- Pericoronary adipose tissue attenuation (PCAT), a novel marker of perivascular inflammation, has not been adequately validated for clinical use and its reporting is optional at this time.
- Any deviation from normal coronary anatomy should be reported, e.g., ectasia, dissection, fistulas, intramural course, etc.
- Table 25.5 lists commonly expected reporting of coronary anatomy details.

Table 25.5 Recommended reporting of coronary arterial anatomy

Typically required	Optional
Origin of left and right coronary arteries	Myocardial bridging
Coronary dominance	Quantified vessel caliber (mm)
Normal variants and anomalies	Pericoronary adipose tissue attenuation
Caliber of main vessels and branches	
Graft anatomy	
Stent location	
Coronary ectasia	
Coronary dissection/intramural hematoma	

25.5.4 Coronary Artery Disease Reporting

25.5.4.1 Introduction

- Details and structure of coronary artery disease (CAD) reporting are subject to controversy [5].
- Traditionally, CAD has been reported by invasive cardiologists based on cardiac catheterization and determination of “significant” CAD.
- “Significant” CAD used to denote atherosclerotic disease which is associated with reduced coronary flow reserve, also described as *hemodynamically* significant.
- Before the availability of intracoronary hemodynamic assessment using coronary flow reserve or fractional flow reserve (FFR), a diameter stenosis of ≥70% by visual assessment or ≥ 50 when quantified using contour detection (visual assessment tends to overestimate stenoses) had been used to describe “significant” or “obstructive” CAD [6].
- “Significant” CAD has been further described as single, dual, triple vessel CAD (involving 1, 2, or 3 coronary arteries) and/or the LM disease with associated implications for management according to practice guidelines.

- Coronary atherosclerotic disease with <50% associated lumen narrowing has been described as insignificant or *nonobstructive* CAD.
- In recent years, however, nonobstructive CAD has been associated with impaired myocardial blood flow reserve and considerable proportion of observed myocardial infarctions in patients with stable atherosclerosis [7], rendering the notion of "insignificant" CAD as obsolete [6].
- The widespread use of CT coronary angiography has further complicated reporting because of the vast additional options for CAD characterization, including atherosclerotic plaque description, atheroma quantification, and discussion of the so-called vulnerable features (see Chap. 13).

25.5.4.2 CAD-RADS

- The CAD Reporting and Data System (CAD-RADS) was introduced in 2016 to establish standardized CAD reporting from CT angiography and it has been used since particularly by radiologists [8].
- CAD-RADS uses seven categories (CAD-RADS 0–5 + N for nondiagnostic) plus several subcategories and qualifiers to describe CAD disease severity and provides general recommendations for each stage (Table 25.6).
- CAD-RADS is much less used by cardiologists because the system is complicated, not intuitive, and unfamiliar to nonradiologists, including most referring providers.

Table 25.6 Revised CAD-RADS Reporting and Data System

CAD-RADS stage	Percent stenosis	Modifiers
0	0	N:Nondiagnostic
1	1–24	HRP:High-risk plaque
2	25–49	I: Ischemia
3	50–69	S: Stent
4A	70–99	G: Graft
4B	LM >50	E: Exceptions
4C	3-vessel ≥70	P1–4: Plaque burden
5	100	

- Specific criticism relates to the insensitivity of CAD-RADS for capturing total CAD burden (including nonobstructive CAD burden), and high-risk coronary anatomy, as well as to questionable recommendations for subsequent testing and interventions [5].
- An updated version of CAD-RADS released in 2022 addressed some of these issues but gained even more complexity with numerous qualifiers and subcategorizations.
- Importantly, CAD-RADS has not been shown to yield superior risk stratification or improved management when compared to simple, traditional CAD reporting [9].
- For these reasons, I do not recommend reporting CAD using CAD-RADS.

25.6 Recommended CAD Reporting

25.6.1 Presence of Atherosclerosis

- Presence or absence of coronary atherosclerosis should be noted for the LM, LAD, LCx, and RCA. If present, atherosclerotic disease should be noted for major side branches, including ramus intermedius, diagonal, OM, and posterolateral branches as well as the posterior descending artery.
- Location of atherosclerosis should be further detailed for the proximal, mid, or distal portion of the affected vessel or branch.
- Atherosclerosis should be denoted as calcified, noncalcified, or partially calcified.
- Severity of calcification may be described as mild, moderate, or severe (dense).
- It should be noted if the atherosclerosis is focal or diffuse.
- Optional description includes remodeling status.
- The so-called high-risk features, e.g., napkin-ring sign, spotty calcification, have not been adequately validated nor have they shown to lead to improved patient management (see Chap. 13) and thus should not be routinely reported to avoid confusion and anxiety.

- Similarly, standards for acquiring and interpreting coronary atheroma volume are lacking and thus its reporting is not recommended at this time (although it is likely that atheroma volume will be a key criterion for CAD grading in the near future).

25.6.2 Coronary Stenosis Grading

- Coronary artery stenoses have been traditionally assessed using diameter stenosis (see Chap. 11) despite major limitations of this method, particularly with noncircular lumen geometry.
- Lumen area measurements or area stenosis evaluation is easily obtainable by CT but adequate reference data are not available, limiting its application.
- Diameter stenosis assessment is typically performed by visual evaluation, although quantification using software tools for contour detection is readily available and may be used to assist grading (note that these values tend to be lower than with visual inspection) [6].
- Given considerable interobserver variability for stenosis quantification, stenosis *ranges* rather than specific values are generally recommended for reporting.
- The stenosis range should be adjusted to the observer confidence, e.g., 0–10% range for high confidence vs. 20–30% range for less confident assessment.
- Stenosis ranges recommended by the SCCT [4] are adequate for most scenarios but its severe stenosis range of 70–99% is wide and we recommend further differentiation (Table 25.6).
- Stenosis grading in bypass grafts and stents typically is less granular and often is confined to normal, <50%, >50%, 100% (Table 25.7).

Table 25.7 Recommended Coronary Artery Stenosis Grading

Percent stenosis	Description	Associated myocardial perfusion abnormality
0	Normal	Highly unlikely
1–24	Very mild or minimal	Very unlikely
25–49	Mild or nonobstructive	Unlikely
50–69	Moderate or borderline severe	Not likely but possible
70–89	Severe or obstructive	Likely
90–99%	Very severe	Very likely
100%	Total occlusion	Highly likely

Table 25.8 Recommended Overall Grading and Reporting of Coronary Artery Disease

CAD Stage	Description	Management recommendation
I	Normal	Risk factor control
II	Limited nonobstructive (<50%) in 1–2 coronary arteries	Additional dedicated prevention and lifestyle modifications
III	Extensive nonobstructive or limited obstructive (≥50%) CAD	Intensive prevention; consideration of PCI or CABG for failed optimal medical therapy
IV	High-risk CAD: Obstructive disease in LM or three arteries	Intensive prevention; consideration of revascularization for improved survival[a]

Stenosis values are based on quantitative assessment. Abbreviations: *CABG* coronary artery bypass grafting, *CAD* coronary artery disease, *LM* left main coronary artery, *PCI* percutaneous coronary intervention

[a] particularly in the setting of diabetes mellitus or reduced left ventricular ejection fraction

25.7 Summary Statement/ Impression

- The report should include a statement summarizing key findings.
- For CAD reporting, the statement should include an overall assessment which includes if disease is nonobstructive or obstructive, limited or extensive, and presence of high-risk features, e.g., obstructive LM disease or three-vessel obstructive CAD.
- Description of whether the disease is predominantly/severely calcified is optional in the summary statement.
- Recommendations regarding further management are optional.
- We recommend a simple grading of CAD and associated recommendations according to Ferraro et al. [10] (Table 25.8).

References

1. Weigold WG, Abbara S, Achenbach S, et al. Standardized medical terminology for cardiac computed tomography: a report of the society of cardiovascular computed tomography. J Cardiovasc Comput Tomogr. 2011;5(3):136–44.
2. Hecht HS, Blaha MJ, Kazerooni EA, et al. CAC-DRS: coronary artery calcium data and reporting system. An expert consensus document of the society of cardiovascular computed tomography (SCCT). J Cardiovasc Comput Tomogr. 2018;12(3):185–91. https://doi.org/10.1016/j.jcct.2018.03.008.
3. Detrano R, Guerci AD, Carr JJ, et al. Coronary calcium as a predictor of coronary events in four racial or ethnic groups. N Engl J Med. 2008;358(13):1336–45.
4. Raff GL, Abidov A, Achenbach S, et al. SCCT guidelines for the interpretation and reporting of coronary computed tomographic angiography. J Cardiovasc Comput Tomogr. 2009;3(2):122–36.
5. Arbab-Zadeh A. The challenge of effectively reporting coronary angiography results from computed tomography. JACC Cardiovasc Imaging. 2018;11(1):90–3.
6. Arbab-Zadeh A, Fuster V. The risk continuum of atherosclerosis and its implications for defining CHD by coronary angiography. J Am Coll Cardiol. 2016;68(22):2467–78.
7. Hoffmann U, Ferencik M, Udelson JE, et al. Prognostic value of anatomic vs. functional diagnostic testing strategies in symptomatic patients with suspected coronary artery disease. Circulation. 2015;132(Suppl 3):A18053.
8. Cury RC, Abbara S, Achenbach S, et al. Coronary artery disease—reporting and data system (CAD-RADS): an expert consensus document of SCCT, ACR and NASCI: endorsed by the ACC. JACC Cardiovasc Imaging. 2016;9(9):1099–113.
9. Xie JX, Cury RC, Leipsic J, et al. The coronary artery disease-reporting and data system (CAD-RADS): prognostic and clinical implications associated with standardized coronary computed tomographic angiography reporting. JACC Cardiovasc Imaging. 2017;11:78.
10. Ferraro R, Latina JM, Alfaddagh A, et al. Evaluation and management of patients with stable angina: beyond the ischemia paradigm: JACC state-of-the-art review. J Am Coll Cardiol. 2020;76(19):2252–66. https://doi.org/10.1016/j.jacc.2020.08.078.

Appendix: Guidelines and Important References for Cardiac CT

Society of Cardiovascular Computed Tomography Related key References

- Leipsic J, Abbara S, Achenbach S, Cury R, Earls JP, Mancini GJ, et al. SCCT guidelines for the interpretation and reporting of coronary CT angiography: a report of the Society of Cardiovascular Computed Tomography Guidelines Committee. J Cardiovasc Comput Tomogr. 2014;8(5):342–58.
- Narula J, Chandrashekhar Y, Ahmadi A, Abbara S, Berman DS, Blankstein R, et al. SCCT 2021 Expert Consensus Document on Coronary Computed Tomographic Angiography: a Report of the Society of Cardiovascular Computed Tomography. J Cardiovasc Comput Tomogr. 2021;15(3):192–217.
- Shaw LJ, Blankstein R, Bax JJ, Ferencik M, Bittencourt MS, Min JK, et al. Society of Cardiovascular Computed Tomography/North American Society of Cardiovascular Imaging -Expert Consensus Document on Coronary CT Imaging of Atherosclerotic Plaque. J Cardiovasc Comput Tomogr. 2021;15(2):93–109.
- Patel AR, Bamberg F, Branch K, Carrascosa P, Chen M, Cury RC, et al. Society of cardiovascular computed tomography expert consensus document on myocardial computed tomography perfusion imaging. J Cardiovasc Comput Tomogr. 2020;14(1):87–100.
- Blanke P, Weir-McCall JR, Achenbach S, Delgado V, Hausleiter J, Jilaihawi H, et al. Computed tomography imaging in the context of transcatheter aortic valve implantation (TAVI)/ transcatheter aortic valve replacement (TAVR): an expert consensus document of the Society of Cardiovascular Computed Tomography. J Cardiovasc Comput Tomogr. 2019;13(1):1–20.
- Hecht HS, Blaha MJ, Kazerooni EA, Cury RC, Budoff M, Leipsic J, et al. CAC-DRS: coronary Artery Calcium Data and Reporting System. An expert consensus document of the Society of Cardiovascular Computed Tomography (SCCT). J Cardiovasc Comput Tomogr. 2018;12(3):185–91.
- Hirshfeld JW, Ferrari VA, Bengel FM, Bergersen L, Chambers CE, Einstein AJ, et al. 2018 ACC/HRS/NASCI/SCAI/SCCT Expert Consensus Document on Optimal Use of Ionizing Radiation in Cardiovascular Imaging-Best Practices for Safety and Effectiveness, Part 1: Radiation Physics and Radiation Biology: a Report of the American College of Cardiology Task Force on Expert Consensus Decision Pathways Developed in Collaboration With Mended Hearts. Catheter Cardiovasc Interv. 2018;92(2):203–21.
- Hecht H, Blaha MJ, Berman DS, Nasir K, Budoff M, Leipsic J, et al. Clinical indications for coronary artery calcium scoring in asymptomatic patients: expert consensus statement from the Society of Cardiovascular Computed Tomography. J Cardiovasc Comput Tomogr. 2017;11(2):157–68.
- Abbara S, Blanke P, Maroules CD, Cheezum M, Choi AD, Han BK, et al. SCCT guidelines for the performance and acquisition of coro-

A. A. Zadeh, J. Hoe (eds.), *Practical Guide to Cardiac CT*,
https://doi.org/10.1007/978-981-97-6919-3

nary computed tomographic angiography: a report of the society of Cardiovascular Computed Tomography Guidelines Committee: Endorsed by the North American Society for Cardiovascular Imaging (NASCI). J Cardiovasc Comput Tomogr. 2016;10(6):435–49.

- Lancellotti P, Nkomo VT, Badano LP, Bergler-Klein J, Bergler J, Bogaert J, et al. Expert consensus for multi-modality imaging evaluation of cardiovascular complications of radiotherapy in adults: a report from the European Association of Cardiovascular Imaging and the American Society of Echocardiography. J Am Soc Echocardiogr. 2013;26(9):1013–32.
- Han BK, Rigsby CK, Hlavacek A, Leipsic J, Nicol ED, Siegel MJ, et al. Computed Tomography Imaging in Patients with Congenital Heart Disease Part I: rationale and Utility. An Expert Consensus Document of the Society of Cardiovascular Computed Tomography (SCCT): Endorsed by the Society of Pediatric Radiology (SPR) and the North American Society of Cardiac Imaging (NASCI). J Cardiovasc Comput Tomogr. 2015;9(6):475–92.
- Han BK, Rigsby CK, Leipsic J, Bardo D, Abbara S, Ghoshhajra B, et al. Computed Tomography Imaging in Patients with Congenital Heart Disease, Part 2: Technical Recommendations. An Expert Consensus Document of the Society of Cardiovascular Computed Tomography (SCCT): Endorsed by the Society of Pediatric Radiology (SPR) and the North American Society of Cardiac Imaging (NASCI). J Cardiovasc Comput Tomogr. 2015;9(6):493–513.
- Raff GL, Chinnaiyan KM, Cury RC, Garcia MT, Hecht HS, Hollander JE, et al. SCCT guidelines on the use of coronary computed tomographic angiography for patients presenting with acute chest pain to the emergency department: a report of the Society of Cardiovascular Computed Tomography Guidelines Committee. J Cardiovasc Comput Tomogr. 2014;8(4):254–71.
- Achenbach S, Delgado V, Hausleiter J, Schoenhagen P, Min JK, Leipsic JA. SCCT expert consensus document on computed tomography imaging before transcatheter aortic valve implantation (TAVI)/transcatheter aortic valve replacement (TAVR). J Cardiovasc Comput Tomogr. 2012;6(6):366–80.
- Patel MR, Bailey SR, Bonow RO, Chambers CE, Chan PS, Dehmer GJ, et al. ACCF/SCAI/AATS/AHA/ASE/ASNC/HFSA/HRS/SCCM/SCCT/SCMR/STS 2012 appropriate use criteria for diagnostic catheterization: American College of Cardiology Foundation Appropriate Use Criteria Task Force Society for Cardiovascular Angiography and Interventions American Association for Thoracic Surgery American Heart Association, American Society of Echocardiography American Society of Nuclear Cardiology Heart Failure Society of America Heart Rhythm Society, Society of Critical Care Medicine Society of Cardiovascular Computed Tomography Society for Cardiovascular Magnetic Resonance Society of Thoracic Surgeons. Catheter Cardiovasc Interv. 2012;80(3):E50–81.
- Voros S, Rivera JJ, Berman DS, Blankstein R, Budoff MJ, Cury RC, et al. Guideline for minimizing radiation exposure during acquisition of coronary artery calcium scans with the use of multidetector computed tomography: a report by the Society for Atherosclerosis Imaging and Prevention Tomographic Imaging and Prevention Councils in collaboration with the Society of Cardiovascular Computed Tomography. J Cardiovasc Comput Tomogr. 2011;5(2):75–83.
- Weigold WG, Abbara S, Achenbach S, Arbab-Zadeh A, Berman D, Carr JJ, et al. Standardized medical terminology for cardiac computed tomography: a report of the Society of Cardiovascular Computed Tomography. J Cardiovasc Comput Tomogr. 2011;5(3):136–44.
- Nagueh SF, Bierig SM, Budoff MJ, Desai M, Dilsizian V, Eidem B, et al. American Society of Echocardiography clinical recommendations for multimodality cardiovascular imaging of patients with hypertrophic cardiomyopathy: Endorsed by the American Society of Nuclear Cardiology, Society for Cardiovascular Magnetic Resonance, and Society of Cardiovascular Computed Tomography. J Am Soc Echocardiogr. 2011;24(5):473–98.
- Patel MR, Calhoon JH, Dehmer GJ, Grantham JA, Maddox TM, Maron DJ, et al. ACC/AATS/

AHA/ASE/ASNC/SCAI/SCCT/STS 2016 Appropriate Use Criteria for Coronary Revascularization in Patients With Acute Coronary Syndromes: A Report of the American College of Cardiology Appropriate Use Criteria Task Force, American Association for Thoracic Surgery, American Heart Association, American Society of Echocardiography, American Society of Nuclear Cardiology, Society for Cardiovascular Angiography and Interventions, Society of Cardiovascular Computed Tomography, and the Society of Thoracic Surgeons. J Nucl Cardiol. 2017;24(2):439–63.

- Taylor AJ, Cerqueira M, Hodgson JM, Mark D, Min J, O'Gara P, et al. ACCF/SCCT/ACR/AHA/ASE/ASNC/NASCI/SCAI/SCMR 2010 Appropriate Use Criteria for Cardiac Computed Tomography. A Report of the American College of Cardiology Foundation Appropriate Use Criteria Task Force, the Society of Cardiovascular Computed Tomography, the American College of Radiology, the American Heart Association, the American Society of Echocardiography, the American Society of Nuclear Cardiology, the North American Society for Cardiovascular Imaging, the Society for Cardiovascular Angiography and Interventions, and the Society for Cardiovascular Magnetic Resonance. J Cardiovasc Comput Tomogr. 2010;4(6):407.e1–33.
- Patel MR, White RD, Abbara S, Bluemke DA, Herfkens RJ, Picard M, et al. 2013 ACCF/ACR/ASE/ASNC/SCCT/SCMR appropriate utilization of cardiovascular imaging in heart failure: a joint report of the American College of Radiology Appropriateness Criteria Committee and the American College of Cardiology Foundation Appropriate Use Criteria Task Force. J Am Coll Cardiol. 2013;61(21):2207–31.
- Cury RC, Leipsic J, Abbara S, Achenbach S, Berman D, Bittencourt M, Budoff M, Chinnaiyan K, Choi AD, Ghoshhajra B, Jacobs J, Koweek L, Lesser J, Maroules C, Rubin GD, Rybicki FJ, Shaw LJ, Williams MC, Williamson E, White CS, Villines TC, Blankstein R. CAD-RADS™ 2.0–2022 Coronary Artery Disease-Reporting and Data System: An Expert Consensus Document of the Society of Cardiovascular Computed Tomography (SCCT), the American College of Cardiology (ACC), the American College of Radiology (ACR), and the North America Society of Cardiovascular Imaging (NASCI). J Cardiovasc Comput Tomogr. 2022;16(6):536–557.
- More related guidelines and expert consensus can be accessed at: https://scct.org/page/Guidelines#anchor_1632511790710.

Reference Values According to Chamber Sizes, Vascular Dimensions (E.G., Aorta, Pulmonary Artery, Pulmonary Veins, Superior and Inferior Vena Cava), Valves, Pericardium, and Miscellaneous

- Ka wel-Boehm N, Maceira A, Valsangiacomo-Buechel ER, Vogel-Claussen J, Turkbey EB, Williams R, et al. Normal values for cardiovascular magnetic resonance in adults and children. J Cardiovasc Magn Reson. 2015;17:29.
- Juneau D, Erthal F, Clarkin O, Alzahrani A, Alenazy A, Hossain A, et al. Mid-diastolic left ventricular volume and mass: normal values for coronary computed tomography angiography. J Cardiovasc Comput Tomogr. 2017;11(2):135–40.
- Massalha S, Almufleh A, Walpot J, Ratnayake I, Qureshi R, Abbass T, et al. Reference values for mid-diastolic right ventricular volume in population referred for cardiac computed tomography: an additional diagnostic value to cardiac computed tomography. J Cardiovasc Comput Tomogr. 2020;14(3):226–32.
- Kawel-Boehm N, Hetzel SJ, Ambale-Venkatesh B, Captur G, Francois CJ, Jerosch-Herold M, et al. Reference ranges ("normal values") for cardiovascular magnetic resonance (CMR) in adults and children: 2020 update. J Cardiovasc Magn Reson. 2020;22(1):87.
- Kou S, Caballero L, Dulgheru R, Voilliot D, De Sousa C, Kacharava G, et al. Echocardiographic reference ranges for normal cardiac chamber

size: results from the NORRE study. Eur Heart J Cardiovasc Imaging. 2014;15(6):680–90.

- Lang RM, Badano LP, Mor-Avi V, Afilalo J, Armstrong A, Ernande L, et al. Recommendations for cardiac chamber quantification by echocardiography in adults: an update from the American Society of Echocardiography and the European Association of Cardiovascular Imaging. J Am Soc Echocardiogr. 2015;28(1):1–39.e14.
- Lin FY, Devereux RB, Roman MJ, Meng J, Jow VM, Jacobs A, et al. Cardiac chamber volumes, function, and mass as determined by 64-multidetector row computed tomography: mean values among healthy adults free of hypertension and obesity. JACC Cardiovasc Imaging. 2008;1(6):782–6.
- Otto CM, Nishimura RA, Bonow RO, Carabello BA, Erwin JP, Gentile F, et al. 2020 ACC/AHA Guideline for the Management of Patients With Valvular Heart Disease: executive summary: A Report of the American College of Cardiology/American Heart Association Joint Committee on Clinical Practice Guidelines. Circulation. 2021;143(5):e35-e71.
- Vahanian A, Beyersdorf F, Praz F, Milojevic M, Baldus S, Bauersachs J, et al. 2021 ESC/EACTS Guidelines for the management of valvular heart disease. Eur Heart J. 2022;43(7):561–632.
- Adler Y, Charron P, Imazio M, Badano L, Barón-Esquivias G, Bogaert J, et al. 2015 ESC Guidelines for the diagnosis and management of pericardial diseases: The Task Force for the Diagnosis and Management of Pericardial Diseases of the European Society of Cardiology (ESC)Endorsed by: The European Association for Cardio-Thoracic Surgery (EACTS). Eur Heart J. 2015;36(42):2921–64.
- Kim YH, Marom EM, Herndon JE, McAdams HP. Pulmonary vein diameter, cross-sectional area, and shape: CT analysis. Radiology. 2005;235(1):43–9; discussion 9–50.
- Hassani C, Saremi F. Comprehensive Cross-sectional Imaging of the Pulmonary Veins. Radiographics. 2017;37(7):1928–54.
- Romberg EK, Stanescu AL, Bhutta ST, Otto RK, Ferguson MR. Computed tomography of pulmonary veins: review of congenital and acquired pathologies. Pediatr Radiol. 2021.
- Sonavane SK, Milner DM, Singh SP, Abdel Aal AK, Shahir KS, Chaturvedi A. Comprehensive Imaging Review of the Superior Vena Cava. Radiographics. 2015;35(7):1873–92.
- Lin FY, Devereux RB, Roman MJ, Meng J, Jow VM, Simprini L, et al. The right sided great vessels by cardiac multidetector computed tomography: normative reference values among healthy adults free of cardiopulmonary disease, hypertension, and obesity. Acad Radiol. 2009;16(8):981–7.
- Smillie RP, Shetty M, Boyer AC, Madrazo B, Jafri SZ. Imaging evaluation of the inferior vena cava. Radiographics. 2015;35(2):578–92.

Chest Pain Guidelines

- Collet JP, Thiele H, Barbato E, Barthélémy O, Bauersachs J, Bhatt DL, et al. 2020 ESC Guidelines for the management of acute coronary syndromes in patients presenting without persistent ST-segment elevation. Eur Heart J. 2021;42(14):1289–367.
- Gulati M, Levy PD, Mukherjee D, Amsterdam E, Bhatt DL, Birtcher KK, et al. 2021 AHA/ACC/ASE/CHEST/SAEM/SCCT/SCMR Guideline for the Evaluation and Diagnosis of Chest Pain: A Report of the American College of Cardiology/American Heart Association Joint Committee on Clinical Practice Guidelines. Circulation. 2021:CIR0000000000001029.
- Visseren FLJ, Mach F, Smulders YM, Carballo D, Koskinas KC, Bäck M, et al. 2021 ESC Guidelines on cardiovascular disease prevention in clinical practice. Eur Heart J. 2021;42(34):3227–337.
- Knuuti J, Wijns W, Saraste A, Capodanno D, Barbato E, Funck-Brentano C, et al. 2019 ESC Guidelines for the diagnosis and management of chronic coronary syndromes. Eur Heart J. 2020;41(3):407–77.

MIX
Papier aus verantwortungsvollen Quellen
Paper from responsible sources
FSC® C105338

If you have any concerns about our products,
you can contact us on
ProductSafety@springernature.com

In case Publisher is established outside the EU,
the EU authorized representative is:
Springer Nature Customer Service Center GmbH
Europaplatz 3, 69115 Heidelberg, Germany

Printed by Libri Plureos GmbH
in Hamburg, Germany